Stem Cell and Gene-Based Therapy

Alexander Battler and Jonathan Leor

Stem Cell and Gene-Based Therapy

Frontiers in Regenerative Medicine

With 62 Figures
including 27 Color Plates

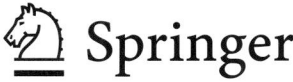 Springer

Alexander Battler, MD, FACC, FESC
Department of Cardiology
Rabin Medical Center, Petach-Tikwa
Sackler Faculty of Medicine
Tel Aviv University
Israel

Jonathan Leor, MD, FACC, FESC
Neufeld Cardiac Research Institute
Sackler Faculty of Medicine
Tel Aviv University
Sheba Medical Center
Tel-Hashomer
Israel

British Library Cataloguing in Publication Data
Stem cell and gene-based therapy: frontiers in regenerative medicine
   1. Stem cells – Research   2. Gene therapy – Research   3. Regeneration (Biology) – Research
I. Battler, Alexander   II. Leor, Jonathan
616'.02774
ISBN-10: 1852339799

Library of Congress Control Number: 2005925974

ISBN-10: 1-85233-979-9   e-ISBN 1-84628-142-3   Printed on acid-free paper
ISBN-13: 978-1-85233-979-1

© Springer-Verlag London Limited 2006

Whilst we have made considerable efforts to contact all holders of copyright material contained in this book, we may have failed to locate some of them. Should holders wish to contact the Publisher, we will be happy to come to some arrangement with them.

Apart from any fair dealing for the purposes of research or private study, or criticism or review, as permitted under the Copyright, Designs and Patents Act 1988, this publication may only be reproduced, stored or transmitted, in any form or by any means, with the prior permission in writing of the publishers, or in the case of reprographic reproduction in accordance with the terms of licences issued by the Copyright Licensing Agency. Enquiries concerning reproduction outside those terms should be sent to the publishers.

The use of registered names, trademarks, etc. in this publication does not imply, even in the absence of a specific statement, that such names are exempt from the relevant laws and regulations and therefore free for general use.

Product liability: The publisher can give no guarantee for information about drug dosage and application thereof contained in this book. In every individual case the respective user must check its accuracy by consulting other pharmaceutical literature.

Printed in the United States of America   (SPI/SB)

9 8 7 6 5 4 3 2 1

Springer Science+Business Media

springeronline.com

Foreword

Regenerative medicine promises to be one of the great future frontiers. Critical to the success of this area is stem cell research, and cell- and gene-based therapy. In this book, a variety of outstanding authors discuss important aspects of these research areas. Important topics include new types of cell therapies and stem cell-based therapy for angiogenesis and cardiac repair. They also include cell-therapy approaches in neurologic areas such as Parkinson's disease, multiple sclerosis, and stroke. A third area that is explored involves the development of cell-based systems for cartilage and bone repair, bladder repair, and kidney regeneration. A fourth area involves important work in the eye, specifically, optic nerve regeneration, retinal repair, and ocular surface regeneration. The potential of using insulin-producing cells or islets is also examined in this book, as are strategies for cord blood transplantation for various hematologic disorders. Finally, important areas of research involving skin regeneration and wound healing are discussed. This book should provide an excellent overview of the important areas in regenerative medicine with respect to cell and gene therapy and hopefully will be a useful guide for scientists doing research in these areas.

Robert Langer
Massachusetts Institute of Technology
Cambridge, MA, USA

Preface

The human body has limited potential to rejuvenate injured organs and tissues. An old dream of scientists and physicians is to be able to rebuild "spare parts" to replace injured or diseased tissues—a notion that was once referred to as the field of science fiction. The new discipline of regenerative medicine aims to help the body heal itself with cells, genes, and bioactive molecules and materials. In the last decade, the notion that stem cells can give rise to mature tissues has made stem cells the focus of intense research designed to explore their promise for the treatment of a variety of diseases.

The aim of our book is to cover key aspects of the promise and existing problems in the emerging field of regenerative medicine. With the contribution of leading figures and pioneers in various disciplines of regenerative medicine and science, the book brings together major approaches of stem cell and gene-based therapy in one text.

The appearance of this book has been made by the willing and corporation of many individuals. We thank our contributors, and section editors Belkin, Dekel, Efrat, Grossman, Melamed, Nagler, Offen, Nevo, and Reisner for generously sharing their expertise and scientific skills on which this book is based. We hope that the book will provide a realistic image of the huge potential, promise and challenges facing the fantastic field of regenerative medicine in its quest to cure disease and prolong life.

Alexander Battler
Jonathan Leor

Acknowledgment

We thank the section editors and coauthors for generously sharing their expertise and skills on which this book is based. We thank Mrs. Elaine Finkelstein from Neufeld Cardiac Research Institute, Tel-Hashomer, Israel, for her unfailing skills that were very helpful in editing and preparing this book.

Alexander Battler, MD, FACC, FESC
Jonathan Leor, MD, FACC, FESC

Contents

Foreword
Robert Langer v

Preface
Alexander Battler and Jonathan Leor vii

Acknowledgment ix

List of Contributors xv

Section 1 Heart

Introduction
Alexander Battler and Jonathan Leor 2

1 Renovation of the Injured Heart with Myocardial Tissue Engineering
Jonathan Leor, Natali Landa, and Smadar Cohen 3

2 Adult Stem Cells for Myocardial Tissue Repair
Dirk Strunk and Christof Stamm 17

3 Regeneration of the Functional Myocardium Using Human Embryonic Stem Cells
Oren Caspi and Lior Gepstien 33

4 Therapeutic Angiogenesis
Shmuel Fuchs and Alexander Battler 45

5 Cell Therapy for Heart Failure
Thorsten Reffelmann and Robert A. Kloner 59

Section 2 Neuro

Introduction
Daniel Offen and Eldad Melamed 72

6 Cell Transplantation for Diseases of Myelin
Tamir Ben-Hur and Ofira Einstein 75

7 Stem Cells as a Source for Cell Replacement in Parkinson's Disease
   Daniel Offen, Yossef S. Levy, and Eldad Melamed 97

8 Cell Replacement Therapy in Acute Stroke: Current State
   Yossi Gilgun-Sherki and Jonathan Y. Streifler 123

9 Gene Therapy to the Nervous System
   Hillel Haim and Israel Steiner 133

Section 3 Musculoskeletal

Introduction
Zvi Nevo and Mark M. Levy 156

10 Mesenchymal Stem Cells: Where Can You Find Them? How Can You Use Them?
   Anna Derubeis, Giuseppina Pennesi, and Ranieri Cancedda 159

11 Basic to Clinical Cartilage Engineering: Past, Present, and Future Discussions
   Mats Brittberg, Tommi Tallheden, and Anders H. Lindahl 169

12 Cartilage
   Rocky S. Tuan and Faye H. Chen 179

13 Bone Regeneration
   A.H. Reddi 195

14 Osteoarthritis and Mesenchymal Cells – The Prospects for Repair of the Disease by Cell Transplantation and Tissue Engineering
   Dror Robinson 203

Section 4 Kidney

Introduction
Benjamin Dekel and Yair Reisner 208

15 Progenitor Cell Therapy for Kidney Regeneration
   Benjamin Dekel and Yair Reisner 209

16 Tissue Engineering – The Bladder
   Anthony Atala 225

Section 5 Eye

Introduction
Michael Belkin 234

17 Neuroprotection in Ophthalmology: A Review
   Yaniv Barkana and Michael Belkin 237

18 Autoimmunity for Central Nervous System Maintenance,
    Regeneration, and Renewal: Development of a T Cell-Based
    Vaccination Against Neurodegeneration
    Michal Schwartz and Jonathan Kipnis 251

19 Retinal Repair by Stem Cell Transplantation
    Jeffrey H. Stern, Sally Temple, and Soma De 259

20 Induction of Ocular Surface Regeneration
    Irina S. Barequet 281

Section 6 Pancreas

Introduction
Shimon Efrat 298

21 Insulin-Producing Cells Generated from Nonpancreatic Tissues
    Shimon Efrat 301

22 Generation of Islets from Pancreatic Progenitor Cells
    *Susan Bonner-Weir, Tandy Aye, Akari Inada,
    Elena Toschi, and Arun Sharma* 309

23 Embryonic Stem Cells as a Source of Pancreatic Precursors
    and Islet Cells In Vitro
    Victoria L. Browning, Brenda W. Kahan, and Jon S. Odorico . . . 321

Section 7 Hematology

Introduction
Arnon Nagler 332

24 Human Umbilical Cord Blood Transplantation: A Viable Option
    for Stem Cell Graft
    Gal Goldstein, Amos Toren, and Arnon Nagler 333

25 Nonmyeloablative Stem Cell Transplantation in the Treatment
    of Hematologic Malignancies
    Avichai Shimoni and Arnon Nagler 351

26 Hematopoietic Stem Cell Transplantation from Human Leukocyte
    Antigen Haploidentical Donor
    Merav Leiba and Arnon Nagler 361

Section 8 Skin

Introduction
Nili Grossman 372

27 Wound Healing and Skin Substitutes
    Adam J. Singer and Marcia Simon 375

28 Skin Regeneration from Multipotent Adult and Embryonic Stem Cells
   Kursad Turksen and Tammy-Claire Troy 395

   Index 407

   Color Insert . . . . following page 206

Contributors

Anthony Atala, MD
The William Boyce Professor and Chair, Department of Urology
Director, Wake Forest Institute for Regenerative Medicine
Wake Forest University School of Medicine
Winston-Salem, NC, USA

Irina S. Barequet, MD
The Goldschleger Eye Institute
Sheba Medical Center Sackler Faculty of Medicine
Tel Aviv University, Tel Aviv, Israel

Alexander Battler, MD, FACC, FESC
Professor and Chair of Cardiology
Rabin Medical Center, Petach-Tikvah
Sackler Faculty of Medicine
Tel Aviv University
Israel

Michael Belkin, MA, MD
Director
Ophthalmic Technologies Laboratory, Eye Research Institute
Sackler School of Medicine, Tel Aviv University
Sheba Medical Center
Tel Hashomer, Israel

Tamir Ben-Hur, MD, PhD
Professor
Neurology
Hadassah Hebrew University Medical Center
Jerusalem, Israel

Susan Bonner-Weir, PhD
Senior Investigator, Joslin Diabetes Center
Associate Professor of Medicine, Harvard Medical School
Boston, MA, USA

Mats Brittberg, MD, PhD
Cartilage Research Unit
Göteborg University
Department of Orthopaedics
Kungsbacka Hospital
Kungsbacka, Sweden

Ranieri Cancedda, MD
Professor
Department of Oncology, Biology and Genetics
University of Genova
Genova, Italy

Benjamin Dekel, MD, PhD
Department of Pediatrics
Safra Children's Hospital
Sheba Medical Center
Tel Hashomer, Israel

Shimon Efrat, PhD
Human Genetics and Molecular Medicine
Sackler School of Medicine
Tel Aviv University
Tel Aviv, Israel

Shmuel Fuchs, MD
Head, Catheterization Laboratory
Department of Cardiology
Rabin Medical Center
Petch-Tikva, Israel

Lior Gepstien, MD, PhD
Department of Biophysics and
 Physiology
The Bruce Rappaport Faculty of
 Medicine
Technion-Israel Institute of
 Technology
Haifa, Israel

Yossi Gilgun-Sherki, PhD
Neuroscientist
Neurology
Laboratory of Neurosciences
Felsenstein Medical Research Center
Petah-Tikva, Israel

Gal Goldstein, MD
Staff Physician
Pediatric Hemato-Oncology
Edmond & Lili Safra's children
 hospital
Tel Hashomer, Israel

Nili Grossman, PhD
Director
Skin Bank and Investigative
 Dermatology Laboratory
 and Department of Microbiology
 and Immunology / Health
 Sciences
Soroka University Medical Center
and Ben Gurion University of the
 Negev
Beer Sheva, Israel

Hillel Haim, MD
Physician
Department of Neurology
Hadassah University Hospital
Jerusalem, Israel

Merav Leiba, MD
Hematology & Bone Marrow
 Transplantation
Chaim Sheba Medical Center
Tel-Hashomer, Israel

Jonathan Leor, MD, FACC, FESC
Director
Neufeld Cardiac Research Institute
Sackler Faculty of Medicine
Tel Aviv University
Sheba Medical Center
Tel Hashomer, Israel

Arnon Nagler, MD, MSc
Director Hematology Division
Hematology
Chaim Sheba Medical Center
Tel Hashomer, Tamat Gan,
 Israel

Zvi Nevo, PhD
ex Department Chairman
Clinical Biochemistry
Sackler School of Medicine
Tel Aviv University
Tel Aviv, Israel

Jon S. Odorico, MD
Assistant Professor, Director –
 Islet Cell Transplantation
 Program
Transplantation Surgery
University of Wisconsin –
 Madison Medical School
Madison, WI, USA

Daniel Offen, PhD
Head of Neurology Laboratory
Felsenstein Medical Research
 Center
Tel Aviv University
Rabin Medical Center
Petha-Tikva, Israel

A. H. Reddi, PhD
Center for Tissue Regeneration
 and Repair
Department of Orthopaedic
 Surgery
University of California, Davis
School of Medicine
Sacramento, CA, USA

Thorsten Reffelmann, MD
Medical Clinic I, University
 Hospital
Department of Cardiology
RWTH Aachen
Aachen, Germany

Dror Robinson, MD, PhD
Chairman
Department of Orthopaedics
Rabin Medical Center
Petah-Tikva, Israel

Contributors

Michal Schwartz, PhD
Professor of Neuroimmunology
Neurobiology
The Weizmann Institute
  of Science
Rehovot, Israel

Avichai Shimoni, MD
Senior Physician
Division of Hematology and Bone
  Marrow Transplantation
Chaim Sheba Medical Center
Tel Hashomer, Israel

Adam J. Singer, MD
Vice Chairman for Research
Emergency Medicine
Stony Brook University
Stony Brook, NY, USA

Christof Stamm, MD
Consultant Surgeon
Department of Cardiac Surgery
University of Rostock
Rostock, Germany

Jeffrey H. Stern, PhD, MD
Retina / Vitreous Surgery
Albany, NY, USA

Rocky S. Tuan, PhD
Branch Chief
Cartilage Biology and
  Orthopaedics Branch
National Institute of Arthritis and
  Musculoskeletal and Skin
  Diseases
Bethesda, MD, USA

Kursad Turksen, PhD
Senior Scientist
Hormones, Growth and
  Development
Ottawa Health Research Institute
Ottawa, Ontario, Canada

Section 1

Heart

Section 1

Heart

Alexander Battler and Jonathan Leor

Despite current pharmacologic and interventional treatment progress, ischemic heart disease and particularly advanced heart failure remains a common and deadly disease. Limited availability of donor organs for heart transplantation has prompted evaluation of alternative therapeutic strategies directed toward patients with advanced heart failure. Intense interest has recently focused on regenerative medicine approach: cell transfer, mobilization of resident stem cells, and tissue engineering as potential strategies for enhancing the repair or regenerative capacity of the injured heart.

In this section, several pioneers and world leaders in the field of cardiac stem cell therapy and tissue engineering describe the incredible progress and achievements in experimental models and initial clinical experience in myocardial tissue repair. They illustrate the promise of new technologies that may provide a new tool for reconstructing damaged hearts that previously would have been irreparable.

Despite the promise of these achievements, challenges lie ahead. A major difficulty persists with regard to identifying appropriate cells and ensuring enough number to repopulate the damaged heart. We should acknowledge that there is still much to be learned before myocardial cell therapy and tissue engineering will be routinely available. However, recent advances in the science of stem cells and biomaterials provide hope for the cure of a variety of myocardial diseases.

1

Renovation of the Injured Heart with Myocardial Tissue Engineering

Jonathan Leor, Natali Landa, and Smadar Cohen

Tissue engineering is a growing area that aims to create, repair, and/or replace tissues and organs by using combinations of cells, scaffolds, biologically active molecules, and physiologic signals. It is an interdisciplinary field that integrates aspects of engineering, chemistry, biology, and medicine. One of the most challenging goals in the field of cardiovascular tissue engineering is the creation of an engineered heart muscle. Unlike heart valves or blood vessels, heart muscle has no replacement alternatives. New discoveries in stem cell biology suggest that stem cells are a potential source of heart muscle cells and blood vessels and can be used to rebuild or replace damaged heart tissue. Recent advances in methods of stem cell isolation, expansion, and culture and the synthesis of new bioactive materials show promise to contribute to the creation of engineered contractile cardiac tissue in vitro and in vivo.

This chapter introduces the basic structural features of myocardium, elucidating the challenges in tissue engineering of a cardiac muscle. It describes the principles of myocardial tissue engineering and reviews various approaches to achieve the ambitious goal of creating contractile heart muscle to treat myocardial infarction and heart failure patients.

The Myocardium

The myocardium is composed mainly of cardiomyocytes, fibroblasts, and the elements of blood vessels: endothelial and smooth muscle cells, macrophages, and extracellular matrix (ECM) (Figure 1.1).[1,2] Cardiomyocytes constitute only one-third of the total cardiac cell number. However, they occupy more than 70% of cardiac volume. Fibroblasts are the dominant cardiac cell and account for 90% to 95% of non-myocyte cell mass.[3,4]

Unlike other somatic tissues, the heart has been viewed as an organ composed of terminally differentiated cardiomyocytes and incapable of regeneration. Recent studies challenge these pre-existing notions regarding cardiac repair/regeneration and suggest that the heart is capable of limited regeneration through the activation and recruitment of a stem/progenitor cell population that is resident in the adult heart.[5]

Cardiomyocytes are tethered in an extensive extracellular network of collagen and other structural proteins, including fibronectins and proteoglycans [Figure 1.2 (see color section)]. The extracellular and intracellular myofibrillar scaffolding is a critical determinant of cardiac shape during normal and abnormal cardiac growth. Collagen is synthesized principally by fibroblasts but also by vascular smooth muscle cells in response to a variety of pathologic stimuli, including increased oxidative and mechanical stress, ischemia, and inflammation.

Of the many collagen types, the major fibrillar collagens are types I (approximately 85%) and III (11%), which constitute the bulk of cardiac ECM. Collagen type I is associated mainly with thick fibers that confer tensile strength and

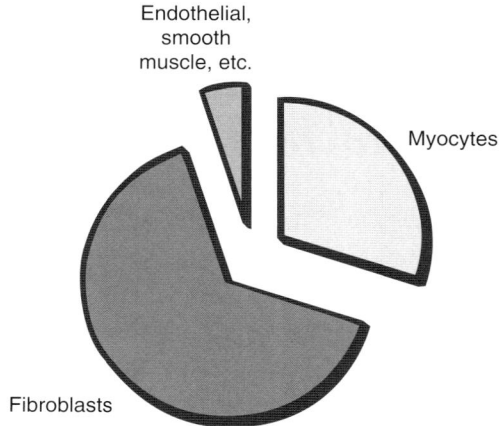

Figure 1.1. Myocardial cells. Cardiomyocytes constitute only one-third of the total cardiac cell number. However, they occupy more than 70% of cardiac volume.[2]

resistance to stretch and deformation, whereas collagen type III is associated with thin fibers that confer resilience.[2]

Cardiomyocytes are tethered to the ECM by membrane-spanning proteins called integrins [Figure 1.2 (see color section)]. The extracellular portion of these molecules binds to fibronectins in the ECM. Perimyocyte extracellular proteins such as dystrophin and dystrophin-related proteins contribute to normal cardiogenesis. When altered in abundance, they can produce a cardiomyopathy.[6]

Myocardial Infarction and Remodeling

Heart failure after myocardial infarction can result from the substantial loss of cardiomyocytes in the infarct zone but more often is precipitated by the delayed and progressive pathologic remodeling of the left ventricle. Cell death in the infarct zone is large in magnitude but short in duration.

When myocardial tissue is injured, normal healing response is initiated through a series of complex events that include acute inflammation, the formation of granulation tissue, and eventual scar formation.[7,8] Cytokines and growth factors are released to recruit white blood cells, mainly neutrophils. Monocytes are then called to the wound site where they differentiate into macrophages. The macrophages are responsible for cleaning the infarcted zone and also for recruiting cells such as fibroblasts, endothelial cells, and stem/progenitor cells creating granulation tissue. The formation of blood vessels is essential to the healing of the infarcted myocardium. The granulation tissue is subsequently replaced by an ECM deposited primarily by fibroblasts. The degree of ECM depends on the extent and location (e.g., anterior or apical) of infarction. In most cases, the granulation tissue is remodeled into scar tissue.

Most of the molecules and signal transduction pathways operant in cardiomyocyte growth have a role in hyperplasia of fibroblasts and in the elaboration of collagen. The resultant fibrosis produces altered myocardial stiffness and arrhythmogenesis in ischemic heart disease, cardiac hypertrophy, and congestive heart failure. Collagen synthesis is continuously and variably offset by ECM resorption mediated by matrix metalloproteinases. The activity of these enzymes is increased in ischemic and dilated cardiomyopathy.[2] Conversely, the activity of a class of enzymes known as tissue inhibitors of matrix metalloproteinases is reduced in this setting. The resultant excessive collagenolyses may induce myofibrillar slippage and contribute to the dilated thin-walled chamber geometry that characterizes acute and chronic heart failure. This process has been termed left ventricular (LV) remodeling.

Myocardial Regeneration

Myocardial regeneration is an exciting novel therapeutic concept.[9] One approach that has received recent attention focuses on repopulation of the injured myocardium by transplantation of healthy cells.[10] Several cell types that might replace necrotic tissue and minimize scarring have been considered (Table 1.1). Fetal cardiomyocytes, skeletal myoblasts, and bone marrow stem cells have all shown limited success in restoring damaged tissues and improving cardiac function. Failure to produce new myocardial fibers in clinically relevant numbers was attributed to cell death occurring after engraftment and inability of engrafted myoblasts to differentiate and integrate within the host myocardium; hence, electromechanical coupling is not likely to occur after in vivo myoblast grafting.

An alternative approach includes mobilization of progenitor or stem cells to the damaged

Table 1.1. Possible cell sources for myocardial tissue engineering
1. Skeletal myoblasts[91,92]
2. Crude bone marrow[93]
3. Endothelial progenitor cells[94]
4. Hematopoietic stem cells[95]
5. Mesenchymal stem cells[96]
6. Smooth muscle cells[78]
7. Umbilical cord cells[97]
8. Fibroblasts[77,98]
9. Human embryonic stem cells[99]
10. Fetal cardiomyocytes[73,74]
11. Myocardial progenitors[13,14,16]
12. Cloned cells[100]

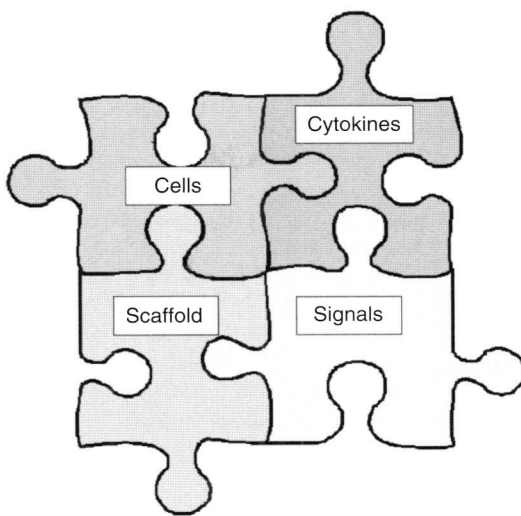

Figure 1.3. The classic paradigm of myocardial tissue engineering. The engineered heart muscle can be produced, ex vivo or in situ based on: (1) cells, such as cardiomyocytes; (2) biomaterial scaffold, such as collagen or alginate; (3) cytokines, such as growth or survival factors; and (4) signals, electric or physiologic, such as pacing or flow. For details, see Tables 1.1, 1.3, and 1.5.

area or stimulation of a regenerative program within the organ.[11] Recent studies have suggested that stem cells residing within the bone marrow or peripheral blood can be mobilized and recruited to the injured heart.[12] In addition, there is now accumulating evidence that the heart contains resident stem cells that can be induced to develop into cardiac muscle and vascular tissue.[13-16] However, cell transplantation approach may be of little clinical benefit when the local cardiac structure cannot support cell seeding because it is absent or seriously damaged. Tissue engineering approach might solve this problem by using three-dimensional (3-D) scaffolds that replace the missing or damaged infrastructure–ECM and provide a temporary support for self or implanted cells.[17]

Tissue Engineering

The aim of tissue engineering is to repair or replace the damaged organ or tissues by delivering functional cells, supporting scaffolds, growth-promoting molecules, or DNA encoding these molecules, and electric or physiologic signals to areas in need (Figure 1.3). The field has already made headway in the synthesis of structural tissues such as skin, cartilage, bone, and bladder.[18] The classic tissue engineering concept is to isolate specific cells through a biopsy from a patient, to grow them on a 3-D biomimetic scaffold under precisely controlled culture conditions, to deliver the construct to the desired site in the patient's body, and to direct new tissue formation into the scaffold that can be degraded over time.[18] To achieve successful regeneration of damaged organs or tissues based on the tissue engineering concept, several critical elements should be considered, including the biomaterial scaffold that serves as a mechanical and biological support for cell growth and differentiation, progenitor cells that can be differentiated into specific cell types, and the inductive growth factors that can modulate cellular activities.

Strategies of tissue engineering can be classified as in vitro and in vivo approaches:

1. In vitro tissue engineering in culture dish or bioreactor
   a. Creation of engineered cardiac graft from cell-seeded scaffold
   b. Creation of cardiac graft from cell culture or expanded stem cells
2. In vivo tissue engineering (in situ generation)
   a. Direct cell transplantation
   b. Cell-seeded scaffold implantation
   c. Nonseeded scaffold implantation and recruiting endogenous cells
   d. Injectable scaffold with or without cells
   e. Promotion of healing and self-repair by active molecules

Myocardial Tissue Engineering Versus Cell Transplantation

The promising results of cardiac cell transplantation in animal models have been partially attributed to reconstruction of the ECM, which maintained the structure, thickness, and elasticity of the LV wall.[19] The concept of tissue engineering using 3-D scaffolds has certain advantages over the direct cell injection (Table 1.2). The 3-D scaffolds can replace the missing or damaged infrastructure (ECM) in the damaged area and provide temporary support for self or implanted cells. With tissue engineering, one can control the size, shape, strength, and composition of the graft in vitro. Tissue engineering may provide a solution to the problem of congenital or acquired heart defects and can be used to replace or reconstruct defective heart parts such as valves or vessels. Actually, these techniques can be complementary. Cellular therapy is applicable when the structure of the failing organ is relatively simple and small and when disease is localized rather than diffuse.

Biomaterials and Scaffolds

The biomaterial scaffold has a key role in most tissue engineering strategies. To guide the organization, growth, and differentiation of cells in tissue engineered constructs, the biomaterial scaffold should be able to provide not only physical support for the cells but also the chemical and biological cues needed in forming functional tissues.[20] The biomaterial should be able to crosstalk, on the molecular level, with the cells in a precise and controlled manner, similarly to the natural interactions existing between cells and the native ECM. At the same time, the basic requirements of a biomaterial should be kept; i.e., the materials and their degradation products must be nontoxic and nonimmunogenic, and their degradation rate should match the rate of new tissue formation (Table 1.3). In cardiac tissue engineering, the material properties, such as flexibility and degradability, need to be adjusted so that they will not interfere with cardiac muscle contractility.

In recent years, the trend has been to design bioactive materials, which on one hand will have the appropriate physical strength as well as the degradation kinetics of synthetic polymers and on the other hand will have the biological specificity of collagen, fibronectin, and laminin – the major ECM components. Such biological resembling biomaterials, termed "biomimetics," should promote cell–matrix interactions, and elicit specific cellular responses and biomolecular recognition.

The approaches for achieving biomimetic materials include synthesis of new materials from scratch or chemical modification of existing materials with bioactive molecules. This approach has the advantages of working with known materials, most of which have been tested and have been proved to be safe in human. The bioactive molecules may be whole ECM molecules or "cell-binding" domain sequences isolated from these proteins. The use of short peptides is advantageous over the whole protein because the protein tends to be randomly folded and the receptor binding domains are not always sterically available. In addition, the short peptide is relatively more stable during the modification process and can be massively synthesized in the laboratory. The most frequently used peptide sequence derived from fibronectin signaling domain is Arg-Gly-Asp (RGD).[21-25] The selection of peptide sequences for modification depends on the cell type seeded onto the matrix or the implanted site of the scaffold and its natural ECM environment and the specific required cellular responses.

Table 1.2. Comparison between myocardial tissue engineering and cell therapy for myocardial repair

	Tissue engineering	Cell transplantation
Cells	Optional	Must
Scaffold	Must	No
Active molecules	Optional	Optional
Controlled drug delivery	Yes	No
Controlled graft shape and size	Yes	No
Angiogenic	Yes	Yes
Myogenic	Yes	Yes
Replace cardiac valves or big vessels	Yes	No
Repair of infarcted myocardium	Yes	Yes
Repair of congenital defects	Yes	No
Injectable	Yes	Yes
Clinical experience	No	Yes

Table 1.3. Biomaterial for myocardial tissue engineering

	References
Natural	
Porous alginate scaffolds	Leor et al.,[74] 2000
Alginate-gelatin-PEG scaffolds	Chandy et al.,[101] 2003
Gelatin scaffolds	Akhyari et al.,[68] 2002
Collagen scaffolds	Zimmermann et al.,[47] 2002
Matrigel	Zimmermann et al.[47]; Kofidis et al.,[90] 2004; Radisic et al.,[60] 2004
Fibrin	Christman et al.,[102] 2004; Ryu et al.,[93] 2005
Synthetic	
PLA-PGA	Stock and Mayer,[103] 2001
Poly-L-lactide-gelatin-PGA	Ozawa et al.,[104] 2002; McDevitt et al.,[65] 2003
Electrically conducting membrane layers composed of PGA, gelatin, alginate, and/or collagen	Shimizu et al.,[48] 2002
ε-Caprolactone-co-L-lactide	Matsubayashi et al.,[78] 2003
Polyurethanes	McDevitt et al.,[65] 2003
TMC-co-ε-caprolactone-co-D,L-lactide	Pego et al.,[105] 2003

Source: Adapted from Zammaretti and Jaconi.[106]
PEG, polyethylene glycol; PLA, polylactic acid; PGA, polyglycolic acid; TMC, 1,3-trimethylene carbonate.

Modification of the material can be performed either in a surface or bulk approach. Surface modification of materials with bioactive molecules is a simple way to make biomimetic materials. In most cases, the goal is to study cell attachment, spreading, proliferation, and differentiation on modified surfaces in 2-D culture, without addressing the effects of the third dimension. Bulk modification of a material, in comparison, should provide a more suitable environment for the cells as it imitates the 3-D environment of the natural ECM. Most of the bulk-modified materials are based on polymers that have been applied before as nonmodified ones for tissue engineering; for example, hyaluronan,[26] polyethylene oxide,[27] poly(N-isopropylacrylamide),[28] polylactic-co-glycolic acid,[29] and alginate.[23] Modification is usually performed through a chemical reaction leading to covalent bond between the polymer backbone and the bioactive peptide. Another method crosslinks the polymer to form a hydrogel using a bifunctional peptide that also has a signaling domain for interactions with cell membrane receptors.[30]

Cell Sources

One of the major challenges of tissue engineering application in human patients is to achieve enough cells to generate significant amount of muscle tissue. The optimal cell source for creating an engineered myocardial patch should be easy to harvest, proliferative, nonimmunogenic, and resistant to ischemia (after transplantation) and have the ability to differentiate into mature, functional cardiomyocyte. Unfortunately, no such cell currently exists. Several cell sources have been proposed (Table 1.1). Donor (allogenic) cells are relatively easier to obtain but entail risky immunosuppression. Autologous cells, however, are more difficult to obtain and to expand but have no immunologic barriers.

Table 1.4 describes the advantages and limitations of various cell sources. Theoretically, the natural electrophysiologic, structural, and contractile properties of cardiomyocytes make them the ideal donor cell type. However, cardiomyocytes are difficult to obtain and to expand, are sensitive to ischemic insults, and are allogenic, e.g., will evoke immune response in the host tissue. Thus, researchers are seeking alternative cells. Although human embryonic stem cells have been shown to have the potential to turn into cardiomyocytes,[31] no studies have demonstrated the controlled differentiation into uniform cell type. Furthermore, unless they are derived from somatic-cell nuclear transfer, human embryonic stem cells will be rejected by a recipient.

Today, the most widely used cell types for cardiac cell therapy in human patients are skeletal

Table 1.4. Advantages and limitations of various cell sources for myocardial tissue engineering

	Autologous	Easily obtainable	Highly expandable	Cardiac myogenesis	Clinical experience	Safety concerns
Fetal cardiomyocytes	No	No	No	Yes	No	No
Embryonic stem cells	No	No	Yes	Yes	No	Yes, teratoma
Skeletal myoblasts	Yes	Yes	Depend on age	Debated	Yes	Yes, arrhythmias
Crude bone marrow cells	Yes	Yes	Depend on age	Debated	Yes	Yes, calcification
Mesenchymal stem cells	Yes	No	Depend on age	Yes	No	Yes, fibrosis
Hematopoietic stem cells	Yes	Yes	Depend on age	Debated	Yes	No
Fibroblasts	Yes	Yes	Depend on age	No	No	No
Smooth muscle cells	Yes	Yes	Yes	No	No	Unknown
Cardiac progenitors	Yes	No	Unknown	Yes	No	Unknown

Source: Adapted from Leor J, Amsalem Y, Cohen S. Cells, scaffolds, and molecules for myocardial tissue engineering. Pharmacol Ther 2005;105:151–163.

muscle-derived progenitors, or myoblasts, and crude bone marrow mononuclear cells.[10] Both cell types share advantages over other cells proposed for cardiac repair in that they are readily available, autologous, and easily expanded in vitro. A limitation of myoblasts is their apparent inability to transdifferentiate into cardiac or endothelial cells. In contrast, bone marrow-derived stem cells are currently gaining favor because of their seeming plasticity, which could allow them to alter their phenotype in response to cues from the target organ, and the possibility of using the patient's own cells. A few recent clinical studies advocate the simple injection of unfractionated autologous bone marrow cells in patients with acute myocardial infarction.[10] However, because such studies have been performed relatively early after the ischemic insult, their relevance to chronically infarcted myocardium remains uncertain.[10]

The use of autologous adult stem cells is particularly restricted by their low recovery from bone marrow, fat, or circulation of elderly patients, and, therefore, it is difficult to obtain in reasonable numbers of suitable cells.[32] In addition, progenitor cells from sick patients, such as type II diabetics, exhibit impaired proliferation, adhesion, and incorporation into vascular structures.[32–34] Furthermore, cell sources are limited by several aspects that are relevant to clinical implications.[35,36] For example, safety issues have been raised regarding the use of various cells for myocardial repair: arrhythmias with skeletal myoblasts,[37] cardiac calcifications with bone marrow mononuclear cells,[38] myocardial scarring with mesenchymal stem cells,[39] and teratoma with human embryonic stem cells.[40] In addition, the search continues for an efficient and reproducible method to control and direct differentiation of stem cells to the desired cell type in vitro.[41,42]

Engineering Beating Construct In Vitro

Zimmermann et al.[43] proposed certain criteria for cardiac tissue construct. The constructs should be (1) contractile, (2) electrophysiologically stable, (3) mechanically robust yet flexible, (4) vascularized or at least quickly vascularized after implantation, and (5) nonimmunogenic. Today, such construct does not exist. Thus, these ambitious criteria illustrate the difficulties in engineering functional myocardial graft.[44,45]

A number of groups reported encouraging results with various techniques for constructing cardiac graft for transplantation.[46–60] They showed that neonatal rat or chick embryo cardiomyocytes can be reconstituted to 3-D myocardial tissue-like constructs. For example, we have shown that cardiomyocyte seeding within porous alginate scaffolds yielded 3-D high-density cardiac constructs with a uniform cell distribution. The hydrophilic nature of the alginate scaffold, its more than 90% porosity, and interconnected pore structure, enabled efficient cell seeding onto the scaffold within a short time, up to 30 minutes. With the aid of a moderate centrifugal force during cell seeding, a uniform cell distribution throughout the alginate scaffolds was achieved, consequently enabling the loading of many cardiomyocytes onto the 3-D scaffolds.[50]

As an alternative to seeding the cells on a preformed scaffold, Zimmermann et al. utilized Matrigel mixed with collagen gel.[43–47,61,62] The cells were mixed with the liquid material, which was solidified by casting in a cylindrical template. After a few days, they moved the tissue patch to a stretching device that simulated the heart's contractions. They demonstrated that collagen type I and ECM proteins when mixed with freshly isolated heart cells join together to a strongly contracting and highly differentiated construct, which they named engineered heart tissue (EHT). The geometric shape of EHT could be altered by utilization of suitable casting molds (square, circular).

An alternative approach has been proposed by Shimizu et al.[48] They grew rat cardiomyocytes on a thin temperature-responsive polymer, PIPAAm [poly(N-isopropylacrylamide)]. The polymer sheet promoted the thin cell layers to detach when the temperature was reduced, thus releasing cardiac myocyte sheets from the dishes without enzymatic or ethylenediaminetetraacetic acid treatment. The researchers laid four of these sheets on top of each other until they fused, and the product was implanted under the skin of rats. Six months later, the researchers observed that the engineered cardiac patches were beating and had been infiltrated by blood vessels. One of the potential advantages of this strategy is the ability to stack other necessary cell sheets between cardiomyocyte sheets as endothelial cells in attempt to cope with the perfusion limitation in thick constructs.

Another technique that may accelerate and optimize engineered myocardial assembly is "organ printing."[63] A cell printer to print gels, single cells, and cell aggregates has been developed. Layer-by-layer sequentially placed and solidified thin layers of a thermo-reversible gel served as "printing paper." This computer-aided, jet-based 3-D tissue engineering of living human organs suggests a new strategy for growing a patch of cardiac muscle.[63]

To achieve better control over the morphology and architecture of engineered constructs, researchers used several modifications. McDevitt et al.[64] laid lanes of laminin, 5–50 micron wide, by microcontact printing onto nonadhesive (bovine serum albumin-coated) surfaces. Adherent cardiomyocytes responded to the spatial constraints by forming elongated, rod-shaped cells whose myofibrils aligned parallel to the laminin lanes. Similar cardiomyocyte patterns were achieved on micropatterned biodegradable polymer polylactic-co-glycolic acid, suggesting that patterned cardiomyocytes could be used in myocardial tissue engineering.[65]

Radisic et al.[59] applied electrical signals, designed to mimic those in the native heart, on cardiac constructs in vitro. After 8 days, electrical field stimulation induced cell alignment and coupling, increased the amplitude of synchronous construct contractions, and resulted in a remarkable ultrastructural organization.[59] In another study, they used an in vitro culture system that maintains efficient oxygen supply to the cells at all times during cell seeding and construct cultivation attempting to mimic convective-diffusive oxygen transport present in vivo. Perfusion resulted in significantly higher numbers of live cells, higher cell viability, and significantly more cells in the S phase compared with dish-grown constructs.[60]

The results of these pioneering experiments provide tools to investigate myocardial physiology, development, and pharmacology ex vivo. In addition, they raise hope for the use of myocardial tissue engineering to repair or replace the infarcted myocardium. Theoretically, the bioengineered cardiac tissue could be used for surgical reconstruction of the infarcted myocardium or repair of congenital cardiac defects.[66]

Bioreactors

One of the major difficulties in cardiac tissue engineering is how to grow 3-D structures that contain more than a few layers of muscle cells. To improve the results of in vitro tissue engineering, researchers have designed several bioreactors, which portray different patterns of fluid dynamics and vessel geometry. A basic fluid-dynamic cultivation vessel is the spinner flask, which is an agitated flask usually at 50 rpm.[51,53] In these vessels, the cell constructs are subjected to turbulently mixed fluid that provides a well-mixed environment around the cell constructs and minimizes the stagnant layer at their surface. It has been shown that cultivation of cardiac cell constructs in spinner flasks produces engineered tissues that are superior, in almost every aspect (e.g., aerobic cell metabolism, DNA content, metabolic activity, and morphologic appearance) to tissues cultivated under static conditions.[51,53,67] The spinner flask may not, however, be the optimal cultivation vessel for cardiac cells. The turbulent fluid flow at the surface of the constructs is usually characterized by eddies that destroy the seeded cells.

Bioreactors combined with mechanical signals, such as under stretching or compression modes, improved the proliferation and distribution of the seeded human heart cells throughout the scaffold volume and further stimulated the formation and organization of the ECM – all of which contributed to the improvement in the mechanical strength of the cardiac graft.[46,47,68] Future bioreactors for cardiac tissue engineering should combine both perfusion and mechanical stimuli, for example, by allowing for adjustable pulsatile flow and varying levels of pressure. Such bioreactors are currently under development for engineering heart valves ex vivo.[69,70]

These encouraging achievements still face significant difficulties. Most bioreactors cannot supply enough nutrients and oxygen to a growing thick tissue. Whereas adult heart muscle is more than 1 cm thick, growth in a bioreactor typically stops once the tissue is about 100 μm, or less than 10 cell layers thick.[71] Beyond this thickness, the innermost cells are too far from the supply of fresh growth medium to thrive. Furthermore, after transplantation, rapid vascularization, adequate perfusion, cell survival, integration, and function of the engineered cardiac patch remain critical steps in the translation of in vitro achievements into effective therapeutic tools.[44,72]

Transplantation of Engineered Myocardial Construct

In their pioneering study, Li et al.[73] reported that bioengineered cardiac grafts can be made of fetal cardiac cells and 3-D gelatin mesh. The cells in the graft formed cardiac-like tissue and contracted spontaneously. However, after transplantation on infarcted myocardium of rat, compared with a control, LV-developed pressure was lower in hearts into which either a cell-seeded or unseeded graft had been implanted. The authors proposed that inappropriate sizing of the grafts interferes with the contractility of the viable myocardium.[73]

We reported successful seeding of rat fetal cardiomyocytes into porous scaffolds composed of alginate sponges.[74] We found that the seeded fetal cardiac cells retained viability within the scaffolds and within 24 hours formed multicellular beating cell clusters. After implantation of the cellular constructs into the infarcted myocardium, some of the cells appeared to differentiate into mature myocardial fibers. The implanted cardiac grafts were supplied by intensive neovascularization, which evidently contributed to the survival of the cells in the grafts. The biografts attenuated LV dilatation and deterioration of heart function. The mechanism behind this beneficial effect remains unclear. A direct contribution of the biograft to contractility is unlikely because only a relatively small fraction of the biograft was composed of myocardial tissue. Attenuation of infarct expansion by virtue of the elastic properties of bioartificial grafts is possible. Restraining the expansion of the left ventricle by a mesh placed over the infarcted myocardium, preserves left ventricle geometry and resting function in a sheep model of myocardial infarction[75] and has now tested in clinical trial.[76] Angiogenesis induced by growth factors secreted from the seeded cells, resulting in improved collateral flow and augmentation of contractility, is also a possible mechanism.[77]

Zimmermann et al.[46] created EHT by mixing cardiac myocytes from neonatal Fischer 344 rats with liquid collagen type I, Matrigel, and serum-containing culture medium. EHTs were designed in circular shapes to fit around the circumference of hearts from syngeneic rats. After 12 days in culture, they were implanted on uninjured hearts. Fourteen days after implantation, EHTs were heavily vascularized and retained a well-organized heart muscle structure as indicated by immunolabeling of actinin, connexin 43, and cadherins. Ultrastructural analysis demonstrated that implanted EHTs surpassed the degree of differentiation reached before implantation. Contractile function of EHT grafts was preserved in vivo, but, compared with baseline values, did not improve LV function as indicated by serial echocardiography studies.[46] In addition, the transplantation results were limited by immune response of the host animal against the biomaterial mixture and the need for continuous immunosuppression.[46]

In another study, Matsubayashi et al.[78] showed that surgical repair with smooth muscle cell-seeded grafts reduced abnormal chamber distensibility and improved LV function after myocardial infarction as compared with unseeded grafts. The authors proposed that bioengineered muscle grafts may be superior to synthetic materials for the surgical repair of LV scar.[78]

Construct Vascularization

The 3-D cell constructs that are developed ex vivo usually lack the vascular network that exists in normal tissues. One of the most important requirements from a tissue engineering scaffold is its ability to support vascular infiltration.[79] Implanted cardiomyocytes are very sensitive to prolonged ischemia and may die by necrosis and apoptosis. Thus, to become clinically relevant, a myocardial tissue engineered graft requires persistent neovascularization, or angiogenesis, for its growth and survival. The extent of angiogenesis is determined by the regulating molecules that grafted cells and host cells release into the microenvironment of the engineered tissue.

Recent advances in our understanding of the process of blood vessel growth have provided significant tools for the neovascularization of bioengineered tissues. Several growth factors serve as stimuli for endothelial cell proliferation and migration as well as the formation of new blood vessels. Vascular epithelial growth factor (VEGF) is a major regulator of neovascularization. VEGF has a major role in the early development of blood cell progenitors.[80,81] Basic fibroblast growth factor (bFGF) is a potent inducer of endothelial cell proliferation and blood vessel growth in vitro and in vivo. VEGF and bFGF have been injected into under-vascularized ischemic myocardial tissues, resulting in new blood vessel formation and tissue perfusion.[80,81] Additional potential therapeutic angiogenic factors are listed in Table 1.5.

Site-specific delivery of angiogenic growth factors from tissue engineered devices should provide an efficient means of stimulating localized vessel recruitment to the cell transplants and would enhance cell survival and function. Local growth factors delivery will avoid serious adverse effects such as hyperpermeability, edema, hypotension, and accelerated atherosclerosis.[82] Angiogenic factors have been incorporated into bioengineered tissues and have facilitated blood vessel growth.[83-85] Richardson et al.[83] moved one step forward by creating a new polymeric system that delivers two or more growth factors, with controlled dose and rate of delivery. The utility of this system was investigated in the context of therapeutic angiogenesis. They showed that dual delivery of VEGF-165 and platelet-derived growth factor-BB, each with distinct kinetics, from a single, structural polymer scaffold results in the rapid formation of a mature vascular network.[83]

Other approaches such as prevascularization of the implanted scaffold before cell seeding[86] and incorporation of endothelial cells into the bioengineered tissues have produced encouraging results[87] and could be applied to myocardial tissue engineering.

In Situ Tissue Engineering

Although in vitro tissue engineering to create an engineered muscle patch in a bioreactor is fascinating and exciting, it faces significant difficulties, such as constructing significant cardiac

Table 1.5. Bioactive molecules to enhance self-repair, neoangiogenesis, and regeneration in animal models

Factor	Stem cell mobilization or recruitment	Myogenesis	Angiogenesis	Anti-apoptosis
Erythropoietin (EPO)[107]	Yes	No	Yes	Yes
Granulocyte colony-stimulating factor (G-CSF)[11,108]	Yes	No	Yes	No
Hepatocyte growth factor (HGF)[109,110]	Yes	Yes	Yes	Yes
Insulin-like growth factor (IGF-1)[111]	Yes	Yes	Yes	Yes
Leukemia inhibitory factor (LIF)[112]	Yes	Yes	Yes	Yes
Stromal-derived growth factor (SDF-1)[113]	Yes	No	Yes	Yes
Thymosin β4[114]	Yes	Yes	Yes	Yes

muscle from scaffold and cells in vitro, and poor graft survival. An alternative to the in vitro tissue engineering is the in situ tissue engineering approach. In this approach, unseeded alginate scaffolds are implanted on the damaged myocardium and, after their vascularization, they create a friendly environment and space for the implanted cells. To accelerate angiogenesis and engraftment, the implanted scaffold may be impregnated with bioactive molecules that improve viability and survival and may enhance stem cell homing and self-repair.

This strategy could be enhanced by bioactive materials (Table 1.3). With this approach, the biomaterial itself or its degradation/dissolution products are used to stimulate local tissue repair. Bioactive materials release chemicals in the form of ionic dissolution products, or growth factors, at controlled rates, by diffusion or network breakdown, that activate the cells in contact with the stimuli. The cells produce additional growth factors that in turn stimulate multiple generations of growing cells to self-assemble into tissues in situ along the biochemical and biomechanical gradients that are present. These materials, once implanted, will help the body heal itself.[88]

Molecular modifications of the biomaterial are intend to elicit specific interactions with cell integrins and thereby direct cell proliferation, differentiation, and ECM production and organization. The mechanism for in situ tissue regeneration involves up-regulation of genes that control the cell cycle, mitosis, and differentiation. Gene activation by controlled ion release provides the conceptual basis for molecular design of a third generation of biomaterials optimized for in situ tissue regeneration.[86]

In situ regeneration in the injured myocardium can be enhanced by direct delivery of several cytokines that potentially stimulate myocardial healing and repair in the setting of myocardial infarction (Table 1.5). Those cytokines may induce recruitment of stem/progenitor cells into the healing infarct, which may differentiate into endothelial cells and even lead to myocardial regeneration.

Injectable Tissue Engineering

Most of the efforts in cardiac tissue engineering focus on the use of implantable scaffolds that deliver cells to the epicardial surface. However, many strategies of cell or gene delivery to repair the infarcted myocardium are shifting toward a catheter-based approach. This semi-invasive approach avoids the risk of open chest surgery and anesthetics and is favored by both patients and physicians. The injectable scaffold facilitates repair after infarction by providing a matrix support within which cells are retained, migrate, and neoangiogenesis takes place.[89,90] Several works suggest that injectable biomaterials can serve as a cell implantation matrix that enhances neovascularization and repair of the infarcted myocardium. An important advantage of this concept of in situ tissue engineering is its feasibility for a catheter-based approach and to avoid the need for surgical thoracotomy.

We have recently presented preliminary data that show that injection of biodegradable alginate solution into the infarcted myocardium stimulates neoangiogenesis and efficiently attenuates infarct expansion, heart dilatation, and dysfunction.[45] Our preliminary work provides a minimally invasive, catheter-based, acellular option to facilitate neovascularization, self-repair, and rejuvenation of the infarcted myocardium. The injectable bioactive material proposes a viable solution to the difficulties in achieving appropriate cells to treat myocardial infarction and a future strategy of catheter-based injectable tissue engineering.

Summary and Future Perspectives

The ability to engineer or regenerate lost myocardial tissue caused by injury, aging, disease, or genetic abnormality holds great promise. The vision is to generate significant mass of functional heart muscle tissue. However, the area of myocardial tissue engineering still faces significant difficulties. Scientists are still searching for cell types other than cardiomyocytes. Novel approaches are warranted for material processing to create bioactive scaffolds, which would allow composition of the evolving myocardial structure. There is a need for development of strategies to promote vascularization and/or innervations within engineered myocardial tissue. Other important goals include achievement of immunologic tolerance for engineered constructs and increased understanding of the basic principles governing tissue formation, function, and failure, including the assembly of multiple cell types and biomaterials into multidimensional structures that mimic the architecture and function of native myocardial tissue.

In addition to laboratory-grown myocardial tissue, more research is warranted in the area of cardiac self-repair and regenerating functional myocardium in situ. If successful, these strategies could be used for surgical repair of the infarcted myocardium or congenital cardiac defects and would have a dramatic impact on the future of cardiovascular medicine and public health.

References

1. Walsh RA. Molecular and cellular biology of the normal, hypertrophied, and failing heart. In: O'Rouke RA, ed. The Heart, Arteries and Veins. 10th ed. New York: McGraw-Hill; 2001:115–118.
2. Jugdutt BI. Ventricular remodeling after infarction and the extracellular collagen matrix: when is enough enough? Circulation 2003;108:1395–1403.
3. Weber KT, Anversa P, Armstrong PW, et al. Remodeling and reparation of the cardiovascular system. J Am Coll Cardiol 1992;20:3–16.
4. Nag AC. Study of non-muscle cells of the adult mammalian heart: a fine structural analysis and distribution. Cytobios 1980;28:41–61.
5. Garry DJ, Martin CM. Cardiac regeneration: self-service at the pump. Circ Res 2004;95:852–854.
6. Lapidos KA, Kakkar R, McNally EM. The dystrophin glycoprotein complex: signaling strength and integrity for the sarcolemma. Circ Res 2004;94:1023–1031.
7. Sun Y, Kiani MF, Postlethwaite AE, Weber KT. Infarct scar as living tissue. Basic Res Cardiol 2002;97:343–347.
8. Nian M, Lee P, Khaper N, Liu P. Inflammatory cytokines and postmyocardial infarction remodeling. Circ Res 2004;94:1543–1553.
9. Etzion S, Kedes LH, Kloner RA, Leor J. Myocardial regeneration: present and future trends. Am J Cardiovasc Drugs 2001;1:233–244.
10. Lee MS, Makkar RR. Stem-cell transplantation in myocardial infarction: a status report. Ann Intern Med 2004;140:729–737.
11. Minatoguchi S, Takemura G, Chen XH, et al. Acceleration of the healing process and myocardial regeneration may be important as a mechanism of improvement of cardiac function and remodeling by postinfarction granulocyte colony-stimulating factor treatment. Circulation 2004;109:2572–2580.
12. Askari AT, Unzek S, Popovic ZB, et al. Effect of stromal-cell-derived factor 1 on stem-cell homing and tissue regeneration in ischaemic cardiomyopathy. Lancet 2003;362:697–703.
13. Beltrami AP, Barlucchi L, Torella D, et al. Adult cardiac stem cells are multipotent and support myocardial regeneration. Cell 2003;114:763–776.
14. Oh H, Bradfute SB, Gallardo TD, et al. Cardiac progenitor cells from adult myocardium: homing, differentiation, and fusion after infarction. Proc Natl Acad Sci USA 2003;100:12313–12318.
15. Matsuura K, Nagai T, Nishigaki N, et al. Adult cardiac Sca-1-positive cells differentiate into beating cardiomyocytes. J Biol Chem 2004;279:11384–11391.
16. Messina E, De Angelis L, Frati G, et al. Isolation and expansion of adult cardiac stem cells from human and murine heart. Circ Res 2004;95:911–921.
17. Leor J, Aboulafia-Etzion S, Dar A, et al. Bioengineered cardiac grafts: a new approach to repair the infarcted myocardium? Circulation 2000;102:III56–61.
18. Vacanti JP, Langer R. Tissue engineering: the design and fabrication of living replacement devices for surgical reconstruction and transplantation. Lancet 1999;354(suppl 1):SI32–34.
19. Etzion S, Battler A, Barbash IM, et al. Influence of embryonic cardiomyocyte transplantation on the progression of heart failure in a rat model of extensive myocardial infarction. J Mol Cell Cardiol 2001;33:1321–1330.
20. Langer R, Tirrell DA. Designing materials for biology and medicine. Nature 2004;428:487–492.
21. Humphries MJ, Akiyama SK, Komoriya A, Olden K, Yamada KM. Identification of an alternatively spliced site in human plasma fibronectin that mediates cell type-specific adhesion. J Cell Biol 1986;103:2637–2647.
22. Griffith LG, Lopina S. Microdistribution of substratum-bound ligands affects cell function: hepatocyte spreading on PEO-tethered galactose. Biomaterials 1998;19:979–986.
23. Rowley JA, Madlambayan G, Mooney DJ. Alginate hydrogels as synthetic extracellular matrix materials. Biomaterials 1999;20:45–53.
24. Tiwari A, Salacinski HJ, Punshon G, Hamilton G, Seifalian AM. Development of a hybrid cardiovascular graft using a tissue engineering approach. FASEB J 2002;16:791–796.
25. Pratt AB, Weber FE, Schmoekel HG, Muller R, Hubbell JA. Synthetic extracellular matrices for in situ tissue engineering. Biotechnol Bioeng 2004;86:27–36.
26. Nguyen H, Qian JJ, Bhatnagar RS, Li S. Enhanced cell attachment and osteoblastic activity by P-15 peptide-coated matrix in hydrogels. Biochem Biophys Res Commun 2003;311:179–186.
27. Koo LY, Irvine DJ, Mayes AM, Lauffenburger DA, Griffith LG. Co-regulation of cell adhesion by nanoscale RGD organization and mechanical stimulus. J Cell Sci 2002;115:1423–1433.
28. Kim MR, Jeong JH, Park TG. Swelling induced detachment of chondrocytes using RGD-modified poly(N-isopropylacrylamide) hydrogel beads. Biotechnol Prog 2002;18:495–500.
29. Mann BK, West JL. Cell adhesion peptides alter smooth muscle cell adhesion, proliferation, migration, and matrix protein synthesis on modified surfaces and in polymer scaffolds. J Biomed Mater Res 2002;60:86–93.
30. Halstenberg S, Panitch A, Rizzi S, Hall H, Hubbell JA. Biologically engineered protein-graft-poly(ethylene glycol) hydrogels: a cell adhesive and plasmin-degradable biosynthetic material for tissue repair. Biomacromolecules 2002;3:710–723.
31. Kehat I, Kenyagin-Karsenti D, Snir M, et al. Human embryonic stem cells can differentiate into myocytes with structural and functional properties of cardiomyocytes. J Clin Invest 2001;108:407–414.
32. Scheubel RJ, Zorn H, Silber RE, et al. Age-dependent depression in circulating endothelial progenitor cells

in patients undergoing coronary artery bypass grafting. J Am Coll Cardiol 2003;42:2073–2080.
33. Rauscher FM, Goldschmidt-Clermont PJ, Davis BH, et al. Aging, progenitor cell exhaustion, and atherosclerosis. Circulation 2003;108:457–463.
34. Dimmeler S, Vasa-Nicotera M. Aging of progenitor cells: limitation for regenerative capacity? J Am Coll Cardiol 2003;42:2081–2082.
35. Leor J, Barbash IM. Cell transplantation and genetic engineering: new approaches to cardiac pathology. Expert Opin Biol Ther 2003;3:1023–1039.
36. Menasche P. Cellular transplantation: hurdles remaining before widespread clinical use. Curr Opin Cardiol 2004;19:154–161.
37. Smits PC, van Geuns RJ, Poldermans D, et al. Catheter-based intramyocardial injection of autologous skeletal myoblasts as a primary treatment of ischemic heart failure. Clinical experience with six-month follow-up. J Am Coll Cardiol 2003;42:2063–2069.
38. Yoon Y-S, Park J-S, Tkebuchava T, Luedeman C, Losordo DW. Unexpected severe calcification after transplantation of bone marrow cells in acute myocardial infarction. Circulation 2004;109:3154–3157.
39. Vulliet PR, Greeley M, Halloran SM, MacDonald KA, Kittleson MD. Intra-coronary arterial injection of mesenchymal stromal cells and microinfarction in dogs. Lancet 2004;363:783–784.
40. Thomson JA, Itskovitz-Eldor J, Shapiro SS, et al. Embryonic stem cell lines derived from human blastocysts. Science 1998;282:1145–1147.
41. Mummery C, Ward-Van Oostwaard D, Doevendans P, et al. Differentiation of human embryonic stem cells to cardiomyocytes: role of coculture with visceral endoderm-like cells. Circulation 2003;107:2733–2740.
42. Takahashi T, Lord B, Schulze PC, et al. Ascorbic acid enhances differentiation of embryonic stem cells into cardiac myocytes. Circulation 2003;107:1912–1916.
43. Zimmermann WH, Melnychenko I, Eschenhagen T. Engineered heart tissue for regeneration of diseased hearts. Biomaterials 2004;25:1639–1647.
44. Leor J, Cohen S. Myocardial tissue engineering: creating a muscle patch for a wounded heart. Ann NY Acad Sci 2004;1015:312–319.
45. Cohen S, Leor J. Rebuilding broken hearts. Biologists and engineers working together in the fledgling field of tissue engineering are within reach of one of their greatest goals: constructing a living human heart patch. Sci Am 2004;291:44–51.
46. Zimmermann WH, Didie M, Wasmeier GH, et al. Cardiac grafting of engineered heart tissue in syngenic rats. Circulation 2002;106:I151–157.
47. Zimmermann WH, Schneiderbanger K, Schubert P, et al. Tissue engineering of a differentiated cardiac muscle construct. Circ Res 2002;90:223–230.
48. Shimizu T, Yamato M, Isoi Y, et al. Fabrication of pulsatile cardiac tissue grafts using a novel 3-dimensional cell sheet manipulation technique and temperature-responsive cell culture surfaces. Circ Res 2002;90:e40.
49. Shimizu T, Yamato M, Akutsu T, et al. Electrically communicating three-dimensional cardiac tissue mimic fabricated by layered cultured cardiomyocyte sheets. J Biomed Mater Res 2002;60:110–117.
50. Dar A, Shachar M, Leor J, Cohen S. Optimization of cardiac cell seeding and distribution in 3D porous alginate scaffolds. Biotechnol Bioeng 2002;80:305–312.
51. Carrier RL, Rupnick M, Langer R, Schoen FJ, Freed LE, Vunjak-Novakovic G. Perfusion improves tissue architecture of engineered cardiac muscle. Tissue Eng 2002;8:175–188.
52. Papadaki M, Bursac N, Langer R, Merok J, Vunjak-Novakovic G, Freed LE. Tissue engineering of functional cardiac muscle: molecular, structural, and electrophysiological studies. Am J Physiol Heart Circ Physiol 2001;280:H168–178.
53. Carrier RL, Papadaki M, Rupnick M, et al. Cardiac tissue engineering: cell seeding, cultivation parameters, and tissue construct characterization. Biotechnol Bioeng 1999;64:580–589.
54. Bursac N, Papadaki M, Cohen RJ, et al. Cardiac muscle tissue engineering: toward an in vitro model for electrophysiological studies. Am J Physiol 1999; 277:H433–444.
55. Akins RE, Boyce RA, Madonna ML, et al. Cardiac organogenesis in vitro: reestablishment of three-dimensional tissue architecture by dissociated neonatal rat ventricular cells. Tissue Eng 1999;5:103–118.
56. Bursac N, Papadaki M, White JA, Eisenberg SR, Vunjak-Novakovic G, Freed LE. Cultivation in rotating bioreactors promotes maintenance of cardiac myocyte electrophysiology and molecular properties. Tissue Eng 2003;9:1243–1253.
57. Kofidis T, Lenz A, Boublik J, et al. Pulsatile perfusion and cardiomyocyte viability in a solid three-dimensional matrix. Biomaterials 2003;24:5009–5014.
58. Kofidis T, Akhyari P, Boublik J, et al. In vitro engineering of heart muscle: artificial myocardial tissue. J Thorac Cardiovasc Surg 2002;124:63–69.
59. Radisic M, Park H, Shing H, et al. Functional assembly of engineered myocardium by electrical stimulation of cardiac myocytes cultured on scaffolds. Proc Natl Acad Sci USA 2004;101:18129–18134.
60. Radisic M, Yang L, Boublik J, et al. Medium perfusion enables engineering of compact and contractile cardiac tissue. Am J Physiol Heart Circ Physiol 2004;286:H507–516.
61. Zimmermann WH, Fink C, Kralisch D, Remmers U, Weil J, Eschenhagen T. Three-dimensional engineered heart tissue from neonatal rat cardiac myocytes. Biotechnol Bioeng 2000;68:106–114.
62. Zimmermann WH, Eschenhagen T. Cardiac tissue engineering for replacement therapy. Heart Fail Rev 2003;8:259–269.
63. Mironov V, Boland T, Trusk T, Forgacs G, Markwald RR. Organ printing: computer-aided jet-based 3D tissue engineering. Trends Biotechnol 2003;21:157–161.
64. McDevitt TC, Angello JC, Whitney ML, et al. In vitro generation of differentiated cardiac myofibers on micropatterned laminin surfaces. J Biomed Mater Res 2002;60:472–479.
65. McDevitt TC, Woodhouse KA, Hauschka SD, Murry CE, Stayton PS. Spatially organized layers of cardiomyocytes on biodegradable polyurethane films for myocardial repair. J Biomed Mater Res 2003;66A: 586–595.
66. Krupnick AS, Kreisel D, Engels FH, et al. A novel small animal model of left ventricular tissue engineering. J Heart Lung Transplant 2002;21:233–243.
67. Papadaki M, Bursac N, Langer R, Merok J, Vunjak-Novakovic G, Freed LE. Tissue engineering of functional cardiac muscle: molecular, structural, and

68. Akhyari P, Fedak PW, Weisel RD, et al. Mechanical stretch regimen enhances the formation of bioengineered autologous cardiac muscle grafts. Circulation 2002;106:I137–142.
69. Sodian R, Sperling JS, Martin DP, et al. Fabrication of a trileaflet heart valve scaffold from a polyhydroxyalkanoate biopolymer for use in tissue engineering. Tissue Eng 2000;6:183–188.
70. Dohmen PM, Ozaki S, Verbeken E, Yperman J, Flameng W, Konertz WF. Tissue engineering of an auto-xenograft pulmonary heart valve. Asian Cardiovasc Thorac Ann 2002;10:25–30.
71. Colton CK. Implantable biohybrid artificial organs. Cell Transplant 1995;4:415–436.
72. Zandonella C. Tissue engineering: the beat goes on. Nature 2003;421:884–886.
73. Li RK, Jia ZQ, Weisel RD, Mickle DA, Choi A, Yau TM. Survival and function of bioengineered cardiac grafts. Circulation 1999;100:II63–69.
74. Leor J, Aboulafia-Etzion S, Dar A, et al. Bioengineered cardiac grafts: a new approach to repair the infarcted myocardium? Circulation 2000;102:III56–61.
75. Kelley ST, Malekan R, Gorman JH 3rd, et al. Restraining infarct expansion preserves left ventricular geometry and function after acute anteroapical infarction. Circulation 1999;99:135–142.
76. Oz MC, Konertz WF, Kleber FX, et al. Global surgical experience with the Acorn cardiac support device. J Thorac Cardiovasc Surg 2003;126:983–991.
77. Kellar RS, Landeen LK, Shepherd BR, Naughton GK, Ratcliffe A, Williams SK. Scaffold-based three-dimensional human fibroblast culture provides a structural matrix that supports angiogenesis in infarcted heart tissue. Circulation 2001;104:2063–2068.
78. Matsubayashi K, Fedak PW, Mickle DA, Weisel RD, Ozawa T, Li RK. Improved left ventricular aneurysm repair with bioengineered vascular smooth muscle grafts. Circulation 2003;108(suppl 1):II219–225.
79. Patel ZS, Mikos AG. Angiogenesis with biomaterial-based drug- and cell-delivery systems. J Biomater Sci Polym Ed 2004;15:701–726.
80. Losordo DW, Dimmeler S. Therapeutic angiogenesis and vasculogenesis for ischemic disease. Part II. Cell-based therapies. Circulation 2004;109:2692–2697.
81. Losordo DW, Dimmeler S. Therapeutic angiogenesis and vasculogenesis for ischemic disease. Part I. Angiogenic cytokines. Circulation 2004;109:2487–2491.
82. Epstein SE, Kornowski R, Fuchs S, Dvorak HF. Angiogenesis therapy: amidst the hype, the neglected potential for serious side effects. Circulation 2001;104: 115–119.
83. Richardson TP, Peters MC, Ennett AB, Mooney DJ. Polymeric system for dual growth factor delivery. Nat Biotechnol 2001;19:1029–1034.
84. Perets A, Baruch Y, Weisbuch F, Shoshany G, Neufeld G, Cohen S. Enhancing the vascularization of three-dimensional porous alginate scaffolds by incorporating controlled release basic fibroblast growth factor microspheres. J Biomed Mater Res 2003;65A:489–497.
85. Peters MC, Isenberg BC, Rowley JA, Mooney DJ. Release from alginate enhances the biological activity of vascular endothelial growth factor. J Biomater Sci Polym Ed 1998;9:1267–1278.
86. Hench LL, Xynos ID, Polak JM. Bioactive glasses for in situ tissue regeneration. J Biomater Sci Polym Ed 2004;15:543–562.
87. Park HJ, Yoo JJ, Kershen RT, Moreland R, Atala A. Reconstitution of human corporal smooth muscle and endothelial cells in vivo. J Urol 1999;162:1106–1109.
88. Hench LL, Polak JM. Third-generation biomedical materials. Science 2002;295:1014–1017.
89. Christman KL, Fok HH, Sievers RE, Fang Q, Lee RJ. Fibrin glue alone and skeletal myoblasts in a fibrin scaffold preserve cardiac function after myocardial infarction. Tissue Eng 2004;10:403–409.
90. Kofidis T, De Bruin JL, Hoyt G, et al. Injectable bioartificial myocardial tissue for large-scale intramural cell transfer and functional recovery of injured heart muscle. J Thorac Cardiovasc Surg 2004;128:571–578.
91. Kamelger FS, Marksteiner R, Margreiter E, et al. A comparative study of three different biomaterials in the engineering of skeletal muscle using a rat animal model. Biomaterials 2004;25:1649–1655.
92. Li RK. Cell transplantation to improve heart function: cell or matrix. Yonsei Med J 2004;45(suppl):S72–73.
93. Ryu JH, Kim IK, Cho SW, et al. Implantation of bone marrow mononuclear cells using injectable fibrin matrix enhances neovascularization in infarcted myocardium. Biomaterials 2005;26:319–326.
94. Wu X, Rabkin-Aikawa E, Guleserian KJ, et al. Tissue-engineered microvessels on three-dimensional biodegradable scaffolds using human endothelial progenitor cells. Am J Physiol Heart Circ Physiol 2004; 287:H480–487.
95. Stamm C, Westphal B, Kleine HD, et al. Autologous bone-marrow stem-cell transplantation for myocardial regeneration. Lancet 2003;361:45–46.
96. Krupnick AS, Kreisel D, Szeto WY, Popma SH, Rosengard BR. A murine model of left ventricular tissue engineering. J Heart Lung Transplant 2001; 20:197–198.
97. Kadner A, Zund G, Maurus C, et al. Human umbilical cord cells for cardiovascular tissue engineering: a comparative study. Eur J Cardiothorac Surg 2004;25:635–641.
98. Li RK, Yau TM, Weisel RD, et al. Construction of a bioengineered cardiac graft. J Thorac Cardiovasc Surg 2000;119:368–375.
99. Kehat I, Khimovich L, Caspi O, et al. Electromechanical integration of cardiomyocytes derived from human embryonic stem cells. Nat Biotechnol 2004;22:1282–1289.
100. Lanza R, Moore MA, Wakayama T, et al. Regeneration of the infarcted heart with stem cells derived by nuclear transplantation. Circ Res 2004;94:820–827.
101. Chandy T, Rao GH, Wilson RF, Das GS. The development of porous alginate/elastin/PEG composite matrix for cardiovascular engineering. J Biomater Appl 2003;17:287–301.
102. Christman KL, Vardanian AJ, Fang Q, Sievers RE, Fok HH, Lee RJ. Injectable fibrin scaffold improves cell transplant survival, reduces infarct expansion, and induces neovasculature formation in ischemic myocardium. J Am Coll Cardiol 2004;44:654–660.
103. Stock UA, Mayer JE Jr. Tissue engineering of cardiac valves on the basis of PGA/PLA co-polymers. J Long Term Eff Med Implants 2001;11:249–260.

104. Ozawa T, Mickle DA, Weisel RD, Koyama N, Ozawa S, Li RK. Optimal biomaterial for creation of autologous cardiac grafts. Circulation 2002;106:I176–182.
105. Pego AP, Siebum B, Van Luyn MJ, et al. Preparation of degradable porous structures based on 1,3-trimethylene carbonate and D,L-lactide (co)polymers for heart tissue engineering. Tissue Eng 2003;9:981–994.
106. Zammaretti P, Jaconi M. Cardiac tissue engineering: regeneration of the wounded heart. Curr Opin Biotechnol 2004;15:430–434.
107. Calvillo L, Latini R, Kajstura J, et al. Recombinant human erythropoietin protects the myocardium from ischemia-reperfusion injury and promotes beneficial remodeling. Proc Natl Acad Sci USA 2003;100:4802–4806.
108. Takano H, Ohtsuka M, Akazawa H, et al. Pleiotropic effects of cytokines on acute myocardial infarction: G-CSF as a novel therapy for acute myocardial infarction. Curr Pharm Des 2003;9:1121–1127.
109. Wang Y, Ahmad N, Wani MA, Ashraf M. Hepatocyte growth factor prevents ventricular remodeling and dysfunction in mice via Akt pathway and angiogenesis. J Mol Cell Cardiol 2004;37:1041–1052.
110. Jayasankar V, Woo YJ, Bish LT, et al. Gene transfer of hepatocyte growth factor attenuates postinfarction heart failure. Circulation 2003;108(suppl 1):II230–236.
111. Musaro A, Giacinti C, Borsellino G, et al. Stem cell-mediated muscle regeneration is enhanced by local isoform of insulin-like growth factor 1. Proc Natl Acad Sci USA 2004;101:1206–1210.
112. Zou Y, Takano H, Mizukami M, et al. Leukemia inhibitory factor enhances survival of cardiomyocytes and induces regeneration of myocardium after myocardial infarction. Circulation 2003;108:748–753.
113. Hiasa K-I, Ishibashi M, Ohtani K, et al. Gene transfer of stromal cell-derived factor-1alpha enhances ischemic vasculogenesis and angiogenesis via vascular endothelial growth factor/endothelial nitric oxide synthase-related pathway: next-generation chemokine therapy for therapeutic neovascularization. Circulation 2004;109:2454–2461.
114. Bock-Marquette I, Saxena A, White MD, Dimaio JM, Srivastava D. Thymosin beta4 activates integrin-linked kinase and promotes cardiac cell migration, survival and cardiac repair. Nature 2004;432:466–472.

2

Adult Stem Cells for Myocardial Tissue Repair

Dirk Strunk and Christof Stamm

The prospect of using adult stem cells for myocardial tissue repair has caused understandably great excitement among cardiovascular physicians and scientists, because it may all but revolutionize treatment of the sequels of ischemic heart disease. The traditional definition of a stem cell requires the capacity for "asymmetric" cell division (i.e., the stem cell divides into one stem cell and one differentiated cell), whereas a classic progenitor cell divides in two differentiated daughter cells. The cells that are used in myocardial regeneration attempts do not always fulfill these criteria; it may therefore be more appropriate to talk about cardiac cell therapy in a more general way. In this context, some biologic principles of stem cells may be worth reiterating: Whereas embryonic stem cells are uncommitted and pluripotent in their differentiation capability, adult stem cells are believed to be committed to differentiate only into specialized cells of the organ or tissue they are derived from. The function of adult stem cells seems to be maintenance and repair of their tissue of origin; they are therefore also termed somatic stem cells. Understanding of adult/somatic stem cells has been upset by recent experimental data indicating that adult stem cells derived from hematopoietic tissue can give rise to non-hematopoietic cells such as cardiomyocytes, hepatocytes, endothelial, and epithelial cells. Initially, this was interpreted to represent trans-differentiation of hematopoietic stem cells (HSCs) by crossing lineage boundaries, the so-called "stem cell plasticity."[1] Alternatively, the existence of non-HSCs or even more immature multipotent types of stem cells in the various transplanted cell sources as well as the phenomenon of fusion of transplanted cells with resident cells in the damaged organ have been taken into consideration.[2,3] To date, the mechanisms underlying adult stem cell-mediated organ regeneration are not clear (Figure 2.1). Various types of progenitors and stem cells with myocardial regenerative potential have been derived from skeletal muscle and myocardium as well as different hematopoietic cell sources including bone marrow (BM), peripheral blood (PB), and umbilical cord blood.

In the following text, we will discuss the pathophysiologic background of ischemic heart failure and the rationale for the use of adult stem cells to regenerate ischemic myocardium. We will further highlight information on contractile muscle-derived regenerative cells as well as adult stem cells from hematopoietic tissue to build a basis for a critical discussion of the ongoing clinical trials.

Ischemic Heart Disease

Despite a better understanding of its etiology, the prevalence of ischemic heart disease remains exceedingly high in industrialized countries, and is on the rise in developing countries. Risk factors for coronary atherosclerosis have long been established, but it remains unclear whether

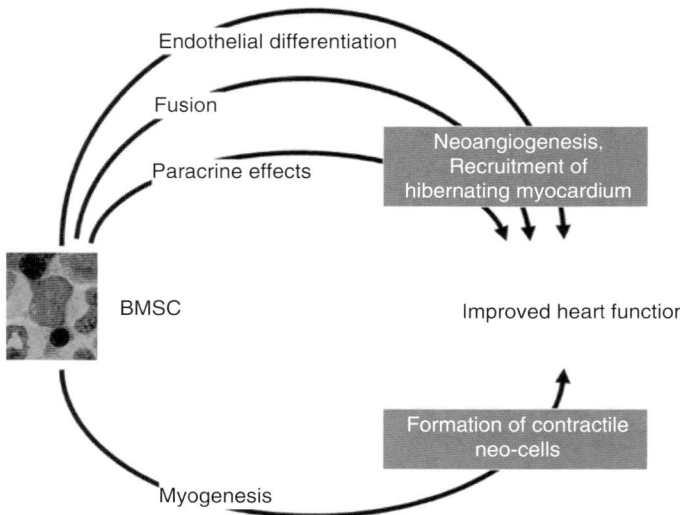

Figure 2.1. Several mechanisms for cell therapy-induced improvement of left ventricular contractility are possible. Neoangiogenesis does not necessarily require true differentiation of adult stem cells in cells of endothelial phenotype. Paracrine effects of transplanted stem cells have been shown to be at least partly responsible for vasculogenesis, and fusion with host tissue cells might also have beneficial effects. In turn, improved perfusion of ischemic myocardium may translate into better contractility via recruitment of hibernating myocardium. However, formation of new contractile tissue would likely require myogenic differentiation of stem or progenitor cells. BMSC, bone marrow stem cell.

there is one unifying mechanism by which atherosclerotic narrowing of the coronary arteries develops. In many patients, sudden rupture of the endothelial surface of a localized atherosclerotic plaque leads to thrombus formation with acute occlusion of the coronary vessel. The resulting myocardial ischemia induces immediate biochemical changes and loss of myocardial contractility. Irreversible necrosis of cardiomyocytes takes approximately 30 minutes to develop, and further extends with time for several hours. Thanks to improvements in primary and secondary prevention as well as therapeutic interventions, both incidence and mortality of acute myocardial infarction (AMI) recently decreased, but the number of individuals suffering AMI is still estimated to exceed 1.5 million per year in the United States and 2 million per year in Western and Central Europe. Many patients develop diffuse atherosclerotic disease of the entire coronary artery tree, and repeated episodes of AMI may result in severely impaired myocardial contractility and heart failure, often described as "ischemic cardiomyopathy." The most problematic consequence – besides the clinical symptoms of angina pectoris – is a net loss of contractile tissue. The myocardium consists of terminally differentiated cells without a clinically relevant potential for regeneration, although the existence of cardiac stem cells has recently been indicated. Hence, large numbers of cardiomyocytes that were subject to necrotic or apoptotic cell death cannot sufficiently be replaced by new contractile cells. Instead, remodeling processes ultimately lead to diffuse interstitial myocardial fibrosis or formation of a transmural fibrous scar. Without invasive treatment, survival of patients with myocardial infarction and considerably reduced left ventricular (LV) contractility [e.g., LV ejection fraction (LVEF) <30%] is less than 40% after 5 years, which illustrates the urgent need for novel therapeutic measures. Surgical or interventional restoration of blood supply to ischemic myocardium effectively treats angina, prevents myocardial infarction, improves function of the remaining viable myocardium, but viability and function of necrotic myocardium cannot be restored with current therapeutic means.

Recently, transplantation of cells into infarcted myocardium has evolved as a strategy to restore myocardial viability and contractility. Initial reports on cell therapy for myocardial tissue repair described the implantation of differentiated cells (i.e., cardiomyocytes) or defined progenitor cells [i.e., skeletal myoblasts or endothelial progenitor cells (EPCs)].[4–6] Contractile cell types such as allogenic cardiomyocytes or skeletal myoblasts have been shown to survive in areas of myocardial necrosis and to improve local contractile function.[4] Because of their ease of isolation, cells from hematopoietic tissue are considered the best available source of adult stem cells.[7] Finally, embryonic stem cells have been used experimentally in the context of myocardial cell therapy, but will not be reviewed in this chapter. The potential to induce both neoangiogenesis and neomyogenesis in infarcted myocardium by transplanting adult stem cells attracted tremendous attention by clinicians and basic researchers. The current understanding of the underlying mechanisms has recently been reviewed in great detail.[8–10] Herein, we will briefly portray the various cell types and their experimental applications, summarize the current clinical experience with myocardial cell therapy, and discuss some of the problems arising in the process of rapid bench-to-bedside translation.

Contractile (Progenitor) Cells

Among the first cells that were implanted in experimental models of myocardial infarction were allogenic or syngenic *cardiomyocytes*. After direct injection of cardiomyocytes into postinfarction scar tissue, they survived, appeared to be integrated into the myocardial syncytium as evidenced by formation of intercalated disks and expression of specific gap-junction proteins, and led to improvement of myocardial contractility.[11] Even though the initial reports were promising, cardiomyocyte transplantation will probably not reach clinical significance for several reasons: First, availability is limited. Neonatal rodent cardiomyocytes can be isolated and cultivated, but adult cardiomyocytes in higher mammals have virtually no capacity for proliferation in cell culture. Theoretically, allogenic or xenogenic cardiomyocytes could be obtained from donors, but would be subject to rejection, unless immunosuppression would be induced as in any other organ transplant patient. Second, transplanted cardiomyocytes are as susceptible to ischemia as the native cardiomyocytes. Implanted in ischemic myocardium, they are therefore prone to succumb to tissue hypoxia just as the native host cells did. Third, ventricular cardiomyocytes spontaneously produce action potentials and contract, albeit slowly. This quality is potentially lifesaving in a patient with bradycardia, but may result in serious ventricular arrhythmia when such cells form an arrhythmogenic focus that cannot be effectively suppressed by the surrounding host myocardium. In fact, cardiomyocytes have been shown to act as pacemakers after implantation in dog hearts once the native conduction system was destroyed.[12] In contrast, *smooth muscle cells* do not contract spontaneously in vitro or after implantation in the heart. They can be isolated from intestine, blood vessel wall, or genitourinary organs, and may readily be expanded in cell culture. Their potential usefulness for restoration of contractile tissue after AMI has been demonstrated in rodent models,[13] but they are currently not as intensively studied as other cell types. The largest body of knowledge has most likely been collected regarding *skeletal myoblasts*. These so-called "satellite cells" reside in the periphery of skeletal muscle fibers and serve to regenerate skeletal muscle tissue after injuries. Skeletal myoblasts can be readily isolated from a small muscle biopsy; in humans, the thigh musculature is often used. The isolation process involves enzymatic digestion and mechanic destruction of myofibers, and the myoblasts are collected and enriched by filtration and plating. No specific surface marker-based cell selection is necessary. There is usually some fibroblast contamination, which can be sufficiently controlled by frequent culture replating, and purity of the final product should exceed 80%. Myoblasts have a robust proliferation capacity and multiply in high-serum concentration for numerous passages without changes in phenotype. Once the serum concentration in the medium is lowered, they rapidly differentiate and fuse to form multinucleated myotubes. Besides their intrinsically preprogrammed differentiation in a myocyte phenotype, their most intriguing quality is resistance to hypoxia, and it has been assumed that myoblasts are able to survive in ischemic myocardium better and longer than cardiomyocytes. Doubt remains, however, as to their ability to functionally integrate into the myocardial syncytium, i.e., to express cardiac-specific connexins and form functioning gap junctions with surrounding viable cardiomyocytes. In principle, undifferentiated myoblasts can express connexin 43 (C×43), the predominant gap-junction protein in ventricular myocardium, and at least some of the myoblasts appear to be able to form functioning cell–cell communications with cocultured cardiomyocytes in vitro.[14] Once they have differentiated and formed myotubes in conventional two-dimensional (2-D) culture, the C×43 expression is markedly down-regulated but may persist to some degree. However, when myoblasts are grown and differentiate in 3-D culture under mechanical stimulation such as longitudinal strain, C×43 expression is preserved or even up-regulated. The situation in vivo after implantation in infarcted myocardium is naturally more difficult to assess. Many reports indicated that skeletal myotubes are not morphologically integrated in the host myocardium; instead they appear to form distinct islets in postinfarct tissue. C×43 expression in transplanted myoblasts has been described in several animal models, but has not been detected in patients who underwent myoblast injection and postmortem histologic studies. In a careful study of myoblast transplantation in mice, Rubart et al.[15] found that the majority of the intramyocardial myoblasts/myotubes are functionally isolated from the surrounding myocardium, and suggested that the remaining cells connect with host cardiomyocytes as a result of cell fusion. Their observations might not only explain the conflicting results of other studies, but also provide an explanation of a significant clinical problem: The durations of calcium transients recorded from intramyocardial skeletal myoblasts were heterogeneous compared with those in neighboring host cardiomyocytes, which may interfere with the propagation of excitation across the ventricular myocardium and pose the heart at risk of ventricular arrhythmia. Rhythm disturbances have indeed been observed in several patients who underwent skeletal myoblast implantation. Whereas the very first patient who underwent myoblast implantation together with a coronary artery bypass grafting (CABG) operation in a pioneering undertaking by Menasché and colleagues[16] had an uneventful postoperative course, several other patients developed life-threatening ventricular arrhythmia a few days after the procedure. Surgical patients were still under close observation and could be treated, but elsewhere patients had undergone transcatheter myoblast implantation with early discharge from the hospital and could not be saved. Therefore, at least in well-structured trials, clinical myoblast implantation for heart failure is currently limited to patients who have an automatic defibrillator device implanted. As to the efficacy of myoblast implantation, numerous small and large animal studies have shown a significant improvement of LV contractility. Results of the early clinical pilot trials were also encouraging, but results of large-scale controlled clinical trials are not yet available.

Marrow, Blood, and Cord Blood Cells

Blood and bone are attractive, readily accessible sources of stem cells (Table 2.1). These cell reservoirs harbor various populations of candidate regenerative cells including hematopoietic progenitor cells (HPCs)[4] and HSCs, EPCs,[5] mesenchymal stem cells (MSCs),[6–8] and multipotent adult progenitor cells (MAPCs).[9,10] In the context of cardiac cell therapy, the term "adult stem cells" usually refers to the application of mixed cell populations obtained from marrow, PB, or cord blood. Other sources of cells with the capacity for asymmetric division and plasticity such as fatty tissue or pancreas have, so far, only occasionally been used in myocardial regeneration attempts. Contradictory findings regarding the regenerative potency of these cells are, at least in part, attributed to the heterogeneity of stem cells present in different sources and preparations. Within BM, at least two distinct populations of progenitor and stem cells have so far been clearly recognized. These are (i) CD34$^+$/45$^+$/133$^+$ HPCs including a small fraction of HSCs as the traditional source of hematopoietic progeny, and (ii) CD34$^-$/45$^-$/133$^-$ MSCs with the capacity to renew marrow stroma, support hematopoiesis, and to differentiate into various mesodermal cell types including connective tissue (chondrocytes, osteocytes), adipocytes, and myocytes.[17,18] The phenotype of in vitro cultured MSCs shows a typical combination of marker molecules CD73 (SH3, SH4), CD90 (Thy1), and CD105 (SH2) with a lack of the HSC markers CD34 and CD133. The homogeneous expression of the otherwise endothelial-specific molecule CD146 (Muc18) may allow for speculations about a certain relation between MSCs and the endothelial lineage (Figure 2.2). In fact, MSCs cultured under standard conditions readily form vascular-like networks after implantation into a 3-D Matrigel matrix [Figure 2.3A (see color section)], although these structures are less complete than that formed by primary vascular endothelial cells

Adult Stem Cells for Myocardial Tissue Repair

Table 2.1. Adult progenitor and stem cells for myocardial repair*

Cord blood	Bone marrow	Peripheral blood	Mobilized peripheral blood	Tissue
Hematopoietic stem cells[52]	Hematopoietic stem cells[52]	Hematopoietic stem cells[52]	Hematopoietic stem cells[52]	Side population[52]
Hemangioblast[53]	Hemangioblast[53]	Blood outgrowth endothelial cell[23]	Hemangioblast[54]	Endothelial progenitor cells[8]
Circulating endothelial progenitor[55]	Marrow endothelial progenitor[21]	Circulating endothelial progenitor[24]	Circulating endothelial progenitor[55]	Mesenchymal stem cells[56]
Universal somatic stem cell[57]	Mesenchymal stem cell[58]	Endothelial progenitor cell[6]	Mesenchymal stem cell[59]	Skeletal myoblast[4]
	Multipotent adult progenitor cell[21]	Circulating endothelial cell[25]		

*Candidate adult stem cell types and possible sources for cell transfer-induced myocardial regeneration. Numerous subpopulations of cells with regenerative capacity have been described. They are mainly defined by expression of surface markers, and some by functional properties such as adhesion to plastic surfaces. Although the list of cell types is growing steadily, the ideal cell has not yet been found. The references are by no means exhaustive. They have merely been selected to allow for a first orientation in the rapidly growing field of adult stem cell research.

[Figure 2.3B (see color section)]. Another hallmark of EPCs, the formation of cord-like structure in liquid cultures, can also regularly be found in early MSC-containing BM explants [Figure 2.3C (see color section)]. Almost complete acquisition of endothelial phenotype and function under optimized culture conditions has recently been reported.[19] A minute subpopulation of cells that copurify with MSCs has been originally described as mesodermal progenitor cells and, because of the wide spectrum of differentiation, renamed as multipotent adult progenitor cells (MAPCs).[20] These CD34⁻/133⁺/Flk1⁺ cells have been postulated to comprise the principle endothelial progenitor in human postnatal BM.[21] Human MAPCs can differentiate into adipocytes, osteoblasts, endothelial cells, and hepatocytes in vitro and, after injection into the tibialis anterior muscle of NOD/SCID mice in vivo, into myocytes.[22]

Endothelial cells can definitively be derived from BM[23] but a conclusive description of an endothelial stem cell in adult BM is still a matter of debate. CD133⁺/VEGFR2⁺ BM-derived cells are currently the most widely used functional EPC.[6] Putative BM-derived progenitors of endothelial cells have been originally recovered from normal PB as CD34⁺/45⁺ cells.[24] The relation between these cells and circulating endothelial cells could not be clarified so far.[25] Various types of cells related to the endothelial lineage have thus far been described in most hematopoietic

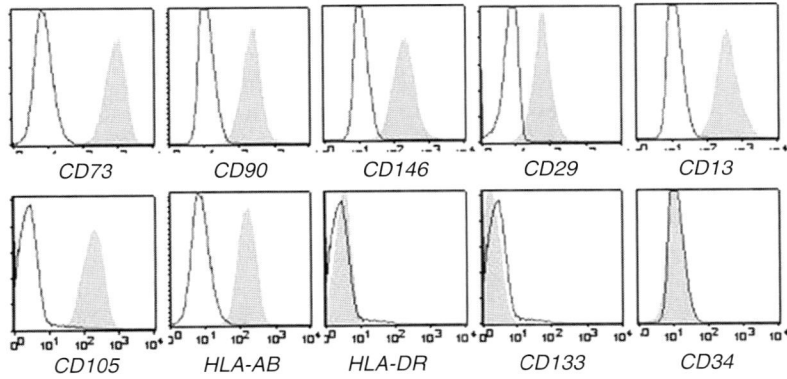

Figure 2.2. Immune phenotype of in vitro cultured adult human bone marrow MSCs. Flow cytometric analysis of typical marker molecules on short-term cultured human adult MSCs. (Courtesy of Christina Malischnik, BSc.)

and nonhematopoietic tissues (Table 2.1). The differences in frequency, phenotype, and function of these endothelial lineage cells clearly need to be analyzed in greater detail. The reactivity of several of these cell types with CD133 and the coexpression of CD133 on the greater part of CD34+ HPCs and HSCs have been taken as a strong argument in favor of positive selection to enrich adult stem cells for clinical use.

Adult Stem Cells for Myocardial Regeneration

Ideally, a stem cell that has been implanted into infarcted myocardium would give rise to new blood vessels *and* new contractile cells (i.e., angiogenesis and myogenesis). Proliferation and differentiation would be guided by local humoral and/or cellular control mechanisms, and no neoplastic growth or differentiation in unwanted noncardiac cell types would occur. So far, neither the ideal source and type of stem cell nor the critical cell number and mode of application have been defined. In 2001, two experimental studies of myocardial repair by adult stem cells from hematopoietic sources after experimental myocardial infarction promoted an unparalleled boost of clinical and experimental regenerative stem cell therapy studies. They also mirror the variety of adult stem cells used for myocardial repair. Kocher et al.[26] found that systemic intravenous infusion of purified human CD34+ cells from granulocyte colony-stimulating factor (G-CSF) mobilized PB can improve rat heart function by generating new blood vessels within the infarct area ("neovasculogenesis"). Our own group has reproduced this phenomenon using human cord blood cells [Figures 2.4 and 2.5 (see color section)]. Orlic et al.[27,28] reported on both neovasculogenesis and transdifferentiation of transplanted cells into cardiomyocytes by either using intramyocardial application of mouse BM-derived Lin^{NEG}/c-Kit+ stem cells or cytokine-induced stem cell mobilization. Many of the initial clinical pilot trials were fueled by the suggestion that early hematopoietic stem cells have a plasticity high enough to enable differentiation into contractile cells of cardiomyocyte phenotype. In fact, such cells were considered to be able to truly regenerate infarcted myocardium by promoting both neoangiogenesis and neomyogenesis. The initial enthusiasm, however, has largely faded. Whereas in situ neoangiogenesis induction by hematopoietic cells, associated with functional improvements, is consistently observed, it proved difficult to find corroborating evidence for true cardiomyocyte differentiation. In fact, two independent groups reported early in 2004 that they did not detect any meaningful evidence of cardiomyocyte differentiation of HSCs in mouse models that were designed to confirm the earlier findings.[29,30] In contrast, the myogenic potential of stroma cell-derived MSCs is much better documented. Several years ago, Wakitani et al.[31] reported the in vitro development of myogenic cells from rat BM MSCs exposed to the DNA-demethylating agent 5-azacytidine, and Makino et al.[32] isolated a cardiomyogenic cell line from murine BM stromal cells that were treated with 5-azacytidine and screened for spontaneous beating. Those cells connected with adjoining cells, formed myotube-like structures, and beat spontaneously and synchronously. They expressed various cardiomyocyte-specific proteins, had a cardiomyocyte-like ultrastructure, and generated several types of sinus node-like and ventricular cell-like action potentials. When isogenic marrow stromal cells are implanted in rat hearts, they appear to become integrated in cardiac myofibers, assume the histologic phenotype of cardiomyocytes, express connexins, and form gap junctions with native cardiomyocytes.[33,34] Again, pretreatment with 5-azacytidine is believed to facilitate differentiation toward a cardiomyocyte phenotype in vivo.[35] Human MSCs derived from the marrow of volunteers have also been injected in hearts of immunodeficient mice, and again it was observed that they assume cardiomyocyte morphology and express various cardiomyocyte-specific proteins.[36]

Taken together, there is quite convincing evidence that MSCs derived from marrow stroma may assume a myocyte-like phenotype under certain conditions, whereas hematopoietic stem and progenitor cell types are primarily involved in angiogenic processes (Figure 2.6). Nevertheless, numerous questions remain to be answered before cell therapy for neovascularization of ischemic myocardium can become clinical routine: First, is the angiogenic potential of human cells sufficient for relevant neovascularization of ischemic myocardial tissue? Second, what are the best surface markers of human adult stem cells with angiogenic potential? Third, how are such cells best delivered to ischemic myocardium? Fourth, what is the molecular mechanism of stem

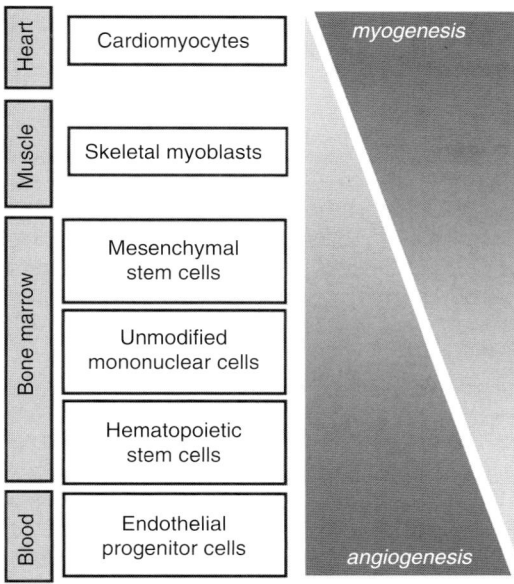

Figure 2.6. Of the clinically relevant cell types, some are primarily myogenic cells, and others have angiogenic characteristics. Some investigators argue that the angiogenic and myogenic properties are mutually exclusive; others claim that several cell types have capacity for both.

the suggested survival rate over days or weeks ranges between 0.1% and 10%. The causality is probably multifactorial. First of all, the ischemic myocardium is obviously a hostile environment, because of local hypoxia, acidosis, lack of substrates, and accumulation of metabolites. Skeletal myoblasts are known to be quite resistant to ischemia, but little is known about the energy requirements of hematopoietic or mesenchymal stem cells. Second, necrotic myocardium is subject to infiltration with phagocytic cells that remove cell debris and initiate the scarring process. Even though the stem/progenitor cells used clinically are autologous, many are probably lost in this "clean-up" process. Third, the mechanic forces that are present in the myocardium may have a role. Transmural pressure is high during systole, and there are shear forces between contracting myofibers and layers. Again, a skeletal myoblast might be able to tolerate this, but a marrow cell is certainly not well equipped to withstand such stress. Fortunately, the rate of cell death can be slowed by targeted manipulation of the cells to be injected. Transfection of marrow stromal cells with a gene encoding for the anti-apoptotic protein AKT has been shown to greatly improve cell survival and regenerative capacity upon injection in infarcted myocardium. Pretreatment of EPCs with endothelial nitric oxide synthase-enhancing substances also seems to have a beneficial conditioning effect. Simple hypoxic preconditioning before cell injection might also help, because it has been shown to activate both antiapoptotic and nitric oxide-related signaling pathways.

cell-endothelial differentiation? Fifth, are there risks of cell-induced neovascularization that outweigh the potential benefit? Finally, can the natural angiogenesis-inducing capacity of adult stem cells, which is obviously not sufficient in many situations, be further augmented?

Cell Survival

When cells are injected into ischemic myocardium, it is likely that most of them do not survive. The cell preparation process is usually well tolerated. Skeletal myoblasts or other ex vivo expanded cells, as well as processed primary cells normally have viability rates higher than 90%. It is often argued that injection of cell suspension through a needle or a catheter significantly compromises cell viability. In our experience, this is not the case. Even injection through a long cardiac catheterization device has very little effect on cell survival. Once the cells have entered the myocardial interstitium, however, many of them appear to succumb to necrotic or apoptotic death. Its magnitude is difficult to determine, but

Functional Effects

To the clinician, the functional effects of myocardial cell therapy matter so much more than histologic evidence of neoangiogenesis or neomyogenesis. The reliability of LV function measurements in experimental models depends both on the animal model and on the method used. Much of the basic experimental work on cell therapy for myocardial regeneration has been done in mouse models. The main reasons for that are the availability of immunodeficient mice (SCID mice) that allow for the use of human cell transplants with immunologic response, the use of GFP, lac-Z, or otherwise labeled cells from genetically modified animals, and the ready availability of antibodies and nucleic acid probes for detailed expression analysis in situ. The possibilities of histologic analysis of mouse heart tissue after cell transfer are virtually unlimited. The problem, however, is the functional analysis. Echocardiographic as well as magnetic resonance imaging of mouse hearts are indeed possible, but given the tiny dimensions and tremendously high heart rate, reliable determination requires highly experienced investigators. The most robust parameter of global LV contractility in mice may be shortening fraction (the extent by which the diameter of the LV cavity decreases during systole), but reproducible data on regional contractility are almost impossible to obtain. The next larger model, the rat, has been used for cardiac cell transplantation with good results. The availability of athymic rats allows for xenogenic transplantation of human cell populations without T cell-mediated acute rejection, and functional studies are much easier. Serial echocardiographic analysis of global LV function and dimensions can be performed with good reproducibility. Moreover, cardiac catheterization is feasible, and by using a multielectrode electromagnetic conductance catheter supplied with a pressure transducer, LV pressure-volume curves can be recorded. Those allow for detailed functional analysis of myocardial contractility and relaxation properties. The rabbit as a model for myocardial cell transfer experiments is being used quite rarely. There is no clear advantage with respect to functional analysis as compared with the rat, and the problems with antibodies and other tools for expression profiling and histology are notorious. Thus, truly reliable analysis of myocardial function after cell therapy requires the use of a large animal model, i.e., porcine, canine, or ovine. Here, both echocardiography and magnetic resonance imaging allow for serial studies of global as well as regional myocardial contractility in the specific area of interest. In acute experiments or set-ups with chronic instrumentation, very reliable sonomicrometry data can be obtained after cardiac implantation of ultrasound crystals. Scintigraphic perfusion scans and coronary angiography can be performed. A major disadvantage of many large animal models is the deficiency of antibodies against stem cell surface markers, and the inevitable immune response when xenogenic, i.e., human cells are used.

The baseline result of most of the published work is that there is some improvement of global and – if appropriate – regional contractility after adult stem/progenitor cell implantation in ischemic myocardium. This has been described for skeletal myoblasts, unfractionated mononuclear BM cells, stroma cell-derived cell lines, and cells selected using markers of HSCs or EPCs. Most frequently, an improvement of regional wall movement and/or systolic wall thickening in the cell-treated area has been described. The improvement of global LV contractility is usually in the range of 5% to 20%, and the size of the infarct area is somewhat smaller on histology than in untreated animals. In several small animal studies, a reduction of postinfarct mortality has also been observed. One particularly important lesson learned from large animal experiments is the notion that one should aim at injecting cells that work primarily via angiogenesis induction into the infarct border zone, rather than in the center of the infarct area. Only by doing so, a relevant improvement of myocardial contractility and perfusion is likely to be induced.[37] When primarily contractile cells, i.e., myoblasts, are used in sufficiently vascularized tissue, this may be less important. To date, no clear advantage of one cell type over another can be seen. Several studies attempted a direct comparison between two or more different cell populations, i.e., skeletal myoblasts versus BM cells, or marrow cells versus EPCs, but the data are not conclusive, yet. The same is to be said regarding the dose-response relationship of a given cell population, as well as the host-related issues such as the infarct size or the interval between myocardial infarction and cell treatment.

Clinical Application

Translation of experimental cell-therapy approaches for myocardial regeneration into the clinical setting has just begun (Table 2.2). Whether the first clinical pilot trials were initiated too early remains subject to very controversial debate. The earliest clinical application was reported by Menasché and colleagues.[16] A patient with significantly reduced LV contractility after myocardial infarction had to undergo CABG to optimize myocardial blood supply. Two weeks before, a muscle sample was

Table 2.2. Clinical cell therapy for myocardial tissue repair*

Reference	Disease	Cell type/Source	Application mode	Patients (n)	Effects	Readout	Additional readout
BOOST Wollert et al.[44]	AMI	BM-MNC (80–120 mL) vs. CTRL; prospective, randomized (30 + 30)	PCI Intracoronary	60	EF↑ Coronary flow reserve↑	Cardiac MRI i.c. Doppler	LVA FCM
TOPCARE-AMI Assmus et al.[60]	AMI	BM-MNC (50 mL) vs. adher. cult. PB-MNC (250 mL) vs. CTRL	PCI Intracoronary	59 (200)	Global and regional EF↑ Viability↑ LVESV↓	LVA, TTE, MRI PET, MRI LVA	FCM
Univ. Düsseldorf Strauer et al.[61]	AMI	BM-MNC (40 mL) vs. CTRL	PCI Intracoronary	60	EF unchanged Hypokinetic area↓ Contract. infarct region↑	MUGA – RNV LVA LVA	DSE RVA
MAGIC Kang et al.[49]	AMI	G-CSF PB-MNC (10^9 ~ Aph.) vs. G-CSF (s.c. 10 μg/mL) vs. CTRL – stopped	PCI Intracoronary vs. s.c G-CSF mobilization	27	Aggravated restenosis↑ EF↑ Perfusion defect↓ LVESV↓ ($P = 0.05$) Exercise capacity↑	LVA D-SPECT Treadmill	i.c. Doppler DSE FCM
NIH Hill et al.[51]	CAD (iAP)	G-CSF (10 μg/kg/d) Pilot study – closed	s.c.	12	2 AMI 1 Cardiac death		
Univ. Rostock Stamm et al.[40]	cIHF post-AMI	CD133+ BM-MNC (85–195 mL)	i.my./CABG	33	EF↑ Perfusion defect↓ LVEDV↓	SPECT	24 h ECG FCM
Texas Heart Perin et al.[41]	cIHF	BM-MNC (50 mL) vs. CTRL; prospective, nonrandomized (14 + 7)	i.my./NOGA (15 × 0.2 cc)	30	EF↑ LVESV↓ Perfusion defect↓ NYHA/ CCSAS↓	LVA SPECT	Clinical/lab. eval.; treadmill; 2-D Doppler; 24 h ECG
Washington, DC; New York; and Israel Fuchs et al.[42,43]	cIHF	BMC (20 mL) Pilot study	i.my./NOGA (12 × 0.2 cc)	27	Stress perfusion defect↓ CCSAS↓ (Exercise capacity non sign↑) No arrhythmia	D-SPECT Treadmill	ECG Clinical/lab. eval. ELISA (VEGF; MCP1)
Univ. Hong Kong Tse et al.[39]	cIHF	BM-MNC (40 mL)	i.my./NOGA	8	Wall motion and thickening↑ Perfusion defect↓; no arrhythmia EF unchanged NYHA↓	MRI (7/8) SPECT; 24 h ECG	ECG; medication use Clinical/lab. eval. CFU-GM; FCM
Paris Menasché et al.[16,62]	cIHF post-AMI EF <35%	Cultured skeletal muscle cells (myoblasts ~8.7×10^8)	i.my./CABG	10	EF↑; wall thick. ↑; NYHA↓ 4 Delay tachycardia → ICD 1 Unrelated death	TTE 24 h ECG	Clinical/lab. eval.

(Continued)

Table 2.2. Clinical cell therapy for myocardial tissue repair*—Cont'd

Reference	Disease	Cell type/Source	Application mode	Patients (n)	Effects	Readout	Additional readout
Univ. Pamplona Herreros et al.[63]	cIHF post-AMI EF <35%	Cultured skeletal muscle cells (myoblasts ~1.8 × 10⁸)	i.my./CABG	12	Perfusion defect↓; no arrhythmia EF↑; wall thick. ↑	¹⁸F FDG PET TTE	ECG; Clinical/lab. eval. ¹³N PET; FCM

*Published studies more than patients all showing feasibility; update AHA 2004 if available.
†Coronary restenosis observed.
cIHF, chronic ischemic heart failure; LVA, RVA, left/right ventricular angiography; LVESV, left ventricular end systolic volume; BMC, filtered heparinized whole bone marrow; DSE, dobutamine stress echo; Aph., apheresis; D-SPECT, dipyridamole/Persantine-SPECT; CAD, severe coronary artery disease; iAP, intractable angina pectoris.

obtained from the thigh, and skeletal myoblasts were cultivated and grown for several passages. During the bypass operation, these cells were directly injected into the infarcted myocardium. The patient tolerated the procedure well, and a distinct improvement of wall thickening and motion in the area of cell injection was noted postoperatively. This procedure has been repeated worldwide ever since, and the reports quite uniformly describe a mild improvement in contractility. Analogous to the experimental experience, however, the myofibers that originated from the transferred myoblasts appear to survive in the infarct tissue but do not fully integrate into the myocardial syncytium (see above). The CABG operation represents a unique opportunity to directly access the infarcted myocardium, but, at the same time, conceals the effects of the cell therapy. Analysis of regional contractility may give some hints regarding the cell-induced functional improvement, but, inevitably, there is always some overlap of the effects of myocardial revascularization and those of the cell injection. Shortly after the advent of combined CABG and myoblast injection, a procedure was developed that enables the cardiologist to delivery myoblasts directly to the myocardium as a stand-alone treatment. By using a novel cardiac catheterization device, the infarcted myocardium can be quite precisely located based on its electrophysiologic properties [Figure 2.7 (see color section)]. A map of the endocardial surface of the LV myocardium is then constructed that clearly depicts the localization of the infarct tissue. A needle is advanced through the endocardial layer into the myocardium at a preset depth, and the cell suspension is injected. This procedure has been performed in patients with severely impaired LV function, and, again, a mild improvement of LV contractility was noted, together with some relief of the symptoms of ischemic heart failure. The myoblast injection, however, seemed to result in a transient period of electrical instability a few days after the injection, which repeatedly led to sustained ventricular arrhythmia. Therefore, myoblast injection as a stand-alone treatment is currently limited to patients who have an automatic defibrillation device implanted. It should also be noted that it is still controversial to what extent the preexisting ischemic heart disease, rather than the cell transfer, is responsible for the observed rhythm disturbances.

Although clinical skeletal myoblast transfer is mainly limited to patients with chronic heart failure, cell therapy with BM or blood-derived cells may evolve in a novel treatment option for both chronic ischemic heart disease and AMI (Table 2.3). In either situation, the angiogenic potential of certain adult stem/progenitor cell types is probably the key to functional improvements, whereas true neomyogenesis is, at present, rather unlikely. Around 2001, a number of clinical trials were initiated, and among the first published was the work by Hamano et al.,[38] who injected BM mononuclear cells intramyocardially during a CABG operation, Tse et al.,[39] who used a catheter-based system for direct intramyocardial delivery of mononuclear cells, and our own group,[40] who injected a purified population of AC133+ BM cells, again in conjunction with a CABG operation. Several other groups have

Table 2.3. Principal "Pros" (+) and "Cons" (−) of clinically usable stem cell sources

	+	−
Skeletal myoblasts	Myocyte phenotype	Arrhythmia Preparation Angiogenesis ?
Crude bone marrow	Instant preparation	Stem cell content ? Inflammation ?
Marrow stroma cells/mesenchymal stem cells	Myogenic potential	Preparation Angiogenesis ?
Hematopoietic marrow stem cells	Rapid preparation Approval (GMP/GLP) Angiogenesis	Myogenesis ?
Circulating progenitor cells	Angiogenesis	Preparation Myogenesis ?
Mobilization (G-CSF)	"Noninvasive"	Systemic inflammation

This simplified summary is based on data and anecdotal experience that are constantly being revised and updated. To date, there is no "ideal" cell type for myocardial regeneration.

reported similar studies since then.[41–43] What these trials have in common is that patients with chronic ischemic heart disease are addressed. The most recent myocardial infarction in those patients usually dates back several weeks, months, or even years. In the infarcted or chronically ischemic myocardium, a substantial net loss of contractile tissue mass has occurred, increased collagen deposition has led to a more or less pronounced, diffuse, or localized scar formation, and blood supply to the myocardium remains impaired although there may have been some collateral vessel growth. Usually, the ischemic myocardium in those patients is not a complete transmural fibrous scar, which would eventually progress into an LV aneurysm, but still vital cardiomyocytes are dispersed within the fibrous network. Theoretically, such "hibernating" cardiomyocytes can be re-recruited for contractile work once sufficient supply of oxygen and nutrients has been reestablished, and stem/progenitor cell-induced growth of microvessels in the infarct borderzone may thus translate into improved myocardial contractility. Nevertheless, it should be kept in mind that the chances to resuscitate hibernating cells in a functionally relevant manner are likely to decrease with time. The longer the interval between myocardial infarction and cell treatment is, the smaller the chance to achieve a beneficial effect becomes. This notion, however, is largely intuitive, and presently not supported by clear-cut data.

The situation in AMI studies is fundamentally different. Here, the onset of myocardial ischemia was usually between several hours and a few days previous. Typically, a patient is admitted with acute chest pain and electrocardiogram shows signs of myocardial ischemia. Laboratory tests indicate the onset of myocardial necrosis and liberation of cardiomyocyte-specific intracellular proteins (i.e., CK-MB, troponin) after loss of cell membrane integrity. If possible, the blocked coronary artery is immediately reopened by emergency catheterization, balloon dilation, and stent placement. The extent of myocardial necrosis and thus the impairment in contractility largely depend on the time that has passed until the infarct vessel is reopened. There is no way to predict the ultimate infarct size in a given patient. Ideally, cardiomyocyte necrosis is completely prevented because the coronary artery has been quickly reopened. In many patients, the necrotic myocardium does not extend across the entire wall thickness (nontransmural infarction), and in some the entire myocardium downstream to the arterial obstruction is subject to complete necrosis (transmural infarction). Analogous to the chronically hibernating myocardium, acutely ischemic cardiomyocytes can still be vital but have temporarily lost much of their capacity for contractile work (myocardial stunning). Tissue infiltration with inflammatory cells is beginning, but fibrous scarring has not yet occurred. In this situation, direct injection of cell suspension into the weakened myocardium is prohibitive, but infusion of stem/progenitor cells into the reopened coronary artery is currently being evaluated.

So far, mainly BM mononuclear cell preparations have been used in such trials. A few days after the onset of myocardial infarction, a second cardiac catheterization is performed and the cell suspension is injected into the infarct vessel while blood is temporarily interrupted by balloon inflation. Pilot studies have demonstrated feasibility and safety of this approach, and controlled efficacy trials are currently on the way. In one of the first of those trials, there was a difference in LV ejection fraction of 6% at 6 months follow-up between 30 patients who received intracoronary cell injection and 30 patients who only had standard infarct treatment. On average, LVEF improved by 6.7% in cell-treated patients as compared with immediately after myocardial infarction, whereas LVEF in control patients remained largely unchanged.[44] Other clinical trials based on the same principle are currently underway, but it is too early to make a definitive judgment about long-term functional efficacy and possible side effects. One of the most interesting questions is how, and to what extent, the intracoronary cell injection leads to stem/progenitor cell extravasation and migration into the myocardial interstitium. Our group has recently established a mouse model that allows for direct visualization of stem cell–endothelial cell interaction and interstitial migration using intravital fluorescence microscopy. This technique will hopefully help to better understand and to optimize the stem cell trafficking to ischemic myocardium.

Stem Cell Mobilization

Another, fundamentally different approach aims at circumventing any invasive procedure for cell delivery while minimizing the interval between the onset of myocardial infarction and cell therapy by mobilizing marrow cells using G-CSF. The idea is that stem/progenitor cells mobilized from marrow will be attracted to the ischemic heart and initiate regeneration events or at least modulate remodeling processes. That the number of circulating progenitor cells can be greatly enhanced by G-CSF stimulation has been well established. However, the number of mature leukocytes also increases markedly, and this has already raised principle concerns regarding the safety of G-CSF treatment. The pathophysiologic equivalent of such reasoning may be the mobilization of EPCs in patients with AMI or various degrees of congestive heart failure.[45–47] Because stem cell mobilization did not result in a favorable outcome in a nonhuman primate model of myocardial infarction, this practicable pharmacologic approach has been viewed with some restraint.[48] Despite safety of G-CSF mobilization with or without consecutive apheresis and favorable short-term results of intracoronary infusion of G-CSF mobilized PB in patients with myocardial infarction after coronary stenting, an unexpectedly high rate of in-stent restenosis has been observed in association with G-CSF.[49] Moreover, restenosis has at least been mentioned in another (TACT) trial for adult stem cell therapy for peripheral occlusive artery disease with unfractionated BM.[50] In a third study in 12 patients with intractable angina, the administration of G-CSF was associated with two AMIs and one cardiac death.[51] Nevertheless, several other clinical pilot studies are currently on the way.

Summary

The fundamentals of myocardial tissue repair based on adult progenitor or stem cells are far from being "textbook knowledge." Knowledge is progressing rapidly, but it is not uncommon that the assumed progression is quickly followed by regression. The unresolved issues are too manifold to list. Despite the surge in cell therapy-related publications, the "facts" that are largely undisputed are few: 1. Contractile cells or their immediate progenitors, obtained from whatever source, can be transferred into ischemic myocardium, and some of them survive and prosper. In many experimental models, this cell transfer indeed leads to an improvement of LV function. 2. Cell types belonging to the hematopoietic–angiogenetic complex, obtained from whatever source, can enhance the vascularization of ischemic tissue, including infarcted myocardium. Again, in many experimental models, this is associated with some improvement of heart function. Having accepted the limitations of our current knowledge, it does not seem inappropriate to state that adult stem/progenitor cell therapy for myocardial tissue repair holds exceedingly great promise. If the translation of experimental approaches in clinical medicine succeeds (Figure 2.8), we will, for the first time, be able to offer patients with heart failure a true cure.

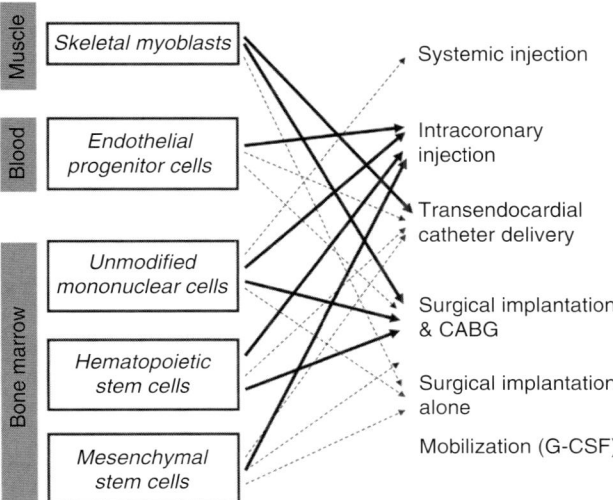

Figure 2.8. Several adult stem cell types can at least theoretically be used in clinical trials of cell therapy for myocardial regeneration. There are also numerous clinically applicable ways to deliver cells to the infarcted heart. The result is a confusing variety of possible trial designs. The solid arrows indicate trials that are currently underway; the results of clinical trials indicated by interrupted arrows have not been reported to date.

References

1. Korbling M, Estrov Z. Adult stem cells for tissue repair: a new therapeutic concept? N Engl J Med 2003;349: 570–582.
2. Goodell MA. Stem-cell "plasticity": befuddled by the muddle. Curr Opin Hematol 2003;10:208–213.
3. Camargo FD, Chambers SM, Goodell MA. Stem cell plasticity: from transdifferentiation to macrophage fusion. Cell Prolif 2004;37:55–65.
4. Menasché P. Cellular transplantation: hurdles remaining before widespread clinical use. Curr Opin Cardiol 2004;19:154–161.
5. Masuda H, Asahara T. Post-natal endothelial progenitor cells for neovascularization in tissue regeneration. Cardiovasc Res 2003;58:390–398.
6. Urbich C, Dimmeler S. Endothelial progenitor cells: characterization and role in vascular biology. Circ Res 2004;95:343–353.
7. Honold J, Assmus B, Lehman R, Zeiher AM, Dimmeler S. Stem cell therapy of cardiac disease: an update. Nephrol Dial Transplant 2004;19:1673–1677.
8. Rafii S, Lyden D. Therapeutic stem and progenitor cell transplantation for organ vascularization and regeneration. Nat Med 2003;9:702–712.
9. Perin EC, Geng YJ, Willerson JT. Adult stem cell therapy in perspective. Circulation 2003;107:935–938.
10. Forrester JS, Price MJ, Makkar RR. Stem cell repair of infarcted myocardium: an overview for clinicians. Circulation 2003;108:1139–1145.
11. Li RK, Jia ZQ, Weisel RD, et al. Cardiomyocyte transplantation improves heart function. Ann Thorac Surg 1996;62:654–661.
12. Ruhparwar A, Tebbenjohanns J, Niehaus M, et al. Transplanted fetal cardiomyocytes as cardiac pacemaker. Eur J Cardiothorac Surg 2003;21:853–857.
13. Li RK, Jia ZQ, Weisel RD, Merante F, Mickle DA. Smooth muscle cell transplantation into myocardial scar tissue improves heart function. J Mol Cell Cardiol 1999;31:513–522.
14. Reinecke H, MacDonald GH, Hauschka SD, Murry CE. Electromechanical coupling between skeletal and cardiac muscle: implications for infarct repair. J Cell Biol 2000;149:731–740.
15. Rubart M, Soonpaa MH, Nakajima H, Field LJ. Spontaneous and evoked intracellular calcium transients in donor-derived myocytes following intracardiac myoblast transplantation. J Clin Invest 2004;114:775–783.
16. Menasché P, Hagege AA, Scorsin M, et al. Myoblast transplantation for heart failure. Lancet 2001;357: 279–280.
17. Pittenger MF, Mackay AM, Beck SC, et al. Multilineage potential of adult human mesenchymal stem cells. Science 1999;284:143–147.
18. Pittenger MF, Martin BJ. Mesenchymal stem cells and their potential as cardiac therapeutics. Circ Res 2004;95:9–20.
19. Oswald J, Boxberger S, Jorgensen B, et al. Mesenchymal stem cells can be differentiated into endothelial cells in vitro. Stem Cells 2004;22:377–384.
20. Reyes M, Lund T, Lenvik T, Aguiar D, Koodie L, Verfaillie CM. Purification and ex vivo expansion of postnatal human marrow mesodermal progenitor cells. Blood 2001;98:2615–2625.
21. Reyes M, Dudek A, Jahagirdar B, Koodie L, Marker PH, Verfaillie CM. Origin of endothelial progenitors in human postnatal bone marrow. J Clin Invest 2002;109:337–346.
22. Muguruma Y, Reyes M, Nakamura Y. In vivo and in vitro differentiation of myocytes from human bone marrow-derived multipotent progenitor cell. Exp Hematol 2003;31:1323–1330.

23. Lin Y, Weisdorf D, Solovey A, Hebbel RP. Origins of circulating endothelial cells and endothelial outgrowth from blood. J Clin Invest 2000;105:71–77.
24. Asahara T, Murohara T, Sullivan A, et al. Isolation of putative progenitor endothelial cells for angiogenesis. Science 1997;275:964–967.
25. Solovey A, Lin Y, Browne P, Choong S, Wayner E, Hebbel RP. Circulating activated endothelial cells in sickle cell anemia. N Engl J Med 1997;337:1584–1590.
26. Kocher AA, Schuster MD, Szabolcs MJ, et al. Neovascularization of ischemic myocardium by human bone-marrow-derived angioblasts prevents cardiomyocyte apoptosis, reduces remodeling and improves cardiac function. Nat Med 2001;7:430–436.
27. Orlic D, Kajstura J, Chimenti S, et al. Bone marrow cells regenerate infarcted myocardium. Nature 2001;410:701–705.
28. Orlic D, Kajstura J, Chimenti S, et al. Mobilized bone marrow cells repair the infarcted heart, improving function and survival. Proc Natl Acad Sci USA 2001;98:10344–10349.
29. Murry CE, et al. Haematopoietic stem cells do not transdifferentiate into cardiac myocytes in myocardial infarcts. Nature 2004;428:664–668.
30. Balsam LB Haematopoietic stem cells adopt mature haematopoietic fates in ischaemic myocardium. Nature 2004;428:668–673.
31. Wakitani S, Saito T, Caplan AI. Myogenic cells derived from rat bone marrow mesenchymal stem cells exposed to 5-azacytidine. Muscle Nerve 1995;18(12): 1417–1426.
32. Makino S, Fukuda K, Miyoshi S, et al. Cardiomyocytes can be generated from marrow stromal cells in vitro. J Clin Invest 1999;103:697–705.
33. Chedrawy EG, Wang JS, Nguyen DM, Shm-Tim D, Chiu RCJ. Incorporation and integration of implanted myogenic and stem cells into native myocardial fibers: anatomic basis for functional improvements. J Thorac Cardiovasc Surg 2002;124:584–590.
34. Wang JS, Shum-Tim D, Galipeau J, Chedrawy E, Eliopoulos N, Chiu RCJ. Marrow stromal cells for cellular cardiomyoplasty: feasibility and potential advantages. J Thorac Cardiovasc Surg 2000;120:999–1006.
35. Bittira B, Kuang JQ, Al-Khaldi A, Shum-Tim D, Chiu RCJ. In vitro preprogramming of marrow stromal cells for myocardial regeneration. Ann Thorac Surg 2002;74:1154–1160.
36. Toma C, Pittenger MF, Cahill KS, et al. Human mesenchymal stem cells differentiate to a cardiomyocyte phenotype in the adult murine heart. Circulation 2002;105:93–98.
37. Hamano K, Li TS, Kobayashi T, et al. Therapeutic angiogenesis induced by local autologous bone marrow cell implantation. Ann Thorac Surg 2002;73(4):1210–1215.
38. Hamano K, Nishida M, Hirata K, et al. Local implantation of autologous bone marrow cells for therapeutic angiogenesis in patients with ischemic heart disease: clinical trial and preliminary results. Jpn Circ J 2001;65:845–847.
39. Tse HF, Kwong YL, Chan JK, Lo G, Ho CL, Lau CP. Angiogenesis in ischaemic myocardium by intramyocardial autologous bone marrow mononuclear cell implantation. Lancet 2003;361:47–49.
40. Stamm C, Westphal B, Kleine HD, et al. Autologous bone-marrow stem-cell transplantation for myocardial regeneration. Lancet 2003;361:45–46.
41. Perin EC, Dohmann HF, Borojevic R, et al. Transendocardial, autologous bone marrow cell transplantation for severe, chronic ischemic heart failure. Circulation 2003;107:2294–2302.
42. Fuchs S, Satler LF, Kornowski R, et al. Catheter-based autologous bone marrow myocardial injection in no-option patients with advanced coronary artery disease: a feasibility study. J Am Coll Cardiol 2003;41:1721–1724.
43. Fuchs S, et al. Transendocardial autologous bone marrow cell transplantation in patients with advanced ischemic heart disease: final results from a multi-center feasibility study. J Am Coll Cardiol 2004;43:99A.
44. Wollert KC, Meyer GP, Lotz J, et al. Intracoronary autologous bone-marrow cell transfer after myocardial infarction: the BOOST randomised controlled clinical trial. Lancet 2004;364:141–148.
45. Shintani S, Murohara T, Ikeda H, et al. Mobilization of endothelial progenitor cells in patients with acute myocardial infarction. Circulation 2001;103:2776–2779.
46. Valgimigli M, Rigolin GM, Fucili A, et al. CD34+ and endothelial progenitor cells in patients with various degrees of congestive heart failure. Circulation 2004;110:1209–1212.
47. Hill JM, Zalos G, Halcox JP, et al. Circulating endothelial progenitor cells, vascular function, and cardiovascular risk. N Engl J Med 2003;348:593–600.
48. Orlic D, et al. Cytokine mobilized CD34+ cells do not benefit rhesus monkeys following induced myocardial infarction. Blood 2002;100:28A–29A.
49. Kang HJ, Kim HS, Zhang SY, et al. Effects of intracoronary infusion of peripheral blood stem-cells mobilised with granulocyte-colony stimulating factor on left ventricular systolic function and restenosis after coronary stenting in myocardial infarction: the MAGIC cell randomised clinical trial. Lancet 2004;363: 751–756.
50. Tateishi-Yuyama E, Matsubara H, Murohara T, et al. Therapeutic angiogenesis for patients with limb ischaemia by autologous transplantation of bone-marrow cells: a pilot study and a randomised controlled trial. Lancet 2002;360:427–435.
51. Hill JM, et al. Efficacy and risk of granulocyte colony stimulating factor administration in patients with severe coronary artery disease. Circulation 2003;108:478.
52. Kondo M, Wagers AJ, Manz MG, et al. Biology of hematopoietic stem cells and progenitors: implications for clinical application. Ann Rev Immunol 2003;21:759–806.
53. Pelosi E, Valtieri M, Coppola S, et al. Identification of the hemangioblast in postnatal life. Blood 2002;100: 3203–3208.
54. Schmeisser A, Strasser RH. Phenotypic overlap between hematopoietic cells with suggested angioblastic potential and vascular endothelial cells. J Hematother Stem Cell Res 2002;11:69–79.
55. Peichev M, Naiyer AJ, Pereira D, et al. Expression of VEGFR-2 and AC133 by circulating human CD34(+) cells identifies a population of functional endothelial precursors. Blood 2000;95:952–958.
56. Pittenger MF, Martin BJ. Mesenchymal stem cells and their potential as cardiac therapeutics. Circ Res 2004;95:9–20.
57. Kogler G, Sensken S, Airey JA, et al. A new human somatic stem cell from placental cord blood with

intrinsic pluripotent differentiation potential. J Exp Med 2004;200:123–135.
58. Pittenger MF, Mackay AM, Beck SC, et al. Multilineage potential of adult human mesenchymal stem cells. Science 1999;284:143–147.
59. Kawada H, Fujita J, Kinjo K, et al. Nonhematopoietic mesenchymal stem cells can be mobilized and differentiate into cardiomyocytes after myocardial infarction. Blood 2004;104:3581–3587.
60. Assmus B, Schachinger V, Teupe C, et al. Transplantation of progenitor cells and regeneration enhancement in acute myocardial infarction (TOPCARE-AMI). Circulation 2002;106:3009–3017.
61. Strauer BE, Brehm M, Zeus T, et al. Repair of infarcted myocardium by autologous intracoronary mononuclear bone marrow cell transplantation in humans. Circulation 2002;106:1913–1918.
62. Menasché P, Hagege AA, Vilquin JT, et al. Autologous skeletal myoblast transplantation for severe postinfarction left ventricular dysfunction. J Am Coll Cardiol 2003;41:1078–1083.
63. Herreros J, Prosper F, Perez A, et al. Autologous intramyocardial injection of cultured skeletal muscle-derived stem cells in patients with non-acute myocardial infarction. Eur Heart J 2003;24:2012–2020.

Regeneration of the Functional Myocardium Using Human Embryonic Stem Cells

Oren Caspi and Lior Gepstien

The introduction of human embryonic stem cell (hESC) lines provided scientists with the means for investigation of early human development and potential tools for tissue replacement therapies.[1] Although research using hESCs suffers from significant restraints, important accomplishments have already been achieved. This review will focus on the derivation of cardiomyocytes from hESCs and their potential applications for the regeneration of functional myocardium.

All stem cells, whether from embryonic or adult sources, share a number of characteristics. First, they are capable of self-renewal, meaning they can generate stem cells with similar properties. Second, the stem cells are clonogenic, meaning that each cell can form a colony in which all the cells are derived from this single cell and have identical genetic constitution. Third, they are capable of differentiation into one or more mature cell types.

These properties of stem cells make them a unique and a powerful tool both for clinicians and basic science researchers. Except for the attractive and promising potential use of stem cells for tissue regeneration, stem cells also provide scientists with a unique insight to developmental stages that were previously out of reach for experimentation, especially in human models. Moreover, better understanding of the mechanisms involved in early stem cell differentiation may be a prerequisite for safe and efficient application of stem cells in regenerative medicine.

Derivation and Differentiation of Embryonic Stem Cells

Embryonic stem cells were initially isolated from mouse blastocysts in 1981 by two independent groups.[2,3] The potential therapeutic applications and the unique opportunity to study early mammalian development exemplified by the murine model motivated researchers to establish similar hESC lines.[1,4] The origin of the hESC lines, similar to the mouse and rhesus models, is from the preimplantation embryo produced by in vitro fertilization for clinical purposes and donated by individuals after informed consent. The blastocyst contains an outer cell layer and an inner cell mass (ICM). Whereas the outer cells become the trophectoderm and subsequently give rise to the placenta and other embryonic supporting tissues, the ICM cells will ultimately create all tissues in the body [Figure 3.1 (see color section)]. The hESC lines were established by isolating the ICM cells after removal of the trophectoderm with specific antibodies (immunosurgery). The cells were then plated on a feeder layer of mitotically inactivated mouse embryonic fibroblasts (MEFs). Plating of the hESCs on top of this feeder layer allows continuous undifferentiated propagation of these cells in cultures, a unique property not shared by adult stem cells. The undifferentiated hESCs were also shown to express specific surface markers, such as stage specific embryonic antigen 3 (SSEA-3), SSEA-4, Tra-1-60 and Tra-1-81, the embryonic transcription factor Oct-4, and alkaline phosphatase. In addition, undifferentiated hESCs express high levels of telomerase activity and retain a normal karyotype for several passages.[1,4]

There are many differences between hESCs and their murine counterparts, as extensively reviewed by Pera and Trounson.[5] Briefly, mouse embryonic stem cell (mESC) colonies are more rounded with a glassy appearance and indistinct cell borders, whereas hESC colonies are flatter and often display more distinct cell borders. In addition, the hESC doubling time is 3 times longer and it lacks the surface antigen SSEA-1 but expresses SSEA-3 and SSEA-4.[6] However, the most important difference between the two cell lines is probably the mechanisms involved in their self-renewal as reviewed by Rao.[7] The maintenance of the undifferentiated state of the ESC is mediated both by differentiation inhibiting signals as well as by the lack of expression of differentiation genes. Among the differentiation inhibiting signals, the well-known leukemia inhibitory factor (LIF) is considered to be a sufficient trigger for the maintenance of pluripotency in the mESC system in the presence of serum. In addition, a recent publication suggests that induction of the expression of inhibitor of differentiation (Id) genes by bone morphogenetic proteins (BMPs) in concert with LIF can maintain in vitro self-renewal capabilities of mESCs in serum-free conditions.[8] However, in the hESC system, LIF is insufficient or even not required for this purpose, and the presence of the MEF feeder layer itself, its conditioned medium[9] or other cell support system such as human fetal fibroblast, adult epithelial cells,[10] or foreskin cells,[11] is required.

Except for the difference in LIF-gp130 signaling between human and mESCs, several key regulators of stem cell self-renewal have been demonstrated to be conserved between the human and mouse systems. Sato et al.[12] elucidated the role of the canonical Wnt pathway in the maintenance of embryonic stem cell self-renewal; this study demonstrated that 6-bromoindirubin-3′-oxime, a specific glycogen synthase kinase 3 inhibitor, is sufficient for the maintenance of "stemness" propagation and pluripotency of both human and mESCs. The homebox-domain containing protein Nanog was recently demonstrated to act parallel to the LIF pathway in maintaining ESC self-renewal both in the mouse and hESC.[13–15] Further studies elucidating the factors participating in ESC self-renewal are crucial for establishing a reproducible, well-defined, animal and serum-free supporting system that may be upscaled and will facilitate research practices and provide a safer alternative for future clinical applications of hESCs.

The most exciting properties of the hESCs lies in their potential to differentiate in vitro to cell derivatives of all three embryonic germ layers. This ability to differentiate to a variety of mature somatic cell types was demonstrated using both spontaneous and directed in vitro differentiation systems. Since the initial report of the derivation of the hESCs, they were shown to differentiate into cardiac tissue,[16] neuronal tissue including dopaminergic cells,[17,18] β islet pancreatic cells,[19] hematopoietic progenitors,[20] keratinocytes,[21] bone tissue,[22] and endothelial cells.[23]

From hESCs to Cardiomyocytes

The generation of a reproducible spontaneous cardiomyocyte differentiating system from the clonal hESC line (H9.2) was originally described by Kehat et al.[16] in our laboratory. The induction of in vitro differentiation of hESCs to cardiomyocytes required their removal from the feeder layer and cultivation in suspension. The hESCs then tend to generate three-dimensional cell aggregates termed embryonic bodies (EBs). The human EBs contain tissue derivatives of endodermal, ectodermal, and mesodermal origin but seem to be less organized from their murine counterparts.[24,25] After 7–10 days in suspension, the EBs are plated on top of gelatin-coated culture dishes and observed microscopically for the appearance of spontaneous contraction. Rhythmically contracting areas appeared at 4–22 days after plating in 8.1% of the EBs.[16] Recently, other groups reinforced our findings and generated hESC-derived cardiomyocytes (hESDCMs) using different clonal and nonclonal cell lines.[26–28]

Structural Properties

Several lines of evidence confirmed the cardiomyocyte phenotype of the contracting areas generated within the EBs. Reverse transcriptase-polymerase chain reaction studies demonstrated that cells isolated from the beating areas express the cardiac transcription factors GATA4 and

Nkx2.5 and cardiac-specific genes, such as cardiac troponin I and T, atrial natriuretic peptide, and atrial and ventricular myosin light chains (MLCs). Immunostaining studies demonstrated the presence of the cardiac-specific sarcomeric proteins such as myosin heavy chain, α-actinin, desmin, cardiac troponin I, and atrial natriuretic peptide. Electron microscopy studies revealed the development of well-aligned sarcomeres accompanied by the development of the known sarcomeric striated pattern with recognizable A, I, and Z bands [Figure 3.2A (see color section)].[16,29] Compared with the murine ESCs,[30,31] the hESCs differentiated in a slower rate and their ultrastructural development was more heterogeneous, lasted longer, and did not reach the same level of maturity.

The degree of structural and functional maturation of the generated cardiomyocytes may be important for the possible utilization in myocardial repair strategies. Although it is possible that the in vivo environment after cell grafting may promote such maturation, an alternative approach may be the application of oscillating mechanical load either in vitro or in vivo. Zimmermann et al.[32] demonstrated that application of phasic mechanical stretch on neonatal rat ventricular cardiomyocytes grown as tissue constructs with collagen and other extracellular matrix factors resulted in significant maturation of the cells. In addition to mechanical stretching, low-frequency magnetic fields have also been demonstrated to affect cardiac differentiation and might also serve to hasten the maturation process.[33] Alternative approaches might be to use certain growth factors or transcription factors to affect cell maturation such as BMP-10,[34] Foxp1,[35] TBX5.[36]

The Electrophysiological Characteristics of hESDCMs

The hESDCMs were demonstrated to have a functional phenotype of early-stage human cardiac tissue including typical extracellular electrical activity, intracellular action potentials and ionic currents [Figure 3.2B (see color section)], calcium transients, and chronotropic response to adrenergic agents [Figure 3.2C (see color section)]. High-resolution activation maps using the multielectrode array system demonstrated the presence of functional electrical syncytium with synchronous action potential propagation and pacemaker activity (Figure 3.2D).[37] Immunostaining studies showed that this functional syncytium results from the presence of gap junctions [comprised both of connexin (Cx)43 and Cx45] between the cells.

According to studies based on the murine differentiation system, the beating EB is populated by cells representing all cardiac phenotypes. The percentage of the different cell types transforms during development from pacemaker-like cell predominance to atrial or ventricular cell predominance in older EBs.[31] Detailed electrophysiological analysis of the developing murine EBs has revealed a developmental cascade of ion channel expression and modulation. The noncontracting precursor cells display voltage-dependent L-type Ca^{+2} channels at very low densities. Cardiomyocytes of an early differentiation stage exhibit a primitive pacemaker action potential generated only by voltage-dependent L-type Ca^{+2} channels and transient outward K^+ channels. Terminally differentiated cardiomyocytes express various additional ion channels according to their various phenotypes. Ventricle-like cells express voltage-dependent Na^+ channels, delayed outward-rectifying K^+ channels, and inward-rectifying K^+ channels. Additional ion channels, such as muscarinic acetylcholine-activated K^+ channels and the hyperpolarization-activated pacemaker channels were demonstrated in atrial-like cells and sinus node-like cells, respectively.[31]

Similar to the mESC model, whole-cell patch clamp studies demonstrated that the hESDCMs also display cardiac-specific action potential morphologies and ion currents. Additional work from our laboratory revealed the basis for the spontaneous automaticity in these cells, at least at the mid-differentiation stages. These studies revealed that, during this stage, the spontaneous electrical activity is mediated by the absence of significant inward-rectifier K^+ current and a prominent Na^+ current sensitive to Tetrodotoxin (TTX) coupled with the presence of the hyperpolarization and cyclic nucleotide-activated ion channels (HCN) pacemaker current (If).[38] The paucity of the inward current creates a high-input resistance state that allows a small inward current to bring the membrane potential to threshold. Further electrophysiological and molecular characterization of the developmental cascade of cardiac ion channels using the hESC model will provide a unique insight to the development of excitability in early human cardiac tissue and will allow engineering of the functional properties of the cell grafts.

Cell Proliferation

Based on animal models, cardiomyocytes switch from hyperplastic to hypertrophic growth soon after birth.[39] In human fetal tissue, the number of cells in the S-phase of cell cycle is estimated to be 16.8%.[40] Interestingly, during the process of ultrastructural maturation of the hESDCMs, the cells start to withdraw from the cell cycle. Using [^{3}H] thymidine incorporation or Ki-67 immunolabeling, the hESDCMs demonstrated a gradual withdrawal from cell cycle with cessation of DNA synthesis after 7 weeks.[41] Several possible reasons may explain the "early" withdrawal of the hESDCMs from the cell cycle. First, disparity may stem from the inherent limitations of an in vitro model, which may be different from the in vivo setting (hemodynamic load, paracrine effect, etc.) and this may alter the cell cycle activity as well as the cell maturation. Second, the fact that the evaluated cells are concentrated in a small area adjacent to nonmyocytic proliferating tissue may also activate contact inhibition signals. Because cell replacement therapy for heart failure is one of the most promising applications of the hESDCMs, the proliferative capacity of the cells is of great importance for planning the amount of cells needed for transplantation. Further studies aimed at evaluating the proliferative capacity of the hESDCMs in vivo after transplantation to the adult heart may provide additional data concerning this issue.

Promoting Stem Cell Differentiation to Cardiomyocytes

The hESC model may provide valuable information regarding the process involved in early lineage commitment, differentiation, and maturation of human cardiac tissue. The currently available cardiomyocyte differentiation system of the hESC is essentially spontaneous, however, and thus characterized by relatively low efficacy and reproducibility. Understanding the mechanisms that drive early-cardiac differentiation of the hESC may also have important clinical implications. One of the major obstacles for the utilization of these cells in future myocardial regeneration strategies is the insufficient number of cardiomyocytes achieved by the currently available differentiation scheme. Therefore, further efforts aimed at developing a more productive cardiomyocyte differentiation system are essential for the generation of the large quantities of cells needed to achieve the successful application of this strategy.

The development of a directed differentiation system is hampered by the relative lack of data regarding the inductive cues that lead to commitment and terminal differentiation of human cardiomyocytes. Thus, strategies for directed differentiation should undoubtedly follow the research conducted in a number of model organisms, most notably the chick, amphibians, zebrafish, and the mouse. The heart arises from cells in the anterior lateral plate mesoderm of the early embryo. The cells of the cardiogenic mesoderm adopt a crescent-like morphology and are therefore termed "the cardiac crescent."[42] The endoderm that is in direct contact with the cardiac crescent is considered to have an obligatory role in the induction of the cardiac fate. Various genetic and biochemical perturbations in several organisms have shown a key role for BMP members of the transforming growth factor β superfamily expressed in endoderm as well as in adjacent ectoderm and extraembryonic tissues in specifying and/or maintaining the myocardial lineage.

Studies from the xenopus and chick models suggested that cardiogenesis is inhibited by Wnt-mediated signals from the underlying neural tube activating the canonical Wnt pathway. Based on the same animal models, cardiac differentiation was induced by Wnt-binding proteins (crescent and Dkk-1) secreted from the anterior endoderm. However, two recent articles suggest that the role of the Wnt family of proteins in cardiomyogenesis is much more complex. Pandur et al.[43] demonstrated that Wnt-11, an activator of the noncanonical Wnt/JNK pathway, is required for cardiogenesis using the xenopus model and the pluripotent mouse embryonic carcinoma stem cell line P19. Nakamura et al.,[44] using the P19 cell line as well, revealed that the canonical β-catenin pathway of Wnt signaling is actually activated very early during mammalian cardiogenesis.

In response to the inductive signal, the cardiac crescent activates several transcriptional regulators of the cardiac program including Gata4/Gata5/Gata6, Nkx 2-5, myocyte enhancer factor (Mef2b/Mef2c), and T-Box 5/20 – and a positive cardiac cross regulatory network is established.[45] A powerful transcription factor termed myocardin was recently identified and shown to coactivate transcription of several cardiac-specific gene promoters in conjunction with serum response factor.[46]

Possible strategies for increasing the cardiomyocyte yield during hESC differentiation may thus include the use of different growth factors, overexpression of cardiac-specific transcription factors, coculturing with feeder layers, and mechanical factors. Directed differentiation of ESCs to the cardiac lineage in the murine model was achieved using a variety of soluble factors including dimethylsulfoxide,[47] retinoic acid,[48] and more recently BMP-2 and transforming growth factor β,[49] and ascorbic acid.[50] Xu et al.[51] demonstrated enhancement of cardiac differentiation in the hESC model by using 5-aza-2′-deoxycytidine but surprisingly not by dimethylsulfoxide or retinoic acid. There is also evidence to suggest that lessons learned from early cardiac differentiation in the model systems, described above, may also be applicable to the hESC.[52] The cardiogenic inductive role of the primitive visceral endoderm was also demonstrated to have a role in the cardiomyocyte differentiation of the hESC line in an elegant study conducted by Mummery et al.[27] Co-culturing of an hESC line (hES2) that does not regularly differentiate spontaneously to cardiomyocytes, with END-2 cells (a visceral endoderm-like cell line) provided the missing trigger for cardiac differentiation.[27]

Myocardial Regeneration Strategies Using hESCs

It is generally believed that adult cardiomyocytes have limited regenerative capacity and that this ability is insufficient to overcome the massive heart cell loss that occurs, for example, during an extensive myocardial infarction leading to the development of progressive heart failure. Congestive heart failure is a growing epidemic in the western world because of the increasing age of the population and the improved postinfarction survival rates. Cardiac transplantation is currently the treatment of choice for end-stage heart failure. However, with the number of available donor organs limiting this treatment to only a minority of the patients, the development of new therapeutic paradigms for heart failure has become imperative. Cell replacement therapy is emerging as an innovative therapeutic approach for the treatment of degenerative heart diseases. This therapeutic approach is based on the assumption that myocardial function may be improved by repopulating diseased areas with a new pool of functional cells. Based on this assumption, a number of myogenic cells have been suggested for tissue grafting including skeletal myoblasts[53]; fetal,[54,55] neonatal,[56,57] and adult[56] cardiomyocytes; smooth muscle cells[58]; murine embryonic stem cells[59-62]; and hematopoietic and mesenchymal bone marrow-derived stem cells.[63]

The ideal donor cell should exhibit the electrophysiological, structural, and contractile properties of cardiomyocytes and should be able to integrate structurally and functionally with host tissue. In addition, it has to retain an initial high proliferative potential that may enable improved colonization of the scar tissue. The ability to undergo genetic manipulation ex vivo in order to promote desirable characteristics such as resistance to ischemia and apoptosis and improved contractile functions may be another advantage of such an ideal cell type. Finally, the optimal candidate cell should have an autologous origin or retain minimal immunogenicity and should be readily available in large quantities for transplantation. Unfortunately, none of the currently available candidate cell sources exhibit all of the aforementioned properties.

The capability of bone marrow-derived stem cells to regenerate the heart by transdifferentiation to cardiomyocytes[63] has been challenged by several studies demonstrating cell fusion of the progenitor cells with the host cells.[64,65] Moreover, recent studies suggest that the bone marrow-derived stem cells continue to differentiate along the hematopoietic lineage[66,67] and the possible left ventricle functional improvement noted may not be related to transdifferentiation into the cardiac lineage but rather may result from indirect mechanisms such as their ability to enhance blood vessel formation.[68]

The autologous origin and the high availability of adult skeletal muscle cells led to their application in recently conducted phase I clinical trials.[69] However, although previous reports suggest that these cell may have the ability to adopt cardiac-like phenotype after cardiac transplantation, it is now clear that they do not possess such a capability.[53,70] Moreover, the relatively high rate of ventricular arrhythmias observed in the initial phase I clinical trials may stem from the differences in the electrophysiological properties between the host cells and the engrafted myotubes and may further limit this approach.

Although a number of cell sources have been used in the aforementioned studies, the inherent electrophysiological, structural, and contractile properties of cardiomyocytes strongly suggest that they may be the ideal donor cell type. The clinical utility of fetal and neonatal cardiomyocytes is hampered, however, by the inability to obtain human cardiomyocytes in sufficient numbers because of practical and ethical reasons. Nevertheless, animal studies using fetal and neonatal cardiomyocytes have been instrumental to establish the proof-of-concept for the possible role of cell-based myocardial repopulation in improving myocardial performance of the injured heart. The fundamental work by Soonpaa et al.[55] demonstrated the ability of fetal cardiomyocytes transplanted into mice hearts to survive, align, and form intercalated disks with host cells. Further studies in animal models of myocardial infarction demonstrated that grafting of cardiomyocytes from fetal and neonatal sources was associated with smaller infarcts,[71] prevented cardiac dilatation and remodeling,[72] and also improved ventricular function.[73] The mechanisms underlying these functional improvements may be multifactorial and may include a direct contribution to contractility by the transplanted cells, attenuation of the remodeling process by changing the architectural and structural properties of the scar, and improvement in the function of viable tissue within the border zone by induction of angiogenesis.

The derivation of the hESC lines offers a number of potential advantages over the currently available candidate donor cells. hESC are currently the only cell source that can potentially provide, ex vivo, an unlimited number of human cardiac cells for transplantation. Second, the ability of the ESCs to differentiate into a plurality of cell lineages may be utilized for transplantation of different cell types such as endothelial progenitor cells for induction of angiogenesis, and even specialized cardiomyocytes subtypes (pacemaking cells, atrial, ventricular, etc.) tailored for specific applications. Third, because of their clonal origin, the ESC-derived cardiomyocytes could lend themselves to extensive characterization and genetic manipulation to promote desirable characteristics such as resistance to ischemia and apoptosis, improved contractile function, and specific electrophysiological properties. Fourth, the embryonic stem-derived cells could also serve as a platform and a cellular vehicle for different gene therapy procedures aiming to manipulate the local myocardial environment by local secretion of growth promoting factors, various drugs, and angiogenic growth factors. Last, the ability to generate potentially unlimited numbers of cardiomyocytes ex vivo from the hESC may also bring a unique value to tissue engineering approaches.

Although hESDCMs could theoretically have the potential to fulfill most of the properties of the ideal donor cell, a number of critical obstacles need to be overcome before clinical application: (1) Studies assessing the ability of the cells to survive and integrate upon transplantation to the normal and diseased myocardial host tissue should be conducted. (2) Strategies need to be developed for directing hESC differentiation into the cardiac lineage (as discussed above). (3) Purification of the cardiomyocyte population should be achieved using selection protocols. (4) Upscaling of the culturing techniques is needed to yield a clinically relevant number of cells for transplantation. (5) A transplantation technique should be developed to enable proper alignment of the graft tissue, high seeding rate of the transplanted cells, and minimal damage to the host tissue. (6) Strategies aimed at preventing immunologic rejection of the cells should be developed.

Optimal functional improvement after cell grafting would require structural, electrophysiological, and mechanical coupling of donor cells to the existing network of host cardiomyocytes. In a recent study, we tested the ability of the hESDCMs to integrate structurally and functionally with host cardiac tissue both in vitro and in vivo. Initially, the ability of the hESDCMs to form electromechanical connections with primary cardiac cultures was assessed in a high-resolution in vitro coculturing system. Primary cultures were created from neonatal rat ventricular myocytes. The contracting areas within the EBs were then mechanically dissected and added to the cocultures. Interestingly, within 24 hours postgrafting, we could detect synchronous contraction in the cocultures that persisted for several weeks. Detailed studies of the hybrid cultures using the multielectrode array mapping technique demonstrated tight electrophysiological coupling between the two tissue types. The electrophysiological assessment was reinforced by demonstrating the development of gap junc-

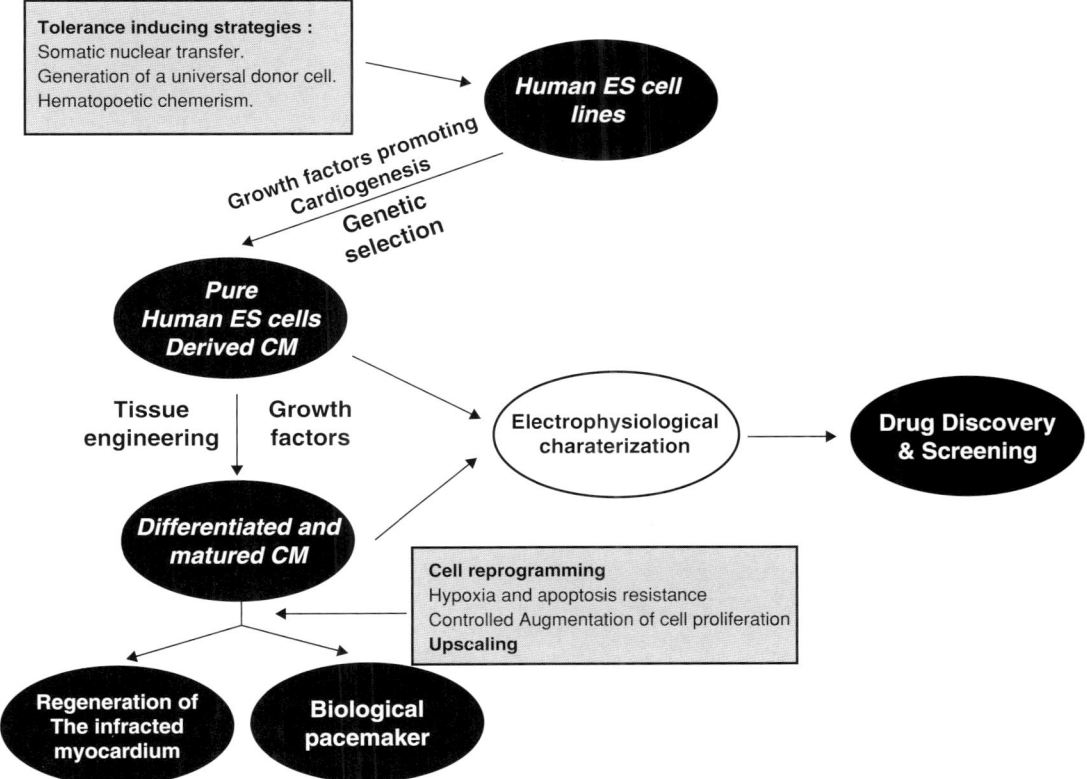

Figure 3.3. Potential applications of human embryonic stem (ES) cell-derived cardiomyocytes. The diagram describes some of the potential applications of hESDCMs as well as the possible obstacles to be overcome. CM, cardiomyocyte.

tions between the human and the rat cells as suggested by Cx43 immunostainings.

To demonstrate the ability of the hESDCMs to survive, function, and integrate also in the in vivo heart, we assessed their ability to pace the heart and to function as a "biological pacemaker." To examine this possibility, the cells were transplanted to the posterolateral region of the left ventricle in a swine model of slow hear rate. After cell grafting, a new ectopic ventricular rhythm was detected in 11 of 13 animals studies, in 6 of which it was characterized by sustained and long-term activity [Figure 3.4A (see color section)]. Pathological studies validated the presence and integration of the grafted hESDCMs at the site of transplantation. [Figure 3.4B (see color section)]. Three-dimensional electrophysiological mapping revealed that this ectopic ventricular rhythm originated from the area of cell transplantation (Figure 3.4C–E (see color section)]. Pathological studies validated the presence and integration of the grafted hESDCMs at the site of transplantation [Figure 3.4D (see color section)].

Cell Selection Strategies

Although the development of directed differentiation systems is essential for increasing cardiomyocyte yield from the hESC, it is unlikely that the degree of purity that will be achieved would be sufficient for clinical purposes. Because the beating EBs are comprise a mixed population of cells, selection strategies are crucial not only for increasing cardiomyocyte numbers but also for preventing the presence of other cell derivatives as well as ensuring the absence of pluripotent stem cells carrying the risk of teratomas. In addition, a similar strategy may aid in selecting specific cardiac cell types.

An elegant selection scheme to generate pure cardiomyocyte populations was suggested by Klug et al.[60] in the mESC model. Undifferentiated mESCs were transfected with a fusion gene coding resistance to neomycin under the regulation of the cardiac specific α-myosin heavy chain promoter. In addition, the transgene also carried sequence encoding hygromycin resistance enabling the selection of the stably transfected undifferentiated mESCs. Differentiation was then induced, and cardiomyocytes were selected based on the resistance for neomycin. A slightly different approach was reported by Muller et al.[73a] using GFP driven by the CMV enhancer and a ventricle specific promoter (MLC-2V). In conjunction with the use of Percoll gradient centrifugation and subsequent fluorescence-activated cell sorter, this strategy yielded a relatively pure (97%) population of ventricular cells. Although achieving high efficiency of stable transfection in the hESC has been difficult to achieve previously, the recent description of successful utilization of lentiviral vectors in these cell[74,75] will foster the application of the selection strategies described above also in the hESC model.

Upscaling

The left ventricle of the human heart contains approximately 5.8×10^9 cardiomyocytes.[76] Given the fact that 25% of the cells are lost during a typical myocardial infarction leading to heart failure, cell transplantation strategies aiming to completely regenerate the myocardium would have to use at least 10^9 cells. Generation of this number of cells can be achieved by increasing the number of ESCs used for cardiomyocyte differentiation, by using directed differentiation systems and enrichment strategies, and by increasing the ability of the cells to proliferate after cardiomyocyte differentiation. Zweigerdt et al.,[77] using the mESC model, combined the aforementioned cardiomyocyte selection strategies with the bioreactor technology to generate more than 10^9 vital cardiomyocytes in a single 2-L bioreactor run.

Genetic and Tissue Engineering

Optimal regeneration of the infarcted myocardium leading to systolic augmentation would undoubtedly depend on the ability of the grafted tissue to form a functional syncytium with the host heart. Thus, any expected functional improvement would require the long-term survival of the grafted cells, the presence of a critical tissue mass, and the appropriate alignment and integration of the donor cells. Increasing the survival of engrafted cells is a critical issue because the hostile ischemic scar tissue may result in significant cell death.[78-80] Because adequate vascularization of the graft tissue is critical to its survival, the potential ability to generate "smart hESDCMs" resistant to apoptosis and ischemia and capable of promoting graft vascularization by secretion of angiogenic growth factors may bring an added value to this. Future studies should also determine the ideal nature of the graft (e.g., individual cells, beating EBs, or combined with scaffolding biomaterials). Additional factors to be determined include the ideal degree of differentiation of the transplanted cells and the appropriate delivery method such as epicardial injections, transendocardial, or via the coronary circulation.

The ability to generate potentially unlimited numbers of cardiomyocytes ex vivo from the hESC may also bring a unique value to tissue engineering approaches. This new discipline combines functional cells with three-dimensional polymeric scaffolds to create tissue substitutes. The possible advantages of this approach versus direct cell transplantation may lie in the ability to control graft shape and size, to control the alignment of the engrafted cells, and to avoid the unpreventable initial cell loss encountered with the latter approach.[81]

Immunogenicity of the hESCs and Strategies Aimed at Achieving Tolerance

A major obstacle for the utilization of hESC derivatives in regeneration of different tissue types is the prevention of their immune rejection. Initial characterization of the immunogenicity of the hESC was conducted by Drukker et al.[82] The hESCs were shown to express a relatively low level of human leukocyte antigens (HLA) class I molecules. This expression was only moderately increased after differentiation in vitro (to EBs) and in vivo (to teratoma cells) but was significantly augmented after interferon-γ treatment. No expression of HLA class II molecules and the ligands for NK cell receptors was detected on the hESCs or their differentiated products. However, this study did not examine in detail the possible effects of the degree of EB maturation and differentiation and the heterogeneity of the cells within the EB on the immunogenicity of the cells. In addition, possible expression of HLA class II molecules should also be assessed in vivo especially in the setting of an inflammatory response such as occurs during graft rejection.

Several strategies aimed at achieving immunologic tolerance were suggested. One of the most promising strategies is based on the generation of isogenic hESC lines tailored specifically for each patient. Recently, Hwang et al.[83] demonstrated that, using somatic nuclear transfer technology, this strategy may become technically possible. The authors derived a hESC line from an enucleated oocyte after somatic nuclear transfer. Although nuclear transfer may be a promising strategy, it might be limited by technical constraints as well as by ethical reasons. Another attractive strategy for inducing tolerance is hematopoietic chimerism. Theoretically, hematopoietic chimerism may be achieved by transplanting hematopoietic stem cells derived from hESCs. After cell engraftment, the host will obtain tolerance because of the negative selection of alloreactive T cells in the thymus. Hence, various differentiated derivative of the specific hESC line could be then safely transplanted without the risk for immune rejection. An alternative strategy might be to establish "banks" of major histocompatibility complex antigen typed hESCs. The optimal solution for prevention of immune rejection may be the generation of a universal donor hESC line. These could be achieved by silencing genes associated with the assembly or transcriptional regulation of the major histocompatibility complexes or by overexpression of FAS ligand in the hESCs and thereby inducing apoptosis of the infiltrating T lymphocytes mediating immune rejection.

Summary and Future Potential Research Directions

The derivation of the hESC lines and the resulting cardiomyocyte differentiation system may bring a unique value to several basic and applied research fields. Research based on the cells may help to elucidate the mechanisms involved in early human cardiac lineage commitment, differentiation, and maturation. Moreover, this research may promote the discovery of novel growth and transcriptional factors using gene trapping techniques, functional genomics, and proteomics as well as providing a novel in vitro model for drug development and testing. Finally, the ability to generate, in vitro for the first time, human cardiac tissue provides an exciting and promising cell source for the emerging discipline of regenerative medicine and myocardial repair.

References

1. Thomson JA, Itskovitz-Eldor J, Shapiro SS, et al. Embryonic stem cell lines derived from human blastocysts. Science 1998;282(5391):1145–1147.
2. Evans MJ, Kaufman MH. Establishment in culture of pluripotential cells from mouse embryos. Nature 1981;292(5819):154–156.
3. Martin G. Isolation of a pluripotent cell line from early mouse embryos cultured in medium conditioned by teratocarcinoma stem cells. Proc Natl Acad Sci USA 1981;78:7634–7638.
4. Reubinoff BE, Pera MF, Fong CY, et al. Embryonic stem cell lines from human blastocysts: somatic differentiation in vitro. Nat Biotechnol 2000;18(4):399–404.
5. Pera MF, Trounson AO. Human embryonic stem cells: prospects for development. Development 2004;131(22): 5515–5525.
6. Odorico JS, Kaufman DS, Thomson JA. Multilineage differentiation from human embryonic stem cell lines. Stem Cells 2001;19(3):193–204.
7. Rao M. Conserved and divergent paths that regulate self-renewal in mouse and human embryonic stem cells. Dev Biol 2004;275(2):269–286.
8. Ying QL, Nichols J, Chambers I, et al. BMP induction of Id proteins suppresses differentiation and sustains embryonic stem cell self-renewal in collaboration with STAT3. Cell 2003;115(3):281–292.
9. Xu C, Inokuma MS, Denham J, et al. Feeder-free growth of undifferentiated human embryonic stem cells. Nat Biotechnol 2001;19(10):971–974.
10. Richards M, Fong CY, Chan WK, et al. Human feeders support prolonged undifferentiated growth of human inner cell masses and embryonic stem cells. Nat Biotechnol 2002;20(9):933–936.
11. Amit M, Margulets V, Segev H, et al. Human feeder layers for human embryonic stem cells. Biol Reprod 2003;68(6):2150–2156.
12. Sato N, Meijer L, Skaltsounis L, et al. Maintenance of pluripotency in human and mouse embryonic stem cells through activation of Wnt signaling by a pharmacological GSK-3-specific inhibitor. Nat Med 2004;10(1):55–63.
13. Bhattacharya B, Miura T, Brandenberger R, et al. Gene expression in human embryonic stem cell lines: unique molecular signature. Blood 2004;103(8): 2956–2964.
14. Mitsui K, Tokuzawa Y, Itoh H, et al. The homeoprotein Nanog is required for maintenance of pluripotency in mouse epiblast and ES cells. Cell 2003;113(5):631–642.
15. Chambers I, Colby D, Robertson M, et al. Functional expression cloning of Nanog, a pluripotency sustaining factor in embryonic stem cells. Cell 2003;113(5):643–655.
16. Kehat I, Kenyagin-Karsenti D, Snir M, et al. Human embryonic stem cells can differentiate into myocytes

16. with structural and functional properties of cardiomyocytes. J Clin Invest 2001;108(3):407–414.
17. Zeng X, Cai J, Chen J, et al. Dopaminergic differentiation of human embryonic stem cells. Stem Cells 2004;22(6):925–940.
18. Reubinoff BE, Itsykson P, Turetsky T, et al. Neural progenitors from human embryonic stem cells. Nat Biotechnol 2001;19(12):1134–1140.
19. Assady S, Maor G, Amit M, et al. Insulin production by human embryonic stem cells. Diabetes 2001;50(8):1691–1697.
20. Kaufman DS, Thomson JA. Human ES cells: haematopoiesis and transplantation strategies. J Anat 2002;200(Pt 3):243–248.
21. Green H, Easley K, Iuchi S. Marker succession during the development of keratinocytes from cultured human embryonic stem cells. Proc Natl Acad Sci USA 2003;100(26):15625–15630.
22. Sottile V, Thomson A, McWhir J. In vitro osteogenic differentiation of human ES cells. Cloning Stem Cells 2003;5(2):149–155.
23. Levenberg S, Golub JS, Amit M, et al. Endothelial cells derived from human embryonic stem cells. Proc Natl Acad Sci USA 2002;99(7):4391–4396.
24. Doetschman TC, Eistetter H, Katz M, et al. The in vitro development of blastocyst-derived embryonic stem cell lines: formation of visceral yolk sac, blood 0islands and myocardium. J Embryol Exp Morphol 1985;87:27–45.
25. Itskovitz-Eldor J, Schuldiner M, Karsenti D, et al. Differentiation of human embryonic stem cells into embryoid bodies compromising the three embryonic germ layers. Mol Med 2000;6(2):88–95.
26. He JQ, Ma Y, Lee Y, et al. Human embryonic stem cells develop into multiple types of cardiac myocytes: action potential characterization. Circ Res 2003;93(1):32–39.
27. Mummery C, Ward-van Oostwaard D, Doevendans P, et al. Differentiation of human embryonic stem cells to cardiomyocytes: role of coculture with visceral endoderm-like cells. Circulation 2003;107(21):2733–2740.
28. Xu C, Police S, Rao N, et al. Characterization and enrichment of cardiomyocytes derived from human embryonic stem cells. Circ Res 2002;91(6):501–508.
29. Snir M, Kehat I, Gepstein A, et al. Assessment of the ultrastructural and proliferative properties of human embryonic stem cell-derived cardiomyocytes. Am J Physiol Heart Circ Physiol 2003;285(6):H2355–H2363.
30. Guan K, Furst DO, Wobus AM. Modulation of sarcomere organization during embryonic stem cell-derived cardiomyocyte differentiation. Eur J Cell Biol 1999;78(11):813–823.
31. Hescheler J, Fleischmann BK, Lentini S, et al. Embryonic stem cells: a model to study structural and functional properties in cardiomyogenesis. Cardiovasc Res 1997;36(2):149–162.
32. Zimmermann WH, Schneiderbanger K, Schubert P, et al. Tissue engineering of a differentiated cardiac muscle construct. Circ Res 2002;90(2):223–230.
33. Ventura C, Maioli M, Asara Y, et al. Turning on stem cell cardiogenesis with extremely low frequency magnetic fields. FASEB J 2005;19(1):155–157.
34. Chen H, Shi S, Acosta L, et al. BMP10 is essential for maintaining cardiac growth during murine cardiogenesis. Development 2004;131(9):2219–2231.
35. Wang B, Weidenfeld J, Lu MM, et al. Foxp1 regulates cardiac outflow tract, endocardial cushion morphogenesis and myocyte proliferation and maturation. Development 2004;131(18):4477–4487.
36. Fijnvandraat AC, Lekanne Deprez RH, Christoffels VM, et al. TBX5 overexpression stimulates differentiation of chamber myocardium in P19C16 embryonic carcinoma cells. J Muscle Res Cell Motil 2003;24(2–3):211–218.
37. Kehat I, Gepstein A, Spira A, et al. High-resolution electrophysiological assessment of human embryonic stem cell-derived cardiomyocytes: a novel in-vitro model for the study of conduction. Circ Res 2002;91(8):659–661.
38. Satin J, Kehat I, Caspi O, et al. Mechanism of spontaneous excitability in human embryonic stem cell derived cardiomyocytes. J Physiol 2004;559(Pt 2):479–496.
39. Li F, Wang X, Capasso JM, et al. Rapid transition of cardiac myocytes from hyperplasia to hypertrophy during postnatal development. J Mol Cell Cardiol 1996;28(8):1737–1746.
40. Whittaker P, Zheng S, Patterson MJ, et al. Histologic signatures of thermal injury: applications in transmyocardial laser revascularization and radiofrequency ablation. Lasers Surg Med 2000;27(4):305–318.
41. Snir M, Kehat I. Assessment of the ultrastructural and proliferative properties of human embryonic stem cell-derived cardiomyocytes. Am J Physiol Heart Circ Physiol 2003;285(6):H2355–H2363.
42. Zaffran S, Frasch M. Early signals in cardiac development. Circ Res 2002;91(6):457–469.
43. Pandur P, Lasche M, Eisenberg LM, et al. Wnt-11 activation of a non-canonical Wnt signalling pathway is required for cardiogenesis. Nature 2002;418(6898):636–641.
44. Nakamura T, Sano M, Songyang Z, et al. A Wnt- and beta-catenin-dependent pathway for mammalian cardiac myogenesis. Proc Natl Acad Sci USA 2003;100(10):5834–5839.
45. Harvey RP. Patterning the vertebrate heart. Nat Rev Genet 2002;3(7):544–556.
46. Harvey RP. Patterning the vertebrate heart. Nat Rev Genet 2002;3(7):544–556.
47. Ventura C, Maioli M. Opioid peptide gene expression primes cardiogenesis in embryonal pluripotent stem cells. Circ Res 2000;87(3):189–194.
48. Wobus AM, Kaomei G, Shan J, et al. Retinoic acid accelerates embryonic stem cell-derived cardiac differentiation and enhances development of ventricular cardiomyocytes. J Mol Cell Cardiol 1997;29(6):1525–1539.
49. Behfar A, Zingman LV, Hodgson DM, et al. Stem cell differentiation requires a paracrine pathway in the heart. FASEB J 2002;16(12):1558–1566.
50. Takahashi T, Lord B, Schulze PC, et al. Ascorbic acid enhances differentiation of embryonic stem cells into cardiac myocytes. Circulation 2003;107(14):1912–1916.
51. Xu C, Police S, Rao N, et al. Characterization and enrichment of cardiomyocytes derived from human embryonic stem cells. Circ Res 2002;91(6):501–508.
52. Mummery CL, van Achterberg TA, van den Eijnden-van Raaij AJ, et al. Visceral-endoderm-like cell lines

induce differentiation of murine P19 embryonal carcinoma cells. Differentiation 1991;46(1):51–60.
53. Murry CE, Wiseman RW, Schwartz SM, et al. Skeletal myoblast transplantation for repair of myocardial necrosis. J Clin Invest 1996;98(11):2512–2523.
54. Leor J, Patterson M, Quinones MJ, et al. Transplantation of fetal myocardial tissue into the infarcted myocardium of rat. A potential method for repair of infarcted myocardium? Circulation 1996; 94(9 suppl):332–336.
55. Soonpaa MH, Koh GY, Klug MG, et al. Formation of nascent intercalated disks between grafted fetal cardiomyocytes and host myocardium. Science 1994;264(5155):98–101.
56. Muller-Ehmsen J, Whittaker P, Kloner RA, et al. Survival and development of neonatal rat cardiomyocytes transplanted into adult myocardium. J Mol Cell Cardiol 2002;34(2):107–116.
57. Reinecke H, Zhang M, Bartosek T, et al. Survival, integration, and differentiation of cardiomyocyte grafts: a study in normal and injured rat hearts. Circulation 1999;100(2):193–202.
58. Yoo KJ, Li RK, Weisel RD, et al. Autologous smooth muscle cell transplantation improved heart function in dilated cardiomyopathy. Ann Thorac Surg 2000;70(3): 859–865.
59. Behfar A, Zingman LV, Hodgson DM, et al. Stem cell differentiation requires a paracrine pathway in the heart. FASEB J 2002;16(12):1558–1566.
60. Klug MG, Soonpaa MH, Koh GY, et al. Genetically selected cardiomyocytes from differentiating embryonic stem cells form stable intracardiac grafts. J Clin Invest 1996;98(1):216–224.
61. Min JY, Yang Y, Sullivan MF, et al. Long-term improvement of cardiac function in rats after infarction by transplantation of embryonic stem cells. J Thorac Cardiovasc Surg 2003;125(2):361–369.
62. Yang Y, Min JY, Rana JS, et al. VEGF enhances functional improvement of postinfarcted hearts by transplantation of ESC-differentiated cells. J Appl Physiol 2002;93(3):1140–1151.
63. Orlic D, Kajstura J, Chimenti S, et al. Bone marrow cells regenerate infarcted myocardium. Nature 2001;410(6829):701–705.
64. Alvarez-Dolado M, Pardal R, Garcia-Verdugo JM, et al. Fusion of bone-marrow-derived cells with Purkinje neurons, cardiomyocytes and hepatocytes. Nature 2003;425(6961):968–973.
65. Terada N, Hamazaki T, Oka M, et al. Bone marrow cells adopt the phenotype of other cells by spontaneous cell fusion. Nature 2002;416(6880):542–545.
66. Murry CE, Soonpaa MH, Reinecke H, et al. Haematopoietic stem cells do not transdifferentiate into cardiac myocytes in myocardial infarcts. Nature 2004;428(6983):664–668.
67. Balsam LB, Wagers AJ, Christensen JL, et al. Haematopoietic stem cells adopt mature haematopoietic fates in ischaemic myocardium. Nature 2004;428(6983):668–673.
68. Kocher AA, Schuster MD, Szabolcs MJ, et al. Neovascularization of ischemic myocardium by human bone-marrow-derived angioblasts prevents cardiomyocyte apoptosis, reduces remodeling and improves cardiac function. Nat Med 2001;7(4):430–436.
69. Menasche P, Hagege AA, Scorsin M, et al. Myoblast transplantation for heart failure. Lancet 2001;357(9252): 279–280.
70. Reinecke H, MacDonald GH, Hauschka SD, et al. Electromechanical coupling between skeletal and cardiac muscle. Implications for infarct repair. J Cell Biol 2000;149(3):731–740.
71. Li RK, Mickle DA, Weisel RD, et al. Natural history of fetal rat cardiomyocytes transplanted into adult rat myocardial scar tissue. Circulation 1997;96(9 suppl): 179–186.
72. Etzion S, Battler A, Barbash IM, et al. Influence of embryonic cardiomyocyte transplantation on the progression of heart failure in a rat model of extensive myocardial infarction. J Mol Cell Cardiol 2001;33(7): 1321–1330.
73. Scorsin M, Hagege AA, Marotte F, et al. Does transplantation of cardiomyocytes improve function of infarcted myocardium? Circulation 1997;96(9 suppl):188–193.
73a. Muller M, Fleischmann BK, Selbert S, et al. Selection of ventricular-like cardiomyocytes from ES cells in vitro. FASEB J 2000;14(15):2540–2548.
74. Ma Y, Ramezani A, Lewis R, et al. High-level sustained transgene expression in human embryonic stem cells using lentiviral vectors. Stem Cells 2003; 21(1):111–117.
75. Gropp M, Itsykson P, Singer O, et al. Stable genetic modification of human embryonic stem cells by lentiviral vectors. Mol Ther 2003;7(2):281–287.
76. Kajstura J, Leri A, Finato N, et al. Myocyte proliferation in end-stage cardiac failure in humans. Proc Natl Acad Sci USA 1998;95(15):8801–8805.
77. Zandstra PW, Bauwens C, Yin T, et al. Scalable production of embryonic stem cell-derived cardiomyocytes. Tissue Eng. 2003; 9(4):767–768.
78. Muller-Ehmsen J, Peterson KL, Kedes L, et al. Rebuilding a damaged heart: long-term survival of transplanted neonatal rat cardiomyocytes after myocardial infarction and effect on cardiac function. Circulation 2002;105(14):1720–1726.
79. Zhang M, Methot D, Poppa V, et al. Cardiomyocyte grafting for cardiac repair: graft cell death and antideath strategies. J Mol Cell Cardiol 2001;33(5):907–921.
80. Watanabe E, Smith DM Jr, Delcarpio JB, et al. Cardiomyocyte transplantation in a porcine myocardial infarction model. Cell Transplant 1998;7(3): 239–246.
81. Zimmermann WH, Eschenhagen T. Cardiac tissue engineering for replacement therapy. Heart Fail Rev 2003;8(3):259–269.
82. Drukker M, Katz G, Urbach A, et al. Characterization of the expression of MHC proteins in human embryonic stem cells. Proc Natl Acad Sci USA 2002;99(15): 9864–9869.
83. Hwang WS, Ryu YJ, Park JH, et al. Evidence of a pluripotent human embryonic stem cell line derived from a cloned blastocyst. Science 2004;303(5664):1669–1674.

4

Therapeutic Angiogenesis

Shmuel Fuchs and Alexander Battler

Atherosclerotic vascular disease is a leading cause of mortality and morbidity in the industrial countries. It is estimated that more than 12,000,000 Americans have angina pectoris[1] and at least 5%–10% of patients who are referred to coronary angiography have advanced disease not amenable for current conventional revascularization.[2] The dearth of effective treatment strategies for this sick patient population together with progress achieved in understanding the complex mechanisms inherent in the development of new blood vessels, has facilitated a new treatment strategy commonly termed as therapeutic myocardial angiogenesis. This chapter summarizes the current clinical experience with this approach with specific focus on cell-based therapy.

Two main postembryonic mechanisms are involved in the complex process of new blood vessel formation. The first, *angiogenesis*, is the main postembryogenesis mechanism and encompasses sprouting of preexisting capillaries to form a new capillary network. The process is tightly regulated by the concerted activity of ample proangiogenic factors, including the family of vascular endothelial growth factor (VEGF), placental growth factor, and fibroblast growth factor (FGF).[3] The process occurs in various physiologic and pathological conditions including diabetic proliferative retinopathy, rheumatoid arthritis, and tumor growth.[4] The second mechanism, *arteriogenesis*, relates to the formation of resistance blood vessel growth via remodeling of preexisting small arterioles into larger conductance vessels. This phenomenon is prompted in part by an increase in shear stress, which occurs in the small, high-resistance arterioles that are in parallel with the main occluded arterial conduit. Endothelial shear-stress responsive elements mediate increased expression of macrophage chemoattractant protein-1, granulocyte-macrophage colony-stimulating factor (GM-CSF), and intercellular adhesion molecule-1 among other genes.[5-7] The process occurs in various conditions associated with arterial narrowing or occlusion including coarctation of the aorta, and peripheral and coronary artery occlusions. These two processes, angiogenesis and arteriogenesis, are complementary and together may be referred to as a recently proposed term: collaterogenesis.[8] In this chapter, angiogenesis, the most common term, is being used in reference to the process of complete reconstitution of a new functioning vascular network.

Growth Factor Proteins and Genes for Myocardial Ischemia

Proteins

The initial attempts of therapeutic angiogenesis advocate the administration of a single angiogenic growth factor protein or gene to promote the development of endogenous collateral vessels in ischemic myocardium. The driven concept to this approach was that VEGF and FGF, among other growth factors, have a major role in the complex process of collateral blood vessel formation, and exogenous administration of these growth factors will facilitate the natural process.[3,9–11] However, the initial excitement, driven by several nonrandomized small phase I studies, was hampered by negative results of subsequent larger randomized trials (Tables 4.1 and 4.2).[12–25] The Vascular endothelial growth factor in Ischemia for Vascular Angiogenesis (VIVA) trial was the first therapeutic angiogenic phase II study.[19] The study enrolled 178 patients who were randomized to placebo, low-, and high-dose intracoronary injection of rhVEGF$_{165}$ protein followed by repeated intravenous infusion at days 3, 6, and 9. The primary endpoint was the change in exercise treadmill test (ETT) time from baseline to day 60. Secondary endpoints included change in ETT time at day 120, myocardial perfusion imaging on day 60, and Canadian Cardiovascular Society (CCS) angina class and quality of life (QOL) measures at days 60 and 120. At 2 months, ETT similarly improved in the three treatment groups (placebo, 48 seconds; low dose, 30 seconds; and high dose, 30 seconds). No differences were noted in angina class at day 60 although a significant improvement was noted in the high rhVEGF$_{165}$ compared with the placebo group. Myocardial perfusion study failed to demonstrate improvement either at rest or at stress. This important study suggested that the systemic administration of VEGF protein is safe but carries limited therapeutic angiogenic benefit. The FGF Initiating RevaScularization Trial (FIRST) assessed the potential efficacy of a single intracoronary injection of escalated doses of rFGF2 a (0, 0.3, 3, or 30 µg/kg) among 337 patients with coronary artery disease considered suboptimal to revascularization.[20] The primary efficacy endpoint was the change in ETT duration from baseline to 90 days follow-up. Secondary efficacy variables included the change in ETT duration from baseline to 180-day follow-up; changes in CCS angina class and QOL variables from baseline to 90- and 180-day

Table 4.1. Clinical trials of VEGF therapy for myocardial angiogenesis

Author	Patients (n)	Angiogenic factor	Route of administration	Results
Nonrandomized				
Rosengart et al.[21]	21	VEGF$_{121}$ gene-Ad	Intramuscular, thoracotomy	Improved
Symes et al.[23]	20	VEGF$_{165}$ plasmid	Intramuscular, thoracotomy	Improved
Losordo et al.[13]	19	VEGF-2 plasmid	Transendocardial via catheter	Improved
Randomized				
Fuchs et al.[28]	10	VEGF$_{121}$ gene-Ad	Transendocardial via catheter	Safe
Henry et al.[19]	178	VEGF$_{165}$ protein	Intracoronary plus intravenous	No effect
Kastrup[29]	80	VEGF$_{165}$ plasmid	Transendocardial via catheter	No effect

Table 4.2. Clinical trials of FGF therapy for myocardial angiogenesis

Author	Patients (n)	Angiogenic factor	Route of administration	Results
Nonrandomized				
Laham et al.[25]	52	bFGF protein	Intracoronary	Improved
Udelson[14]	59	bFGF protein	Intracoronary	Improved
Randomized				
Schumacher et al.[22]	40	aFGF protein	Intramuscular, thoracotomy	Improved
Laham et al.[24]	24	bFGF-protein pellets	Intramuscular, thoracotomy	Improved
Unger et al.[16]	25	bFGF protein	Intracoronary	Safe
FIRST trial[20]	337	bFGF protein	Intracoronary	1º endpoint: negative
AGENT trial[18]	79	FGF-4 Gene-Ad	Intracoronary	1º endpoint: negative

follow-up; QOL as measured by the Seattle Angina Questionnaire (SAQ), and the changes in myocardial rest and stress perfusion from baseline to 90 and 180 days. Similarly to the VIVA study, the improvement noted in ETT duration (approximately 40–60 seconds) did not differ among the four groups. CCS angina class and angina frequency significantly improved in the mid-dose FGF group at 90 days. However, this benefit was lost at 180 days follow-up. In accord with the VIVA trial, nuclear study failed to demonstrate any change in myocardial perfusion.

Genes

Given the complexity of the processes of functional new blood vessel formation, these negative results may suggest that the single growth factor approach may be too simplistic. However, interpretation of the negative results suggests that several study design-related parameters may also have a role. For example, an essential concern is whether the failure of the single growth factor approach is attributable to the insufficient intramyocardial level/concentration of the injected growth factor. After intracoronary infusion of radioactive-labeled FGF, Laham et al.[26] reported that pick myocardial activity was only 0.12%, which was lower than the liver activity. It is conceivable, therefore, that after intracoronary injection of protein, both intramyocardial pick and trough levels may be insufficient.

Several subsequent studies attempted to overcome the above potential hurdles. The Angiogenic Gene Therapy (AGENT) study was the first randomized trial to evaluate the safety and potential anti-ischemic effects of five escalating doses of replication defective adenovirus encoding FGF4 in patients with angina pectoris.[18] The study's driven hypothesis was that gene administration would allow achieving intramyocardial critical level of angiogenic growth factor for the minimal duration needed for promoting an effective collateral vessel formation, thus overcoming some of the potential limitations of the protein-based approach. The primary objectives of the trial were safety and selecting effective doses for subsequent study. Seventy-nine patients with chronic stable angina CCS class 2 or 3 were randomized to single intracoronary injection of placebo (n = 19) or Ad5-FGF4 (five ascending doses, n = 60). The study demonstrated safety whereas no virus was detected in the urine and no FGF protein was detected in the plasma of the patients. Three patients had increased temperature after the procedure; all received the highest viral dose. At follow-up, two patients who received active treatment were diagnosed with malignancy, concluded as probably not related to the treatment. Change in ETT duration between baseline and 4 and 12 weeks was similar between active treatment and control groups. In a prespecified post hoc analysis, patients enrolled in group 4 had a higher rate of substantial improvement in ETT duration at 4 weeks compared with placebo. After this study, a 400-patient phase II study was initiated. In this study, patients with coronary artery disease who did not need urgent revascularization were randomized to single intracoronary administration of Ad5-FGF4 or placebo. The study was put on hold after enrolling approximately 200 patients because of lack of efficacy (unpublished data).

After the failure of the above randomized studies to demonstrate efficacy of intracoronary injection of angiogenic growth factors, a new injection method – direct, catheter-based intramyocardial injection has become an attractive mode of delivery. Its potential advantages, compared with intracoronary and systemic administration, include a reduced systemic distribution, thus allowing delivery of a higher concentration of angiogenic compound, and to approach myocardial territories supplied by severely diseased coronary arteries, often not suitable for intracoronary injection. Currently, most of the clinical experience is with a nonfluoroscopic guided system (Biosense, Johnson & Johnson).[27] The safety of this approach was tested in two small phase I studies. Fuchs et al.[28] assessed the safety of transendocardial injection of adenovirus encoding for $VEGF_{121}$ in 10 patients who were randomized (2:1) to active treatment or placebo. Losordo et al.[13] assessed the safety of similar catheter-based delivery of VEGF2 plasmid in 19 patients. Both studies demonstrated safety and feasibility and paved the way for larger phase II studies (see below). The first phase II double-blind randomized study to assess this approach was the EUROINJECT trial.[29] In this study, 80 patients with CCS class of 3 or higher were randomized to transendocardial injection of plasmid encoding $VEGF_{165}$ or empty plasmid (10 injections, 0.3 mL each). The primary and secondary endpoints were change in myocardial perfusion (SPECT) and CCS class, nitrogen consumption, SAQ, and ETT, respectively. There was an improvement in myocardial perfusion in 44% of the treated patients. However, no statistically significant change was noted between the active treatment and the placebo groups. Although CCS class similarly improved in both groups (approximately 1 class), only patients who received $VEGF_{165}$ also experienced less anginal attacks at 3 months compared with baseline.

Despite the negative results of the EUROINJECT study, the questions whether the administration of a gene encoding for a single angiogenic growth factor will turn to be a valid therapeutic approach is still open – one may assume that with a more potent angiogenic growth factor, or with the use of adenovirus rather than plasmid as a vector, the results of this strategy would be different. Two new studies, one European based and one United States based are on the way. Losordo et al. have initiated a United States phase II double-blind randomized study evaluating the efficacy of transendocardial injection of plasmid encoding to VEGF2. The NOGA Delivery of VEGF for Angina (NOVA) trial is a European/Israeli multicenter, double-blind randomized study evaluating the efficacy of $AD_{GV}VEGF121$ delivered by the Biosense injection platform in 120 "no option" patients with class 2–4 CCS angina to be initiated Q1 2005.

Cell-Based Therapy for Myocardial Ischemia

General Concept and Principles

The overall disappointing results from the single growth factor approach led to intensive investigation for alternative strategies. Assuming that the complex process of angiogenesis required a large array of growth factors and administration of such a large number of cytokines will not be feasible, several alternatives were investigated. One approach involves the administration of a master switch gene such as hypoxia inducible factor 1 in order to regulate activation of multiple genes necessary for vascular bed formation. Several clinical studies were initiated; however, currently, no results are available. An attractive concept is that the administration of bone marrow (BM)-derived cells (or peripheral blood-derived mononuclear and progenitor cells) will result in therapeutically meaningful collateral vessel development. The potential angiogenic activity of BM cells can broadly be divided into two type. The first and highly debatable mechanism is their capability to *differentiate* into cellular constituents that physically contribute to the developing collaterals. The second is their *secretory* capacity. Many of the growth factors and cytokines required to stimulate and coordinate the complex processes involved in the remodeling of preexisting small collaterals have been shown to be secreted by cultured BM cells.[30-33]

BM-Derived Cell Differentiation

In vitro studies demonstrated that several BM-derived cells are able to differentiate into one or more of the cellular components of the vascular bed. The mechanisms by which the local milieu affects the differentiation pathway of these stem cells are yet unknown. It is agreed, however, that several BM cell subpopulations are the precursors of endothelial cells.[34-37] Animal and human studies suggest that endothelial progenitor cells and angioblasts are present in the peripheral circulation in the resting state. After tissue ischemia, these cells are preferentially released, migrate, and actively participate in newly forming capillaries.[38-40] Thus, direct administration of BM cells into ischemic tissue may augment the natural responses to ischemia, optimizing restoration of tissue perfusion. A wide variety of BM-derived cells was tested at the bench and in various animal models (Table 4.3). There is no direct comparison between the efficacy of the wide variety of the cell types, and the magnitude of response varied substantially among studies (3%–56%). Differences in animal models [myocardial infarction (MI) versus ischemia, myocardial versus hindlimb ischemia, and coronary ligation versus cryo-injury], number of injected cells, and mode of delivery (systemic versus intramyocardial versus intraventricular) preclude any meaningful comparison between studies. Recently, the issue of adult stem cell plasticity has been questioned. Several groups proposed that spontaneous cell fusion and generation of hybrid cells with subsequent adoption of recipient cell phenotype accounted

Table 4.3. BM-derived cells used in various animal models

Cell type	Reference	Animal model	Route of administration	Cell Incorporation into blood vessels	Tissue perfusion	Myocardial function	Comments
Nonisolated cells							
Unfractionated BM	Fuchs et al.[44]	Pig, chronic ischemia	Transendocardial	NA[§]	Improved	Improved	Improved collaterals on angiography
BMNCs*	Kamihata et al.[45]	Pig, ischemia-reperfusion	Transepicardial	Yes, incorporated into ~31% of neocapillaries	Improved	Lower end-diastolic pressure	Increased capillary density, ↑ VEGF, FGF, Angiop-1 intramyocardial mRNA
Isolated cells							
Side population (CD34−/kit+/Sca+)	Jackson et al.[69]	Irradiated mouse ischemia-reperfusion	Transepicardial	Yes, 3.3% of vascular cells were from SP cell origin	NA[§]	NA[§]	Low rate of engraftment to cardiomyocytes (0.02%) ↑ Capillary density
CD31+	Kawamoto et al.[70]	Pig, chronic ischemia	Transendocardial	Yes	NA[§]	Improved	↑ Angiographic collaterals
CD34+ (CD34+/Ckit+)	Kocher et al.[71]	Rat, MI[†]	Systemic (IV)	Yes, accounted for 20%–25% of total capillary vasculature	NA[§]	Improved	Increased capillary density, reduced scar area, reduced peri-infarct apoptosis
Lineage negative/c-kit+	Orlic et al.[72]	Mouse, MI[†]	Transepicardial		NA[§]		Regeneration of myocytes and vascular network
Mesenchymal stem cells	Davani et al.[73]	Rat, MI[†]	Transepicardial	Yes	NA[§]	Improved	Differentiation into SM and endothelial cells (CD31+), ↑ Vascular density

*BMNC, bone marrow nuclear cells; [§]NA, not available; [†]MI, myocardial infarction.

for what was originally thought to be a "pure" cell transdifferentiation.[41,42] In addition, others suggested that hematopoietic stem cells injected into myocardium adopt only a mature hematopoietic fate.[43] It is thus evident that several fundamental issues remain unresolved and their addressing is crucial for optimizing cell-based therapies.

Secretory Capacity

The improved tissue perfusion observed in preclinical[44,45] and clinical studies[46-50] using heterogeneous nonselected BM cell populations, which contain very few stem cells (<0.01% of total cells) suggest the importance of the secretory mechanism.

BM cells can secrete an entire array of growth factors that are involved in the initiation and coordination of angiogenesis. These cytokines are secreted by several cellular components of the marrow population including lymphocytes, monocytes, megakaryocytes, platelets, as well as mesenchymal stem cells and early attached cells.[30-33] After direct myocardial delivery of these cells, increases in cardiac mRNA expression of VEGF, FGF, and angiopoietin-1 were demonstrated suggesting localized in vivo secretion of angiogenic growth factors by the injected cells.[45] The marrow stromal cells, via secretion of multiple growth factors and cytokines, support hematopoiesis. Several of these mediators also regulate angiogenesis including interleukin-1, interleukin-6, colony-stimulating factors, erythropoietin, and hepatocyte cell growth factor.[37] The humoral angiogenic potential of stromal cells was examined in a series of in vitro studies. The monocyte fraction of freshly aspirated and filtered porcine[44] and human[48,49] BM was cultured for 4 weeks and the effect of the conditioned medium on endothelial proliferation, migration, and tube formation was measured. Results showed that cultured BM cells continuously secrete VEGF and macrophage chemoattractant protein-1 and administration of BM-derived conditioned media (CM)-enhanced endothelial cell proliferation and migration and endothelial and smooth muscle tube formation. Recently, intramuscular stromal cell injection was reported to improve ischemic hindlimb perfusion.[51,52] Histopathology assessment revealed an islet of marked stromal cells in the interstitium of the muscle fibers but not in blood vessel wall. Interestingly, in situ hybridization revealed localized secretion of VEGF and FGF by these cells, supporting the importance of the secretory mechanism. Finally, in a similar mouse ischemic hindlimb model, administration of BM-derived conditioned medium improved tissue perfusion (T. Kinnaird, personal communication).

Route of Administration

Route of administration may have a crucial role in optimizing cell therapy. The least invasive – intravenous injection – allows repeated treatments with minimal risk. The efficiency of this approach largely depends on the transpulmonary first-pass effect on the injected cells, as well as on the homing efficiency of the circulating cells to target the ischemic myocardial tissue. A recent MI small animal study suggested a significant cell trapping within the pulmonary vascular bed that was associated with reduced efficacy of intravenous compared with intraventricular injection of BM-derived cells to augment myocardial perfusion and function.[53] Also, evidence suggests that these cells distribute widely after intravenous injection, although tissue ischemia may enhance localization.[38,39] Intracoronary delivery may improve tissue localization, and the safety, feasibility, and potential efficacy of this approach was recently demonstrated in several small clinical trials in patient who underwent primary target vessel angioplasty.[54-60] In this group of patients, the injection is performed via patent artery; therefore, the safety and feasibility of this approach in patients with severely narrowed/occluded coronary arteries are yet to be tested. Potential tradeoffs of this approach are discussed below.

Direct intramyocardial delivery approaches are the most invasive, and include: 1) transepicardial injections as an adjunctive therapy to coronary bypass grafting surgery, 2) transepicardial injections as a sole therapy via mini-thoracotomy or thoracoscopy, and 3) catheter-based percutaneous transendocardial injection. The main potential advantage of the surgical procedure is "injection under direct visualization" allowing anatomical identification of the target area and even distribution of the injections. Limitations of this approach include inability for repeat procedures and difficulties in accessing septal and posterior segments.

Transendocardial injection is a less invasive, catheter-based approach. Current clinical experience is greatest with the electromechanical mapping-guided technique. The three-dimensional left ventricular (LV) map serves as an anatomical navigation platform, allowing identification of catheter-tip location and orientation, injection within a prespecified delineated zone, and avoidance of undesirable areas such as the mitral valve apparatus or thinned infarcted myocardium, annotation of each injection site, and even injection distribution [Figure 4.1 (see color section)]. Using fluoroscopic, electromechanical, and electrocardiographic parameters to assure catheter stability and needle penetration, the delivery efficiency is approximately 95%.[61] Limitation of this approach include the need for intraventricular catheter manipulation with the resultant irritation of the myocardium and the induction of ventricular premature beats. In certain cases, this precludes injection in highly arrhythmogenic zones and can extend significantly the duration of the procedure. No sustained ventricular tachycardia (VT) or ventricular fibrillation (VF) was reported, but a careful monitoring is mandatory.[13,46–50] The procedure also required specific technical skills with a relatively long training period. However, a fast mapping technology, currently in clinical evaluation, seems to shorten learning curve, ease of performance, and overall procedure time.

Clinical Studies with BM and Peripheral Blood-Derived Cells

Surgical Approach

The first clinical study was performed in Japan in 1999.[62] Five patients who underwent coronary artery bypass graft (CABG) received an adjunctive transepicardial injection of mononuclear fraction of ABM cells directly into the ungraftable myocardial zone. Postoperative evaluation revealed no adverse effects and clinical follow-up was performed for a minimum of 1 year. Perfusion in the target area improved in three of the five patients.

A similar approach with injection of isolated AC133+ progenitor cells was recently examined in six patients.[63] In this study, patients with recent MI who underwent routine CABG surgery received 10 direct intramyocardial injections of 1×10^5 AC133+ cells into the infarcted territory. During the 6–9 months' follow-up, no malignant neoplasms or ventricular arrhythmias were noted. SPECT study revealed significant improvement in the injected territory.

These studies suggest feasibility and safety of transepicardial injection of BM-derived cells in adjunct to CABG. As an adjunctive therapy, the true efficacy of such strategy cannot be assessed as it would be when implemented as a sole therapy. Nevertheless, the long follow-up provides an additional safety level for the BM-derived cell transplantation approach.

Catheter-Based Transendocardial Approach

The safety and feasibility of transendocardial injection of autologous BM cells were assessed in three phase I studies (Tables 4.4 and 4.5).[46–50] The studies share several similarities – patient population comprised individuals with symptomatic coronary artery disease not amenable to conventional revascularization; injections were delivered into ischemic/viable (noninfarcted) myocardial territory using the NOGA™ electromechanical-guided system and only freshly aspirated and filtered BM or its isolated mononuclear fraction was injected. The studies' results demonstrate safety, feasibility, and practicality of this approach. All patients underwent BM aspiration followed within 2–4 hours by electromechanical mapping and injections, and were discharged the following day. At 3 months, CCS angina class improved by an average of 1 or higher class and myocardial perfusion improved significantly compared with baseline in all three studies. One-year follow-up was reported in two of the studies, suggesting sustained clinical improvement. Of note, the study by Perin et al.[46] included patients with low ejection fraction – at 3 months, a significant improvement was noted in LV function in the BM-treated group, compare with no change among nonrandomized controls. This beneficial effect, however, was lost at 12 months. Fuchs et al.[49] followed 27 patients for 1 year. During this period, 25% of the patients underwent revascularization procedures because of late restenosis and disease progression. Interventions were to vascular conduits supplying remote noninjected territories. The observations obtained form the 1-year follow-up of these studies underscores the

Table 4.4. Clinical studies: Design and injected cell profile

Study	Patient population	Patients (n)	Design	BM-derived cells	Ex vivo expansion	Injected cells (n × 10⁶)	Injected CD34+ (% or n)	Injected AC133+ (% or n)
Transendocardial								
Tse et al.[50]	Chronic ischemia	8	R (−) Control (−)	BMMN	No	10–22	2.1 ± 28	0.65 ± 0.4
Perin et al.[46,47]	Low EF, chronic ischemia	14 BMMN, 7 controls	R (−) Control (+)	BMMN	No	26–34	2.4 ± 1.3	NA[§]
Fuchs et al.[48,49]	Chronic ischemia	27	R (−) Control (−)	Unfractionated BM	No	62 ± 59	2.2 ± 1.4	NA[§]
Intracoronary								
Strauer et al.[54]	Acute MI[†]	10	R (−) Control (−)	BMMN	No	9–28	2.1 ± 0.28	0.65 ± 0.4
TOPCARE MI[55,56†]	Acute MI[†]	9	R (−) Control (+)	BMNC*	No	238 ± 79	5.5 ± 2.8 × 10⁶	0.7 ± 0.4 × 10⁶
TOPCARE MI[55,56†]	Acute MI[†]	11	R (−) Control (+)	CPC	3-day culture: VEGF+ atorvastatin	13 ± 12	—	>90% EPCs character.
BOOST[57]	Acute MI[†]	30 BMMN, 30 controls	R (+) Control (+)	BMMN	No	2460 ± 940	~0.38 ± 0.25	NA[§]
MAGIC[58]	Acute MI[†]	10 BM, 10 G-CSF	R (−) Control (−)	PBC (apheresis)	No (apheresis)	1500	8.3 ± 10.2	NA[§]
Fernandez-Aviles et al.[59]	Acute MI[†]	20	R (−) Control (−)	BMMN	No (overnight culture)	78 ± 41	1 ± 0.6	0.6 ± 0.3
Chen et al.[60]	Acute MI[†]	69	R (−) Control (−)	MSC	Culture for 10 days (MSC)	48,000–60,000	—	–
CABG (adjunct)								
Stamm et al.[63]	Recent MI[†], CABG	6	R (−) Control (−)	AC133+ enriched MN	No	1.75 ± 0.84	80.6 ± 8.7	80.6 ± 8.7

*BMNC, bone marrow nuclear cells; [§]NA, not available; [†]MI, myocardial infarction.

recombinant fibroblast growth factor-2: double-blind, randomized, controlled clinical trial. Circulation 2002; 105:788–793.
21. Rosengart TK, Lee LY, Patel SR. Angiogenesis gene therapy: phase I assessment of direct intramyocardial administration of an adenovirus vector expressing VEGF121 cDNA to individuals with clinically significant severe coronary artery disease. Circulation 1999;100:468–474.
22. Schumacher B, Pecher P, von Specht BU, Stegmann T. Induction of neoangiogenesis in ischemic myocardium by human growth factors: first clinical results of a new treatment of coronary heart disease. Circulation 1998; 97:645–650.
23. Symes JF, Losordo DW, Vale PR, et al. Gene therapy with vascular endothelial growth factor for inoperable coronary artery disease. Ann Thorac Surg 1999; 68:830–836.
24. Laham RJ, Sellke FW, Edelman ER, et al. Local perivascular delivery of basic fibroblast growth factor in patients undergoing coronary bypass surgery: results of a phase I randomized, double-blind, placebo-controlled trial. Circulation 1999;100:1865–1871.
25. Laham RJ, Chronos NA, Pike M, et al. Intracoronary basic fibroblast growth factor (FGF-2) in patients with severe ischemic heart disease: results of a phase I open-label dose escalation study. J Am Coll Cardiol 2000; 36:2132–2139.
26. Laham RJ, Rezaee M, Post M, Xu X, Sellke FW. Intrapericardial administration of basic fibroblast growth factor: myocardial and tissue distribution and comparison with intracoronary and intravenous administration. Catheter Cardiovasc Interv 2003;58: 375–381.
27. Kornowski R, Fuchs S, Tio FO, Pierre A, Epstein SE, Leon MB. Evaluation of the acute and chronic safety of the Biosense injection catheter system in porcine hearts. Catheter Cardiovasc Interv 1999;48:447–453.
28. Fuchs S, Dib N, Cohen B, Okubagzi P, et al. A randomized, double blind, placebo controlled, multicenter, pilot study of the safety and the feasibility of AdGVVEGF121.10 via an intramyocardial injection catheter in patients with advanced coronary artery disease [abstract]. J Am Coll Cardiol 2003;41:21A.
29. Kastrup J. Gene Therapy With phVEGF-A 165 in Severe Ischemic Heart Disease: The Euroinject One Trial. Late Breaking Clinical Trials Presentation; ACC 2003.
30. Mohle R, Green D, Moore MA, et al. Constitutive production and thrombin-induced release of vascular endothelial growth factor by human megakaryocytes and platelets. Proc Natl Acad Sci USA 1997;94:663–668.
31. Bikfalvi A, Han ZC. Angiogenic factors are hematopoietic factors and vice versa. Leukemia 1994;8:523–529.
32. Sensebe L, Deschaseaux M, Li J, et al. The broad spectrum of cytokine gene expression by myoid cells from the human marrow microenvironment. Stem Cells 1997;15:133–143.
33. Rohde D, Wickenhauser C, Denecke S, et al. Cytokine release by human bone marrow cells: analysis at the single cell level. Virchows Arch 1994;424:389–395.
34. Solovey A, Lin Y, Browne P, Choong S, Wayner E, Hebbel RP. Circulating activated endothelial cells in sickle cell anemia. N Engl J Med 1997;337:1584–1590.
35. Asahara T, Murohara T, Sullivan A, et al. Isolation of putative progenitor endothelial cells for angiogenesis. Science 1997;275:964–967.
36. Kalka C, Masuda H, Takahashi T, et al. Transplantation of ex vivo expanded endothelial progenitor cells for therapeutic neovascularization. Proc Natl Acad Sci USA 2000;97:3422–3427.
37. Takahashi T, Kalka C, Masuda H, et al. Ischemia-, and cytokine-induced mobilization of bone marrow-derived endothelial progenitor cells for neovascularization. Nat Med 1999;5:434–438.
38. Bittira B, Shum-Tim D, Al-Khaldi A, Chiu RC. Mobilization and homing of bone marrow stromal cells in myocardial infarction. Eur J Cardiothorac Surg 2003;24:393–398.
39. Ceradini DJ, Kulkarni AR, Callaghan MJ, et al. Progenitor cell trafficking is regulated by hypoxic gradients through HIF-1 induction of SDF-1. Nat Med 2004;10:858–864.
40. Quaini F, Urbanek K, Beltrami AP, et al. Chimerism of the transplanted heart. N Engl J Med 2002;346:5–15.
41. Nygren JM, Jovinge S, Breitbach M, et al. Bone marrow-derived hematopoietic cells generate cardiomyocytes at a low frequency through cell fusion, but not transdifferentiation. Nat Med 2004;10:494–501.
42. Murry CE, Soonpaa MH, Reinecke H, et al. Haematopoietic stem cells do not transdifferentiate into cardiac myocytes in myocardial infarcts. Nature 2004;428:664–668.
43. Balsam LB, Wagers AJ, Christensen JL, Kofidis T, Weissman IL, Robbins RC. Haematopoietic stem cells adopt mature haematopoietic fates in ischaemic myocardium. Nature 2004;428:668–673.
44. Fuchs S, Baffour R, Zhou YF, et al. Transendocardial delivery of autologous bone marrow enhances collateral perfusion and regional function in pigs with chronic experimental myocardial ischemia. J Am Coll Cardiol 2001;37:1726–1732.
45. Kamihata H, Matsubara H, Nishiue T, et al. Implantation of bone marrow mononuclear cells into ischemic myocardium enhances collateral perfusion and regional function via side supply of angioblasts, angiogenic ligands, and cytokines. Circulation 2001;104:1046–1052.
46. Perin EC, Dohmann HF, Borojevic R, et al. Transendocardial, autologous bone marrow cell transplantation for severe, chronic ischemic heart failure. Circulation 2003;107:2294–2302.
47. Perin EC, Dohmann HF, Borojevic R, et al. Improved exercise capacity and ischemia 6 and 12 months after transendocardial injection of autologous bone marrow mononuclear cells for ischemic cardiomyopathy. Circulation 2004;110(11 suppl 1):II213–II218.
48. Fuchs S, Satler LF, Kornowski R, et al. Catheter-based autologous bone marrow myocardial injection in no-option patients with advanced coronary artery disease: a feasibility study. J Am Coll Cardiol 2003;41:1721–1724.
49. Fuchs S, Kornowski R, Weisz G, et al. Transendocardial autologous bone marrow cell transplantation in patients with advanced ischemic heart disease: final results from a multi-center feasibility study [abstract]. J Am Coll Cardiol 2004;43:864A.
50. Tse H-F, Kwong Y-L, Chan JKF, Lo G, Ho C-L, Lau C-P. Angiogenesis in ischaemic myocardium by intramyocardial autologous bone marrow mononuclear cell implantation. Lancet 2003;361:47–49.
51. Kinnaird T, Stabile E, Burnett MS, et al. Marrow-derived stromal cells express genes encoding a broad spectrum of arteriogenic cytokines and promote

52. Kinnaird T, Stabile E, Burnett MS, et al. Local delivery of marrow-derived stromal cells augments collateral perfusion through paracrine mechanisms. Circulation 2004;109:1543–1549.
53. Barbash IM, Chouraqui P, Baron J, et al. Systemic delivery of bone marrow-derived mesenchymal stem cells to the infarcted myocardium: feasibility, cell migration, and body distribution. Circulation 2003;108:863–868.
54. Strauer BE, Brehm M, Zeus T, et al. Repair of infarcted myocardium by autologous intracoronary mononuclear bone marrow cell transplantation in humans. Circulation 2002;106:1913–1918.
55. Assmus B, Schachinger V, Teupe C, et al. Transplantation of progenitor cells and regeneration enhancement in acute myocardial infarction (TOPCARE-AMI). Circulation 2002;106:3009–3017.
56. Britten MB, Abolmaali ND, Assmus B, et al. Infarct remodeling after intracoronary progenitor cell treatment in patients with acute myocardial infarction (TOPCARE-AMI): mechanistic insights from serial contrast-enhanced magnetic resonance imaging. Circulation 2003;108:2212–2218.
57. Wollert KC, Meyer GP, Lotz J, at al. Intracoronary autologous bone-marrow cell transfer after myocardial infarction: the BOOST randomised controlled clinical trial. Lancet 2004;364:141–148.
58. Kang HJ, Kim HS, Zhang SY, et al. Effects of intracoronary infusion of peripheral blood stem-cells mobilised with granulocyte-colony stimulating factor on left ventricular systolic function and restenosis after coronary stenting in myocardial infarction: the MAGIC cell randomised clinical trial. Lancet 2004;363:751–756.
59. Fernandez-Aviles F, San Roman JA, Garcia-Frade J, et al. Experimental and clinical regenerative capability of human bone marrow cells after myocardial infarction. Circ Res 2004;95:742–748.
60. Chen SL, Fang WW, Ye F. Effect on left ventricular function of intracoronary transplantation of autologous bone marrow mesenchymal stem cell in patients with acute myocardial infarction. Am J Cardiol 2004;94:92–95.
61. Kornowski R, Leon MB, Fuchs S, et al. Electromagnetic guidance for catheter-based transendocardial injection: a platform for intramyocardial angiogenesis therapy. Results in normal and ischemic porcine models. J Am Coll Cardiol 2000;35:1031–1039.
62. Hamano K, Nishida M, Hirata K, et al. Local implantation of autologous bone marrow cells for therapeutic angiogenesis in patients with ischemic heart disease: clinical trial and preliminary results. Jpn Circ J 2001;65:845–847.
63. Stamm C, Westphal B, Kleine HD, et al. Autologous bone-marrow stem-cell transplantation for myocardial regeneration. Lancet 2003;361:45–46.
64. Yoon YS, Park JS, Tkebuchava T, Luedeman C, Losordo DW. Unexpected severe calcification after transplantation of bone marrow cells in acute myocardial infarction. Circulation 2004;109:3154–3157.
65. Epstein SE, Stabile E, Kinnaird T, et al. Janus phenomenon: the interrelated tradeoffs inherent in therapies designed to enhance collateral formation and those designed to inhibit atherogenesis. Circulation 2004;109:2826–2831.
66. Vulliet PR, Greeley M, Halloran SM, MacDonald KA, Kittleson MD. Intra-coronary arterial injection of mesenchymal stromal cells and microinfarction in dogs. Lancet 2004;363:783–784.
67. Kawamoto A, Murayama T, Kusano K, et al. Synergistic effect of bone marrow mobilization and vascular endothelial growth factor-2 gene therapy in myocardial ischemia. Circulation 2004;110:1398–1405.
68. Iwaguro H, Yamaguchi J, Kalka C, et al. Endothelial progenitor cell vascular endothelial growth factor gene transfer for vascular regeneration. Circulation 2002;105:732–738.
69. Jackson KA, Majka SM, Wang H, et al. Regeneration of ischemic cardiac muscle and vascular endothelium by adult stem cells. J Clin Invest 2001;107:1395–1402.
70. Kawamoto A, Tkebuchava T, Yamaguchi J, et al. Intramyocardial transplantation of autologous endothelial progenitor cells for therapeutic neovascularization of myocardial ischemia. Circulation 2003;107:461–468.
71. Kocher AA, Schuster MD, Szabolcs MJ, et al. Neovascularization of ischemic myocardium by human bone-marrow-derived angioblasts prevents cardiomyocyte apoptosis, reduces remodeling and improves cardiac function. Nat Med 2001;7:430–436.
72. Orlic D, Kajstura J, Chimenti S, et al. Bone marrow cells regenerate infarcted myocardium. Nature 2001;410:701–705.
73. Davani S, Marandin A, Mersin N, et al. Mesenchymal progenitor cells differentiate into an endothelial phenotype, enhance vascular density, and improve heart function in a rat cellular cardiomyoplasty model. Circulation 2003;108(suppl 1):II253–II258.

5
Cell Therapy for Heart Failure

Thorsten Reffelmann and Robert A. Kloner

Developing New Treatment Strategies for Heart Failure: A Challenge in the New Millennium

Different Models of Heart Failure as a Guide to Therapy

"Heart failure is the state of any heart disease in which ... the heart is unable to pump blood at a rate adequate for satisfying the requirements of the tissues."[1] This basic definition of heart failure represents the fundamental approach to the clinical syndrome of cardiac failure and many treatment strategies are aimed at enhancing myocardial contractility and increasing cardiac index. However, in the light of recent investigations, this definition may not be sufficient to explain some relevant characteristics of "heart failure." Whereas the traditional cardiorenal or cardiocirculatory model of congestive cardiac failure emphasized salt and water retention in combination with the altered cardiac pumping capacity, the insidious disease progression accompanied by left ventricular dilation and alterations in left ventricular geometry are now regarded as crucial steps in the development of heart failure. These observations gave rise to a novel, so-called "progressive" model of heart failure,[2] in which several biochemical molecules, such as hormone-like substances and chemokines, have been put forward as potential mediators of left ventricular remodeling, in effect leading to deterioration in ventricular function and symptoms over time.[3] Moreover, in the last decades, convincing investigations demonstrated beneficial effects of treatment strategies, derived from this "progressive" or "neurohormonal" model, such as angiotensin-converting enzyme inhibition,[4,5] angiotensin II receptor inhibition,[6] β-adrenoreceptor-blocking interventions,[7] and aldosterone antagonism.[8,9] A significant benefit with respect to mortality, morbidity, and also quality of life could be achieved in large-scale trials using these pharmacologic classes or a combination of them. Therefore, any novel therapy targeting symptoms and prognosis of heart failure, including the novel techniques of cellular cardiomyoplasty, will be compared with and/or added to the current state of medical (and also interventional) treatment.

Cell Therapy: Inspired by the Cardiocirculatory Model of Heart Failure

As a new potential treatment strategy, transplantation of cells with the potential of forming contractile elements has been extensively evaluated in experimental investigations. The principal idea was to replace scar tissue after myocardial infarction by transplanting immature cardiomyocytes, skeletal myoblasts, or stem cells of various origin (embryonic or mesenchymal), which should proliferate and thereafter form contractile tissue (Figure 5.1). Therefore, the main principles of cardiac cell

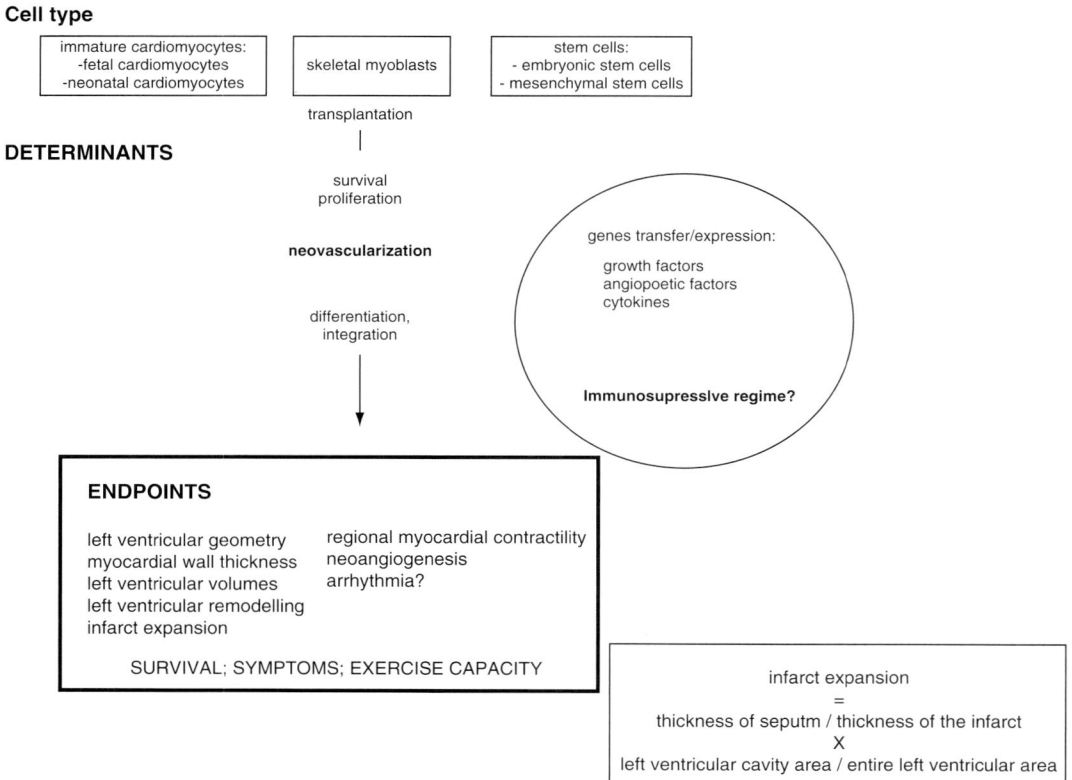

Figure 5.1. Schematic on important determinants for the success of cell therapy for heart failure, and possible endpoints in experimental investigations and clinical studies.

transplantation are derived from a cardiocirculatory model of heart failure, emphasizing the altered pumping capacity of the heart as the main therapeutic target of the disease. The initial goal of cell therapy was to completely rebuild the infarcted part of the heart by actively and synchronously contracting myocardium-like tissue, finally restoring cardiac pumping capacity. As discussed in the following paragraphs, this goal has not yet completely been accomplished: In recent years, several studies demonstrated the feasibility of various techniques of transplanting cells of different origin and state of differentiation.[10] Some specific techniques and cell types have already been tested in clinical trials.[11,12] Moreover, in a wide range of basic science models, important prerequisites for successful cell engraftment could be demonstrated[13]: Survival of the transplant with the formation of a viable graft within the myocardial tissue was obvious in various experimental studies with observational periods for up to 6–12 months after transplantation.[14–17] Vascularization of the graft tissue with effective regional blood flow appears to develop under certain conditions,[18,19] and also some degree of differentiation of immature cell types seems to be achievable in different experimental settings, which could be demonstrated as morphologic signs at histologic examination and on the basis of the expression of biochemical markers.[13–15,20] Important issues requiring further investigations in this field are related to the improvement of integration of grafted tissue into its host, which on the one hand means the spatial distribution of the grafted cells within the host and on the other hand meaning the development of effective cell-to-cell contacts, unifying both parts – the host and the graft.[14,15,21] Nonetheless, after all these basics of experimental research, some pivotal questions, regarding not only the effects on regional and global contractile function, but also the influence on disease progression and remodeling need to be answered[10,13] (Figure 5.1): Does the transplanted tissue contribute to contractile myocardial performance? How does transplantation affect ventricular geometry and hemodynamics over time? Can progression of heart failure be attenuated? Does the procedure relieve symptoms of heart failure, and is survival in transplanted individuals significantly different from nontransplanted controls?

Some Basics

Different Cell Types

The main sources of cells for transplantation that have been studied in models of myocardial damage are firstly immature cardiomyocytes (i.e., embryonic or fetal cardiac cells, harvested in utero at a specified gestational age) that conserve a certain potential of proliferation, secondly skeletal myoblasts, harvested from fully differentiated skeletal muscles, the so-called satellite cells, and thirdly stem cells, either derived from the bone marrow or as embryonic stem cells.[10] These various sources for myocardial regeneration are characterized by numerous differences with respect to stage of differentiation, proliferative capacity, plasticity of phenotype, etc. However, a prerequisite for these cells to generate a graft, which actively contributes to contractile force, is at least in theory, a certain degree of differentiation into a "contractile phenotype." The following discussion of the potential of these cells for treatment of heart failure will therefore focus on transplantation of immature cardiomyocytes, which – in our opinion – can be regarded as the basic scientific model of what can be achieved by cell therapy. In practice, the greater availability of cells from other sources and for some cell types also their autologous character without need for immunosuppression may be the most important arguments for using other cells than cardiomyocytes for cellular cardiomyoplasty when reaching the level of clinical application.

Survival and Proliferation After Transplantation

In most experimental cell grafting studies, a suspension of the cells was injected into the myocardium or the infarcted/cryoinjured part of the left ventricle via an epicardial approach. Pilot studies had shown that, for example, injection of fetal or neonatal cardiomyocytes into a rat hindlimb resulted in a spontaneously contracting tissue that increased in size over the first 2 weeks and developed sarcomeres.[22] The feasibility of direct intramyocardial injection of cultured fetal cardiomyocytes into normal mice hearts, was first demonstrated by Soonpaa et al.[23] The grafted cells survived more than 8 weeks, and formed intercalated disks, as shown by electron microscopy. In the rat, the injected suspension of immature cardiomyocytes formed a "pocket" of packed cells within the myocardium right after transplantation. Thereafter, they tended to form clusters of cells with increasingly organized pattern and signs of differentiation. Using a quantitative analysis (based on the detection of the Sry gene on the Y chromosome after transplantation of male cells into female recipients), Müller-Ehmsen et al.[24] reported a survival rate of 15% 12 weeks after transplantation of neonatal cardiomyocytes into normal myocardium. In contrast, 6 months after transplantation of neonatal cardiomyocytes into infarcted myocardium (permanent coronary artery ligation), approximately 60% of the initially injected number of cells was still detectable.[15] One might speculate that transplanted cells in normal myocardium are more likely to be lost through the intact vasculature, whereas cells injected into an ischemic zone are more likely to stay in place.

The success of engraftment depends on the type of injected cells and also on the time between myocardial injury and transplantation. As shown by Reinecke et al.,[25] cultured fetal and neonatal cardiomyocyte suspensions transplanted into normal hearts, acutely cryoinjured hearts, and 6-day-old cryoinjured hearts ("granulation tissue") survived up to 8 weeks after transplantation, whereas transplanted adult cardiomyocytes showed evidence of coagulation necrosis already by 1 day after transplantation. Better survival of the graft was also demonstrated when transplantation was performed 2 weeks after cryoinjury (granulation tissue) in comparison with transplantation early after myocardial injury,[26] when the acute inflammatory response after myocardial necrosis had calmed down.[27]

However, the degree of proliferation after transplantation might also determine the final size of the graft and its spatial distribution and integration within the host tissue. Only cardiomyocytes in the stage of hyperplastic growth, such as fetal and neonatal cardiomyocytes (in contrast to adult cardiomyocytes), survive after transplantation.[25] In the investigations by Reinecke et al.,[25] neonatal cardiomyocytes were positive for PCNA (proliferating cell nuclear antigen) only during the first 2 weeks after transplantation with a peak at day 6. Labeling with tritiated thymidine in mice cardiomyocytes (as an indicator for DNA synthesis) demonstrated 29% positive embryonic donor cardiomyocytes before transplantation (gestational day 15), but 19 days after transplantation only 0.6% of the surviving cells showed evidence of DNA synthesis.[23] Thus, proliferative growth of the transplanted cells might significantly contribute to colonization of the host, but it decreases substantially within the first weeks after transplantation.

Although the mentioned investigations on survival and proliferation mainly apply to fetal and neonatal cardiomyocytes, the same aspects are to be considered for other cell types as well, and enhancing survival or proliferation could improve the outcome. For optimizing the success of transplantation, several techniques, such as stimulation of proliferation by altered expression of selected genes (e.g., overexpression of fibroblast growth factor-2 isoforms,[28] overexpression of cyclin D1[29]), modifying the culturing technique, or new methods of tissue processing before transplantation, have been suggested. For example, pretreatment of skeletal muscles before harvesting skeletal myoblasts (e.g., preinjecting of bupivacaine as a pharmacologic stressor to activate satellite cells) was proposed by Pouzet et al.[30] for improving skeletal myoblast transplantation. Heat shock treatment or antiapoptosis interventions were also tested to reduce posttransplantation death.[26,31] Culturing the cells in three-dimensional scaffolds of various materials, so-called tissue engineering, seems to be a promising approach to overcome some of the current problems of limited survival, engraftment, and integration.[32]

Differentiation and Integration

Depending on the type of cell used for transplantation, development of the "contractile phenotype" requires a certain period of differentiation. Although methods and obstacles of inducing differentiation in stem cells will be discussed in other chapters of this book,[33] immature cardiomyocytes also require a significant period of time to develop morphologic signs of differentiation (increase in diameter, decrease of nucleus-to-cytoplasm ratio, the development of sarcomeric striation, etc.) and biochemical and ultrastructural markers of differentiation (myofibrils, desmosomes, connexin 43, etc.). A short look at Figure 5.2 (see color section), comparing normal myocardium (left) and graft tissue, 4 weeks after transplantation of neonatal cardiomyocytes into a permanent occlusion infarct (right), illustrates incomplete differentiation and integration at first sight. There is substantial disarray in the overall orientation of the cells within the graft and sarcomeric striations are less organized in comparison with normal myocardium.

The temporal development of differentiation after transplantation of immature myocytes in the experiments by Reinecke et al.[25] was characterized by a progressive increase in graft-cell diameter up to 8 weeks posttransplantation, without reaching the range of host myocyte diameters. These results indicate a switch from hyperplastic to hypertrophic growth, which parallels the observations on graft proliferative activity. Li et al.[34] compared cultured fetal cardiomyocytes with cardiomyocytes 4 weeks after transplantation into cryoinjured heart by light and electron microscopy. Initially, the cells were spherical and the myofilaments were disorganized without sarcomeres, but, after 4 weeks, the grafts contained sarcomeres and cellular junctions composed of desmosomes and fascia adherens. Electron microscopy studies in the transplant experiments (into normal hosts) by Soonpaa et al.[23] demonstrated a high degree of differentiation with myofibrillae forming complete sarcomeres, numerous junctional complexes between cells, and abundant mitochondria, which obviously did not allow distinguishing them from host cardiomyocytes. However, various studies reported that transplanted fetal tissue was positive for α-actin (fetal heart isoform) up to 65 days after transplantation.[20,35] Therefore, differentiation remains incomplete with respect to morphologic and biochemical markers.

Integration into the host is another unresolved issue. For cardiac systolic function with synchronous contractions of the myocardium, it is crucial to form a mechanical and electrical syncytium. Whereas transplanting immature cardiomyocytes into a normal (noninfarcted) myocardium seems to result in relatively effective host-to-graft coupling with the formation of intercalated disks between the myocytes,[23] the results in injured hearts with scar formation are less promising.

In the aforementioned study by Reinecke et al.,[25] neonatal cardiomyocytes expressed the adherens junction protein N-cadherin and connexin 43, initially circumferential and thereafter restricted to intercalated disks. Host and graft cells showed a close spatial approximation early after transplantation, but by 2 and 8 weeks, most grafts were separated from the host by granulation or scar tissue. Contact sites between host and graft were demonstrated in 40% of the hearts only at the peripheral sites of the graft. Using confocal microscopy, in some (rare) cases gap junctions between host and graft were detectable. Connold et al.[36] reported similar results with respect to the development of cell-to-cell coupling in a study transplanting fetal cardiomyocytes with a follow-up period of up to 7 months. In a short-term follow-up after fetal cardiomyocyte transplantation, connexin 43, desmoplakin, and cadherin were demonstrated to be localized between grafted cardiomyocytes, which tended to align parallel to host cardiomyocytes, and between grafted and host cardiomyocytes.[37] Thus, coupling between grafted and host cells occurs, but within a scar, separation of the graft from remote tissue, in particular later after transplantation, might hinder effective integration of the graft.

At 6 months after transplantation, Müller-Ehmsen et al.[15] described the graft as "large confluent clusters of myocardial cells in the scar." Figure 5.3 (see color section) shows an example from our laboratory showing the graft 4 weeks after transplantation of neonatal cardiomyocytes into the infarcted tissue, produced by permanent coronary artery occlusion in the rat. A significant separation of the graft from host tissue develops by the disposition of collagen and connective tissue [Figure 5.3 (see color section)].

Despite positive immunostaining for connexin 43 at junctions between grafted cells in the study by Müller-Ehmsen et al., no gap junctions between host and graft were demonstrated in this 6 months follow-up.[15] Although Connold et al.[36] suggested a certain degree of migration of the transplanted cells over the surface of the left ventricle after 5–7 months, the majority of the graft was found at the site of the injection. In summary, the integration of grafted cells appears to remain incomplete, mainly because of separation by scar tissue with longer periods of follow-up, despite the principal possibility of cell-to-cell connections between host and graft.

Vascularization of the Graft

In early transplant studies, when fetal cardiac tissue was transplanted into a nonphysiological environment, such as the anterior eye chamber,[38] it was remarkable that the development and growth of the hearts in these investigations was always accompanied by vascularization of the tissue. In long-term studies on transplantation of embryonic cardiomyocytes into the heart, an increased vascularization of the graft was shown up to 53 days.[35] Another transplant investigation demonstrated a markedly increased capillary density along with a non-significant improvement of regional myocardial blood flow after cardiomyocyte grafting into 3-week-old scars, created by cryoinjury. Transfection of the donor cells with a plasmid encoding vascular endothelial growth factor further enhanced angiogenesis in this study.[39] Recently, we measured regional myocardial blood flow by radioactive microspheres and capillary density in a permanent coronary artery occlusion model with transplantation of neonatal cardiomyocytes. Four weeks after transplantation, a significantly higher regional blood flow in the infarcted tissue was demonstrated in the transplant group (see Table 5.1), showing that neovascularization in response to cell therapy results in effective enhancement of tissue perfusion. Counting of perfused capillaries in the scar clearly demonstrated that neovascularization was confined to regions of successful engraftment, whereas scar tissue in the transplant and medium group contained the same number of capillaries.[18] Therefore, the grafted cells seem to induce a vasculature to nourish them, which effectively increases directed regional flow.

Effects on Left Ventricular Performance

Although, as discussed above, important prerequisites for success of cell therapy have been demonstrated, the central question of how and

Table 5.1. Regional myocardial blood flow and capillary density in the infarcted tissue (permanent coronary artery occlusion) four weeks after transplantation of neonatal cardiomyocytes in rats (according to reference 18)

		Control group	Transplantation group
Regional myocardial blood flow (ml/g/min)	scar	0.61 ± 0.11	0.97 ± 0.18 ($p < 0.05$)
	normal myocardium	2.73 ± 0.39	2.90 ± 0.48
Capillary density (perfused capillaries/mm^2)	scar	125 ± 10	156 ± 62
	normal myocardium	1788 ± 83	1924 ± 114
Capillary density in the graft (perfused capillaries/mm^2)		—	1217 ± 114

Source: According to Reffelmann et al.[18]

to what extent the graft contributes to cardiac contractile force is much more difficult to answer. Looking at the marked disarray in the organization of the graft in Figure 5.2 (see color section) or the huge amount of connective tissue separating the host and the graft in Figure 5.3 (see color section), it is difficult to conceive how these grafts could effectively contribute to synchronous contractions of the heart.[40]

However, it is likely that the graft created by the described techniques of transplantation has the principal capacity of contracting.[41] When the tissue formed 4 weeks after transplantation of fetal cardiomyocytes into cryoinjured hearts was excised, it "appeared to beat spontaneously and regularly at the time of explantation."[42] Because the function depends crucially on synchronous contractions of the cells, it is important to mention a recent study, which was the first to show synchronized and organized propagation of calcium-transients from host to graft cells in mice experiments of transplanting cardiomyocytes in noninjured myocardium.[43] Although not absolutely proving synchronous contractions of the host and the graft, this is, nonetheless, a very strong argument in favor of the efficacy of host and graft coupling via intercalated disks. However, these studies were performed in noninjured hearts, where host and graft might be much more juxtaposed than in scarred parts of the left ventricle.

After transplantation of cells into scar tissue or infarcted myocardium, the integration into the host, especially in studies with longer follow-up, remains incomplete. Already Reinecke et al.[25] reported the tendency of separation by collagen with longer periods of observation after transplantation. Table 5.2 illustrates the comparative results of three studies from our laboratory using similar techniques, in which either fetal or neonatal cells were transplanted into permanent occlusion infarcts. The follow-up after transplantation ranged between 4 weeks and 6–7 months.[14,15,18]

Left ventricular volumes in systole and diastole were assessed by intravenous ventriculography in vivo. In all these studies, there was a strong tendency to less left ventricular dilation after transplantation of cells. This was most obvious in a study of 4 weeks' observational time after transplantation.[18] When calculating left ventricular ejection fraction, however, there was no difference in this study between the transplant and medium-injected hearts. Interestingly, the other studies with longer follow-up demonstrated a slight and significant improvement in ejection fraction in the cell groups. One might speculate that the longer the time after transplantation the more differentiated are the cells with respect to the "contractile phenotype." However, we could only speculate about potential mechanisms of increasing ejection fraction in the cell group: 1. Some rare cell-to-cell contacts may have triggered active contraction of the graft in these studies, 2. the grafted cells may also contract independently from the host, 3. contraction of transplanted cells during systole are triggered by wall stress, or 4. the effects observed are solely a consequence of scar thickening and stiffening by the transplanted cells reducing systolic wall stress and on the long-term reducing left ventricular remodeling.

Regional wall motion analysis by ventriculography in the 6-month study mainly revealed that the transplanted group was characterized by less dyskinesia in the area of the scar, which, on the contrary, was a prominent feature in the medium hearts (Table 5.3). Therefore, it was proposed that the main effects of cell transplantation in this

Table 5.2. Parameters of left ventricular contractile performance, left ventricular dimensions from intravenous ventriculography, and postmortem morphometric analysis in three studies[14,15,18] using a similar rat model of transplantation of immature cardiomyocytes with different periods of follow-up

	Permanent coronary occlusion, transplantation of *neonatal* cardiomyocytes, 4 weeks of follow-up[18]		Permanent coronary occlusion, transplantation of *neonatal* cardiomyocytes, 6 months of follow-up[15]		Permanent coronary occlusion, transplantation of *fetal* cardiomyocytes, 6–7 months of follow-up[14]	
	Control	Transplant	Control	Transplant	Control	Transplant
Analysis of intravenous contrast ventriculography						
Diastolic LV volume (µL)	300.9 ± 10.5	256.0 ± 10.4*	286.0 ± 26.6	268.4 ± 20.4	417 ± 26	390 ± 26
Systolic LV volume (µL)	174.2 ± 11.1	146.2 ± 8.7*	214.8 ± 20.5	172.0 ± 18.4	286 ± 27	238 ± 19
Ejection fraction (%)	43.2 ± 1.7	42.6 ± 2.0	25 ± 2	36 ± 3*	33 ± 2	39 ± 2*
Postmortem morphometric analyses						
Scar thickness (mm)	0.75 ± 0.04	0.93 ± 0.07*	0.32 ± 0.07	0.53 ± 0.07*	0.33 ± 0.01	0.69 ± 0.05*
Expansion index	0.83 ± 0.06	0.64 ± 0.07*	—	—	2.41 ± 0.10	1.17 ± 0.10*
Infarct size (%)	38.2 ± 2.2	36.0 ± 2.5	34.2 ± 2.8	31.5 ± 1.7	38 ± 1	35 ± 2

LV, left ventricular.
*Significant versus control group.

Table 5.3. Regional wall motion analysis from intravenous ventriculograms in a rat model of permanent coronary occlusion six months after intramyocardial injection of neonatal cardiomyocytes or medium

	Control group	Transplantation group
Zone of dyskinesia (% of infarct)	55.1 ± 7.3	29.5 ± 8.3*
Zone of dyskinesia (% of perimeter)	24.4 ± 3.9	11.1 ± 3.3*

Source: Modified according to Müller-Ehmsen[15]; data from a lateral projection of intravenous ventriculography.
Dyskinesia, zone of paradoxic systolic movement of the endocardium.
*Significant versus control group.

study were attributable to a (maybe passive) stiffening of the infarcted area with less bulging during systole and by reducing left ventricular dilation during the remodeling process.

Additionally, morphometric analyses confirmed the (to a certain extent unexpected) beneficial effect on left ventricular remodeling. The scars after cell transplantation were significantly thicker (in all three studies) and this resulted (together with less left ventricular dilation) in a significant reduction of infarct expansion [see table, infarct expansion index according to Hochman and Choo,[44] summarizing infarct thinning and left ventricular dilation in one index; Figures 5.1 and 5.4 (see color section)]. One might conjecture that stiffening and thickening the infarcted wall by grafting the cells results in reduced wall stress, thereby leading to less ventricular dilation and remodeling after myocardial infarction.

Thus, cell transplantation exhibited a significant effect on left ventricular performance in these studies, but the main effect of cell transplantation seemed to be the result of less dilation, and favorable effects on the remodeling process. Even if ejection fraction was improved in the studies with longer follow-up, synchronous and effective contractions could not be proven in these investigations.

Similarly, results were observed in a permanent coronary occlusion model with extensive scarring, where scar thinning and left ventricular dilation was prevented by transplantation of fetal cardiomyocytes.[35] Importantly, a study in which fetal cardiomyocytes were transplanted 4 weeks after coronary artery ligation, a period in which major steps of ventricular remodeling have already developed, did not show reversal of the remodeling process.[45] Nonetheless, the type of cell (fibroblasts or contractile cells) seems to be important with respect to the efficacy, as suggested in comparative studies of various cell types.[46,47]

Therefore, cell therapy, a treatment strategy initially developed from the cardiocirculatory model of heart failure and aimed at enhancing contractile systolic force, surprisingly exhibited its most convincing effects by reducing remodeling and progression of heart failure over time in these studies, a characteristic of therapies derived from the progressive-neurohumoral model of cardiac failure.

However, another experimental study using infarcted mouse hearts demonstrated pronounced improvement of echocardiographic parameters after transplantation and higher force development, as measured in isolated muscle strips.[48] Additionally, a preserved electrical excitability of the transplanted cells was shown, and the authors suggested that direct development of contractile force was the main mechanism of improved ventricular performance.

Interestingly, a study using skeletal myoblast transplantation demonstrated less left ventricular dilation along with increased ex vivo parameters of systolic force, which mainly seemed to be attributable to favorable effects on the remodeling process rather than active systolic contractions.[49] Similarly, investigations on transplantation of embryonic and mesenchymal stem cells were performed, and differential effects on remodeling, active force development, and also enhancement of angiogenesis, which also may contribute to improved healing of the scar and favorable effects on remodeling, remain to be evaluated.[49,50,51]

Symptoms of Heart Failure, Exercise Capacity, and Survival: The Parameters to Decide for or Against Cell Therapy

Cell therapy has the potential to exhibit favorable effects on left ventricular remodeling and performance, and there are many clinical and experimental studies suggesting that this might transfer into improvement of symptoms and survival. However, there are only a few studies addressing these issues in experimental investigations. Indeed, most frequently used models of coronary artery ligation (e.g., in the rat, in the mouse) do not result in a high percentage of animals that develop clinically overt heart failure. The study by Roell et al.,[48] performed in a mouse model of coronary artery ligation, which reported a pronounced increase in echocardiographic parameters of left ventricular performance after cardiomyocyte transplantation, also reported a marked improvement in survival after cell transplantation. However, most of the animals in the control group died early after transplantation, and the follow-up was relatively short in this study. Jain et al.[49] reported an improvement of exercise capacity after transplantation of skeletal myoblasts parallel to favorable remodeling effects. Other studies examined effects on diastolic function, which may equally contribute to symptoms and capacity to exercise.[52] Importantly, Pouzet et al.[53] investigated whether beneficial effects might occur in addition to angiotensin-converting enzyme inhibition, which is especially important for the translation into clinical practice. Any new therapy for heart failure will be tested against a control group of best medical treatment according to the current state of medical therapy. In their experimental study, they found an additional effect of cell therapy with angiotensin-converting enzyme inhibitors. Apart from this, studies addressing these important questions are rare, but will become most relevant in the phase of clinical testing.

Heart Failure Attributed to Systolic Contractile Dysfunction

Especially when talking about potential clinical applications, we must emphasize that using the term "heart failure" in this chapter as well as in many publications on these topics is a simplification, which needs to be specified. The first step in evaluating a patient with clinical signs of heart failure is undoubtedly a detailed search for potential causes, including valvular heart disease, diastolic dysfunction, pericardial effusion, restrictive filling pattern, etc., any of which may require specific treatment. The majority of studies on cellular cardiomyoplasty (and also on medical treatment) were aimed at cardiac failure attributed to *regional systolic* left ventricular dysfunction. In the clinical realm, regional systolic dysfunction will be most frequently the consequence of myocardial infarction. In experimental investigations, coronary artery ligation, temporary coronary artery occlusion, or even epicardial application of cryoinjury to the left ventricle have been used to mimic this situation. There are also some experimental investigations using models of dilated cardiomyopathy for the evaluation of cell therapy. All these models may be adequate for studying the basic mechanisms and the overall potential of the technique. However, when transferring the results to the patient with heart failure, the terminology will need to be used more precisely, and (among others) a clear differentiation between systolic and diastolic dysfunction, global and regional contractile dysfunction, as well as ischemic and nonischemic cardiac disease will be necessary when estimating the therapeutic potential of cell therapy.

Summary

Cell therapy is a relatively novel approach to the treatment of heart failure. Although the initial aims of completely rebuilding scarred myocardium by contractile tissue, thereby completely restoring cardiac pumping capacity, have not yet been accomplished, many experimental studies reported beneficial effects on left ventricular performance, most of them attributed to less ventricular dilation, scar thickening, and reduction of infarct expansion. Synchronous beating of the graft in the infarcted territory with the host has not been undoubtedly proven, although it seems to be likely that effective cell-to-cell coupling between the host and graft with propagation of calcium transients and in consequence propagation of contraction is possible after transplantation. A major obstacle in completely restoring regional contractile force seems to be the incomplete integration of the graft into the host and the separation from host cells by connective tissue and the scar. For effectively restoring regional contractile function, this will be the most important issue to be solved.

Nonetheless, transplantation appears to exhibit beneficial effects on myocardial performance that can at least in part be ascribed to less ventricular remodeling. Thus, it is likely that progression of heart failure over time can be attenuated to a certain degree by cell therapy. Paradoxically, the fundamental idea of restoring pumping capacity of the heart by cell therapy originates in a cardiocirculatory model of cardiac failure, but many effects of cellular cardiomyoplasty may be attributed to beneficial effects on the remodeling process of the ventricle, resembling other therapeutical approaches derived from a progressive model of heart failure.

Whether less ventricular dilation and less infarct expansion translate into better outcome over time and survival, improved symptoms, and exercise capacity remains to be investigated. Most importantly, for potential clinical applications, cell therapy will need to be compared with the best medical and interventional treatment strategies when evaluating its potential benefit for the patient with heart failure.

References

1. Denolin H, Kuhn H, Krayenbuehl HP, et al. The definition of heart failure. Eur Heart J 1983;4:445–448.
2. Mann DL. Mechanisms and models of heart failure. A combinatorial approach. Circulation 1999;100:999–1008.
3. Packer M. The neurohormonal hypothesis: a theory to explain the mechanism of disease progression in heart failure. J Am Coll Cardiol 1992;20:248–254.
4. Rutherford JD, Pfeffer MA, Moye LA, et al. Effects of captopril on ischemic events after myocardial infarction. Results of the survival and ventricular enlargement trial SAVE investigators. Circulation 1994;90:1731–1738.
5. The SOLVD Investigators. Effects of enalapril on survival in patients with reduced left ventricular ejection fraction and congestive heart failure. N Engl J Med 1991;325:293–302.
6. Pitt B, Segal R, Martinez FA, et al. Randomised trial of losartan versus captopril in patients over 65 with heart failure (Evaluation of Losartan in the Elderly Study, ELITE). Lancet 1997;349:747–752.
7. Packer M, Bristow WR, Cohne JN, et al. The effect of carvedilol on morbidity and mortality in patients with chronic heart failure. N Engl J Med 1996;334:1350–1355.
8. Pitt B, Zannad F, Remme WJ, et al. The effect of spironolactone on morbidity and mortality in patients with severe heart failure. N Engl J Med 1999;341:709–717.
9. Pitt B, Williams G, Remme W, et al. The EPHESUS trial: eplerenone in patients with heart failure due to systolic dysfunction complicating acute myocardial infarction. Cardiovasc Drugs Ther 2001;15:79–87.
10. Reffelmann T, Kloner RA. Cellular cardiomyoplasty: cardiomyocytes, skeletal myoblasts, or stem cells for regenerating myocardium and treatment of heart failure? Cardiovasc Res 2003;58:358–368.
11. Menasché P, Hagege A, Scorsin M, et al. Myoblast transplantation for heart failure. Lancet 2001;357:279–280.
12. Strauer BE, Brehm M, Zeus T, et al. Repair of infarcted myocardium by autologous intracoronary mononuclear bone marrow cell transplantation in humans. Circulation 2002;106:1913–1918.
13. Reffelmann T, Leor J, Müller-Ehmsen J, et al. Cardiomyocyte transplantation into the failing heart: new therapeutic approach for heart failure? Heart Fail Rev 2003;8:201–211.
14. Yao M, Diterle T, Hale SL, et al. Long-term outcome of fetal cell transplantation on postinfarction ventricular remodeling and function. J Mol Cell Cardiol 2003;35:661–670.
15. Müller-Ehmsen J, Peterson KL, Kedes L, et al. Rebuilding a damaged heart: long-term survival of transplanted neonatal rat cardiomyocytes after myocardial infarction and effect on cardiac function. Circulation 2002;105:1720–1726.
16. Al Attar N, Carrion C, Ghostine S, et al. Long-term (1 year) functional and histological results of autologous skeletal muscle cells transplantation in rat. Cardiovasc Res 2003;58:142–148.
17. Ghostine S, Carrion C, Souza LC, et al. Long-term efficacy of myoblast transplantation on regional structure and function after myocardial infarction. Circulation 2002;106(suppl I):I131–136.
18. Reffelmann T, Dow JS, Dai W, et al. Transplantation of neonatal cardiomyocytes after permanent coronary artery occlusion increases regional blood flow of infarcted myocardium. J Mol Cell Cardiol 2003;35:607–613.
19. Yau TM, Fung K, Weisel RD, et al. Enhanced myocardial angiogenesis by gene transfer with transplanted cells. Circulation 2001;104(suppl I):I218–222.
20. Leor J, Patterson M, Quiniones MJ, et al. Transplantation of fetal myocardial tissue into the infarcted myocardium of rats. A potential method for repair of infarcted myocardium? Circulation 1996;94(suppl II):II332–336.
21. Leobon B, Garcin I, Menasche P, et al. Myoblasts transplanted into rat infarcted myocardium are functionally isolated from their host. Proc Natl Acad Sci USA 2003;100:7808–7811.
22. Li RK, Mickle DA, Weisel RD, et al. In vivo survival and function of transplanted rat cardiomyocytes. Circ Res 1996;78:283–288.
23. Soonpaa MH, Koh GY, Klug MG, et al. Formation of nascent intercalated disks between grafted fetal cardiomyocytes and host myocardium. Science 1994;264:98–101.
24. Müller-Ehmsen J, Whittaker P, Kloner RA, et al. Survival and development of neonatal rat cardiomyocytes transplanted into adult myocardium. J Mol Cell Cardiol 2002;34:107–116.
25. Reinecke H, Zhang M, Bartosek T, et al. Survival, integration, and differentiation of cardiomyocyte grafts: a study in normal and injured rat hearts. Circulation 1999;100:193–202.
26. Zhang M, Methot D, Poppa V, et al. Cardiomyocyte grafting for cardiac repair: graft cell death and antideath strategies. J Mol Cell Cardiol 2001;33:907–921.
27. Li RK, Mickle DA, Weisel RD, et al. Optimal time for cardiomyocyte transplantation to maximize myocardial function after left ventricular injury. Ann Thorac Surg 2001;72:1957–1963.
28. Sheikh F, Fandrich RR, Kardami E, et al. Overexpression of long or short FGFR-1 results in FGF-2-mediated

proliferation in neonatal myocyte cultures. Cardiovasc Res 1999;42:696–705.
29. Soonpaa MH, Koh GY, Pajak L, et al. Cyclin D1 overexpression promotes cardiomyocyte DNA synthesis and multinucleation in transgenic mice. J Clin Invest 1997;99:2644–2654.
30. Pouzet B, Vilquin JT, Hagege AA, et al. Intramyocardial transplantation of autologous myoblasts: can tissue processing be optimized? Circulation 2000;102(suppl III):III210–215.
31. Suzuki K, Smolenski RT, Jayakumar J, et al. Heat shock treatment enhances graft cell survival in skeletal myoblast transplantation to the heart. Circulation 2000;102(suppl III):III216–221.
32. Leor J, Aboulafia-Etzion S, Dar A, et al. Bioengineered cardiac grafts. A new approach to repair the infarcted myocardium? Circulation 2000;102(suppl III):III56–61.
33. Murry CE, Soonpaa MH, Reinecke H, et al. Haematopoietic stem cells do not transdifferentiate into cardiac myocytes in myocardial infarcts. Nature 2004;428:664–668.
34. Li RK, Mickle DAG, Weisel RD, et al. Natural history of fetal rat cardiomyocytes transplanted into adult rat myocardial scar tissue. Circulation 1997;96(suppl II):II179–187.
35. Etzion S, Battler A, Barbash IM, et al. Influence of embryonic cardiomyocyte transplantation on the progression of heart failure in a rat model of extensive myocardial infarction. J Mol Cell Cardiol 2001;33:1321–1330.
36. Connold AL, Frischknecht R, Dimitrakos M, et al. The survival of embryonic cardiomyocytes transplanted into damaged host rat myocardium. J Muscle Res Cell Motil 1997;18:63–70.
37. Matsushita T, Oyamada M, Kurata H, et al. Formation of cell junctions between grafted and host cardiomyocytes at the border zone of myocardial infarction. Circulation 1999;100(suppl II):II262–268.
38. Bishop SP, Anderson PG, Tucker DC. Morphological development of the rat heart growing in oculo in the absence of hemodynamic work load. Circ Res 1990;66:84–102.
39. Yau TM, Fung K, Weisel RD, et al. Enhanced myocardial angiogenesis by gene transfer with transplanted cells. Circulation 2001;104(suppl I):I218–222.
40. Whittaker P, Müller-Ehmsen J, Dow JS, et al. Development of abnormal tissue architecture in transplanted neonatal rat myocytes. Ann Thorac Surg 2003;75:1450–1456.
41. Dai W, Hale SL, Kloner RA. Implantation of immature neonatal cardiac cells into the wall of the aorta in rats: a novel model for studying morphological and functional development of heart cells in an extracardiac environment. Circulation 2004;110:324–329.
42. Sakai T, Li RK, Weisel RD, et al. Fetal cell transplantation: a comparison of three cell types. J Thorac Cardiovasc Surg 1999;118:715–725.
43. Ruhart M, Pasumarthi KB, Nakajima H, et al. Physiological coupling of donor and host cardiomyocytes after cellular transplantation. Circ Res 2003;92:1217–1224.
44. Hochman JS, Choo H. Limitation of myocardial infarct expansion by reperfusion independent of myocardial salvage. Circulation 1987;75:299–306.
45. Sakakibara Y, Tambara K, Lu F, et al. Cardiomyocyte transplantation does not reverse cardiac remodeling in rats with chronic myocardial infarction. Ann Thorac Surg 2002;74:25–30.
46. Sakai T, Li RK, Weisel RD, et al. Fetal cell transplantation: a comparison of three cell types. J Thorac Cardiovasc Surg 1999;118:715–724.
47. Li RK, Jia ZQ, Weisel RD, et al. Smooth muscle cell transplantation into myocardial scar tissue improves heart function. J Mol Cell Cardiol 1999;31:513–522.
48. Roell W, Lu ZJ, Bloch W, et al. Cellular cardiomyoplasty improves survival after myocardial injury. Circulation 2002;105:2435–2441.
49. Jain M, DerSimonian H, Brenner DA, et al. Cell therapy attenuates deleterious ventricular remodeling and improves cardiac performance after myocardial infarction. Circulation 2001;103:1920–1927.
50. Min JY, Yang Y, Converso KL, et al. Transplantation of embryonic stem cells improves cardiac function in postinfarcted rats. J Appl Physiol 2002;92:288–296.
51. Kamihata H, Matsubara H, Nishiue T, et al. Implantation of bone marrow mononuclear cells into ischemic myocardium enhances collateral perfusion and regional function via side supply of angioblasts, angiogenic ligands, and cytokines. Circulation 2001;104:1046–1052.
52. Atkins BZ, Hueman MT, Meuchel J, et al. Cellular cardiomyoplasty improves diastolic properties of injured heart. J Surg Res 1999;85:234–242.
53. Pouzet B, Ghostine S, Vilquin JT, et al. Is skeletal myoblast transplantation clinically relevant in the era of angiotensin-converting enzyme inhibitors? Circulation 2001;104(suppl I):I223–228.

Section 2

Neuro

Section 2

Neuro

Daniel Offen and Eldad Melamed

Despite the protection of the central nervous system (CNS) provided by the skull and vertebral column, it remains vulnerable to a variety of injuries and neurodegenerative diseases. Generally, head trauma or stroke are associated with extensive damage and may involve multiple cell types. Most neurodegenerative disorders follow a progressive disease course, and result in the loss of specific neuronal populations. Effective therapy that would delay disease progression or offer any significant recovery is yet to be found.

It has been suggested that neuronal replacement therapy using stem cell transplants may be one possible answer. Currently, there is much enthusiasm for the therapeutic potential of stem cells. Recent experiments have indicated that several stem cell populations have the ability to replace lost neurons and to repair damaged ones.

Stem cells are self-renewing, multi-, or pluripotent cells capable of differentiating into a wide range of cell types. This property makes stem cells a potentially invaluable source of transplantable cells, which could provide the basis for cell replacement therapy. Stem cells have four different sources: embryonic stem cells from the blastocyst, neural stem cells from the embryonic or adult brain, or stem cells in other tissues, e.g., bone marrow.

Attention has been focused on the use of embryonic stem cells for research purposes and for the development of treatment for various diseases. The recent isolation of human embryonic stem cells is offering great hope for their future utilization in effective treatment of a wide range of human neurodegenerative disorders.

The potential for tissue repair and regeneration in the CNS is encouraging, as recent research has provided solid evidence for the continuous generation of many types of stem cells in various adult tissues, where they differentiate to assorted derivatives. For example, cells from bone marrow have been shown to migrate to various tissues, and take part in the normal physiological process of regeneration. In addition, a line of evidence has been accumulating, indicating that adult bone marrow stem cells might possess pluripotent properties similar to those of embryonic stem cells. Efforts should be made to identify natural factors that could augment this normal process of mobilization and homing of bone marrow stem cells to target tissues in various degenerative diseases.

Important sources for stem cells include the developing embryo and adult CNS. It has already been shown experimentally that neural as well as non-neural stem cells can be used for structural brain repair.

In this section, the prospects for using grafted stem cells or recruiting endogenous stem cells to treat various neurologic injuries and diseases are examined.

Parkinson's disease is a progressive neurodegenerative disorder characterized by the degeneration of the dopamine producing neurons projecting from the substantia nigra into the corpus striatum. Current medical therapy is limited and cannot stop or reverse the degeneration. Because this disorder may be a good candidate for cell replacement, attempts were made to change the course of the disease by replacing the lost neurons with grafts from various sources. Although results of controlled clinical trials of fetal cell transplantation in Parkinson's disease have been unsatisfactory, researchers are now trying alternative cell sources. Indeed, animal studies with stem cells show great promise (see Chapter 7 by Offen, Levy, and Melamed).

Because mortality is very high after strokes, there is much enthusiasm about the therapeutic potential of stem cells for this condition. Although there is no convincing evidence that neuronal replacement can work in stroke patients, much thought and work have been invested in attempts to repair the damaged area via grafts of neuronal or non-neuronal stem cells (see Chapter 8 by Gilgun-Sherki and Streifler).

Stem cell transplantation could promote remyelination in demyelinative disorders such as multiple sclerosis. It is now well established that spontaneous remyelination occurs in the CNS of patients with multiple sclerosis. However, this process is not robust enough to promote a functional and stable recovery of the myelin architecture. Recent efforts are described by Ben-Hur and Einstein (see Chapter 6).

New perspectives for the use of stem cells in gene therapy, as a possible strategy for addressing diseases in the CNS, are being studied. New methods of gene transfer and delivery to the CNS by cells or viruses are discussed by Haim and Steiner (see Chapter 9).

The prospects for using grafted stem cells or recruiting endogenous stem cells to treat neurologic injury or disease offers hope. However, to enable the translation of this novel biomedical field to the clinic, a few essential issues must be settled. The ideal stem cell source for transplantation should be determined, and the most appropriate route of stem cell administration ascertained. Last but not least, the best approach for achieving an appropriate, functional, and long-lasting integration of transplanted stem cells into the host should be established, to ensure a long-term therapeutic effect.

6

Cell Transplantation for Diseases of Myelin

Tamir Ben-Hur and Ofira Einstein

Recent advances in stem cell biology have ignited enthusiastic expectations to heal central nervous system (CNS) diseases by transplantation of regenerating cells. In this chapter, we will review the potential application of stem cell transplantation (cell-based therapy) in demyelinating disorders, with special reference to multiple sclerosis (MS) and mention some problematic issues that still face this therapeutic approach.

Stem Cells and Lineage Restricted Progenitors in the Developing and Adult CNS

Stem cells are defined as precursor cells that have the potential for continuous self-renewal and are multipotent in their ability to generate progeny cells of different lineages.[1] Neural stem cells (NSCs) that proliferate in the ventricular zone and later in the subventricular zone (SVZ) of the developing brain, give rise to the three neural lineages of the CNS, i.e., neurons, astrocytes, and oligodendrocytes.[2] The identification of NSCs, as well as progenitor cells of specific lineages, in the adult CNS,[3-11] has changed considerably the past view of the adult brain as an organ with no ability for cell renewal. NSCs that were isolated from the adult rodent CNS showed similar characteristics to their embryonic counterparts in regard to their response to mitogenic factors and potential to generate the three neural lineages.[12] Precursor cells have been identified in several specific regions of the adult rodent CNS where they continue to generate neural progeny. New neurons are continuously generated in the anterior SVZ from which they migrate via the rostral migratory stream to the olfactory epithelium.[13-17] Additionally, there is ongoing neuronogenesis in the adult rodent and human hippocampus.[18,19] Precursor cells in the dentate gyrus generate hippocampal granular neurons throughout life.[20] One specific population of cells that has been suggested to consist of NSCs is the ventricular and spinal ependymal cell layer, which may represent the residua of the embryonic ventricular zone.[21] In addition to their potential to generate neurons, spinal ependymal cells react to traumatic injury by increased proliferation and migration into the lesion and participate in formation of the glial scar.[21,22] In the adult human brain, similar precursors may exist in the ventricular wall.[23] Glial precursor cells exist in the adult brain as well. Oligodendrocyte progenitor cells (OPCs) have been isolated from various adult rodent CNS regions.[24-26] Similar adult human OPCs were grown in vitro[27] and identified in the adult human brain[28-30] and spinal cord[31] in vivo (Figure 6.1A–C).

Current Treatment of MS Does Not Promote Tissue Repair

MS is the most common cause of neurologic disability in young adults, characterized by chronic inflammatory, demyelinating multifocal lesions

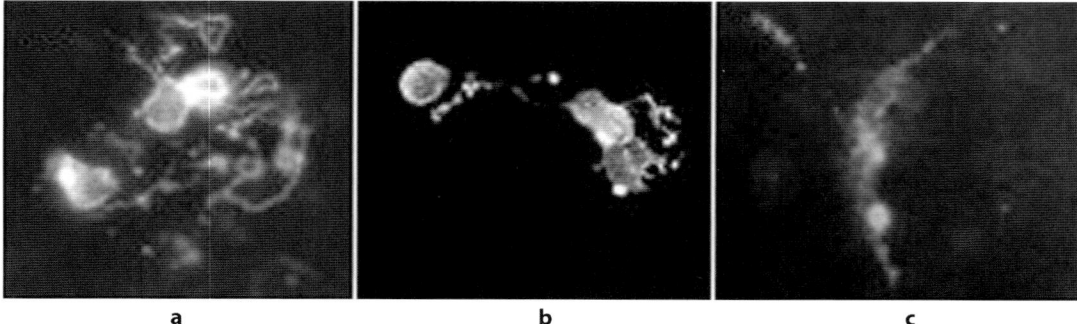

Figure 6.1. Oligodendrocyte progenitor cells that were isolated from the adult human brain display similar morphologic and antigenic characteristics as their rodent counterparts. These cells are O4+ **a** PDGFRα + **b** and NG2+ **c**. They incorporate BrdU into their DNA in culture, indicating their proliferative state (not shown).

within the CNS[32-35] and heterogeneous pathology.[36,37] MS etiology is multifactorial, including an interplay between environmental factors and susceptibility genes. These factors trigger a cascade of events, involving engagement of the immune system, acute inflammatory injury of axons and glia, and demyelination.[38-43] Demyelinated areas can undergo partial remyelination, leading to structural repair and recovery of function.[44-49] However, the most frustrating aspect is the inadequacy of the healing response of remyelination. Eventually, remyelination fails, contributing to the progression of demyelination and axonal damage, postinflammatory gliosis, and neurodegeneration.[50,51] Several studies have indicated that axonal pathology is the best correlate of chronic neurologic impairment in experimental autoimmune encephalomyelitis (EAE) and MS.[52-58] The sequential involvement of these processes underlies the clinical course, characterized by episodes of relapses, which after full remissions early in the course of disease, eventually leave persistent deficits, and finally deteriorate into a secondary chronic progressive phase.

The aim of current treatment is to relieve symptoms, reduce the relapse frequency, and limit the lasting effects of relapses.[59,60] Current conventional immunosuppressive and immunomodulating treatments in MS have only mild efficacy in terms of preventing long-term disability.[59] Thus, it is clear that novel therapeutic approaches need to be developed to promote tissue repair.

Animal Models of Myelin Diseases

There are various experimental models of genetic dysmyelinating diseases and of acquired demyelination in the adult animals. The most commonly used experimental models of genetic deficiency in myelin include the myelin-deficient (*md*) rat, which carries a point mutation in the gene for proteolipid protein (PLP), leading to failure in myelination of the developing postnatal brain,[61] the shaking (*sh*) pups,[62] a canine model of PLP gene deficiency, representing the human X-linked Pelizaeus-Merzbacher disease, and the shiverer (*shi*) mouse that lacks a functional myelin basic protein (MBP) gene.[63] Experimental demyelination has been induced in the CNS of adult animals by a variety of means, including physical injury, toxic, immune-mediated, and viral-induced demyelination. Injection of myelinotoxic chemicals, such as lysolecithin, cuprizone, or ethidium bromide (EB),[64-66] or injection of anti-galactocerebroside antibodies combined with complement,[67] to normal animals, causes a focal, persistent, demyelinating lesion in the white matter of the CNS, usually performed in the spinal cord. Demyelination occurs after injection and all subsequent events are associated with the regenerative response, providing a useful means of separating demyelination from remyelination. To prevent host remyelination, focal X-irradiation of the lesion is performed to kill endogenous cells capable of reforming myelin. Widespread, disseminated demyelination has been achieved by providing cuprizone in the drinking water[68] and also by viral infection. Strains of Theiler's virus, a picornavirus, induce in susceptible strains of mice a biphasic disease – an early acute disease resembling encephalomyelitis, followed by late chronic multifocal demyelinating disease.[69–71] The A-59 and JHM strains of mouse hepatitis viruses also produce multifocal demyelination in mice.[72,73]

The animal model that is considered to best represent human MS is EAE. EAE is a T cell-mediated disease of the CNS that shares many features with MS, both clinically and pathologically, and has proved to be especially useful in studies on pathogenesis and treatment of MS.[74–76] EAE is induced in rodents by sensitizing the animals to myelin antigens, either actively by direct antigen exposure or passively by the adoptive transfer of myelin-specific T cells. This results in inflammation in the CNS that is often accompanied by demyelination and axonal damage.[77,78] Acute EAE is a transient monophasic paralytic disease from which most animals spontaneously recover. It is characterized pathologically by disseminated inflammatory foci throughout the CNS with just a minor component of demyelination.[79] Neurologic symptoms are believed to be the result of the inflammation and reversible conduction blocks caused by edema. Chronic EAE is a chronic paralytic disease, characterized pathologically by inflammation, demyelination, and axonal damage.[69,80–82] These animals do not recover and remain with fixed neurologic defects.

Precursor Cells in the Adult CNS Are Capable of Regenerating Oligodendrocytes and Myelin

In different experimental models of focal demyelination, it has been shown that endogenous cells in the adult rodent CNS have the potential for regenerating oligodendrocytes and myelin.[83–85] Several studies have investigated the nature of the cells that remyelinate the adult CNS after induction of demyelinated lesions. The lack of spontaneous remyelination in experimentally chemical demyelinated lesions that were X-irradiated to kill proliferating cells, suggests that cell division is an absolute prerequisite for myelin regeneration.[86,87] Although differentiated oligodendrocytes may survive within such lesions, they are unable to rebuild myelin sheaths.[87–89] Although mature astrocytes retain the potential to react to injury and divide, there is no convincing evidence that fully differentiated oligodendrocytes are able to revert into a proliferating state. Therefore, it is thought that remyelination depends mainly on proliferating OPCs, identified by expression of NG2 or platelet-derived growth factor receptor-α (PDGFRα) on their cell surface, and are probably the major cycling cell population that reacts to demyelination.[83–85,90–94] The adult SVZ contains neural precursor cells (NPCs) that express the embryonic-polysialated form of the neural cell adhesion molecule (PSA-NCAM). Such SVZ PSA-NCAM+ cells also react to inflammation and demyelination by proliferation and differentiation, generating astrocytes, and remyelinating oligodendrocytes.[85,95,96]

Myelin Regeneration Fails in MS

Attempts to regenerate myelin can be also recognized pathologically in brains of MS patients by the existence of shadow plaques, which are partially remyelinated lesions.[44–47,49] The process of spontaneous functional remyelination is often incomplete and limited, leading to permanent axonal loss and fixed neurologic disability. The ultimate reason why remyelination fails over time in MS remains unknown, as reviewed by Franklin.[51] Failure of remyelination could stem either from insufficiency of endogenous remyelinating cells or from lack of environmental support for this process. Data from experimental models of demyelination and from human brain tissue indeed suggest that several factors may have a role in limiting myelin regeneration in the adult brain and its subsequent failure. In experimental focal demyelination, it has been shown that only a subpopulation of local progenitor cells react to injury and generate new oligodendrocytes and myelin.[91] Although the existence of progenitor cells was demonstrable in acute and chronic MS lesions, they did not exhibit reactive increase in cell number as compared with normal white matter.[28,97,98] This suggests that the response of the progenitor cell population to the demyelinating process in the human brain is deficient. It has also been suggested that repeated demyelinating episodes in chronic and relapsing MS causes a depletion in the endogenous pool of progenitor cells. Although progenitor cells decrease in number after experimental focal demyelination,[91,99] this was not observed in pathological specimens of chronic MS lesions.[28,44,98] Analysis of brain tissue from MS patients suggested that there are several different pathological patterns of demyelination.[36] In some patients, there was progressive loss of oligodendrocytes and myelin without reactive remyelination, whereas in others, who exhibited strong T cell and macrophage activity, there was robust remyelination, indicating the important role of tissue support to the remyelinating response.[100]

Cell migration seems to be another limiting factor in myelin regeneration. It has been shown that only progenitor cells that reside at the margins of experimental lesions migrate into the lesion core and remyelinate it, whereas long-distance migration of progenitor cells does not occur in the brain parenchyma.[85,101,102] The limited recruitment of OPCs in the adult CNS may be related to their apparent dormant state. Adult OPCs have a considerably slower cell cycle than progenitor cells of the developing brain and they require prolonged exposure to multiple growth factors before they convert into rapidly proliferating cells.[103] Therefore, another aspect of the limited tissue support may be that mobilization of the adult progenitor cells is limited by insufficient supply of environmental signals in the brain.

Bidirectional trophic interactions between oligodendrocytes and axons are necessary for their long-term survival. The chronic and supposedly irreversible neurologic disability in MS patients is thought to correlate best with the degree of axonal loss in the CNS.[52–55,58] Moreover, there is evidence that extensive axonal transection occurs already in acute MS lesions.[42] If so, it is clear that remyelination is hampered. Therefore, achieving remyelination before development of axonal damage is crucial in any therapeutic strategy. It has been suggested that CNS regeneration and specifically remyelination are closely linked to the acute inflammatory phase of the disease, whereas in the chronic stage, regeneration does not occur.[104]

In conclusion, both environmental factors and basic properties of endogenous adult progenitor cells limit the degree of spontaneous remyelination. The apparent linkage between the acute inflammatory phase and myelin regeneration and the necessity to remyelinate before axonal damage occurs, may define a narrow time window when remyelination is feasible. Although this time window may be too narrow for adequate endogenous progenitor cell mobilization, it may also determine the window of opportunity for therapeutic cell transplantation.

Rationale for Cell Transplantation into the CNS to Repair Myelin

Basically, there are two therapeutic approaches to induce remyelination in MS and both have shown promising results in experimental animals:

1. Promotion of endogenous remyelination by growth factors therapy.[105,106] In acquired demyelinating diseases, such as MS, growth factor therapy has proven effective in enhancing the endogenous brain's capacity for repair. Insulin-like growth factor-1 (IGF-1) and glial growth factor-2 (GGF2) are neurotrophic factors that promote survival and proliferation in the oligodendrocyte lineage. Treatment with these factors was beneficial clinically and pathologically in animals with EAE.[107–109]

2. Transplantation of myelin-forming cells is a mode of delivering the entire "cell factory" that manufactures myelin. This approach may be advantageous over other modes of gene therapy,[110] in which targeting the gene to specific cells and tissues and controlling its degree of expression may be problematic or even detrimental.[111–114] Experimental transplantation has been performed in several animal models of myelin disease. Transplanted myelin-forming cells remyelinated focal lesions in the optic nerve and spinal cord and restored normal conduction properties, indicating fully functional regenerated myelin.[115,116] Transplantation of various cell populations into the CNS has been suggested for genetic dysmyelinating disorders as well as for acquired demyelinating diseases.[115–128]

Remyelination by Various Myelin-Forming Cells

The traditional primary condition for any cell type to be a candidate for therapeutic cell transplantation in myelin disorders has been its ability to remyelinate and to restore nerve function (Table 6.1). Neural transplantation for

Table 6.1. Potential use of different cell populations for transplantation

Cell Type	Advantages	Disadvantages	Experimental models
Embryonic stem (ES) cells	Totipotent, self-renewing	Teratoma formation, uncommitted	1. Rat ES cells in 1-week-old *md* rats[202] 2. Mouse ES cells in EB or LPC-induced spinal cord demyelination in adult rats and *shi* mice[204] 3. Mouse embryonic (E16) NPCs in postnatal and adult *shi* mouse[205]
Neural precursor cells (NPCs)	Multipotential, self-renewing	Uncommitted	1. Human adult NPCs in EB-induced lesion in adult rats[191] 2. Rat postnatal striatal NPCs in SCH-induced EAE rats[126,189,190] 3. Mouse adult SVZ NPCs in MOG35-55-induced EAE mice[125]
Glial committed precursor cells	PSA-NCAM+, earliest glial committed precursors	Restricted to glia, probably limited source	1. Rat postnatal CNS glial cells in EB-induced lesion in adult rats[117] 2. Mouse postnatal glial cells in EB-induced lesion in adult rats[252] 3. Rat postnatal and adult CNS glial cells in EB-induced lesion in adults rats[133]
Oligodendrocyte progenitor cells (OPCs)	The "classical" remyelinating cell	Probably less efficient than earlier glial precursors, limited source	1. Rat adult O-2A progenitor cells in EB-induced lesion in adult rats[115] 2. Mouse adult oligodendroglial lineage cells in adult *shi* mice[118] 3. Human adult and fetal oligodendroglial lineage cells in adult *shi* mice[127]
Schwann cells	Autograft possible	Restricted to myelin-forming cells	1. Rat adult Schwann cells in EB-induced lesion in adult rats[139] 2. Monkey perinatal and adult Schwann cells in LPC-induced demyelination of the dorsal funiculus of the spinal cord of adult monkeys[144] 3. Human adult Schwann cells in EB-induced lesion in adult rats[142]
Olfactory nerve ensheathing cells (OECs)	Autograft possible	Restricted to myelin-forming cells	1. Rat adult clonal OEC line in EB-induced lesion in adult rats[150] 2. Rat postnatal OECs in EB-induced lesion in adult rats[151] 3. Canine adult OECs in EB-induced lesion in adult rats[153] 4. Human adult OECs in EB-induced lesion in adult rats[157] 5. Pig adult OECs in EB-induced lesion in adult rats[152]
Bone marrow stromal cells (BMSCs)	Autograft possible	Uncommitted	1. Rat adult BMSCs in EB-induced spinal lesion in adult rats[122,225]

remyelination has been studied for more than 25 years, following early work by several researchers.[129-132] Various cell populations were shown to myelinate efficiently after transplantation into experimental animals.

The Oligodendrocyte Lineage

Studies designed to identify the oligodendrocyte lineage cells that had best myelinating potential showed that when focally injected to chemically induced demyelinated lesions, postmitotic oligodendrocytes had poor remyelinating capacity,[133] whereas OPCs showed greater mitotic, migratory, and regenerative properties.[115,118,134,135] Interestingly, transplanted OPCs were found to be more efficient in remyelination than endogenous OPCs.[136] When glial cells were transplanted into the spinal cord of *md* rats, they myelinated nude axons and restored nerve conduction velocity to near normal values.[137] Similarly, transplantation of canine OPCs resulted in repair of large areas in the *sh* pup.[134]

Schwann Cells

Remyelination of CNS axons has been achieved by other myelin-forming cells as well. Schwann cells, the peripheral myelin-forming cells, have excellent myelinating properties in the CNS.[132,138-140] They produce thick and compact myelin after transplantation into the CNS[140,141] and can restore normal conduction velocity in the dorsal columns of the spinal cord, indicating functional recovery.[138,142-145] The main advantage of using these peripheral nervous system myelin-forming cells is that Schwann cells can be isolated from a sural nerve biopsy of patients affected with a myelin disorder of the CNS, cultured and expanded in vitro under appropriate conditions, cryopreserved, and finally serve for autologous transplantation into demyelinated CNS areas. Another potential advantage of transplanted autologous Schwann cells is that they might escape the autoimmune attack in MS that is directed against central myelin antigens.

The impressive animal experimental results has led to the first clinical trial of Schwann cell transplantation, performed in patients with MS between July 2001 and April 2002 in Yale University. Autologous Schwann cells were transplanted intracranially into single demyelinating lesions in three different MS patients. In this first-ever attempt to transplant myelin-producing cells in the human CNS, the Yale trial showed the surgical procedure to be safe, with none of the patients experiencing adverse side effects from the transplantation. However, the study was discontinued in early 2003, after brain biopsies performed 5 months after transplantation did not show any evidence of either Schwann cell survival or new myelin formation. These negative results have dampened some of the expectations raised during the last 25 years of successful experimental Schwann cell-based approach.

Olfactory Nerve Ensheathing Cells

Olfactory nerve ensheathing cells (OECs) display properties of both astrocytes and Schwann cells (Figure 6.2A). These cells are unique in that they continue to develop in the olfactory epithelium throughout life from which they migrate to the olfactory bulb.[146–148]

Studies have shown that although these cells do not normally make myelin, they are able to do so when transplanted to areas of demyelination in the brain or spinal cord.[145,149–156] These cells have a capacity to grow in vitro and to remyelinate large axons with a Schwann-cell-like pattern of myelin and improve conduction properties after transplantation into the demyelinated adult rat CNS.[150–153,157] These cells seem also to promote axonal growth[158–161] and secrete neurotrophic molecules.[162,163] Thus, the relative availability of these cells, their apparent myelinating properties, and their trophic effect on axonal growth make them another promising candidate for autologous therapeutic transplantation. However, it is not yet clear whether OECs can be expanded in sufficient amounts for human transplantation and whether they will need to be isolated only from the olfactory bulb, located intracranially, or also more easily from the olfactory mucosa, situated at the back of the nose outside the cranium.[164]

Neural Stem Cells

The main advantage of stem cells is that they are nontransformed precursors that are potentially able to self-renew indefinitely, allowing their expansion in large quantities.

As discussed previously, mammalian multipotential NSCs support neurogenesis and gliogenesis within specific areas of the CNS during development and throughout adulthood and can be isolated from fetal and adult brains.[6,165,166] NSCs can be expanded in vitro, maintain their capacity for self-renewal, and generate a progeny of the three neural cell lineages[11,167] (Figure 6.2B). NSCs retain their functional plasticity after in vitro passaging and after several freezing-thawing cycles and they can still be modulated in vitro by exposure to different growth factors.[166,168] These uncommitted NSCs can integrate and repair the damaged CNS[169–172] and thus might represent a renewable source of cells that can be used for transplantation procedures. Stem cells can adapt their lineage fate and function according to environmental needs.

Transplanted NSCs of various origins improved the clinical outcome in experimental models of stroke,[171,172] spinal cord trauma,[169,170] and proved to have good myelinating properties as well. Intraventricularly transplanted clonal NSCs in the newborn *shi* mouse disseminated in widespread brain areas and participated in myelination.[173] Some recipient animals showed a decrease in their symptomatic tremor. In adult animals with traumatic spinal cord injury, rat NSCs migrated in the spinal cord and differentiated into myelinating oligodendrocytes.[174,175] Recently, it was also shown that intraventricular, as well as intravenous, transplantation of stem cells into mice with chronic EAE, resulted in clinical improvement.[125] This was correlated by graft-derived and endogenous remyelination and by reduction in axonal pathology. These data suggest that cell transplantation in de- and dysmyelinated human disease may have therapeutic potential for functional restoration.

In the process of neural development, there is continuous functional and lineage potential specification of the stem cell, before entering the

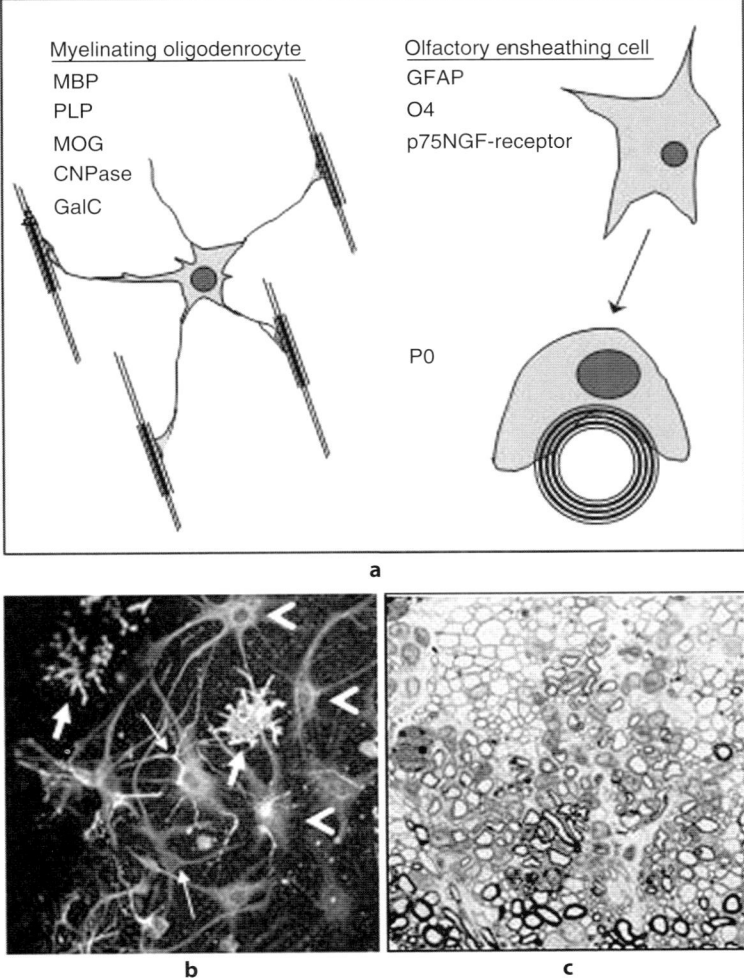

Figure 6.2. a Schematic representation of myelinating cells. An oligodendrocyte typically myelinates several axons and expresses specific antigens of CNS myelin, such as myelin basic protein (MBP), proteolipid protein (PLP), myelin-oligodendrocyte-glycoprotein (MOG), and galactocerebroside (GalC). Olfactory nerve enshealthing cells (OECs) have mixed features when cultured in vitro, such as expression of glial fibrillary acidic protein (GFAP) (similar to astrocytes), O4 (as in oligodendrocytes), and the p75 low affinity nerve growth factor receptor (p75NGFR, typical for Schwann cells). Remyelination by OECs has the typical characteristics of Schwann cells, with the "signet ring" appearance and one cell–one axon ratio. **b** PSA-NCAM+ neural stem cells that were grown in spheres generate cells of the three neural lineages, including astrocytes (arrowheads), oligodendrocytes (short arrows), and neurons (long thin arrows). Originally, the cells were identified by triple immunofluorescence for GFAP (astrocytes), O4 (oligodendrocytes), and neurofilament (neurons). **c** After transplantation of neurospheres into the demyelinated adult rat spinal cord, they fully remyelinate the lesion (upper part of the image). In remyelinated axons, the myelin is morphologically normal, but typically thinner than regular myelin (lower part of the image).

neuronal, oligodendroglial, or astroglial lineage. The exact developmental stage that is optimal for therapeutic transplantation is not clear. Although early NSCs in the developing cortical plate expand very rapidly, they are not migratory cells. In the SVZ of the CNS reside stem cells that generate mainly glia progeny. Donor-derived myelin was observed after SVZ precursor cells were propagated in culture with epidermal growth factor (EGF) and transplanted into the spinal cords of *md* rat and *sh* pup[176,177] and to the retinas of young mice.[178,179] SVZ precursors, grown with neuroblastoma-conditioned medium, myelinated also the brains of *shi* mice,[180–182] the embryonic telencephalic ventricles[183] and postnatal spinal cords of *md* rats.[90,184]

Expression of PSA-NCAM on the cell membrane has been associated with stem cell commitment to neuronal or glial fate, depending on time and place in development[185,186] and with especially good migratory and regenerative properties, as reviewed by Kleene and Schachner.[187] Such PSA-NCAM+ glial committed precursors, growing as neurospheres and termed also oligospheres,[181,184,185] remyelinated 95%–100% of the axons in the dorsal columns of rats[188] (Figure 6.2C), as compared with only 70% remyelinated axons that is expected from OPCs, and migrated efficiently along inflamed white matter tracts of rats with EAE.[126,189,190] Similarly, PSA-NCAM-enriched OPCs from fetal or adult human brain, xenografted to newborn *shi* mice brains, dispersed throughout the white matter, differentiated into oligodendrocytes, and remyelinated nude axons.[127] Also, adult human SVZ precursors remyelinated the demyelinated adult rat spinal cord.[191]

Embryonic Stem Cells

Embryonic stem (ES) cells are derived from the inner cell mass of blastocyst-stage embryos and are the totipotent stem cells that generate the entire repertoire of cells in the body. ES cell lines can actually be established from virtually all mammals[192–194] and can be banked and propagated in vitro almost indefinitely, with maintenance of a normal karyotype and totipotency, as was shown by the culturing of mouse ES cell lines in the presence of leukemia inhibitory factor.[166,168,195–197] Mouse ES cells can be induced to differentiate in vitro into neurons.[198–201] The sequential use of growth factors, such as fibroblast growth factor-2 (FGF2), EGF, and platelet-derived growth factor (PDGF), in a program that mimics embryonic development, has been successful to derive glial precursors from mouse ES cells.[202–204] The myelinogenic potential of mouse ES-derived OPCs, that were expanded in vitro, was demonstrated in the embryonic *md* rat brains, when these cells extensively myelinated the brain and spinal cord.[202] When transplanted in a rodent model of chemically induced demyelination and in spinal cords of *shi* mice, mouse ES-derived progenitors cells were also able to differentiate into glial cells and remyelinate demyelinated axons in vivo.[204,205] Since the isolation of human ES cells,[206,207] it has been possible to generate an endless source of transplantable human ES-derived neural precursors.[208,209] Transplanted human ES-derived neural progenitors into newborn mice differentiated into all three neural lineages, including oligodendrocytes.[208,209] Currently, there are close to 150 lines of human ES cells available.

The most important potential hazard in stem cell (and especially ES cell) transplantation is the risk of tumor formation. By definition, ES cells are capable of forming teratomas after transplantation. These teratomas contain cells of the three embryonic layers, i.e., ectoderm, mesoderm, and endoderm. When undifferentiated mouse ES cells were transplanted into the brain, they could generate brain cells, but at the expense of teratoma formation.[210,211] Clearly, the commitment to a restricted neural lineage should be complete before transplantation in order to eliminate this problem. Indeed, transplantation of mouse and human ES-derived neural precursors, obtained after multiple in vitro passages and exposure to various growth factors, did not result in teratoma formation.[202,208,209]

Another problem in stem cell transplantation is the possibility of graft rejection. In most studies of xeno-transplantation of human cells into rodents, graft rejection did not pose a significant problem. However, there is no long-term systematic follow-up of the survival of these cells in the brain. If graft rejection will prove to be a major obstacle, then in the future nuclear transfer from somatic cells to oocyte or stem cells may be attempted in order to generate the patient's own stem cell line for syngeneic transplantation.

Ethical Considerations

The promise of stem cell therapy has ignited public dispute on the ethics of using aborted embryos for medical purposes. Individual attitudes are usually influenced by religious and liberal views but also by concerns that the practice of embryonic tissue transplantation will increase the pressure to perform abortions and create a black market in which pregnancy and aborted tissues will be sold to the highest bidder. The regulated banking of stem cell lines may solve some of the ethical issues. As in other cases in which medical and scientific advances found society without the means to deal with their ethical, legal, and social consequences, it is impor-

Bone Marrow Stromal Cells

A central issue in the field of stem cell biology is the suggestion that plasticity of stem cells is marked to the degree of promiscuity, where stem cells of one tissue may generate cells of other tissues.[212–215] It has been shown that adult mouse and human bone marrow stromal cells (BMSCs) can differentiate in vitro into other cell types, including muscle, skin, liver, lung, and neural cells.[216–219] In humans affected by hematologic malignancies, peripherally injected BMSCs enter the brain and produce new neurons and microglia.[218–220] Recent reports suggest that these cells could contribute to the generation of new neural cells in the adult brain by a direct conversion of transplanted BMSCs into neurons or oligodendroglial cells, referred to as transdifferentiation[217–219,221–223] and/or assimilation of transplanted cells or their progeny into existing neurons and formation of heterokaryons, referred to as cell fusion.[219,224] In rats with a demyelinated lesion of the spinal cord, intravenous or brain injection of isolated mononuclear BMSCs resulted in varying degrees of remyelination.[225,226] In addition, bone marrow-derived stromal cells from transgenic green fluorescent protein (GFP) mice that were injected directly into the demyelinated spinal cord of immunosuppressed rats, produced myelin and improved axonal conduction velocity.[122] These observations stress the notion that it may not be mandatory to introduce glial committed cells for remyelination in vivo, as the developing and acutely demyelinated CNS may instruct other cells to differentiate into the required lineage. Accordingly, BMSCs might be useful as a therapeutic tool for brain repair by autologous transplantation.

Problematic Issues in Cell Transplantation for Demyelinating Diseases

Most experimental data on cell transplantation for remyelination has been obtained from genetic dysmyelinating models, where transplanted cells integrate into the normal developmental program of the CNS, or in models of acquired focal demyelination. However, the chronic and multifocal nature of MS raises several crucial issues that need to be considered in order to bring the therapeutic cell transplantation approach closer to clinical reality.

When to Transplant

The timing of transplantation is an important consideration. In the developing brain, the targeted migration and lineage fate of transplanted cells are directed by the normal pattern of development, occurring at the time of transplantation. Accordingly, human multipotential NSCs that were transplanted into the embryonic rat brain generated mostly neurons,[227] but when transplanted into the newborn brain, a stage in which neuronogenesis is complete and gliogenesis is in action, the stem cells generated mostly glia.[228] In contrast, the adult CNS does not support the survival of transplanted cells.[229] This may be attributed to the especially low abundance of trophic factors in normal adult brain tissue that maintains the survival of resident cells, but is insufficient for supporting the survival of transplanted cells. Transplanted cells may integrate significantly better in acutely lesioned tissue. When oligodendrocyte progenitor cells were transplanted into the spinal cord of animals with experimental EAE and an ongoing inflammatory process, they survived much better in vivo.[230] Because MS is a chronic and relapsing disease, it would be necessary to maintain long-term survival of transplanted cells both through phases of inflammation and remissions. Moreover, because the time window for remyelination is considered to be narrow, it may be best to introduce remyelinating cells as early as possible, in a form that will keep their survival independent of tissue support and ready for immediate mobilization upon tissue demand.

Route of Cell Delivery

Another key issue for cell transplantation in MS is the route of cell delivery. Because MS is a multifocal disease, it is impossible to introduce regenerating cells into all foci of disease. Moreover, it is

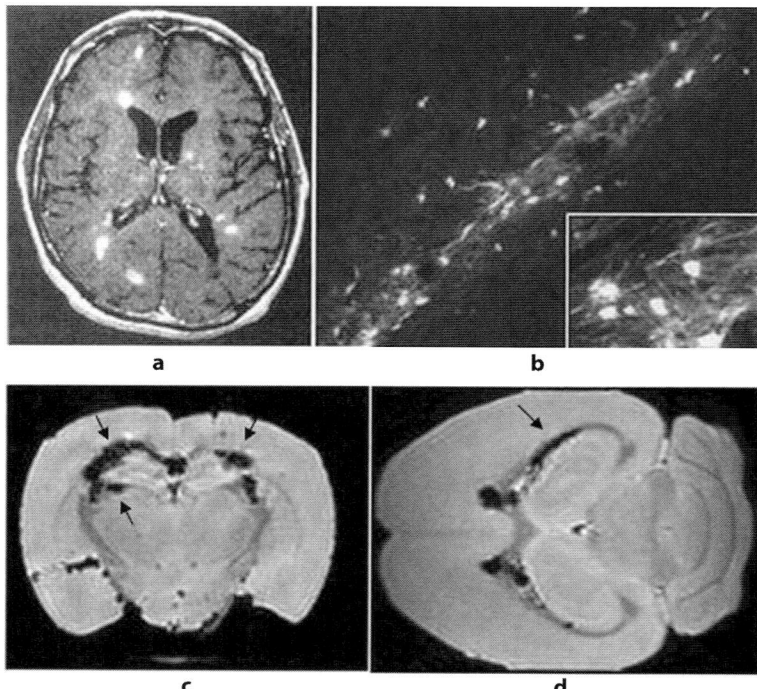

Figure 6.3. a MRI of an MS patient showing multiple lesions, mainly in the periventricular area. This ventricular space may therefore serve as the best accessible route to deliver cells in close proximity to the multiple foci of disease. b Green fluorescent protein (GFP)+, PSA-NCAM+ neurospheres were transplanted into the ventricles of chronic EAE mice. The transplanted GFP+ cells migrated along white matter tracts, especially in the corpus callosum, as shown here. A higher magnification of the fluorescing cells is shown in the inset. c and d Magnetically labeled mouse PSA-NCAM+ cells can be observed in the brain in vivo as hypointense signals on MRI. Coronal (C) and transverse (D) MRIs show the cells (arrows) migrating in the corpus callosum and fimbria.

often difficult to determine which of the multiple foci observed in the brain by magnetic resonance imaging (MRI) is most important clinically. Also, current neuroimaging techniques do not identify the specific pathological pattern of the lesion, and whether it is amenable for effective remyelination. Therefore, it is necessary to contemplate the optimal route of cell delivery that will promote efficient targeted migration of transplanted cells into multiple lesions for repair. Because most white matter tracts that are involved in MS are in close proximity to ventricular and spinal subarachnoid spaces (Figure 6.3A), then intraventricular and intrathecal transplantation may serve as an efficient route of delivering remyelinating cells. After intracerebroventricular injection, transplanted cells may disseminate throughout the neuroaxis without a separating barrier from the CNS white matter. Intraventricular transplantation of OPCs and stem cells led to widespread myelination in the genetic dysmyelinating models of the *shi* mouse[173] and the *md* rat.[183] In the adult brain, intraventricularly transplanted neurosphere cells disseminated along inflamed white matter tracts of EAE rats[126,189,190] (Figure 6.3B–D).

In recent experiments, different therapeutic cells were also injected into the blood stream (intravenously).[125,226,231] The specific homing of NSCs to the brain was explained in part by the constitutive expression of a wide array of adhesion molecules (integrins, selectins, etc.) and chemokine receptors by the transplanted cells.[125,232,233] In particular, integrins promote selective CNS homing through the interaction between transplanted cells and integrin receptor-expressing activated endothelial and ependymal cells surrounding inflamed brain tissues.[234,235] A recent study demonstrated a selective homing of intravenously and intracerebroventricularly injected NSCs to the EAE inflamed brain, via membrane expression of CD44 and very late antigen-4, resulting in functional recovery of myelin sheaths.[125] Although intravenous transplantation is an exciting novel approach for cell delivery, it is still unclear whether injected NSCs efficiently cross the blood-brain barrier in the intact and the inflamed brain and whether the cells home specifically to disease foci.

Migration of Transplanted Cells in the Brain

A crucial feature of transplanted cells is their ability to migrate into inflamed brain areas, integrate, and differentiate. The regenerative potential of transplanted cells is dependent on their ability to arrive to the active inflammatory-demyelinated lesions.

Cell migration is a major limiting factor in remyelination. In the lesioned CNS, spontaneous remyelination is a local event because of the limited migration of endogenous remyelinating cells.[85,101,102] As mentioned before, the adult brain may prove much more problematic in supporting transplanted cell migration and integration. Whereas transplanted multipotential NSCs migrate and integrate in the embryonic and newborn rodent CNS and adopt cellular identity according to local and temporal cues,[227,236,237] the normal adult brain does not permit large-distance migration and does not support transplanted neural cell survival.[229]

Transplanted precursors were found to possess superior migratory capabilities.[119] We have recently studied the response of PSA-NCAM+ NPC sphere cells to inflammation in EAE.[189] We found that, after intraventricular transplantation of spheres, cells migrated almost exclusively into inflamed periventricular white matter tracts, but not into gray matter (Figure 6.3B). There was a general correlation between the severity of the inflammatory response and the degree of transplanted cell migration into the brain. After transplantation into EAE rats, the majority of the precursor cells differentiate into glia cells (30% oligodendrocytes, 25% astrocytes). Similarly, the survival and migration of transplanted CG4 OPCs in the spinal cord were promoted by the inflammatory process.[230] Because MS is a multifocal relapsing disease, these findings exemplified the potential use of an intraventricular transplantation as a route of cell delivery in MS, bringing cells close to white matter tracts and enabling their inflammation-induced targeted migration. These studies are in accordance with recent observations on the reaction of subventricular PSA-NCAM+ cells to EAE.[95,96]

These findings suggest a linkage between parenchymal inflammation and setting regenerative mechanisms in motion. As such, the inflammatory process that develops in disease foci during clinical relapses of demyelinating diseases may serve to attract remyelinating cells. Thus, the brain inflammatory process may have a dual, contrasting action in inflicting brain injury and recruiting the regenerative process simultaneously. This stresses the notion that combination of cell transplantation and immunomodulation for MS in the future will need to be developed as nonreciprocally antagonistic modes of treatments. To this end, it is important to dissect the pro-regenerative components in the inflammatory process and target the immunomodulatory treatment without inhibiting regenerative processes.

Tracking Transplanted Cells Can Be Performed Noninvasively

To develop successful clinical (stem) cell-based therapies, it will be important to develop methods that can assess the fate and distribution of cells noninvasively. It is obvious that traditional histopathological methods for cell detection used in animal studies, which requires the removal of tissue, cannot be applied to patients in most cases. Among the various noninvasive imaging techniques that are currently available, MRI stands out in terms of resolution and whole-body imaging capability. When cells are magnetically labeled in vitro before their administration to a living organism, they can be potentially traced in vivo by MRI to study how certain lesions target cell migration, at what speed cells migrate, and for how long they persist in the target organ. Superparamagnetic iron oxides (SPIOs) are composed of biocompatible iron that provides the targeted cell with a large magnetic moment. A combination of SPIOs with transfection agents has resulted in efficient internalization and stable, nontoxic presence of iron particles in the cells.[238] A wide variety of cells from different species can be labeled, without affecting cell viability and proliferation capacity. The amount of cellular iron uptake (in the range of 10–20 pg Fe per cell) allows the detection of single cells by high-resolution

MRI.[238] Thus, because of their biocompatibility and strong effects on T2(*) relaxation, iron oxide nanoparticles seem to be the contrast agent of choice, and several methods now exist to shuttle a sufficient amount of these compounds into cells.

A series of recent studies indicate that MRI seems ideally suitable as a monitoring tool to follow the biodistribution and migration of cells after transplantation into the CNS.[239] OPCs were magnetically labeled using anti-transferrin monoclonal antibodies and transplanted in the spinal cord of 7-day-old *md* rats.[240] Ten to fourteen days later, the spinal cord was removed and imaged ex vivo at 4.7 Tesla at 78-μm resolution. Migration of labeled cells was easily identified on the MRIs as streaks of hypointensity, primarily along the dorsal column, over a distance of up to 10 mm away from the injection site. Immunohistochemical analysis of newly formed myelin showed an excellent match between the MR contrast and staining for PLP, an essential component of myelin. The density of magnetically labeled cells as evaluated by Prussian Blue staining was far less than the density of myelinated axons, which can be explained by the fact that one oligodendrocyte myelinates several axons in its surrounding. This study showed that magnetically labeled OPCs responded adequately to the normal developmental signals in the postnatal myelinating CNS and retained their capacity to myelinate axons in vivo. Turnbull and colleagues showed a similar example for the normal response of magnetically labeled cells to tissue cues, when CLIO-tat-labeled NSCs could be detected migrating along the rostral migratory stream after transplantation into the embryonic mouse brain. Whereas the ex vivo imaging that was performed in this study provided a basic proof of concept, the ability to image and perform temporal monitoring of labeled progenitor cells in vivo was demonstrated shortly thereafter. OPCs were derived from NSCs, labeled with magnetodendrimers, and transplanted in the ventricles of neonatal Long Evans shaker (*les*) rats.[241] Migration of labeled cells into the brain parenchyma could be observed already at the earliest studied time points (2–3 weeks) throughout the latest time point of imaging (6 weeks). A good agreement was observed between the hypointense MR contrast and expression of *LacZ* that was transfected into cells to serve as a reporter gene for β-galactosidase. In these areas, new myelin was formed as demonstrated by anti-MBP immunolabeling, proving that the cells were still functional after labeling. Labeled cells could also be readily identified when a clinical 1.5 Tesla scanner was used. The contrast appeared to fade out somewhat at the later time points, presumably through biodegradation of the iron oxide particles.

The migration of bromodeoxyuridine (BrdU)-tagged, magnetically labeled neurosphere cells has been recently examined after intraventricular transplantation into acute EAE rats at the peak of their disease.[190] Magnetic labeling of NPCs was employed using two approaches, one through internalization of anti-rat transferrin monoclonal antibodies covalently linked to dextran-coated iron oxide nanoparticles (MION-46LOX-26),[240] and one through nonspecific internalization of dendrimer-coated iron oxides (MD-100).[241] Both contrast agents labeled cells equally well and resulted in their visualization on the obtained MRIs. Ex vivo MRI confirmed that whereas the transplant disseminated in the ventricular system of both naive and EAE brains, widespread migration into white matter tracts occurred only in EAE rats. A good correlation was found between the histologic distribution of iron-labeled cells (by Prussian Blue staining) and BrdU immunostaining, indicating that the magnetic label was retained within labeled cells and not transferred to other cells in vivo.

Mouse neural spheres and human ES cell-derived neural spheres were transplanted in a mouse model of MOG35-55 chronic EAE, and transplanted cell fate and migration were studied by consecutive in vivo MRIs. In this study, both mouse and human cells responded to brain inflammation by migrating exclusively into the involved white matter tracts[242] (Figure 6.3C,D). This is the first indication that human ES-derived neural precursors respond to tissue signals in an MS model similar to rodent cells, a prerequisite for exhibiting myelin-regenerating properties. The observation that the greatest degree of migration occurred very early in the course of disease highlights the narrow time window in which transplantation of remyelinating cells may be effective for obtaining clinical results.

In conclusion, with its excellent spatial resolution and the ability to track labeled cells over prolonged periods of time, MR monitoring of cell therapy is likely to become an important technique in the foreseeable future.

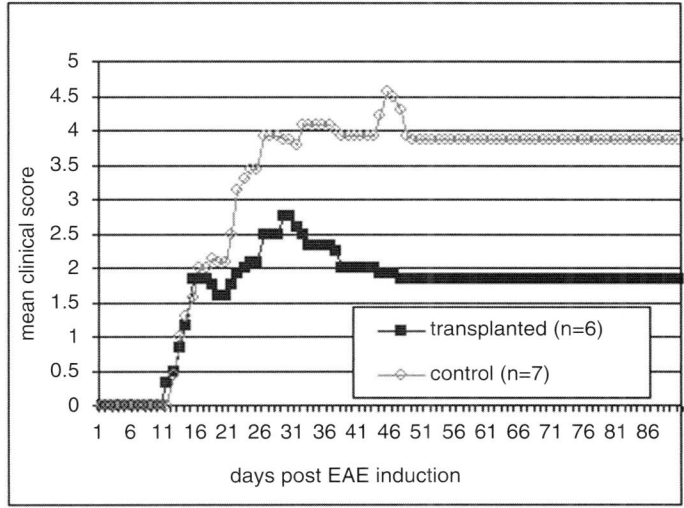

Figure 6.4. Intraventricular transplantation of neurospheres in chronic EAE leads to significant attenuation of the clinical course of disease. This is associated with significant reduction in axonal pathology and in loss of myelin.

Stem Cells Improve the Clinical Course of EAE by Several Mechanisms of Action

An important step toward the future application of stem cell therapy in MS has been made recently with the observation that stem cell transplantation attenuates the clinical course of chronic EAE, a reliable model of MS[125,243] (Figure 6.4). The mechanisms by which transplanted cells affect brain recovery are not fully understood. The vast majority of research has focused until recently on their own regenerative potential as cell-replacement therapy. Recently, it was suggested that transplanted stem cells also enhance endogenous brain repair systems.[244,245] Accordingly, in NSC-transplanted EAE mice, only 20% of remyelination was donor cell-derived.[125] Thus, a neurotrophic effect may underline at least part of the beneficial action of transplanted NSCs. Neural precursors produce a variety of neurotrophic factors that may protect the brain from injury.[246] Transplanted NSCs that remained in an undifferentiated state may continue to release neurotrophins, including FGF2, brain-derived neurotrophic factor, and glial cell line-derived neurotrophic factor.[125,246]

Our recent studies suggest an additional mechanism of stem cell action in the EAE brain. We showed that neural sphere transplantation inhibited the clinical and pathological features of acute EAE, an experimental model for brain inflammation with a minor demyelinating component.[126] Specifically, neurosphere transplantation reduced the inflammatory process in the brain, as determined by several pathological criteria. Similarly, the immune-mediated demyelination and axonal injury were reduced in neurosphere-transplanted chronic EAE mice.[243] Cell transplantation inhibited the cellular inflammatory process in the brain and increased the number of regulatory CD25+ cells and NK-T cells in the brain. Moreover, in transplanted mice, there was a decrease in local cellular inflammatory-associated axonal injury. These findings suggest that the beneficial clinical and pathological effects of NPC transplantation were related, in part, to their immunomodulatory and antiinflammatory properties. Because the autoimmune process is a major determinant of tissue injury in EAE and MS, its local suppression by cell transplantation decreases the pathological and clinical consequences of disease. This has major importance for a transplantation approach in immune-mediated diseases, because the down-regulation of the inflammatory process may protect the graft from future immune attacks. Bidirectional interactions between NSCs and the immune system are largely unknown. NSCs can directly inhibit the specific response of lymph node cells to a myelin antigen.[126] In addition, neurotrophins that may be released by stem cells and inhibit EAE not only by enhancing oligodendrocyte survival,[247,248] but also by decreasing neuroinflammation.[109,249–251]

In conclusion, stem cells may exert their therapeutic effects via different, interacting mechanisms, including their own myelinating qualities, their neurotrophic properties, and their immune regulatory functions.

Stem Cell Therapy in MS May Be Getting Closer

Current research is progressing rapidly, and below are a few examples of unpublished data, presented according to the issues raised in this review.

Transplantation in Clinically Relevant Models of MS

Beneficial effects of cell transplantation in subhuman primates will provide strong support for this novel mode of therapy. To this end, Dr. Gianvito Martino and colleagues at San Raffaele Scientific Institute in Milano, transplanted human NSCs in marmosets with EAE. The donor cells, derived from a renewable cell line developed by Dr. Vescovi, were genetically manipulated to express GFP and transplanted intrathecally in four monkeys and intravenously in five monkeys. Another six monkeys served as controls. All animals receive daily treatment with cyclosporine, an immune-suppressing drug, to prevent rejection of the transplanted cells. Dr. Anne Baron-Van Evercooren and colleagues at the Salpêtrière Hospital in Paris are conducting a similar experiment, pursuing the autologous transplantation of GFP-labeled Schwann cells in marmosets with EAE. In a separate experiment, Dr. Baron is developing a model in which lesions are targeted to the caudal cerebellar peduncle, an area of the brain that controls voluntary movement, in the *Macaca fascicularis* monkey. In this model, the animals should mimic the tremors experienced by MS patients. Cells will be transplanted into these lesions, to ascertain whether they remyelinate the nerves and restore function in the monkeys.

Optimal Site of Transplantation Within the CNS

Dr. Ian Duncan of the University of Wisconsin-Madison and colleagues are transplanting OPCs into different sites of the CNS of the *md* rats. When transplanted into a single site in the spinal cord of 28 rats, OPCs migrated as far as 23 mm from the site of implant and produced extensive myelination of dysmyelinated nerve tracts. By transplanting OPCs at two sites in the spinal cord, the researchers have been able to achieve the same amount of remyelination in half the time compared with transplantation at a single site. In an attempt to obtain greater remyelination, the researchers have begun transplanting OPCs into four different sites, two in the brain and two in the spinal cord. Some animals transplanted at several locations of both the brain and spinal cord showed the most widespread migration ever reported, with myelin-producing cells found along the upper and middle spinal cord, as well as in the sacral area. The researchers plan to confirm these results in a rat model that is longer-lived than the *md* strain and to identify factors that influence the type of migration as well as the distance the cells migrate.

Candidate Cells for Transplantation

At Cambridge University in England, Dr. Robin Franklin has found that the olfactory mucosa is a readily accessible source of stem cells, from which it may be possible to derive OECs. Importantly, the stem cells obtained from this region may potentially provide a source of other cells, such as OPCs. He plans a transplant study in rodents to demonstrate that stem cells from the olfactory mucosa can generate cells that will produce myelin. Dr. Su-Chun Zhang from Cambridge has succeeded in deriving oligodendrocyte precursors from mouse ES cells, and is transplanting them into the *shi* mice. A laboratory test in two transplanted mice was positive for myelin. Several laboratories, including our own in collaboration with Dr. Benjamin Reubinoff, are pursuing the derivation of oligodendrocyte lineage cells from human ES cells, as a possible endless source of cells for transplantation.

Summary

Neural precursor cells that reside in the adult brain, a potential source of myelin-forming cells, do not produce effective remyelination in MS. The transplantation of exogenous cells, as an alternative source of remyelinating cells, has been pursued as a very active research area over the last decade and remarkable progress has been obtained. New sources of myelinating cells were characterized and different transplantation strategies have been proposed. Better understanding of the pros and cons of using each of the various remyelinating cell types, of the different routes of cell delivery, and of methods for cell tracking, form the basis for designing cell transplantation strategies in the clinic. Better understanding of the process of remyelination and insights into the mechanism of action of transplanted cells are still needed to optimize cell therapy in demyelinating diseases.

References

1. McKay R. Stem cells in the central nervous system. Science 1997;276(5309):66–71.
2. Garcia-Verdugo JM, Ferron S, Flames N, Collado L, Desfilis E, Font E. The proliferative ventricular zone in adult vertebrates: a comparative study using reptiles, birds, and mammals. Brain Res Bull 2002;57(6):765–775.
3. Gritti A, Parati EA, Cova L, et al. Multipotential stem cells from the adult mouse brain proliferate and self-renew in response to basic fibroblast growth factor. J Neurosci 1996;16(3):1091–1100.
4. Reynolds BA, Weiss S. Generation of neurons and astrocytes from isolated cells of the adult mammalian central nervous system. Science 1992;255(5052):1707–1710.
5. Arsenijevic Y, Villemure JG, Brunet JF, et al. Isolation of multipotent neural precursors residing in the cortex of the adult human brain. Exp Neurol 2001;170(1):48–62.
6. Nunes MC, Roy NS, Keyoung HM, et al. Identification and isolation of multipotential neural progenitor cells from the subcortical white matter of the adult human brain. Nat Med 2003;9(4):439–447.
7. Rao M. Stem and precursor cells in the nervous system. J Neurotrauma 2004;21(4):415–427.
8. Schaffer DV, Gage FH. Neurogenesis and neuroadaptation. Neuromolecular Med 2004;5(1):1–9.
9. Picard-Riera N, Nait-Oumesmar B, Baron-Van Evercooren A. Endogenous adult neural stem cells: limits and potential to repair the injured central nervous system. J Neurosci Res 2004;76(2):223–231.
10. Gritti A, Bonfanti L, Doetsch F, et al. Multipotent neural stem cells reside into the rostral extension and olfactory bulb of adult rodents. J Neurosci 2002;22(2):437–445.
11. Bottai D, Fiocco R, Gelain F, et al. Neural stem cells in the adult nervous system. J Hematother Stem Cell Res 2003;12(6):655–670.
12. Johe KK, Hazel TG, Muller T, Dugich-Djordjevic MM, McKay RD. Single factors direct the differentiation of stem cells from the fetal and adult central nervous system. Genes Dev 1996;10(24):3129–3140.
13. Lois C, Garcia-Verdugo JM, Alvarez-Buylla A. Chain migration of neuronal precursors. Science 1996;271(5251):978–981.
14. De Marchis S, Fasolo A, Puche AC. Subventricular zone-derived neuronal progenitors migrate into the subcortical forebrain of postnatal mice. J Comp Neurol 2004;476(3):290–300.
15. Pencea V, Bingaman KD, Freedman LJ, Luskin MB. Neurogenesis in the subventricular zone and rostral migratory stream of the neonatal and adult primate forebrain. Exp Neurol 2001;172(1):1–16.
16. Garcia-Verdugo JM, Doetsch F, Wichterle H, Lim DA, Alvarez-Buylla A. Architecture and cell types of the adult subventricular zone: in search of the stem cells. J Neurobiol 1998;36(2):234–248.
17. Alvarez-Buylla A, Herrera DG, Wichterle H. The subventricular zone: source of neuronal precursors for brain repair. Prog Brain Res 2000;127:1–11.
18. Eriksson PS, Perfilieva E, Bjork-Eriksson T, et al. Neurogenesis in the adult human hippocampus. Nat Med 1998;4(11):1313–1317.
19. Roy NS, Wang S, Jiang L, et al. In vitro neurogenesis by progenitor cells isolated from the adult human hippocampus. Nat Med 2000;6(3):271–277.
20. Kuhn HG, Dickinson-Anson H, Gage FH. Neurogenesis in the dentate gyrus of the adult rat: age-related decrease of neuronal progenitor proliferation. J Neurosci 1996;16(6):2027–2033.
21. Johansson CB, Momma S, Clarke DL, Risling M, Lendahl U, Frisen J. Identification of a neural stem cell in the adult mammalian central nervous system. Cell 1999;96(1):25–34.
22. Namiki J, Tator CH. Cell proliferation and nestin expression in the ependyma of the adult rat spinal cord after injury. J Neuropathol Exp Neurol 1999;58(5):489–498.
23. Johansson CB, Svensson M, Wallstedt L, Janson AM, Frisen J. Neural stem cells in the adult human brain. Exp Cell Res 1999;253(2):733–736.
24. Wolswijk G, Noble M. Identification of an adult-specific glial progenitor cell. Development 1989;105(2):387–400.
25. Reynolds R, Hardy R. Oligodendroglial progenitors labeled with the O4 antibody persist in the adult rat cerebral cortex in vivo. J Neurosci Res 1997;47(5):455–470.
26. Dawson MR, Polito A, Levine JM, Reynolds R. NG2-expressing glial progenitor cells: an abundant and widespread population of cycling cells in the adult rat CNS. Mol Cell Neurosci 2003;24(2):476–488.
27. Scolding NJ, Rayner PJ, Sussman J, Shaw C, Compston DA. A proliferative adult human oligodendrocyte progenitor. Neuroreport 1995;6(3):441–445.

28. Scolding N, Franklin R, Stevens S, Heldin CH, Compston A, Newcombe J. Oligodendrocyte progenitors are present in the normal adult human CNS and in the lesions of multiple sclerosis. Brain 1998;121(pt 12):2221–2228.
29. Roy NS, Wang S, Harrison-Restelli C, et al. Identification, isolation, and promoter-defined separation of mitotic oligodendrocyte progenitor cells from the adult human subcortical white matter. J Neurosci 1999;19(22):9986–9995.
30. Horner PJ, Thallmair M, Gage FH. Defining the NG2-expressing cell of the adult CNS. J Neurocytol 2002;31(6–7):469–480.
31. Horner PJ, Power AE, Kempermann G, et al. Proliferation and differentiation of progenitor cells throughout the intact adult rat spinal cord. J Neurosci 2000;20(6):2218–2228.
32. Wingerchuk DM, Lucchinetti CF, Noseworthy JH. Multiple sclerosis: current pathophysiological concepts. Lab Invest 2001;81(3):263–281.
33. Compston A, Coles A. Multiple sclerosis. Lancet 2002;359(9313):1221–1231.
34. Dyment DA, Ebers GC. An array of sunshine in multiple sclerosis. N Engl J Med 2002;347(18):1445–1447.
35. Noseworthy JH, Lucchinetti C, Rodriguez M, Weinshenker BG. Multiple sclerosis. N Engl J Med 2000;343(13):938–952.
36. Lucchinetti C, Bruck W, Parisi J, Scheithauer B, Rodriguez M, Lassmann H. Heterogeneity of multiple sclerosis lesions: implications for the pathogenesis of demyelination. Ann Neurol 2000;47(6):707–717.
37. Lassmann H. Classification of demyelinating diseases at the interface between etiology and pathogenesis. Curr Opin Neurol 2001;14(3):253–258.
38. Lassmann H, Raine CS, Antel J, Prineas JW. Immunopathology of multiple sclerosis: report on an international meeting held at the Institute of Neurology of the University of Vienna. J Neuroimmunol 1998;86(2):213–217.
39. Trapp BD, Bo L, Mork S, Chang A. Pathogenesis of tissue injury in MS lesions. J Neuroimmunol 1999;98(1):49–56.
40. Lassmann H. Mechanisms of demyelination and tissue destruction in multiple sclerosis. Clin Neurol Neurosurg 2002;104(3):168–171.
41. Lassmann H. Neuropathology in multiple sclerosis: new concepts. Mult Scler 1998;4(3):93–98.
42. Trapp BD, Peterson J, Ransohoff RM, Rudick R, Mork S, Bo L. Axonal transection in the lesions of multiple sclerosis. N Engl J Med 1998;338(5):278–285.
43. Kornek B, Storch MK, Weissert R, et al. Multiple sclerosis and chronic autoimmune encephalomyelitis: a comparative quantitative study of axonal injury in active, inactive, and remyelinated lesions. Am J Pathol 2000;157(1):267–276.
44. Chang A, Tourtellotte WW, Rudick R, Trapp BD. Premyelinating oligodendrocytes in chronic lesions of multiple sclerosis. N Engl J Med 2002;346(3):165–173.
45. Barkhof F, Bruck W, De Groot CJ, et al. Remyelinated lesions in multiple sclerosis: magnetic resonance image appearance. Arch Neurol 2003;60(8):1073–1081.
46. Prineas JW, Barnard RO, Kwon EE, Sharer LR, Cho ES. Multiple sclerosis: remyelination of nascent lesions. Ann Neurol 1993;33(2):137–151.
47. Raine CS, Wu E. Multiple sclerosis: remyelination in acute lesions. J Neuropathol Exp Neurol 1993;52(3):199–204.
48. Compston A. Remyelination of the central nervous system. Mult Scler 1996;1(6):388–392.
49. Compston A. Remyelination in multiple sclerosis: a challenge for therapy. The 1996 European Charcot Foundation Lecture. Mult Scler 1997;3(2):51–70.
50. Chari DM, Blakemore WF. New insights into remyelination failure in multiple sclerosis: implications for glial cell transplantation. Mult Scler 2002;8(4):271–277.
51. Franklin RJ. Why does remyelination fail in multiple sclerosis? Nat Rev Neurosci 2002;3(9):705–714.
52. De Stefano N, Matthews PM, Fu L, et al. Axonal damage correlates with disability in patients with relapsing-remitting multiple sclerosis. Results of a longitudinal magnetic resonance spectroscopy study. Brain 1998;121(pt 8):1469–1477.
53. Trapp BD, Ransohoff R, Rudick R. Axonal pathology in multiple sclerosis: relationship to neurologic disability. Curr Opin Neurol 1999;12(3):295–302.
54. Steinman L. Multiple sclerosis: a two-stage disease. Nat Immunol 2001;2(9):762–764.
55. Hemmer B, Cepok S, Nessler S, Sommer N. Pathogenesis of multiple sclerosis: an update on immunology. Curr Opin Neurol 2002;15(3):227–231.
56. Bjartmar C, Kidd G, Mork S, Rudick R, Trapp BD. Neurological disability correlates with spinal cord axonal loss and reduced N-acetyl aspartate in chronic multiple sclerosis patients. Ann Neurol 2000;48(6):893–901.
57. Bjartmar C, Yin X, Trapp BD. Axonal pathology in myelin disorders. J Neurocytol 1999;28(4–5):383–395.
58. Wujek JR, Bjartmar C, Richer E, et al. Axon loss in the spinal cord determines permanent neurological disability in an animal model of multiple sclerosis. J Neuropathol Exp Neurol 2002;61(1):23–32.
59. Rudick RA, Cohen JA, Weinstock-Guttman B, Kinkel RP, Ransohoff RM. Management of multiple sclerosis. N Engl J Med 1997;337(22):1604–1611.
60. Tullman MJ, Lublin FD, Miller AE. Immunotherapy of multiple sclerosis: current practice and future directions. J Rehabil Res Dev 2002;39(2):273–285.
61. Gordon MN, Kumar S, Espinosa de los Monteros A, et al. Developmental regulation of myelin-associated genes in the normal and the myelin deficient mutant rat. Adv Exp Med Biol 1990;265:11–22.
62. Griffiths IR, Duncan ID, McCulloch M. Shaking pups: a disorder of central myelination in the spaniel dog. II. Ultrastructural observations on the white matter of the cervical spinal cord. J Neurocytol 1981;10(5):847–858.
63. Readhead C, Hood L. The dysmyelinating mouse mutations shiverer (shi) and myelin deficient (shimld). Behav Genet 1990;20(2):213–234.
64. Ludwin SK. Central nervous system demyelination and remyelination in the mouse: an ultrastructural study of cuprizone toxicity. Lab Invest 1978;39(6):597–612.
65. Blakemore WF. Ethidium bromide induced demyelination in the spinal cord of the cat. Neuropathol Appl Neurobiol 1982;8(5):365–375.
66. Waxman SG, Kocsis JD, Nitta KC. Lysophosphatidyl choline-induced focal demyelination in the rabbit corpus callosum. Light-microscopic observations. J Neurol Sci 1979;44(1):45–53.
67. Carroll WM, Jennings AR, Mastaglia FL. Experimental demyelinating optic neuropathy induced by intra-neural injection of galactocerebroside antiserum. J Neurol Sci 1984;65(2):125–135.

68. Blakemore WF. Remyelination of the superior cerebellar peduncle in old mice following demyelination induced by cuprizone. J Neurol Sci 1974;22(1): 121–126.
69. Tsunoda I, Fujinami RS. Two models for multiple sclerosis: experimental allergic encephalomyelitis and Theiler's murine encephalomyelitis virus. J Neuropathol Exp Neurol 1996;55(6):673–686.
70. Oleszak EL, Chang JR, Friedman H, Katsetos CD, Platsoucas CD. Theiler's virus infection: a model for multiple sclerosis. Clin Microbiol Rev 2004;17(1): 174–207.
71. Pirko I, Ciric B, Gamez J, et al. A human antibody that promotes remyelination enters the CNS and decreases lesion load as detected by T2-weighted spinal cord MRI in a virus-induced murine model of MS. FASEB J 2004;18(13):1577–1579.
72. Woyciechowska JL, Trapp BD, Patrick DH, et al. Acute and subacute demyelination induced by mouse hepatitis virus strain A59 in C3H mice. J Exp Pathol 1984;1(4):295–306.
73. Sorensen O, Perry D, Dales S. In vivo and in vitro models of demyelinating diseases. III. JHM virus infection of rats. Arch Neurol 1980;37(8):478–484.
74. Lassmann H. Chronic relapsing experimental allergic encephalomyelitis: its value as an experimental model for multiple sclerosis. J Neurol 1983;229(4):207–220.
75. Gold R, Hartung HP, Toyka KV. Animal models for autoimmune demyelinating disorders of the nervous system. Mol Med Today 2000;6(2):88–91.
76. Swanborg RH. Experimental autoimmune encephalomyelitis in rodents as a model for human demyelinating disease. Clin Immunol Immunopathol 1995; 77(1):4–13.
77. Izikson L, Klein RS, Luster AD, Weiner HL. Targeting monocyte recruitment in CNS autoimmune disease. Clin Immunol 2002;103(2):125–131.
78. Kuchroo VK, Anderson AC, Waldner H, Munder M, Bettelli E, Nicholson LB. T cell response in experimental autoimmune encephalomyelitis (EAE): role of self and cross-reactive antigens in shaping, tuning, and regulating the autopathogenic T cell repertoire. Annu Rev Immunol 2002;20:101–123.
79. Karussis DM, Lehmann D, Slavin S, et al. Inhibition of acute, experimental autoimmune encephalomyelitis by the synthetic immunomodulator linomide. Ann Neurol 1993;34(5):654–660.
80. Mendel I, Kerlero de Rosbo N, Ben-Nun A. A myelin oligodendrocyte glycoprotein peptide induces typical chronic experimental autoimmune encephalomyelitis in H-2b mice: fine specificity and T cell receptor V beta expression of encephalitogenic T cells. Eur J Immunol 1995;25(7):1951–1959.
81. Slavin A, Ewing C, Liu J, Ichikawa M, Slavin J, Bernard CC. Induction of a multiple sclerosis-like disease in mice with an immunodominant epitope of myelin oligodendrocyte glycoprotein. Autoimmunity 1998; 28(2):109–120.
82. Oliver AR, Lyon GM, Ruddle NH. Rat and human myelin oligodendrocyte glycoproteins induce experimental autoimmune encephalomyelitis by different mechanisms in C57BL/6 mice. J Immunol 2003;171(1):462–468.
83. Frost EE, Nielsen JA, Le TQ, Armstrong RC. PDGF and FGF2 regulate oligodendrocyte progenitor responses to demyelination. J Neurobiol 2003;54(3):457–472.
84. Redwine JM, Armstrong RC. In vivo proliferation of oligodendrocyte progenitors expressing PDGFalphaR during early remyelination. J Neurobiol 1998;37(3): 413–428.
85. Gensert JM, Goldman JE. Endogenous progenitors remyelinate demyelinated axons in the adult CNS. Neuron 1997;19(1):197–203.
86. Targett MP, Sussman J, Scolding N, O'Leary MT, Compston DA, Blakemore WF. Failure to achieve remyelination of demyelinated rat axons following transplantation of glial cells obtained from the adult human brain. Neuropathol Appl Neurobiol 1996;22(3):199–206.
87. Keirstead HS, Blakemore WF. Identification of postmitotic oligodendrocytes incapable of remyelination within the demyelinated adult spinal cord. J Neuropathol Exp Neurol 1997;56(11):1191–1201.
88. Wolswijk G. Oligodendrocyte survival, loss and birth in lesions of chronic-stage multiple sclerosis. Brain 2000;123(pt 1):105–115.
89. Wolswijk G. Oligodendrocyte precursor cells in the demyelinated multiple sclerosis spinal cord. Brain 2002;125(pt 2):338–349.
90. Zhang SC, Ge B, Duncan ID. Adult brain retains the potential to generate oligodendroglial progenitors with extensive myelination capacity. Proc Natl Acad Sci USA 1999;96(7):4089–4094.
91. Keirstead HS, Levine JM, Blakemore WF. Response of the oligodendrocyte progenitor cell population (defined by NG2 labelling) to demyelination of the adult spinal cord. Glia 1998;22(2):161–170.
92. Levine JM, Reynolds R. Activation and proliferation of endogenous oligodendrocyte precursor cells during ethidium bromide-induced demyelination. Exp Neurol 1999;160(2):333–347.
93. Di Bello IC, Dawson MR, Levine JM, Reynolds R. Generation of oligodendroglial progenitors in acute inflammatory demyelinating lesions of the rat brain stem is associated with demyelination rather than inflammation. J Neurocytol 1999;28(4–5): 365–381.
94. Reynolds R, Dawson M, Papadopoulos D, et al. The response of NG2-expressing oligodendrocyte progenitors to demyelination in MOG-EAE and MS. J Neurocytol 2002;31(6–7):523–536.
95. Nait-Oumesmar B, Decker L, Lachapelle F, Avellana-Adalid V, Bachelin C, Van Evercooren AB. Progenitor cells of the adult mouse subventricular zone proliferate, migrate and differentiate into oligodendrocytes after demyelination. Eur J Neurosci 1999;11(12): 4357–4366.
96. Picard-Riera ND, Delarasse L, Goude C, et al. Experi-mental autoimmune encephalomyelitis mobilizes neural progenitors from the subventricular zone to undergo oligodendrogenesis in adult mice. Proc Natl Acad Sci USA 2002;99(20): 13211–13216.
97. Wolswijk G. Chronic stage multiple sclerosis lesions contain a relatively quiescent population of oligodendrocyte precursor cells. J Neurosci 1998;18(2):601–609.
98. Chang A, Nishiyama A, Peterson J, Prineas J, Trapp BD. NG2-positive oligodendrocyte progenitor cells in adult human brain and multiple sclerosis lesions. J Neurosci 2000;20(17):6404–6412.
99. Mason JL, Toews A, Hostettler JD, et al. Oligodendrocytes and progenitors become progressively depleted within chronically demyelinated lesions. Am J Pathol 2004;164(5):1673–1682.

100. Lucchinetti C, Bruck W, Parisi J, Scheithauer B, Rodriguez M, Lassmann H. A quantitative analysis of oligodendrocytes in multiple sclerosis lesions. A study of 113 cases. Brain 1999;122(pt 12):2279–2295.
101. Franklin RJ, Gilson JM, Blakemore WF. Local recruitment of remyelinating cells in the repair of demyelination in the central nervous system. J Neurosci Res 1997;50(2):337–344.
102. Franklin RJ, Blakemore WF. To what extent is oligodendrocyte progenitor migration a limiting factor in the remyelination of multiple sclerosis lesions? Mult Scler 1997;3(2):84–87.
103. Wolswijk G, Noble M. Cooperation between PDGF and FGF converts slowly dividing O-2Aadult progenitor cells to rapidly dividing cells with characteristics of O-2Aperinatal progenitor cells. J Cell Biol 1992;118(4):889–900.
104. Sharief MK. Cytokines in multiple sclerosis: pro-inflammation or pro-remyelination? Mult Scler 1998;4(3):169–173.
105. Woodruff RH, Franklin RJ. Growth factors and remyelination in the CNS. Histol Histopathol 1997;12(2):459–466.
106. Milner R, Anderson HJ, Rippon RF, et al. Contrasting effects of mitogenic growth factors on oligodendrocyte precursor cell migration. Glia 1997;19(1):85–90.
107. Yao DL, Liu X, Hudson LD, Webster HD. Insulin-like growth factor-I given subcutaneously reduces clinical deficits, decreases lesion severity and upregulates synthesis of myelin proteins in experimental autoimmune encephalomyelitis. Life Sci 1996;58(16):1301–1306.
108. Li W, Quigley L, Yao DL, et al. Chronic relapsing experimental autoimmune encephalomyelitis: effects of insulin-like growth factor-I treatment on clinical deficits, lesion severity, glial responses, and blood brain barrier defects. J Neuropathol Exp Neurol 1998;57(5):426–438.
109. Cannella B, Hoban CJ, Gao YL, et al. The neuregulin, glial growth factor 2, diminishes autoimmune demyelination and enhances remyelination in a chronic relapsing model for multiple sclerosis. Proc Natl Acad Sci USA 1998;95(17):10100–10105.
110. Baker D, Hankey DJ. Gene therapy in autoimmune, demyelinating disease of the central nervous system. Gene Ther 2003;10(10):844–853.
111. Scherer SS, Chance PF. Myelin genes: getting the dosage right. Nat Genet 1995;11(3):226–228.
112. Winter CG, Saotome Y, Saotome I, Hirsh D. CNTF overproduction hastens onset of symptoms in motor neuron degeneration (mnd) mice. J Neurobiol 1996;31(3):370–378.
113. Rubio F, Kokaia Z, Arco A, et al. BDNF gene transfer to the mammalian brain using CNS-derived neural precursors. Gene Ther 1999;6(11):1851–1866.
114. Inoue K, Osaka H, Imaizumi K, et al. Proteolipid protein gene duplications causing Pelizaeus-Merzbacher disease: molecular mechanism and phenotypic manifestations. Ann Neurol 1999;45(5):624–632.
115. Groves AK, Barnett SC, Franklin RJ, et al. Repair of demyelinated lesions by transplantation of purified O-2A progenitor cells. Nature 1993;362(6419):453–455.
116. Kocsis JD. Restoration of function by glial cell transplantation into demyelinated spinal cord. J Neurotrauma 1999;16(8):695–703.
117. Blakemore WF, Crang AJ. Extensive oligodendrocyte remyelination following injection of cultured central nervous system cells into demyelinating lesions in adult central nervous system. Dev Neurosci 1988;10(1):1–11.
118. Warrington AE, Barbarese E, Pfeiffer SE. Differential myelinogenic capacity of specific developmental stages of the oligodendrocyte lineage upon transplantation into hypomyelinating hosts. J Neurosci Res 1993;34(1):1–13.
119. Franklin RJ, Blakemore WF. Transplanting oligodendrocyte progenitors into the adult CNS. J Anat 1997;190(pt 1):23–33.
120. Zhang SC, Duncan ID. Remyelination and restoration of axonal function by glial cell transplantation. Prog Brain Res 2000;127:515–533.
121. Blakemore WF, Franklin RJ. Transplantation options for therapeutic central nervous system remyelination. Cell Transplant 2000;9(2):289–294.
122. Akiyama Y, Radtke C, Kocsis JD. Remyelination of the rat spinal cord by transplantation of identified bone marrow stromal cells. J Neurosci 2002;22(15):6623–6630.
123. Halfpenny C, Benn T, Scolding N. Cell transplantation, myelin repair, and multiple sclerosis. Lancet Neurol 2002;1(1):31–40.
124. Franklin RJ. Remyelination of the demyelinated CNS: the case for and against transplantation of central, peripheral and olfactory glia. Brain Res Bull 2002;57(6):827–832.
125. Pluchino S, Quattrini A, Brambilla E, et al. Injection of adult neurospheres induces recovery in a chronic model of multiple sclerosis. Nature 2003;422(6933):688–694.
126. Einstein O, Karussis D, Grigoriadis N, et al. Intraventricular transplantation of neural precursor cell spheres attenuates acute experimental allergic encephalomyelitis. Mol Cell Neurosci 2003;24(4):1074–1082.
127. Windrem MS, Nunes MC, Rashbaum WK, et al. Fetal and adult human oligodendrocyte progenitor cell isolates myelinate the congenitally dysmyelinated brain. Nat Med 2004;10(1):93–97.
128. Kocsis JD, Akiyama Y, Radtke C. Neural precursors as a cell source to repair the demyelinated spinal cord. J Neurotrauma 2004;21(4):441–449.
129. Duncan ID, Aguayo AJ, Bunge RP, Wood PM. Transplantation of rat Schwann cells grown in tissue culture into the mouse spinal cord. J Neurol Sci 1981;49(2):241–252.
130. Lachapelle F, Gumpel M, Baulac M, Jacque C, Duc P, Baumann N. Transplantation of CNS fragments into the brain of shiverer mutant mice: extensive myelination by implanted oligodendrocytes. I. Immunohistochemical studies. Dev Neurosci 1983;6(6):325–334.
131. Harrison BM. Remyelination by cells introduced into a stable demyelinating lesion in the central nervous system. J Neurol Sci 1980;46(1):63–81.
132. Blakemore WF, Crang AJ. The use of cultured autologous Schwann cells to remyelinate areas of persistent demyelination in the central nervous system. J Neurol Sci 1985;70(2):207–223.
133. Crang AJ, Gilson J, Blakemore WF. The demonstration by transplantation of the very restricted remyelinating potential of post-mitotic oligodendrocytes. J Neurocytol 1998;27(7):541–553.
134. Archer DR, Cuddon PA, Lipsitz D, Duncan ID. Myelination of the canine central nervous system by

glial cell transplantation: a model for repair of human myelin disease. Nat Med 1997;3(1):54–59.
135. Windrem MS, Roy NS, Wang J, et al. Progenitor cells derived from the adult human subcortical white matter disperse and differentiate as oligodendrocytes within demyelinated lesions of the rat brain. J Neurosci Res 2002;69(6):966–975.
136. Blakemore WF, Gilson JM, Crang AJ. Transplanted glial cells migrate over a greater distance and remyelinate demyelinated lesions more rapidly than endogenous remyelinating cells. J Neurosci Res 2000;61(3):288–294.
137. Utzschneider DA, Archer DR, Kocsis JD, Waxman SG, Duncan ID. Transplantation of glial cells enhances action potential conduction of amyelinated spinal cord axons in the myelin-deficient rat. Proc Natl Acad Sci USA 1994;91(1):53–57.
138. Blakemore WF. Remyelination of CNS axons by Schwann cells transplanted from the sciatic nerve. Nature 1977;266(5597):68–69.
139. Blakemore WF, Crang AJ, Patterson RC. Schwann cell remyelination of CNS axons following injection of cultures of CNS cells into areas of persistent demyelination. Neurosci Lett 1987;77(1):20–24.
140. Baron-Van Evercooren A, Gansmuller A, Duhamel E, Pascal F, Gumpel M. Repair of a myelin lesion by Schwann cells transplanted in the adult mouse spinal cord. J Neuroimmunol 1992;40(2–3):235–242.
141. Baron-Van Evercooren A, Avellana-Adalid V, Lachapelle F, Liblau R. Schwann cell transplantation and myelin repair of the CNS. Mult Scler 1997;3(2):157–161.
142. Kohama I, Lankford KL, Preiningerova J, White FA, Vollmer TL, Kocsis JD. Transplantation of cryopreserved adult human Schwann cells enhances axonal conduction in demyelinated spinal cord. J Neurosci 2001;21(3):944–950.
143. Honmou O, Felts PA, Waxman SG, Kocsis JD. Restoration of normal conduction properties in demyelinated spinal cord axons in the adult rat by transplantation of exogenous Schwann cells. J Neurosci 1996;16(10):3199–3208.
144. Avellana-Adalid V, Bachelin C, Lachapelle F, Escriou C, Ratzkin B, Baron-Van Evercooren A. In vitro and in vivo behaviour of NDF-expanded monkey Schwann cells. Eur J Neurosci 1998;10(1):291–300.
145. Imaizumi T, Lankford KL, Kocsis JD. Transplantation of olfactory ensheathing cells or Schwann cells restores rapid and secure conduction across the transected spinal cord. Brain Res 2000;854(1–2):70–78.
146. Barnett SC, Hutchins AM, Noble M. Purification of olfactory nerve ensheathing cells from the olfactory bulb. Dev Biol 1993;155(2):337–350.
147. Barnett SC. Olfactory ensheathing cells: unique glial cell types? J Neurotrauma 2004;21(4):375–382.
148. Barnett SC, Roskams AJ. Olfactory ensheathing cells. Isolation and culture from the rat olfactory bulb. Methods Mol Biol 2002;198:41–48.
149. Barnett SC, Alexander CL, Iwashita Y, et al. Identification of a human olfactory ensheathing cell that can effect transplant-mediated remyelination of demyelinated CNS axons. Brain 2000;123(pt 8):1581–1588.
150. Franklin RJ, Gilson JM, Franceschini IA, Barnett SC. Schwann cell-like myelination following transplantation of an olfactory bulb-ensheathing cell line into areas of demyelination in the adult CNS. Glia 1996;17(3):217–224.
151. Imaizumi T, Lankford KL, Waxman SG, Greer CA, Kocsis JD. Transplanted olfactory ensheathing cells remyelinate and enhance axonal conduction in the demyelinated dorsal columns of the rat spinal cord. J Neurosci 1998;18(16):6176–6185.
152. Imaizumi T, Lankford KL, Burton WV, Fodor WL, Kocsis JD. Xenotransplantation of transgenic pig olfactory ensheathing cells promotes axonal regeneration in rat spinal cord. Nat Biotechnol 2000;18(9):949–953.
153. Smith PM, Lakatos A, Barnett SC, Jeffery ND, Franklin RJ. Cryopreserved cells isolated from the adult canine olfactory bulb are capable of extensive remyelination following transplantation into the adult rat CNS. Exp Neurol 2002;176(2):402–406.
154. Franklin RJ. Remyelination by transplanted olfactory ensheathing cells. Anat Rec 2003;271B(1):71–76.
155. Keyvan-Fouladi N, Li Y, Raisman G. How do transplanted olfactory ensheathing cells restore function? Brain Res Brain Res Rev 2002;40(1–3):325–327.
156. Santos-Benito FF, Ramon-Cueto A. Olfactory ensheathing glia transplantation: a therapy to promote repair in the mammalian central nervous system. Anat Rec 2003;271B(1):77–85.
157. Kato T, Honmou O, Uede T, Hashi K, Kocsis JD. Transplantation of human olfactory ensheathing cells elicits remyelination of demyelinated rat spinal cord. Glia 2000;30(3):209–218.
158. Li Y, Carlstedt T, Berthold CH, Raisman G. Interaction of transplanted olfactory-ensheathing cells and host astrocytic processes provides a bridge for axons to regenerate across the dorsal root entry zone. Exp Neurol 2004;188(2):300–308.
159. Li Y, Field PM, Raisman G. Repair of adult rat corticospinal tract by transplants of olfactory ensheathing cells. Science 1997;277(5334):2000–2002.
160. Ramon-Cueto A, Plant GW, Avila J, Bunge MB. Long-distance axonal regeneration in the transected adult rat spinal cord is promoted by olfactory ensheathing glia transplants. J Neurosci 1998;18(10):3803–3815.
161. Ramon-Cueto A, Cordero MI, Santos-Benito FF, Avila J. Functional recovery of paraplegic rats and motor axon regeneration in their spinal cords by olfactory ensheathing glia. Neuron 2000;25(2):425–435.
162. Lipson AC, Widenfalk J, Lindqvist E, Ebendal T, Olson L. Neurotrophic properties of olfactory ensheathing glia. Exp Neurol 2003;180(2):167–171.
163. Woodhall E, West AK, Chuah MI. Cultured olfactory ensheathing cells express nerve growth factor, brain-derived neurotrophic factor, glia cell line-derived neurotrophic factor and their receptors. Brain Res Mol Brain Res 2001;88(1–2):203–213.
164. Franklin RJ. Obtaining olfactory ensheathing cells from extra-cranial sources a step closer to clinical transplant-mediated repair of the CNS? Brain 2002;125(pt 1):2–3.
165. Weissman I, Spangrude G, Heimfeld S, Smith L, Uchida N. Stem cells. Nature 1991;353(6339):26.
166. Vescovi AL, Parati EA, Gritti A, et al. Isolation and cloning of multipotential stem cells from the embryonic human CNS and establishment of transplantable human neural stem cell lines by epigenetic stimulation. Exp Neurol 1999;156(1):71–83.

167. Galli R, Gritti A, Bonfanti L, Vescovi AL. Neural stem cells: an overview. Circ Res 2003;92(6):598–608.
168. Vescovi AL, Gritti A, Galli R, Parati EA. Isolation and intracerebral grafting of nontransformed multipotential embryonic human CNS stem cells. J Neurotrauma 1999;16(8):689–693.
169. Teng YD, Lavik EB, Qu X, et al. Functional recovery following traumatic spinal cord injury mediated by a unique polymer scaffold seeded with neural stem cells. Proc Natl Acad Sci USA 2002;99(5):3024–3029.
170. McDonald JW, Liu XZ, Qu Y, et al. Transplanted embryonic stem cells survive, differentiate and promote recovery in injured rat spinal cord. Nat Med 1999;5(12):1410–1412.
171. Modo M, Stroemer RP, Tang E, Patel S, Hodges H. Effects of implantation site of stem cell grafts on behavioral recovery from stroke damage. Stroke 2002;33(9):2270–2278.
172. Veizovic T, Beech JS, Stroemer RP, Watson WP, Hodges H. Resolution of stroke deficits following contralateral grafts of conditionally immortal neuroepithelial stem cells. Stroke 2001;32(4):1012–1019.
173. Yandava BD, Billinghurst LL, Snyder EY. "Global" cell replacement is feasible via neural stem cell transplantation: evidence from the dysmyelinated shiverer mouse brain. Proc Natl Acad Sci USA 1999;96(12):7029–7034.
174. Wu S, Suzuki Y, Kitada M, et al. New method for transplantation of neurosphere cells into injured spinal cord through cerebrospinal fluid in rat. Neurosci Lett 2002;318(2):81–84.
175. Wu S, Suzuki Y, Kitada M, et al. Migration, integration, and differentiation of hippocampus-derived neurosphere cells after transplantation into injured rat spinal cord. Neurosci Lett 2001;312(3):173–176.
176. Hammang JP, Archer DR, Duncan ID. Myelination following transplantation of EGF-responsive neural stem cells into a myelin-deficient environment. Exp Neurol 1997;147(1):84–95.
177. Milward EA, Lundberg CG, Ge B, Lipsitz D, Zhao M, Duncan ID. Isolation and transplantation of multipotential populations of epidermal growth factor-responsive, neural progenitor cells from the canine brain. J Neurosci Res 1997;50(5):862–871.
178. Ader M, Meng J, Schachner M, Bartsch U. Formation of myelin after transplantation of neural precursor cells into the retina of young postnatal mice. Glia 2000;30(3):301–310.
179. Ader M, Schachner M, Bartsch U. Transplantation of neural precursor cells into the dysmyelinated CNS of mutant mice deficient in the myelin-associated glycoprotein and Fyn tyrosine kinase. Eur J Neurosci 2001;14(3):561–566.
180. Avellana-Adalid V, Nait-Oumesmar B, Lachapelle F, Baron-Van Evercooren A. Expansion of rat oligodendrocyte progenitors into proliferative "oligospheres" that retain differentiation potential. J Neurosci Res 1996;45(5):558–570.
181. Vitry S, Avellana-Adalid V, Hardy R, Lachapelle F, Baron-Van Evercooren A. Mouse oligospheres: from pre-progenitors to functional oligodendrocytes. J Neurosci Res 1999;58(6):735–751.
182. Vitry S, Avellana-Adalid V, Lachapelle F, Evercooren AB. Migration and multipotentiality of PSA-NCAM+ neural precursors transplanted in the developing brain. Mol Cell Neurosci 2001;17(6):983–1000.
183. Learish RD, Brustle O, Zhang SC, Duncan ID. Intraventricular transplantation of oligodendrocyte progenitors into a fetal myelin mutant results in widespread formation of myelin. Ann Neurol 1999;46(5):716–722.
184. Zhang SC, Lipsitz D, Duncan ID. Self-renewing canine oligodendroglial progenitor expanded as oligospheres. J Neurosci Res 1998;54(2):181–190.
185. Ben-Hur T, Rogister B, Murray K, Rougon G, Dubois-Dalcq M. Growth and fate of PSA-NCAM+ precursors of the postnatal brain. J Neurosci 1998;18(15):5777–5788.
186. Mayer-Proschel M, Kalyani AJ, Mujtaba T, Rao MS. Isolation of lineage-restricted neuronal precursors from multipotent neuroepithelial stem cells. Neuron 1997;19(4):773–785.
187. Kleene R, Schachner M. Glycans and neural cell interactions. Nat Rev Neurosci 2004;5(3):195–208.
188. Keirstead HS, Ben-Hur T, Rogister B, O'Leary MT, Dubois-Dalcq M, Blakemore WF. Polysialylated neural cell adhesion molecule-positive CNS precursors generate both oligodendrocytes and Schwann cells to remyelinate the CNS after transplantation. J Neurosci 1999;19(17):7529–7536.
189. Ben-Hur T, Einstein O, Mizrachi-Kol R, et al. Transplanted multipotential neural precursor cells migrate into the inflamed white matter in response to experimental autoimmune encephalomyelitis. Glia 2003;41(1):73–80.
190. Bulte JW, Ben-Hur T, Miller BR, et al. MR microscopy of magnetically labeled neurospheres transplanted into the Lewis EAE rat brain. Magn Reson Med 2003;50(1):201–205.
191. Akiyama Y, Honmou O, Kato T, Uede T, Hashi K, Kocsis JD. Transplantation of clonal neural precursor cells derived from adult human brain establishes functional peripheral myelin in the rat spinal cord. Exp Neurol 2001;167(1):27–39.
192. Smith AG. Embryo-derived stem cells: of mice and men. Annu Rev Cell Dev Biol 2001;17:435–462.
193. Evans M, Hunter S. Source and nature of embryonic stem cells. C R Biol 2002;325(10):1003–1007.
194. Nakatsuji N, Suemori H. Embryonic stem cell lines of nonhuman primates. ScientificWorldJournal 2002;2:1762–1773.
195. Smith AG, Heath JK, Donaldson DD, et al. Inhibition of pluripotential embryonic stem cell differentiation by purified polypeptides. Nature 1988;336(6200):688–690.
196. Heath JK, Smith AG, Hsu LW, Rathjen PD. Growth and differentiation factors of pluripotential stem cells. J Cell Sci Suppl 1990;13:75–85.
197. Carpenter MK, Cui X, Hu ZY, et al. In vitro expansion of a multipotent population of human neural progenitor cells. Exp Neurol 1999;158(2):265–278.
198. Bain G, Kitchens D, Yao M, Huettner JE, Gottlieb DI. Embryonic stem cells express neuronal properties in vitro. Dev Biol 1995;168(2):342–357.
199. Finley MF, Kulkarni N, Huettner JE. Synapse formation and establishment of neuronal polarity by P19 embryonic carcinoma cells and embryonic stem cells. J Neurosci 1996;16(3):1056–1065.

200. Xian HQ, Gottlieb DI. Peering into early neurogenesis with embryonic stem cells. Trends Neurosci 2001;24(12):685–686.
201. Lang KJ, Rathjen J, Vassilieva S, Rathjen PD. Differentiation of embryonic stem cells to a neural fate: a route to re-building the nervous system? J Neurosci Res 2004;76(2):184–192.
202. Brustle O, Jones KN, Learish RD, et al. Embryonic stem cell-derived glial precursors: a source of myelinating transplants. Science 1999;285(5428):754–756.
203. Billon N, Jolicoeur C, Ying QL, Smith A, Raff M. Normal timing of oligodendrocyte development from genetically engineered, lineage-selectable mouse ES cells. J Cell Sci 2002;115(pt 18):3657–3665.
204. Liu S, Qu Y, Stewart TJ, et al. Embryonic stem cells differentiate into oligodendrocytes and myelinate in culture and after spinal cord transplantation. Proc Natl Acad Sci USA 2000;97(11):6126–6131.
205. Mitome M, Low HP, van den Pol A, et al. Towards the reconstruction of central nervous system white matter using neural precursor cells. Brain 2001;124(pt 11):2147–2161.
206. Thomson JA, Itskovitz-Eldor J, Shapiro SS, et al. Embryonic stem cell lines derived from human blastocysts. Science 1998;282(5391):1145–1147.
207. Reubinoff BE, Pera MF, Fong CY, Trounson A, Bongso A. Embryonic stem cell lines from human blastocysts: somatic differentiation in vitro. Nat Biotechnol 2000;18(4):399–404.
208. Reubinoff BE, Itsykson P, Turetsky T, et al. Neural progenitors from human embryonic stem cells. Nat Biotechnol 2001;19(12):1134–1140.
209. Zhang SC, Wernig M, Duncan ID, Brustle O, Thomson JA. In vitro differentiation of transplantable neural precursors from human embryonic stem cells. Nat Biotechnol 2001;19(12):1129–1133.
210. Deacon T, Dinsmore J, Costantini LC, Ratliff J, Isacson O. Blastula-stage stem cells can differentiate into dopaminergic and serotonergic neurons after transplantation. Exp Neurol 1998;149(1):28–41.
211. Bjorklund LM, Sanchez-Pernaute R, Chung S, et al. Embryonic stem cells develop into functional dopaminergic neurons after transplantation in a Parkinson rat model. Proc Natl Acad Sci USA 2002;99(4):2344–2349.
212. Vescovi A, Gritti A, Cossu G, Galli R. Neural stem cells: plasticity and their transdifferentiation potential. Cells Tissues Organs 2002;171(1):64–76.
213. Bjornson CR, Rietze RL, Reynolds BA, Magli MC, Vescovi AL. Turning brain into blood: a hematopoietic fate adopted by adult neural stem cells in vivo. Science 1999;283(5401):534–537.
214. Horwitz EM. Stem cell plasticity: the growing potential of cellular therapy. Arch Med Res 2003;34(6):600–606.
215. Wagers AJ, Weissman IL. Plasticity of adult stem cells. Cell 2004;116(5):639–648.
216. Kondo M, Wagers AJ, Manz MG, et al. Biology of hematopoietic stem cells and progenitors: implications for clinical application. Annu Rev Immunol 2003;21:759–806.
217. Mezey E, Chandross KJ, Harta G, Maki RA, McKercher SR. Turning blood into brain: cells bearing neuronal antigens generated in vivo from bone marrow. Science 2000;290(5497):1779–1782.
218. Mezey E, Key S, Vogelsang G, Szalayova I, Lange GD, Crain B. Transplanted bone marrow generates new neurons in human brains. Proc Natl Acad Sci USA 2003;100(3):1364–1369.
219. Weimann JM, Charlton CA, Brazelton TR, Hackman RC, Blau HM. Contribution of transplanted bone marrow cells to Purkinje neurons in human adult brains. Proc Natl Acad Sci USA 2003;100(4):2088–2093.
220. Priller J, Persons DA, Klett FF, Kempermann G, Kreutzberg GW, Dirnagl U. Neogenesis of cerebellar Purkinje neurons from gene-marked bone marrow cells in vivo. J Cell Biol 2001;155(5):733–738.
221. Cogle CR, Yachnis AT, Laywell ED, et al. Bone marrow transdifferentiation in brain after transplantation: a retrospective study. Lancet 2004;363(9419):1432–1437.
222. Bonilla S, Alarcon P, Villaverde R, Aparicio P, Silva A, Martinez S. Haematopoietic progenitor cells from adult bone marrow differentiate into cells that express oligodendroglial antigens in the neonatal mouse brain. Eur J Neurosci 2002;15(3):575–582.
223. Tao H, Ma DD. Evidence for transdifferentiation of human bone marrow-derived stem cells: recent progress and controversies. Pathology 2003;35(1):6–13.
224. Alvarez-Dolado M, Pardal R, Garcia-Verdugo JM, et al. Fusion of bone-marrow-derived cells with Purkinje neurons, cardiomyocytes and hepatocytes. Nature 2003;425(6961):968–973.
225. Akiyama Y, Radtke C, Honmou O, Kocsis JD. Remyelination of the spinal cord following intravenous delivery of bone marrow cells. Glia 2002;39(3):229–236.
226. Inoue M, Honmou O, Oka S, Houkin K, Hashi K, Kocsis JD. Comparative analysis of remyelinating potential of focal and intravenous administration of autologous bone marrow cells into the rat demyelinated spinal cord. Glia 2003;44(2):111–118.
227. Brustle O, Choudhary K, Karram K, et al. Chimeric brains generated by intraventricular transplantation of fetal human brain cells into embryonic rats. Nat Biotechnol 1998;16(11):1040–1044.
228. Flax JD, Aurora S, Yang C, et al. Engraftable human neural stem cells respond to developmental cues, replace neurons, and express foreign genes. Nat Biotechnol 1998;16(11):1033–1039.
229. O'Leary MT, Blakemore WF. Oligodendrocyte precursors survive poorly and do not migrate following transplantation into the normal adult central nervous system. J Neurosci Res 1997;48(2):159–167.
230. Tourbah A, Linnington C, Bachelin C, Avellana-Adalid V, Wekerle H, Baron-Van Evercooren A. Inflammation promotes survival and migration of the CG4 oligodendrocyte progenitors transplanted in the spinal cord of both inflammatory and demyelinated EAE rats. J Neurosci Res 1997;50(5):853–861.
231. Mahmood A, Lu D, Chopp M. Intravenous administration of marrow stromal cells (MSCs) increases the expression of growth factors in rat brain after traumatic brain injury. J Neurotrauma 2004;21(1):33–39.
232. Tran PB, Ren D, Veldhouse TJ, Miller RJ. Chemokine receptors are expressed widely by embryonic and adult neural progenitor cells. J Neurosci Res 2004;76(1):20–34.

233. Coulombel L, Auffray I, Gaugler MH, Rosemblatt M. Expression and function of integrins on hematopoietic progenitor cells. Acta Haematol 1997;97(1–2):13–21.
234. Prestoz L, Relvas JB, Hopkins K, et al. Association between integrin-dependent migration capacity of neural stem cells in vitro and anatomical repair following transplantation. Mol Cell Neurosci 2001;18(5):473–484.
235. Brocke S, Piercy C, Steinman L, Weissman IL, Veromaa T. Antibodies to CD44 and integrin alpha4, but not L-selectin, prevent central nervous system inflammation and experimental encephalomyelitis by blocking secondary leukocyte recruitment. Proc Natl Acad Sci USA 1999;96(12):6896–6901.
236. Brustle O, Maskos U, McKay RD. Host-guided migration allows targeted introduction of neurons into the embryonic brain. Neuron 1995;15(6):1275–1285.
237. Flax JD, Aurora S, Yang C, et al. Engraftable human neural stem cells respond to developmental cues, replace neurons, and express foreign genes. Nat Biotechnol 1998;16(11):1033–1039.
238. Frank JA, Miller BR, Arbab AS, et al. Clinically applicable labeling of mammalian and stem cells by combining superparamagnetic iron oxides and transfection agents. Radiology 2003;228(2):480–487.
239. Bulte JW, Duncan ID, Frank JA. In vivo magnetic resonance tracking of magnetically labeled cells after transplantation. J Cereb Blood Flow Metab 2002;22(8):899–907.
240. Bulte JW, Zhang S, van Gelderen P, et al. Neurotransplantation of magnetically labeled oligodendrocyte progenitors: magnetic resonance tracking of cell migration and myelination. Proc Natl Acad Sci USA 1999;96(26):15256–15261.
241. Bulte JW, Douglas T, Witwer B, et al. Magnetodendrimers allow endosomal magnetic labeling and in vivo tracking of stem cells. Nat Biotechnol 2001;19(12):1141–1147.
242. Ben-Hur T, et al. In-vivo MRI tracking of magnetically labeled neural spheres transplanted in animal models of multiple sclerosis. Neurology 2004;62[suppl5(7)]:A112.
243. Ben-Hur, et al. Attenuation of chronic experimental autoimmune encephalomyelitis by intraventricular transplantation of neural spheres. Neurology 2004;62[suppl 5(7)]:A438.
244. Ourednik J, Ourednik V, Lynch WP, Schachner M, Snyder EY. Neural stem cells display an inherent mechanism for rescuing dysfunctional neurons. Nat Biotechnol 2002;20(11):1103–1110.
245. Park KI, Ourednik J, Ourednik V, et al. Global gene and cell replacement strategies via stem cells. Gene Ther 2002;9(10):613–624.
246. Lu P, Jones LL, Snyder EY, Tuszynski MH. Neural stem cells constitutively secrete neurotrophic factors and promote extensive host axonal growth after spinal cord injury. Exp Neurol 2003;181(2):115–129.
247. Linker RA, Maurer M, Gaupp S, et al. CNTF is a major protective factor in demyelinating CNS disease: a neurotrophic cytokine as modulator in neuroinflammation. Nat Med 2002;8(6):620–624.
248. Butzkueven H, Zhang JG, Soilu-Hanninen M, et al. LIF receptor signaling limits immune-mediated demyelination by enhancing oligodendrocyte survival. Nat Med 2002;8(6):613–619.
249. Villoslada P, Hauser SL, Bartke I, et al. Human nerve growth factor protects common marmosets against autoimmune encephalomyelitis by switching the balance of T helper cell type 1 and 2 cytokines within the central nervous system. J Exp Med 2000;191(10):1799–1806.
250. Flugel A, Matsumuro K, Neumann H, et al. Anti-inflammatory activity of nerve growth factor in experimental autoimmune encephalomyelitis: inhibition of monocyte transendothelial migration. Eur J Immunol 2001;31(1):11–22.
251. Ruffini F, Furlan R, Poliani PL, et al. Fibroblast growth factor-II gene therapy reverts the clinical course and the pathological signs of chronic experimental autoimmune encephalomyelitis in C57BL/6 mice. Gene Ther 2001;8(16):1207–1213.
252. Crang AJ, Blakemore WF. Remyelination of demyelinated rat axons by transplanted mouse oligodendrocytes. Glia 1991;4(3):305–313.

7

Stem Cells as a Source for Cell Replacement in Parkinson's Disease

Daniel Offen, Yossef S. Levy, and Eldad Melamed

Parkinson's disease (PD) is a progressive neurodegenerative disease of the basal ganglia (BG), consisting of a remarkable diversity of neuroactive substances, organized into functional subsystems. Pathologically, it is characterized by continuous dopaminergic cell loss in the nigrostriatal and other dopaminergic systems that are found outside the extrapyramidal system, and its main classic triad of signs involves resting tremor, rigidity, and bradykinesia. The disease affects about 1% of the population more than 50 years of age. Current treatment regimes for PD consist primarily of pharmacologic supplementation of the dopaminergic loss with dopamine (DA) agonist and L-3-4-dihydroxyphenylalanine (L-DOPA, levodopa), a precursor of DA. Levodopa that can readily cross the blood-brain barrier is the most effective agent controlling the symptoms of PD. Most PD patients have a good initial response to levodopa, but, after a few years, become subject to adverse effects, which include dyskinesia, fluctuations of efficacy (on-off effect), freezing, mental changes, and loss of efficacy.

Functional replacement of specific neuronal populations through transplantation of neural tissue represents an attractive therapeutic strategy for treating neurodegenerative disorders such as PD. Given that most neurodegenerative diseases affect the neuronal populations of specific neurochemical phenotypes, an ideal source material for transplantation would be a reproducible cell that could be instructed to assume the desired neuronal phenotype upon differentiation. The strategy of cell replacement therapy seeks to replace the loss in synaptic signaling caused by neuronal degeneration. In late 1970s, Bjorklund and collaborators demonstrated that the transplantation of embryonic DA neural tissue, obtained from the fetal ventral mesencephalon, could reverse the symptoms of DA depletion in the unilateral 6-hydroxydopamine (6-OHDA)-treated rat model of PD.[1,2] Encouraged by these findings in animal models, Lindvall and Hagell[3] launched a clinical program in 1984–1985 to attempt transplantation of embryonic neural tissues into the brains of PD patients. Clinical trials with transplantation of human embryonic mesencephalic tissue into the caudate and putamen (striatum) of PD patients were initiated in 1987, and about 350 patients have since undergone transplantation.[3] These clinical tests showed that grafts of fetal ventral mesencephalon successfully survive and reduce motor symptoms.[4-10] Although transplantation is a promising treatment for PD, it requires as many as 5–10 fetal brains for only one PD patient, thus causing ethical and practical problems and limiting its clinical application. The mammalian adult brain is a very plastic system that is capable of incorporating transplanted stem cells into functional neurotransmission. In recent years, the questionable benefit and safety of this procedure has been raised, as a control study pointed to the high risk of adverse signs such as tardive dyskenesis.[11-13] The challenge of cell replacement in PD is huge and efforts to find the best cell source are still being continued with high priority. To overcome this problem, researchers are turning to stem cell biology for materials to use in the therapeutic transplantation of PD. Many researchers have investigated the use of a wide variety of candidate cells as possible transplantation donor cells for PD therapy. Our group has investigated bone marrow stromal cells (BMSc) for experimental therapeutics in PD animal models. However, the complete and coordinated induction of specific neuronal phenotype in multipotent neural precursors in vitro has proved elusive.[14,15] The initial success of levodopa treatment for PD suggested the feasibility of DA-replacement therapy by neural transplantation, and the small size of striatum (or caudate putamen in human beings), which becomes DA-denervated in PD, makes it an easily accessible target for transplantation.[16] Transplantation of DA-producing tissue has received considerable attention as an alternative therapy that delivers DA directly to the striatum, sparing other tissues from adverse effects of DA stimulation and metabolism, and avoiding the drug peaks and valleys of pharmacologic administration by providing a relatively constant source. Much of the scientific efforts during the past 15 years have therefore had to provide proof-of-principle that (i) the grafted DA neurons can survive and form connections in the PD patient's brain; (ii) the patient's brain can integrate and use the grafted neurons; and (iii) the grafts induce a measurable clinical improvement.[17] The aim of this chapter is to describe and illustrate current research strategies for generating tyrosine hydroxylase (TH) cells and/or DA neurons from embryonic and adult stem cells, and to discuss the possible role of this technology to further develop cell replacement therapy in PD.

Role of DA in PD

DA Biosynthesis

Dopaminergic neurons can be identified by the expression of proteins required for the biosynthesis, transport, synaptic packaging, release, and reuptake of DA. DA is produced from the amino acid tyrosine in two steps: TH catalyses the conversion of tyrosine to L-DOPA followed by decarboxylation to DA via the aromatic L-amino acid decarboxylase (AADC). The striatum contains a dense arborization of the fine terminals derived from the DA-containing neurons of the substantia nigra pars compacta (SNpc). Because these structures contain TH, the DA can be synthesized directly at the terminal varicosities. TH requires iron and tetrahydrobiopterine in order to oxidize tyrosine to L-DOPA. Only small amounts of L-DOPA are found in the tissue; however, it is readily decarboxylated by AADC. This enzyme is present in many tissues, including serotonergic neurons, where it decarboxylates 5-hydroxytryptophan to form serotonin. Similar to other amino acid decarboxylases, AADC requires pyridoxal phosphate as its coenzyme. DA synthesis in the nerve terminals is accelerated during depolarization-induced release of the neurotransmitter.

Two types of transporters are essential to DA neurotransmission: the plasma membrane DA transporter (DAT)[18] and the vesicular monoamine transporter 2 (VMAT2).[19] VMAT2 loads cytoplasmic DA, as well as all other monoaminergic neurotransmitters from the presynaptic nerve terminal into vesicles for storage and subsequent release. DA is rapidly taken up into storage vesicles by an energy-dependent transporter-mediated process. It accumulates extremely high concentrations within the storage vesicle by complexing with adenosine triphosphate and vesicular proteins. When the nerve terminal is depolarized by the arrival of a potential action, calcium enters the nerve terminal through voltage-dependent calcium channels. Local increases in calcium promote vesicle fusion to the nerve membrane and DA is released into the extracellular space.[20] DAT is found exclusively in DA neurons where it terminates the action of DA by rapidly removing it from the synapse.[21,22]

Specific DA Pathways in the Mammalian Brain

DA is widely distributed throughout the brain, with particularly high concentrations in the striatal areas.[23] Indeed, although DA accounts for about half of the total catecholamines in the brain, more than 80% of brain DA is in the BG.

DA neurons, one of the many types in the brain of higher vertebrates, are located in the midbrain within the lateral groups of retrorubral field (A8) and the substantia nigra pars compacta (A9), as well as the medially located ventral tegmental area (A10). DA neurons are projected to different forebrain areas, forming the mesotelenecephalic system, where the target neurons are localized in the striatal, limbic, and cortical areas. The substantia nigra pars compacta neurons are connected to the dorsolateral striatum, the caudate putamen, forming the nigrostriatal pathway that is the principal dopaminergic fiber system in the brain and involved in the control of voluntary movement. The neurons of the ventral tegmental area project via the median forebrain bundle to the ventromedial striatum and the subcortical and cortical areas, forming the mesolimbocortical system, which is involved in emotional behavior and mechanisms of natural motivation and reward. Finally, retrorubral field neurons are connected to the substantia nigra and ventral tegmental area and seem to be involved in interconnecting these two areas. They also project to the dorsal striatum via the nigrostriatal pathway.[21,24,25] In addition, there are also DA-containing neurons and terminals in other brain regions, in the retina, and in the spinal cord. The loss of dopaminergic neurons, mainly in the substantia nigra pars compacta and the nigrostriatal pathway seems to have a critical role in Parkinson's and other neurodegenerative diseases.

Stem Cells in the Central Nervous System

Neuronal Stem Cells

The adult vertebrate central nervous system (CNS) consists of four major differentiated cell types: neurons, astrocytes, oligodendrocytes, and ependymal cells. Neuronal stem cells (NSCs) are the self-renewing multipotent stem cells derived from the nervous system with a capacity to give rise to cells belonging to all lineages in the nervous system, namely, neurons, oligodendrocytes, and astrocytes.[26] The long-held belief that we are born with a certain number of nerve cells and that the brain cannot generate new neurons and renew itself has been inverted.[27] Neurogenesis has been shown to occur throughout adulthood in the adult mammalian brain and new neurons are generated continuously in some regions of the adult CNS.[28,29] The forebrain subventricular zone (SVZ) and dentate gyrus are considered to be the major sources of self-renewing, multipotent NSCs.[27] NSCs in the adult SVZ form a cellular continuum with the core of the olfactory bulb (OB) through an extension called the rostral migratory stream (RMS). Cells that originate from the anterior SVZ migrate within the RMS to reside within the OB. Results from in vitro studies with material from human surgical specimens has shown that NSCs can be isolated from regions of the adult human brain, including the wall of the lateral ventricle, cerebral white matter, and the hippocampus.[30,31] The rate of adult neurogenesis is affected by intrinsic and extrinsic factors. There is no direct evidence for generation of new neurons in response to acute injury, but the fact that younger patients have better recovery from ischemic stroke than older ones might be partly attributed to a more dynamic stem cell population existing in younger patients.[32] The self-repairing activity of the adult mammal is poor despite the presence of endogenous NSCs. This could be explained by the microenvironmental factors present in most of the areas of the adult CNS that may inhibit neuronal differentiation of endogenous NSCs, or by the number of endogenous NSCs that may be too small for effective self-repair.[33]

Stem Cells in Embryonic Brain

Three different methods have been successfully used to induce dopaminergic neurons from NSCs of embryo brain. Studer et al.[34] reproduced committed mesencephalic DA neuron precursors from rat embryos in culture. Upon elimination of the mitogen basic fibroblast growth factor (bFGF, FGF2), some cells differentiated into TH-positive, assuming dopaminergic neurons. The extended cells survived transplantation to the rat striatum but the survival of the grafted TH-positive cells was poor. Yan et al.[35] reported that the existence of ascorbic acid promotes dopaminergic differentiation when the mesencephalic precursors are proliferated for extended periods in vitro. Moreover, when the predifferentiation of the precursors was performed in cultures with low oxygen, both proliferation and dopaminergic differentiation were enhanced.[36] It is not yet known, however, whether ascorbic acid and low oxygen will increase the yield of surviving dopaminergic neurons after transplantation in vivo.[17,26]

Carvey et al.[37] described a method of inducing TH expression by reproducing mesencephalic progenitors from rat embryos with B27 and epidermal growth factor (EGF) in neurosphere cultures. Differentiation was achieved by further treatment with interleukin-11, leukemia inhibitory factor, and glial cell line-derived neurotrophic factor (GDNF). This treatment increased the number of TH+ cells to 20%–25% of the overall cell population. More recently, the same in vitro approach combined with low oxygen has also been used to generate cells expressing dopaminergic markers and releasing DA from human embryonic mesencephalic precursors.[38]

In the third approach, Wagner et al.[39] induced a dopaminergic phenotype in an immortalized multipotent mouse neural stem cell line by overexpressing nuclear receptor related-1 (Nurr1), in a mixture with as yet unidentified factors derived from type 1 astrocytes of a ventral mesencephalic source. Most of the Nurr1 transduced cells expressed the TH enzyme as well as aldehyde dehydrogenase-2 (Aldh2) and c-ret, two markers of midbrain mesencephalic dopaminergic neurons. The engineered neurons survived transplantation to the mouse striatum but the yield was very small.

Differentiation of NSCs from the embryonic brain to dopaminergic neurons in vitro (Table 7.1) and in vivo (Table 7.2) as demonstrated above, may offer an effective approach for studying the regulation of cell phenotypes. The plasticity of these cells suggests that they can respond to appropriate cues and may be an effective tool to study the progenitor event necessary to generate dopaminergic neurons. However, we do not foresee the use of NSCs from the embryonic brain as cell therapy in PD because of ethical problems and the complexity of producing these stem cells from the embryo.

NSCs in Adult Brain

During development, neuronal differentiation is influenced by a variety of extracellular signaling molecules that act through nuclear receptors or through one of several cell surface receptor-mediated signal cascades. The use of retinoic acid and forskolin in conjunction with neurotrophic factors such as brain-derived neurotrophic factor (BDNF) or neurotrophin-3 (NT3) has been tested for converting adult hippocampal precursors into dopaminergic neurons. The yield of TH+ neurons under these conditions remains very modest (< 2%) and no evidence of dopaminergic neuron function has been reported.[40]

Expression of Nurr1 in adult NSCs derived from the hippocampus (HC7 or C31), or treatment of these cells with retinoic acid or forskolin, was sufficient to induce TH expression.[41] Interestingly, in this study, Nurr1 was found to bind to the TH promoter and to activate the expression of a green florescence protein (GFP) reporter, indicating that Nurr1 promotes transactivation of the TH gene. However, because the induction of TH does not take place in other Nurr1-expressing NSCs, it seems likely that TH induction requires that additional factors be present in HC7 or C31 cells, and that they would have to be induced in c17.2 cells. In addition, overexpression of pituitary homeobox 3 (Pitx3) in the same system did not cause an increase in TH+ cells.

Daadi and Weiss[42] produced a low number of TH-expressing cells from adult mouse forebrain subependyma (SE) in vitro by exposure to FGF2 and glial cell conditioned media (CM). They labeled the SE precursor of the adult mouse forebrain in vivo by six injections of bromodeoxyuridine (BrdU), a thymidine analog and marker of newly synthesized DNA, given at 2-hour intervals. Thirty minutes after the last BrdU injection, the SE was dissected and cultured in the absence or presence of FGF2 + CM. In control conditions, many cells were labeled with BrdU, but none were TH immunoreactive. However, cultures treated with FGF2 + CM for 1–3 days showed newly generated TH immunoreactivity (0.23% of the total number of cells plated). Of those cells exhibiting TH immunoreactivity, 63% were BrdU-immunoreactive, suggesting that they were derived from the proliferating cells of the adult SE and were born during the 12 hours that preceded the primary culture. Other properties of these cells are unknown.

Akerud et. al.[43] used c17.2 mouse NSCs engineered to release GDNF, which support the nigral dopaminergic neurons.[44] The cells

Table 7.1. In vitro differentiation of stem cells to dopaminergic neural lineages

Population of cells	Induction of differentiation	Gene expression of neuronal lineage	Protein markers of neuronal lineage	Dopaminergic markers (Protein/RNA)	HPLC for DA	% of TH	Reference
Rodent embryonic stem (ES) cells							
Mouse	Five stage protocol. Stage 4: bFGF, Shh, FGF8; Stage5: AA	nestin, Otx1, Otx2	Nestin, β-tubulin III	TH, DA, Nurr1, Pax2, Pax5, Wnt1, En1	+	35	66,90
Mouse transfected with Nurr1	By a five stage protocol. FGF2 after Shh, FGF8	En1	β-Tubulin III, En1, Pax2, Otx2	TH, DA, Nurr1, DAT, Ptx3, AADC	+	78	146
Mouse transfected with Bcl-XL	Differentiated using a five-stage in vitro method	Pax2, Pax5, Wnt1	Nestin, β-tubulin III, calbindin, GFAP	En1, Nurr1, Pitx3, DAT, AADC, TH	+	31	69
Mouse	SDIA and GMEM, KSR, pyruvate, glutamine, ME, nonessential amino acid		β-Tubulin III, NCAM, nestin, synaptophysin	TH, Nurr1, Ptx3, DA	+	30	71
Mouse	SDIA and late BMP4 exposure or Shh	NCAM	β-Tubulin III, NCAM	TH, En2	No	65	77
Mouse nuclear transfer	FGF2, Shh, FGF8, AA		β-Tubulin III	TH	+	>50	89
Mouse nuclear transfer	5 d: SDIA; 2 d: SHH, FGF8, SRM; 4 d: N2, SHH, FGF8 bFGF; 3 d: ascorbic acid, BDNF	Nestin, β-tubulin III, MAP2	Nestin, β-tubulin III	TH, DAT, Pitx3, Nurr1, Lmx1b, En1	+	50	75
Mouse	IL-1β, GDNF, TGF-β₃, NTN, cAMP		Nestin, synaptophysin, GFAP	TH, DAT, D2R, Nurr1, En-1	+	40	76
Mouse transfected with Nurr1 and GFP	Shh, FGF8, AA		β-Tubulin III, nestin, GalC, GFAP	TH, AADC, DAT, Nurr1, calretinin, calbindin, Aldh2, Ptx3	+	62	147
Primate ES cells							
Human embryoid bodies	RA for 10 d	NF-L	NF-H	DRD1, AADC	No	NT	83
Human embryoid bodies	EGF, FGF2, PDGF, IGF1 (3 d) then NT3, BDNF (14–16 d)		β-Tubulin III, nestin, NCAM, MAP2, A2B5, GFAP, synaptophysin	TH	No	3	78
Human ES spheres	RA for 14–21 d (±PDGF, bFGF, EGF)	Nestin, MBP, GFAP, NSE, NF-M	NCAM, vimentin, nestin, β-tubulin III, synaptophysin, NF-L, NF-M, MAP2, synaptophysin, GFAP, O4	TH, Pax6	No	<1	79

(Continued)

Table 7.1. In vitro differentiation of stem cells to dopaminergic neural lineages—Cont'd

Population of cells	Induction of differentiation	Gene expression of neuronal lineage	Protein markers of neuronal lineage	Dopaminergic markers (Protein/RNA)	HPLC for DA	% of TH	Reference
Human embryoid bodies	Cultured on ornithine/laminin substrate in a medium consisting of DMEM/F12, N2 supplement, cAMP, BDNF		NCAM, nestin, musashi1, β-tubulin III, NF-H, GFAP, O4	TH	No	<1	82
Human cell line (MB03)	N2, FGF2, TGF-α		GFAP, NF-200, NF-M	TH	+	20	84
Human cell line (BG01)	SDIA + GDNF or SDIA + astrocytes originating from either embryonic striatum or embryonic rat ventral mesencephalon			TH, DAT, En1, Pitx3	No	934 cells per well	85
Human cell line (H1, H9, HES-3)	sequential application of SDIA, Shh, FGF8, BDNF, GDNF, TGF-β₃, cAMP, AA	MAP2	Nestin, β-tubulin III	TH, VMAT2, AADC, En1, Lmx1b, Nurr1, Nurr1, Aldh1	+	79	86
Cynomolgus monkey	SDIA		β-Tubulin III, NCAM, NeuN	TH, DA, Nurr1, Lmx1b	+	35	72
Cynomolgus monkey	SDIA and late BMP4 exposure or Shh		β-Tubulin III	TH	No	5	77
Macaca fascicularis monkey parthenogenesis	FGF2, Shh, FGF8, AA		β-Tubulin III	TH	+	25	92
Human embryonal carcinoma cell line NT2	RA for 5 wk then LiCl or FGF1 + TEPA + DA + IBMX + forskolin		β-Tubulin III, tau, GAP43	TH, DAT, D2R, Nurr1, Aldh2	+	up to 75	148–154
Bone marrow stromal cells (BMSc)							
Rat	BHA, forskolin, DMSO, heparin, K252a, KCl, valproic acid, bFGF, PDGF	NF-M, tau, synaptophysin	β-Tubulin III, synaptophysin, tau	TH	No	few	102
Rat	Vectors construct consisting of the TH gene and GC gene separated by an internal ribosome entry site	NT	NT	TH, GC, L-DOPA	L-DOPA	most of the cells	118
Rat/human transfected with NICD	bFGF, CNTF, forskolin (7 d) BDNF + NGF or GDNF (11 d)		Nestin, MAP2, β-tubulin III, NF-M	TH, Nurr1, Lmx1b, Pitx3	+	41	114

Source	Culture conditions	Markers	Markers	DA phenotype	+after BH₄	Ref
Human	EGF + bFGF then BDNF + RA	nestin, NeuroD1, Neurog2, musashi1, MBP, β-tubulin III, α-synuclein	MAP2, β-tubulin III	TH	11	115
Human	EGF, bFGF, cAMP, and several growth factors	NEGF2, NSE, glipican 4, necdin, NF-H, NF-M, CD90, nestin	β-Tubulin III, NSE, NF-H, nestin, NeuN, α-synuclein	TH, AADC, D2DR, VMAT2, Nurr1, Pitx3, Aldh1, En1	L-DOPA, DA, DOPAC	60	109
Multipotent adult progenitor cells (MAPCs)						
Rat and mouse	Sequentially with bFGF, FGF8, BDNF for 7 d	Otx2, Otx1, Pax2, Pax5, nestin	GFAP, GalC, NF-H,tau, MAP2	AADC, TH	No	30	123
Mouse	Sequentially with bFGF, FGF8, Shh, BDNF for 7 d, coculturing with astrocytes	Sox1, Otx1, Otx2, Pax2, Pax5, En1, Nestin, GFAP, MBP, GABA	Nestin, NF-H, MBP, GFAP, tau	AADC, TH, DAT, DBH, DA, Nurr1	No	23	122
Adult neuronal stem cells (NSCs)						
Adult rat hippocampus	Sequentially with FGF2, RA, FBS + NGF or BDNF or NT3	trkA, trkB, trkC	MAP2, β-tubulin III, calbindin, GFAP, Gal-C	TH	No	1	40
Adult rat hippocampus	Vectors construct consisting of Nurr1, Pitx3, Shh-N. Sequentially with FGF2, RA or froskolin or FGF8	NT	MAP2	TH, AADC	No	1.5	41
Adult mouse subependyma of lateral ventricle of forebrain	FGF2, glial cell conditioned medium	NT	NT	TH	No	0.23	42
Adult rat substantia nigra progenitor cells	Sequentially DMEM/F12 + N2 supplement + FGF8 or FGF2, DMEM/F12 + FBS + RA for 7 d	NT	Nestin, A2B5, NG2, GFAP, RIP, β-tubulin III	NT	No	NT	52

Acetylcholine esterase (AChE); aldehyde dehydrogenase 1/2 (Aldh1/2); L-amino acid decarboxylase (AADC); ascorbic acid (AA); basic fibroblast growth factor (bFGF, FGF2); brain-derived neurotrophic factor (BDNF); butylated hydroxyanisole (BHA); choline acetyltransferase (ChAT); chondroitin sulfate proteoglycan (NG2); ciliary neurotrophic factor (CNTF); CNPase (marker of oligodendrocytes); dihydroxyphenylacetic acid (DOPAC); 3,4-dihydroxyphenylalanine (L-DOPA); dimethylsulfoxide (DMSO); dopamine (DA); dopamine β-hydroxylase (DBH); dopamine receptor 2 (D2R); dopamine transporter (DAT); Engrailed 1 (En1); Engrailed 2 (En2); fetal bovine serum (FBS); fetal calf serum (FCS); γ-aminobutyric acid (GABA); galactocerebroside (GalC); glasgow minimum essential media (GMEM); glial acidic fibrillary protein (GFAP); glial cell line-derived neurotrophic factor (GDNF); glutamate (Glu); glutamate decarboxylase (GAD); glutamate transporter (GluT); green fluorescence protein (GFP); growth-associated protein (GAP43); high-performance liquid chromatography (HPLC); insulin-like growth factor-1 (IGF1); interleukin-1β (IL-1β); isobutyl-methylxanthine (IBMX); knockout serum replacement (KSR); LIM homeobox transcription factor 1 beta (Lmx1b); lithium chloride (LiCl); microtubule-associated protein 2 (MAP2); 2-mercaptoethanol (ME); myelin basic protein (MBP); neural cell adhesion molecule (NCAM); neurite growth-promoting factor 2 (NEGF2); neurofilament heavy (NF-H); neurofilament light (NF-L); neurofilament medium (NF-M); nerve growth factor (NGF); neurogenic differentiation 1 (NeuroD1); neurogenin 2 (Neurog 2); neuron specific enolase (NSE); neuronal nuclei (NeuN); neurotrophin-3 (NT3); neurturin (NTN); Noch intracellular domain (NICD); not tested (NT); nuclear receptor related-1 (Nurr1); phorbol 12-myristate 13-acetate (TPA); platelet-derived growth factor (PDGF); receptor interacting protein (RIP); all-trans retinoic acid (RA); serum replacement medium (SRM); sonic hedgehog (Shh); stromal cell-derived inducing activity (SDIA); tetrahydrobiopterin (BH₄); transforming growth factor-α or β₃ (TGF-α or β₃); tyrosine hydroxylase (TH); vesicular acetylcholine transporter (VAChT); unified PD rating scale (UPDRS).

Table 7.2. In vivo differentiation of stem cells to neural lineages after transplantation

Population of Cells/Source	Differentiation	Animal model	Dopaminergic and neuronal markers (surviving TH+ cells)	Behavioral test	Behavioral recovery	Reference
Embryonic stem (ES) cells						
Mouse	With or without RA	6-OHDA-lesioned nigrostriatal, rat model for PD	TH (14,500), NSE, NF-H	NT	NT	64
Mouse	Small number of undifferentiated cells	Lesioned the median forebrain bundle by 6-OHDA, rat model for PD	TH (2100), NeuN, DAT, AACD, AHD2, calretinin, calbindin, serotonin	Rotation, PET	+	65
Mouse transfected with Nurr1	By a five-stage protocol	Lesioned striatum by 6-OHDA, rat model for PD	TH (NT), calbindin	Rotation, step, paw-reaching, cylinder	+	146
Mouse	Differentiated using a five-stage in vitro method	6-OHDA-lesioned striatum, mouse model for PD	TH (NT)	Rotational	+	70
Mouse transfected with Bcl-XL	Differentiated using a five-stage in vitro method	Lesioned substantia nigra by 6-OHDA, rat model for PD	TH (18,310)	Rotational, step	+	69
Mouse	ES colonies were cultured on PA6 cells (12 d)	6-OHDA lesioned striatum, mouse model for PD	TH (13,000), β-tubulin III	NT	NT	71
Mouse	ES colonies were cultured on PA6 cells (12 d)	6-OHDA lesioned striatum, mouse model for PD	TH, β-tubulin III	NT	NT	73
Cynomolgus monkey	ES cells were cultured on PA6 cells for 3 wk	6-OHDA lesioned striatum, mouse model for PD	TH (830)	NT	NT	72
Mouse or nuclear transfer	5 d: coculture on stromal cell line 2 d: SHH, FGF8, SRM 4 d: N2, SHH, FGF8, bFGF 3 d: N2, AA, BDNF	6-OHDA lesioned striatum, mouse model for PD	TH (23,000), DAT, AADC	Rotational	+	75

Cell type	Treatment	Model	Markers	Behavioral test	Improvement	Ref.
Human embryonal carcinoma cell line NT2	LiCl pretreated hNT-DA neurons	6-OHDA lesioned nigrostriatal, rat model for PD	TH (few)	Rotational	No	155
Bone marrow stromal cells (BMSc) Mouse	Undifferentiated	MPTP mouse model of PD; cells grafted in striatum 1 wk later	TH (52)	Rotorod	+	121
Mouse	Vectors construct consisting of the GDNF gene	MPTP mouse model of PD; cells grafted intravenously 6 wk before	TH	Locomotor activity	+	119
Rat	Vectors construct consisting of the TH and GC genes	6-OHDA rat model for PD	TH, GC, L-DOPA	Rotation	+	117
Rat/human transfected with NICD	bFGF, CNTF, forskolin (7 d) GDNF (11 d)	6-OHDA rat model for PD	TH (45%), DAT	Rotation, step, paw-reaching	+	114
Neural stem cells (NSCs) c17.2 mouse	NSCs engineered to release GDNF	6-OHDA lesioned striatum, mouse model for PD	Nestin, NeuN, GFAP, CNPase, TH (350)	Rotation	+	43
c17.2 mouse	Undifferentiated	6-OHDA lesioned striatum, rat model for PD	β-Tubulin III, NSE, NeuN, TH, AADC	Rotation	No	156
Human	Differentiation medium (not described)	Human PD	Not relevant	UPDRS	+	55,56

engrafted well in the host striatum, incorporated, and differentiated into neurons (neuronal nuclei, NeuN), astrocytes (glial acidic fibrillary protein, GFAP), and oligodendrocytes (CNPase), 1 month after grafting, and produced high stable levels of GDNF. The percentage of animals showing engraftment at 4 months reached 12.5% in animals receiving GDNF-c17.2 grafts. However, grafting GDNF-c17.2 cells in adult nude mice resulted in the engraftment of cells in 100% of the animals after 4 months. Double TH and GDNF immunohistochemistry clearly showed that GDNF immunoreactivity was contained both in the substantia nigra neurophil and within dopaminergic neurons, suggesting that GDNF was efficiently transported in a retrograde manner by dopaminergic neurons from the striatum to the substantia nigra. GDNF-expressing NSCs decreased the loss of substantia nigra dopaminergic neurons, and increased levels of TH immunoreactivity in the striatum in a 6-OHDA mouse model of PD and showed improvement in behavioral tests.

Yang et al.[45] have shown that undifferentiated NSCs from newborn mouse cerebellum, transplanted into the rat intact or 6-OHDA-lesioned striatum, migrated within the host striatum, and expressed markers associated with neuronal [β-tubulin III, NeuN, and neuron specific enolase (NSE)] but not glial [GFAP−, myelin basic protein (MBP−), A2B5−] differentiation. In 70% of cases, the vast majority of these cells expressed the DA-synthesizing enzymes TH and AADC, 2–5 weeks postgraft. In contrast, no NSCs stained for DA β-hydroxylase (DBH), choline acetyltransferase, glutamate decarboxylase (GAD), or serotonin. Because NSCs were capable of migration and differentiation into TH-expressing cells when grafted directly into a 6-OHDA-lesioned striatum, the response of cells if placed either at a distance from the site of DA denervation or in the absence of DA depletion, was examined. Thus, in this study, NSCs were implanted in the striatum on the side contralateral to a previous 6-OHDA lesion or into the striatum of an intact (unlesioned) rat. When animals were sacrificed 2–4 weeks later, it was observed that the NSCs placed contralaterally as well as those in the intact brain behaved identically to those placed ipsilaterally. It was concluded that, after transplantation into the intact or 6-OHDA-lesioned rat, the adult brain contains intrinsic cues sufficient to direct the specific expression of dopaminergic traits in immature multipotential NSCs. Apparently, the loss of a particular cell type signals the brain to elicit differentiation factors capable of instructing transplanted stem cells in the appropriate phenotypic choices. Natural cues available in the brain can constitutively direct the integration and differentiation of not only some, but virtually all, transplanted NSCs, resulting in their development into neuronal-like cells expressing DA traits. These preliminary data suggest that the TH expressed in engrafted NSCs may produce some measure of DA, a prospect that could improve as TH-expressing NSCs mature, may extend a more extensive neuritic network, and integrate more fully into the host brain.

The most active neurogenic regions are the dentate gyrus (DG) of the hippocampus and the OB. It has been estimated that approximately 10,000 new neurons are added each day to the adult rat DG,[46] and the rate of neurogenesis in the OB is likely to be several-fold higher. In addition to the neurogenesis in the OB and DG, low numbers of new neurons have been suggested to be generated in other parts of the hippocampus as well as in the cortex,[47,48] although the latter remains controversial.[49] Moreover, recent studies in an animal model of stroke have demonstrated neurogenesis in several additional regions in response to injury.[50,51] Obviously, such self-repair mechanisms, if they are in operation in the adult SNpc, are insufficient and need to be more effective.

The question whether the dopaminergic neurons in the SNpc can be divided locally is still unresolved. Lie et al.[52] have shown that the adult rat SNpc contains a population of actively dividing progenitor cells, which in situ give rise only to new mature glial cells but not to neurons. Zhao et al.[53] reported a slow turnover of dopaminergic projection neurons in the adult rodent brain, and that neurogenesis is increased after a partial injury. However, using similar methodologic procedures, Frielingsdorf et al.[54] argue that they found no evidence of new dopaminergic neurons in the SNpc, either in normal or 6-OHDA-lesioned hemi-parkinsonian rodents, or even after growth factor treatment. Furthermore, they claim that there is no evidence of NSCs emanating from the cerebroventricular system and migrating to the substantia nigra. They conclude that it is unlikely that dopaminergic neurons are generated in the adult mammalian substantia nigra.

Human NSCs have been suggested for use in transplantation. This alternative graft source seems to avoid host immune responses and their ready availability and multipotentiality are just a few of their advantages over primary fetal tissues. Levesque and Neuman[55,56] discovered that adult NSCs harvested from a patient's own tissue can be used as a source of dopaminergic neurons to aid in the treatment of PD. The researchers' methodology included isolating adult human NSCs, expanding them in vitro, inducing them to differentiate into DA-secreting neurons, and selectively delivering them back to targets within the patients. Two years after the procedure was performed, the patients showed no symptoms of PD. Autologous stem cell transplantation has numerous advantages in the treatment of PD. The approach eliminates immune reactions at the site of implantation and improves the likelihood of survival of surgically implanted cells. It also minimizes risks of transmission of infectious disease, and does not require immunosuppressants or steroids. Finally, it does not involve the controversial use of fetal tissue or embryonic cell lines. A major finding is that adult NSCs harvested from a patient's own tissue can be used as a source of dopaminergic neurons. But the key advantage is that the restorative procedure seems safe and effective, with the PD patient experiencing a regression in motor symptoms. The finding that adult human brain contains NSCs have raised the hope that the patient's own NSCs could be used to generate DA neurons for neurodegenerative diseases such as PD.

Embryonic Stem Cells as a Source for Dopaminergic Neurons

Embryonic Stem Cells

Embryonic stem (ES) cells are pluripotent cells isolated from the inner cell mass, a cluster of a few hundred identical cells in the blastocyte, which is formed in the early stage of embryonic development. ES cells were first isolated from mouse embryos more than 20 years ago.[57,58] More recently, monkey ES cells were isolated first from the rhesus monkey and then from the marmoset and cynomolgous.[59–62] Shortly after, the same methods were used to isolate human ES cells from in vitro fertilized human embryos and their potential clinical applications became evident.[61,63] ES cells can proliferate extensively in an undifferentiated state and can provide an unlimited source of many tissue types. The isolation of ES cells from monkey and human embryos has generated great interesting in using these cells as a basis of cell replacement therapies for degenerative diseases, especially in PD.

Rodent ES Cells

Differentiation of ES Cells to Dopaminergic Neuron In Vivo

To assess the potential of ES cells to undergo neuronal differentiation in vivo, totipotent stem cells from mouse blastocysts were transplanted, with (0.5 mM) or without *all-trans* retinoic acid (RA) pretreatment, into adult mouse brain and adult lesioned rat brain.[64] Intracerebral grafts survived in 61% of cyclosporine immunosuppressed rats and 100% of mouse hosts, exhibited variable size and morphology, and developed large numbers of cells exhibiting neuronal morphology and immunoreactivity for neurofilament, NSE, TH, serotonin, and cells immunoreactive for GFAP. Although graft size and histology were variable, typical grafts of 5–10 mm^3 contained 10–20,000 TH$^+$ neurons, whereas DBH$^+$ cells were rare. Both TH$^+$ and serotonergic axons from intracerebral grafts grew into regions of the DA-lesioned host striatum. These findings demonstrate that transplantation to the brain can induce a significant fraction of totipotent ES cells to become putative dopaminergic or serotonergic neurons and that, when transplanted to the brain, these neurons are capable of innervating the adult host striatum.

Björklund et al.[65] also demonstrated that undifferentiated mouse ES cells grafted in small numbers into the striatum of a 6-OHDA-lesioned rat survived for 14–16 weeks, and developed into normal midbrain-like DA neurons that expressed dopaminergic and neuronal markers, such as TH, NeuN, DAT, and AADC. All TH-positive neurons coexpressed calretinin, which normally is coexpressed with TH in both A9 and A10 regions of the ventral midbrain, and some TH-positive neurons coexpressed calbindin, which is found primarily in A10 dopaminergic neurons. In addition, the differentiated ES cells developed numerous serotonergic neurons and small amount of γ-aminobutyric acid (GABA) as well as choline acetyltransferase (ChAT) neurons. Numerous astrocytes stained for the astrocyte marker GFAP within the grafts were found. Moreover, the animals with ES cell-derived DA neurons recovered from amphetamine-induced turning behavior, and position emission tomography (PET) imaging of presynaptic markers such [11C]CFT found an increase in binding in the grafted striatum (Table 7.2). These results must be reviewed with caution because of teratoma formation and lack of cell survival seen in some rats.

Induction of ES Cells to Dopaminergic Neurons In Vitro and Function in an Animal Model of PD

Although the in vivo experiments demonstrated that dopaminergic-like cells can be developed or differentiate by the environmental factor presence in the transplanted niche, much effort is invested to induce differentiation to dopaminergic cells in cultures. McKay and his group at the National Institutes of Health described a five-step procedure.[66,90,146] Clusters of ES cells were separated into single cells, and plated for 4 days in the presence of serum. This treatment generated embryoid bodies, floating ES cell aggregates that contain ectodermal, mesodermal, and endodermal derivatives. The embryoid bodies were then plated on adhesive tissue culture plates for 24 hours in the presence of serum and transferred to serum-free medium for 4–6 days to be select for NSCs. These cells were dissociated and cultured for 6 days on an adhesive substrate in the presence of FGF8, sonic hedgehog (Shh), and bFGF. Even though they are essential for the development of midbrain DA neurons in vivo,[67] exogenously added Shh and FGF8 were not essential for the generation of DA neurons from ES cells and only doubled the yield of ES-derived DA neurons. bFGF was then removed, and ascorbic acid was added for a further 6–15 days. The resulting neurons expressed markers that characterize the embryonic midbrain such as Pax2, Pax5, Wnt1, and Engrailed 1 (En1), as well as the dopaminergic neuronal markers Nurr1 and TH. Furthermore, these neurons produced DA and released their DA upon depolarization with potassium or exposure to the neurotransmitter GABA. Under optimal culture conditions, 72% of the ES cells assumed a neuronal morphology, 34% of the neurons were dopaminergic, and 11% were serotonergic. Serotonin and TH were not coexpressed.

An important step forward to increase the proportion of TH+ neurons was achieved by introducing the Nurr1 gene.[68] When cells were treated with FGF8 and Shh, the yield of these cells increased dramatically. Moreover, depolarization markedly increased the DA released in the cultured Nurr1 ES cells. Animals grafted with wild-type ES cells showed a slight recovery in rotation behavior in rats lesioned unilaterally with 6-OHDA whereas the group grafted with Nurr1 ES cells showed a marked improvement. Interestingly, no teratomas were observed in animals that had received grafts of Nurr1 ES cells. These cells also developed functional synapses and demonstrated electrophysiological properties typical to mesencephalic neurons. Shim et al.[69] generated mouse ES cells that constitutively express Bcl-XL, an antiapoptotic protein of Bcl-2 family. In vitro, Bcl-XL overexpressing ES cells resulted in higher expression of genes relating to midbrain dopaminergic neuron development and increased the number of ES-derived neurons expressing midbrain DA markers (TH+, 31%), pronouncing the reversal of behavior in the animal model of PD. However, it is as yet unknown if the cells give rise to a functional reinnervation of the striatum, and their efficacy compared with primary embryonic DA neurons. Additional questions are of long-term safety and whether this type of ES genetic modification of the ES cells is acceptable in a clinical setting.[17]

Nishimura et al.[70] used a similar five-step procedure to differentiate ES cells, carrying the enhanced GFP gene, in a mouse model of PD induced by 6-OHDA. Immunocytochemical evaluations revealed that microtubule-associated protein 2 (MAP2), TH+, GFAP+, and nestin+ cells comprised approximately 80%, 30%, 10%, and 5%, respectively, of the whole cells at stage 5. Furthermore, DA and levodopa were detected in the culture supernatants by high-performance liquid chromatography (HPLC) after a 10-day culture in stage 5. These differentiated ES cell-derived cells were used as allografts in mice after administration of 6-OHDA injections. Four weeks after 6-OHDA injection, mice were transplanted with 10^5 ES-GFP cells into their DA-denervated striata. Improved rotational behavior was observed 2 weeks after transplantation. TH+ cells were found at the grafted sites 8 weeks after transplantation, some of which were immunopositive to GFP, demonstrating the presence of dopaminergic neurons derived from the ES cells.

Kawasaki et al.[71,72] screened for DA neuronal differentiation of ES cells after coculture with various cell lines and discovered that the bone marrow (BM)-derived stromal cell line, PA6, is a potent inducer of neuronal differentiation. This was termed stromal cell-derived inducing activity (SDIA). After coculture with PA6 cells, 16% of the total cell population represents DA neurons. Whereas coculture of ES cells with the PA6 cell line induces neural differentiation, CM from PA6 cells does not. However, SDIA is also not blocked by a 0.4-μm membrane barrier, suggesting that the inducing activity is secreted, but may be labile. When transplanted, SDIA-induced dopaminergic neurons integrate into mouse striatum, previously treated with 6-OHDA, and remain positive for TH and β-tubulin III expression. These cells survive at a reasonable rate (20%) 2 weeks after implantation in mouse striatum and extend dopaminergic neurites into the target tissue. No teratoma formation was observed in the grafted cells by histologic analyses. Morizane et al.[73] optimize the transplantation efficiency and found that the ratio of the number of surviving TH-positive cells to the total number of grafted cells was highest when ES cells were treated with SDIA for 12 days before transplantation. The SDIA method has several advantages in producing neurons, compared with previous embryoid body methods. First, the SDIA method is technically simple. ES cells are grown in a flat culture from single cells into colonies. Second, neural differentiation of ES cells is not only efficient but also speedy; the postmitotic neuron marker, β-tubulin III, appears on day 4 or 5. Finally and most importantly, SDIA-treated ES cells differentiate into midbrain dopaminergic neurons at a high frequency: 30% of neurons derived from mouse ES cells are dopaminergic and produce significant amounts of DA.

Ying et al.[74] monitored the production of neurons during monolayer differentiation of mouse ES cells. Undifferentiated ES cells were dissociated and plated onto gelatin-coated tissue culture plastic at a density of $0.5-1.5 \times 10^4/cm^2$ in N2-B27 medium. Many of the neurons formed in N2-B27 are immunopositive for GABA, with few TH-positive cells. However, replating and the addition of FGF2, FGF8, and Shh resulted in significant numbers of TH-immunoreactive neurons. Therefore, neural precursors generated by monolayer differentiation are malleable and can be directed into particular neuronal fates. They can also produce both astrocytes and oligodendrocytes.

Barberi et al.[75] improved techniques for in vitro differentiation of mouse ES cells into several subtypes by providing a set of coculture conditions that allows rapid and efficient derivation of most CNS phenotypes. The conditions induced neural differentiation by coculturing ES cells with murine BM-derived stromal feeder cell lines. After 5 days of coculture ES cells on stromal cell line, Shh and FGF8 were added to the serum replacement medium, and then the medium was changed to N2 supplemented with Shh and FGF8 in the presence of bFGF (days 8–11). At day 11, terminal differentiation was induced by withdrawal of Shh, FGF8, and bFGF and the addition of ascorbic acid and BDNF. These cells expressed TH, and the midbrain-specific transcription factors En1, Nurr1, Pitx3, and LIM homeobox transcription factor 1 beta (Lmx1b), as well as the DAT. Compared with earlier techniques, this system exhibited minimal variability in obtaining neural cells from a wide range of fertilization cell-derived cells. Neuronal function of ES cell-derived dopaminergic neurons was shown in vitro by electron microscopy, the measurement of neurotransmitter release, and intracellular recording.

Using a different approach with pluripotent mouse ES cells, Rolletscheka et al.[76] used an efficient protocol for growth factor-mediated lineage selection of neuronal cells. The protocol includes proliferation and maintenance of neural precursor cells in the presence of bFGF and EGF. Differentiation was induced by withdrawal of bFGF/EGF, and the combined addition of neurobasal medium plus B27, fetal calf serum, and the survival-promoting factors (SPF). Interleukin-1β was added daily and adenosine 3′,5′-cyclic monophosphate (cAMP) at every 4 days for 30 days. GDNF and transforming growth factor (TGF)-$β_3$ were applied beginning at day 4 and at day 7 of the differentiation, respectively, and neurturin (NTN) was applied on day 7. Four days after plating, 58% of ES cell-derived neural precursor cells were labeled by the nestin and the application of SPF between days 14 and 30 resulted in a significant increase in the frequency of TH (43%) and DAT (39%) positive cells.

Primates' ES Cells

Nonhuman Primate ES Cells

Stromal feeder (SDIA-based) protocols were tested in nonhuman primate ES cell lines. Unlike the embryoid bodies or neural default protocols mentioned above, SDIA also induced primate ES cells to differentiate into TH$^+$ neurons.[77] In addition, Kawasaki et al.[72] also reported that SDIA induces efficient neural differentiation in ES cells derived from *Macaca fascicularis* (cynomolgus monkey), which is frequently used in preclinical studies.

Development of Dopaminergic Neurons from Human ES Cells

Production of tyrosine hydroxylase-positive neurons. Since the derivation of human ES cell lines from preimplantation embryos in 1998 by Thomson et al., considerable research is centered on their biology, and how differentiation can be encouraged toward particular cell lineages. Various studies have described the potential of human ES cells to differentiate into multiple lineages such as neural progenitor,[78–80] hematopoietic precursors,[81] and insulin-secreting cells (Assady et al., 2001).

Differentiation protocols in primate ES cells to neuron are based on the concepts developed for mouse ES cell differentiation. Multistage embryoid bodies-based differentiation protocols for human ES cells have been reported achieving efficient derivation of neuronal and astrocytic fates.[78,82] Carpenter et al.[78] described that human ES cells were maintained for more than 6 months in vitro (more than 100 population duplications) before their ability to differentiate into the neural lineage was evaluated. Differentiation was induced by the formation of embryoid bodies that were subsequently plated onto appropriate substrates in defined medium containing mitogens. These populations contained cells that showed positive immunoreactivity to nestin, polysialylated neural cell adhesion molecule and A2B5. After further maturation, these cells expressed additional neuron-specific antigens and TH. In addition, calcium imaging demonstrated that these cells responded to neurotransmitter application. Electrophysiological analyses showed that cell membranes contained voltage-dependent channels and that action potential was triggered by current injection.

An alternative strategy is based on the manual "lineage selection" in mixed populations of differentiating human ES cells. Neural precursors are generated by default in the absence of any specific extrinsic differentiation cues. Reubinoff et al.[63,79] reported the generation of enriched and expandable preparations of proliferating neural progenitors from human ES cells. The neural progenitors could differentiate in vitro into the three neural lineages – astrocytes, oligodendrocytes, and mature neurons. The differentiated cells expressed markers of mature neurons such as neurofilament medium (NF-M), MAP2, and synaptophysin. Furthermore, the cultures contained cells synthesized glutamate, expressed GAD, GABA, and serotonin, and expressed TH. Cells producing TH and serotonin were relatively rare (<1%). These four studies[78–80,83] demonstrated that human ES cells differentiated to mature neuron-like cells expressing mRNA and proteins that were necessary for dopaminergic neuron-like TH, and AADC for production of DA.

In addition, Zhang et al.[82] described the in vitro differentiation, enrichment, and transplantation of neural precursor cells from human ES cells. Upon aggregation to embryoid bodies, differentiating ES cells formed large numbers of neural tube-like structures in the presence of FGF2. Neural precursors within these formations were isolated by selective enzymatic digestion and further purified on the basis of differential adhesion. After withdrawal of FGF2, they differentiated into neurons, astrocytes, and oligodendrocytes. A small number of neurons (approximately 1%) were found to express TH. After transplantation into the neonatal mouse brain, human ES cell-derived neural precursors were incorporated into a variety of brain regions, where they differentiated into both neurons and astrocytes. No teratoma formation was observed in transplant recipients. These studies may serve as a platform for further manipulations with growth and differentiating factors that may eventually enable the derivation of specific dopaminergic neural cells from human ES cells.

Derivation of midbrain dopaminergic neurons. Despite considerable in vitro and in vivo data on human ES-derived neural precursors, differentiation into specific neuronal subtypes such as DA, serotonin, or other motor neurons has not yet been reported. For human ES cells to be used for transplantation into patients with PD, they must be differentiated into DA neurons with no residual ES cells. Although protocols[78–80,82,83] have been developed for the directed differentiation of human ES to TH-positive neuron, even up to 20% TH-positive cells reported,[84] but there was no confirmation of midbrain DA neuron identity. The first step through achieving derivation of midbrain DA neurons from human ES cells was demonstrated by Buytaert-Hoefen et al.[85] TH-positive neurons with neuronal morphology were generated from human ES cells, after 3–4 weeks in culture, by coculturing on PA6 stromal cells and addition of GDNF to the differentiated media. Moreover, there was RNA expression of En1, Pitx3, and DAT, several factors involved in the development of DA neurons.

Another experiment was directed toward showing that TH-positive cells produced from human ES cells are authentic midbrain DA neurons.[86] Perrier et al.[86] described that midbrain dopaminergic neuron differentiation of human ES was triggered by four stages: 1. Form ES to rosette neural precursors by stromal feeder cells (MS5 stromal cells) for 28 days; 2–3. committed DA precursors was achieved under sequential application of Shh, FGF8, BDNF, and ascorbic acid 7–9 days (two passage); 4. DA neuron differentiation required withdrawal of Shh/FGF8 and exposure to BDNF, GDNF, TGF-β_3, cAMP, and ascorbic acid for 7–9 days. Progression toward a midbrain DA neuron fate was monitored by the sequential expression of key transcription factors, including Pax2, Pax5, Lmx1b, Aldh1, Nurr1, and En1; 30%–50% of the total cells were β-tubulin III-positive neurons, and among them 64%–79% of the cells expressed TH; measurements of DA release by HPLC; the presence of tetrodotoxin-sensitive action potentials; and the electron microscopic visualization of TH-positive synaptic terminals. One important application of the reported midbrain DA neuron derivation protocol will be transplantation into preclinical animal models of PD.

Khaner et al.[87] have developed protocols that allow differentiation of human ES cell-derived neural progenitors toward enriched populations of dopaminergic neurons. The expression of the midbrain marker genes En1 and En2 and the dopaminergic markers TH and AADC was up-regulated in the neural progenitors at an early passage stage, suggesting that they have acquired the potential to adopt a midbrain fate at an early stage of propagation. Based on these data, the neural progenitors have been treated during a specific time window at an early passage stage with FGF8 together with ascorbic acid. Immunofluorescent analysis revealed that this treatment directed the differentiation of the neural progenitors into cultures enriched for TH$^+$ neurons (approximately 30% of the total neurons generated). The TH$^+$ neurons that were generated could secrete DA into the culture medium.

The potential of human ES cells to induce functional recovery in an animal model of Parkinsonism was reported for the first time by Reubinoff et al.[88] They generated highly enriched cultures of neural progenitors from hES cells and grafted the progenitors into the striatum of parkinsonian rats. The grafts survived for at least 12 weeks, the transplanted cells stopped proliferating, and teratomas were not observed. The grafted cells differentiated in vivo into DA neurons, although at a low prevalence similar to that observed after spontaneous differentiation in vitro. Transplanted rats exhibited significant improvement in rotational behavior, and in stepping and placing nonpharmacologic behavioral tests.

The availability of unlimited numbers of midbrain DA neurons is a first step toward exploring the potential of human ES cells in preclinical models of PD. Further developments for the potential use of human ES cells in the treatment of PD are needed. Obtaining functional in vivo data using primate ES cells in animal models of PD will be the next major milestone on the road toward future clinical trials with human ES cells.

Nuclear Transfer and Parthenogenesis ES Cells

Transplantation of allogenic or xenogenic tissues and cells raises immunologic concerns. The need for immunosuppression in neural transplantation remains a controversial issue given the proposed "immunoprivileged" status of the brain. However, it is well established that xenografted cells undergo rapid rejection in the brain without immunosuppression. Nuclear transfer and parthenogenesis are procedures

Dopaminergic Neuron Differentiation of ES Cells Generated from Adult Somatic Cells by Nuclear Transfer

Functional DA neurons were obtained from mouse ES cells established via nuclear transfer from adult tail tip or cumulus cells as described by Wakayama et al.[89] They derived 35 ES cell lines via nuclear transfer (ntES) from adult mouse somatic cells of inbred, hybrid, and mutant strains. ntES embryoid bodies have been induced to differentiate in vitro to produce dopaminergic neurons as described previously[90] with the following minor modifications. Cells were cultured for a longer period during stage III (CNS selection stage), ranging from 9 to 16 days and the concentrations of FGF2, Shh, FGF8, and ascorbic acid were changed. One ES cell line yielded dopaminergic neurons in excess of 50% of the total cell number. The functional nature of these neurons was confirmed by HPLC determination of DA release. Serotonergic neurons were also detected histochemically, although in smaller numbers, and serotonin release was confirmed by HPLC. In combining ES and nuclear transfer theologies, the feasibility of the first steps required for application of cloning to transplant therapy was demonstrated.[66,89,90]

Barberi et al.[75] demonstrated that mouse ntES cell-derived neurons by multistage differentiation protocols have electrophysiological evidence of synapse. Therefore, cloning and long-term expansion of undifferentiated ntES cells do not interfere with the functionality of their differentiated progeny. The ultrastructural detection of typical large, dense-core vesicles suggests that these are dopaminergic neurons. There has been great interest in developing a renewable cell source for the generation of DA neurons in the experimental treatment of PD. Their study demonstrates the functionality of ntES cell-derived neurons in 6-OHDA-lesioned mice, without the requirement of exogenous Nurr1 expression. The transplantation results using ntES cell-derived DA neurons in parkinsonian mice demonstrate the efficacy of therapeutic cloning in an animal model of CNS disease. Earlier work has shown in vivo functionality of bovine DA neurons extracted from cloned fetuses.[91] However, the use of cloned fetuses as cell donors raises ethical barriers that preclude applications in human disease. Notably, the DA neuron survival rate in vivo was higher in ntES than in ES cell-derived grafts (80% versus 40%, 8 weeks after transplantation). The results show the potential of therapeutic cloning in mouse models of PD. Future therapeutic applications may require extensive work to adapt these protocols to human ES cells.

Dopaminergic Neuron Differentiation of Parthenogenesis Stem Cells

Parthenogenesis is the process by which an egg can develop into an embryo in the absence of sperm. Broad differentiation capabilities of non-human primate (*M. fascicularis*) pluripotent stem cells derived by parthenogenesis have been reported.[92,93] Neural differentiation of Cyno-1 cells (one stable cell line from blastocyte's inner cell mass) was induced with a multistep culture procedure,[66,90] and astrocytes and neurons were obtained. Up to 25% of dopaminergic (TH) neurons could be obtained, as judged by immunocytochemical criteria. Neuronal identity and function were confirmed by HPLC analysis, which showed in vitro release of the neurotransmitters DA and serotonin. The in vitro differentiation of these cells to well-characterized dopaminergic neurons is of particular interest, because of their potential to replace lost neurons in PD. The proposal of human therapeutic cloning describes the generation of autologous ES cells through somatic cell nuclear transfer.[94] This study suggests an alternative to human cloning for therapy. Differentiated cell types derived in vitro by parthenogenesis eliminate the requirement to produce or disaggregate a normal, competent embryo and may circumvent the ethical concerns voiced by some, with a positive impact on the debate in stem cell research. Future studies will have to provide a proof-of-principle application of both nuclear transfer and parthenogenesis in animal models of PD.

Generation of DA Neurons from Adult Stem Cells

Adult stem cells are found in different tissues of the adult organism that remain in an undifferentiated, or nonspecialized, state. Adult stem cells possess the ability to self-renew, and can differentiate into at least one tissue-committed cell type. The main function of stem cells in adult tissue is to regenerate the tissue in which they reside. By a traditional developmental paradigm, adult stem cells are able to differentiate only to the tissue in which they reside. Recent data challenge the committed fate of the adult stem cells and present evidence for their plasticity.

Plasticity of the adult stem cells may offer valuable therapy for a broad spectrum of diseases, especially neurodegenerative diseases and brain injuries. The use of cells originating from the patient's BM, skin, or fat cells may provide an autologous transplantation strategy that obviates the introduction of foreign material, circumvents many ethical issues, and significantly reduces the need for immunosuppression. Herein, we will review the potential application of BM-derived stem cell transplantation in PD, although several researchers suggest using skin, fat cells, or other tissues for clinical use.

Bone Marrow Stromal Cells

BMSc were described by Friedenstein and his associates in the 1970s.[95,96] They demonstrated that a small fraction of cells from BM adhere to tissue culture surfaces and that the adherent cells can be differentiated both in culture and in vivo into osteoblasts, chondrocytes, and adipocytes. It was shown that these stromal cells, known also as mesenchymal stem cells, further differentiate into mature connective tissue, muscle, bone, cartilage, and fat cells.[97–99]

Induction of Dopaminergic Neuron-Like Cells from BMSc In Vitro

A series of studies on human, rat, and mouse BMSc found evidence that these cells can be induced to differentiate to neuron-like cells in cultures.[100–116]

The first and most critical step to get neuron-like cells is to isolate the BM-derived multipotent progenitor cells. One of the methods to isolate multipotent cells with broad differentiation potential is based on the size and adherent capacity of the BMSc.

To increase the efficiency of differentiation of neuron-like cells, raising the cAMP levels by dibutyryl cyclic AMP and isobutylmethylxanthine,[104] or addition of the antioxidant butylated hydroxyanisole and dimethylsulfoxide have been used.[101] Another study has suggested that neuronal cells are isolated after induction with noggin, 5-azacytidine, and the neurotrophic factors such as nerve growth factor (NGF), NT3, and BDNF or the combination of FGF2, EGF, NGF, and retinoic acid.[105]

The evidence for differentiation of BMSc into dopaminergic neuron-like cells is limited. Woodbury et al.[102] reported a method for inducing rat BMSc to differentiate into neuron-like cells that express genes associated with neurotransmission. Rat BMSc maintained in induction medium for 10 days were significantly heterogeneous in the level of tau expression, which often correlated with the degree of neuronal morphologic differentiation. β-Tubulin III, an intermediate filament characteristic of mature neurons, was present in virtually all cells. Analysis by reverse transcriptase-polymerase chain reaction (RT-PCR) indicated that synaptophysin mRNA, which is associated with synaptic vesicles and transmission, was not present in undifferentiated BMSc but was detected after 24 hours of neuronal differentiation and continued to increase thereafter. The synaptophysin protein was detected in cell bodies as well as varicose, putative transmitter release sites along processes. Moreover, at 10 days of rat BMSc differentiation, a large population of the neuron-like cells expressed ChAT, which catalyzes the synthesis of the excitatory transmitter acetylcholine. A smaller subpopulation of rat BMSc-derived neuron-like expressed TH. Nevertheless, they did not report a production of DA or other catecholamine neurotransmitters.

An additional study by Hermann et al.[115] described the efficient conversion of human BMSc into a neural stem cell-like population. These cells grow in neurosphere-like structures, express high levels of early neuroectodermal markers, such as the proneural genes neurogenic differentiation 1 (NeuroD1), neurogenin 2 (Neurog2), musashi 1, as well as orthdenticle homolog 1 (OTX1) and nestin, and lose the characteristics of mesodermal stromal cells. The authors used growth factors such as EGF and FGF2 and later exposed the cells to BDNF and retinoic acid. Marker mRNA levels of mature neural cell types (GFAP, MBP, β-tubulin III, and TH) were significantly increased. They obtained 42% of differentiated human BMSc with early neuronal characteristics (β-tubulin III expression) and 6% expressing the marker molecule for mature neurons (MAP2). Moreover, 11% ± 7% of cells expressed TH, and DA was detectable in the media of the differentiated cells, by HPLC, only after supplemented with tetrahydrobiopterin (BH_4).

In our laboratory, Levy et al.[109] induced differentiation of mouse BMSc to neuron-like cells, without any gene introduction, and observed the activation of the tissue-specific promoter of NSE. We used transgenic (Tg) mice that carry the antiapoptotic human bcl-2 gene, expressed only in neurons under the NSE promoter. We found that, after induction, the mouse BMSc demonstrate neuronal phenotype and express the neuronal markers and the human Bcl-2. Furthermore, we also demonstrated that human BMSc might change their designation after induction in culture.[110] The differentiation of human BMSc into neuron-like cells was associated with dramatic morphologic changes. Before treatment, human BMSc displayed a flat, fibroblastic morphology, whereas, after 24 hours of treatment, the cells were rounded, exhibited highly retractile cell bodies, and displayed prominent process-like extensions. The neuron-like morphology of the cells was retained up to 26 days of culture. The structural changes were accompanied by the expression of the tissue-specific neuronal marker, NeuN, as indicated by nuclear immunostaining. We also demonstrated, using RT-PCR methods, that the differentiated human BMSc expressed Nurr1, Aldh1, Pitx3, and EN1, the transcription factors that regulate the midbrain of the DA neuron. Moreover, the DA-related genes AADC, D2 DA receptor, and DAT were increased during the differentiation induction.[110]

Gene Manipulations and Dopaminergic-Like Cells and Functional Assay in an Animal Model of PD

Because the induction of differentiation BMSc into dopaminergic neuron-like cells is limited, gene manipulations were performed to increase the efficiency and quality of the dopaminergic-like cells. Rat BMSc were engineered by transgene to express human TH type 2, and GTP cyclohydrolase I (GC), the enzyme providing the BH_4 cofactor for TH.[117] The gene-engineered rat BMSc synthesized and released L-DOPA. When the rat BMSc that synthesized L-DOPA were transplanted into the rat model of PD, L-DOPA was converted to DA metabolites, and behavioral recovery was observed. However, the ameliorative effect of transplanted rat BMSc was short-lived (up to 7 days), presumably because of inactivation of transgenes introduced into the brain with retroviruses. In the experiments, BMSc were transduced sequentially with two separate retroviruses, each containing TH or GC driven by the cyto megalovirus (CMV) promoter.[117] In addition, they have created a 3.4 kb bicistronic construct consisting of the TH gene and GC gene separated by an internal ribosome entry site (TH-IRES-GC) to avoid the use of two separate retroviruses.[118] Moreover, a small number of rat BMSc producing L-DOPA continued expressing transgenes after a massive expansion in culture by simple low-density plating of approximately 3 months in vitro. However, the BMSc in these studies did not differentiate into neuron-like cells.

Park et al.[119] demonstrated that retroviral transduction of mouse marrow cells with the GDNF cDNA followed by intravenous delivery of these engineered cells results in marrow-derived GDNF-expressing cells within the brain parenchyma. Furthermore, this ex vivo gene transfer strategy performed 6 weeks before exposure to the dopaminergic neurotoxin 1-methyl-4-phenyl-1,2,3,6-tetrahydropyridine (MPTP) results in clear protection of nigral neurons and their striatal terminals. The histochemical protection (TH immunoreactive) correlates with behavioral hyperactivity in GDNF-mouse BMSc-transplanted mice compared with control BMSc-transplanted animals. The observed behavioral changes are reminiscent of the reported increased locomotion in mice after intrastriatal injection of GDNF.[120]

Dezawa et al.[114] demonstrated the highly efficient and specific induction of cells with neuronal characteristics, without glial differentiation, from both rat and human BMSc using gene transfection with Notch intracellular domain (NICD) and subsequent treatment with bFGF, forskolin, and ciliary neurotrophic factor. MSCs expressed markers relating to neural stem cells after transfection with NICD, and subsequent trophic factor administration induced neuronal cells. Some of them showed voltage-gated fast sodium and delayed rectifier potassium currents and action potentials compatible with characteristics of functional neurons. Further treatment of the induced neuronal cells with GDNF increased the proportion of TH-positive and DA-producing cells. The cells released a significant amount of DA (1.1 pmol/10^6 cells) after induced depolarization. Transplantation of these GDNF-treated cells showed improvement in apomorphine-induced rotational behavior and adjusting step and paw-reaching tests after intrastriatal implantation in a 6-OHDA rat model of PD.

The risks of virus-associated gene transfer, although low, are not imaginary (given the evidence of secondary malignancy in children after stem cell transplantation). It is also clear that the limited availability of ES cell sources and the uncertainties regarding the safety of therapeutic viral-based gene transfer have generated interest in alternative approaches, including the use of somatic stem cells. We believe that a key ingredient for implementing a regenerative approach is the ability to epigenetically drive stem cell differentiation by ex vivo regulation of the local cellular environment rather than by genetic alteration. Modulation of the microenvironment would help provide the framework for multipotent cells to recapitulate tissue growth and organogenesis in a postnatal setting, circumvent the risks of exogenous gene transfer, and may lead to a multifaceted and cost-effective approach with enormous translational implications.

Differentiation of BMSc to Dopaminergic-Like Neurons In Vivo

The therapeutic potential of BMSc for the treatment of PD was highlighted by a publication from Li et al.[121] Mouse BMSc prelabeled with BrdU were grafted into the striatum of an MPTP mouse model of PD. The grafted MPTP-treated mice exhibited a significant improvement on the Rotorod test at 35 days after transplant, compared with nongrafted controls. Immunohistochemistry revealed BrdU-reactive cells in the striatum of the grafted MPTP-treated mice at least 4 weeks after transplantation. Double staining showed that approximately 0.8% of BrdU-reactive cells expressed TH immunoreactivity. Although the mouse BMSc injected intrastriatally survive, express TH immunoreactivity, and promote some functional recovery, further investigation is required to understand the mechanism used for this recovery. It is not known whether the grafted cells increase production of DA or whether other processes, such as the secretion of neurotrophic factors by the marrow-derived cells, mediate the improvement in motor function.

Multipotent Adult Progenitor Cells

Jiang et al.[122] recently described that, similar to mouse ES cells, mouse multipotent adult progenitor cells (MAPCs) can also be induced to differentiate in vitro into cells with biochemical, anatomical, and electrophysiological characteristics of midbrain neuronal cells. The population of the MAPCs, a rare cell within human and rat BM mesenchymal stem cultures, can be multiplied more than 120-fold.[123–125] It was demonstrated that cells capable of differentiating in vitro to cells of the three germ layers could be selected from rodent BM.

Mouse MAPC differentiation to neurons was achieved after sequential culture for 7 days with bFGF, FGF8, Shh, and BDNF. Quantitative RT-PCR demonstrated that, by days 10 and 14, levels of GABA, TH, and tryptophan hydroxylase (TPH) mRNA increased between 1.7- and 120-fold. Immunophenotypic analysis on day 21 showed that 25% of cells expressed markers of dopaminergic neurons (AADC and TH), 18% expressed markers of serotonergic (TPH), and 52% of GABAergic (GABA) neurons. Double immunohistochemistry showed that GABA, TPH, and TH were never detected together in the same cell. Mouse MAPC-derived neuron-like cells cultured in the presence of fetal brain astrocytes demonstrated that the cells continued to express markers of dopaminergic neurons (25% TH), serotonergic neurons (25% TPH), and GABAergic neurons (50% GABA) and acquired a much more mature neural morphology with more elaborate array axons.[122] However, despite the ability of mouse MAPCs to differentiate into neuroectoderm-like cells ex vivo, no significant engraftment of mouse MAPCs was seen in the brain after intravenous infusion, and rare donor cells found in the brain did not colabel with neuroectodermal markers.[123]

Marrow-Isolated Adult Multilineage Inducible Cells

D'Ippolito et al.[126] described the marrow-isolated adult multilineage inducible (MIAMI) method. They isolated a population of non-transformed pluripotent human cells from BM with a procedure that was designed to provide conditions resembling the in vivo microenvironment that is home for the most primitive stem cells. Marrow-adherent and -nonadherent cells were cocultured on fibronectin, at low oxygen tension (3%), for 14 days and colonies of small adherent cells were isolated and further expanded on fibronectin at low density, low oxygen tension with 2% fetal bovine serum. The cells expressed markers found among ES cells as well as mesodermal-, endodermal- and ectodermal-derived lineages including neural cells. Neural differentiation was induced by exposing the MIAMI cells to NT3, NGF, and BDNF for 3–7 days. At the end of the differentiation, cells expressed NeuN and NF-M, whereas the expression of nestin was not detected, consistent with mature neuronal phenotype. In addition, after a novel neuronal induction protocol, Montero-Menei et al.[127] were able to first obtain cells expressing neural stem cell markers (nestin and β-tubulin III) and at a later stage of differentiation expressing mature neuronal markers such as NeuN and neurofilaments. Moreover, using an improved four-step in vitro protocol combining NT3 and retinoic acid together with dopaminergic-inducing molecules (SHH and FGF8), TH-expressing neurons were demonstrated. Moreover, to be able to maintain the differentiated functional phenotype and appropriate number of cells after grafting, a new tool for cell therapy has been developed termed pharmacologically active microcarriers (PAM). PAM assembles biodegradable and biocompatible matrix elements and controlled-release technology that provides the needed environment for supporting the functionality and viability of the implanted cells. The efficacy of the PAM was demonstrated in an animal model of PD using a cell lineage and is currently being studied in this same paradigm with fetal mesencephalic cells conveyed by GDNF-releasing PAM. In the near future, this unique technology will be utilized to produce GDNF-releasing PAM conveying the MIAMI-derived physiologically competent DA-releasing neurons designed for the sustained clinical improvement of the Parkinson's animal model.[127]

Possible Mechanisms for Adult BMSc Plasticity into Neurons

What are the proposed mechanisms for adult cell plasticity? Cells have been sorted into unpredicted cellular phenotypes: A. Existence of primitive stem cells in the mature tissue; B. the presence of multiple progenitor/stem cells not derived from the same embryonic germ layers in the tissue; C. direct and indirect dedifferentiation; D. transdifferentiation; and E. cell fusion. It is of essential importance to keep an open mind about these proposals. This does not mean lower scientific standards.

The potential of the BM to differentiate into neurons was first demonstrated in experiments with rodents. Transplanted BM-derived cells were shown to migrate into various brain regions and develop neuron-like features.[128–131] Furthermore, Mezey et al.[132] found Y chromosomes in the human brains of females after transplantation of male BM. Donor cells were found in several selective brain regions, especially in the hippocampus and cerebral cortex. However, other researchers claim that bone-to-brain transdifferentiation may not be general phenomena but may reflect fusion with neurons or transient expression of many proteins including neuronal markers.[133–135] In a recent report, Cogle et al.[136] demonstrated that human hemopoietic cells can transdifferentiate into neurons, astrocytes, and microglia in a long-term setting without fusion. They found that hippocampal cells containing a Y chromosome were present up to 6 years posttransplant in 1% of all neurons and there was no evidence of fusion. In addition, it was demonstrated that rat BMSc were infused into 1.5- to 2-day-old chick embryos.[137] After 4 days, the rat cells had expanded 1.3- to 33-fold in one-third of surviving embryos. The cells engrafted into many tissues, and no multinuclear cells were detected. The most common site of engraftment was the heart, apparently because the cells were infused just above the dorsal aorta. Some of the cells in the heart expressed cardiotin, and α-heavy-chain myosin. GFP+ cells reisolated from the embryos had a rat karyotype. Therefore, the cells engrafted and partially differentiated without evidence of cell fusion.[137]

Chopp et al.[144] reported that transplantation of undifferentiated BMSc in rats revealed therapeutic benefit after traumatic brain injury,[138–141] ischemic brain injury,[121,142,143] or spinal cord injury. In these postinjury transplantation studies, generally less than 20% of transplanted cells were immunoreactive for CNS antigens, raising the possibility that the remaining cells contributed to the clinical benefits.

Although many researchers observed the conversion of BM cells into neurons and glia, several fundamental questions remain for future consideration. First, what is the origin of the pluripotent stem cells found in adult BM? Are they related to primordial germ cells that arrive in the tissue early in development and retain the ability to differentiate into neuron-like cells under experimental conditions, or they are rare, but integrate in the population of the adult BM? Second, does the transformation of grafted BM cells into the neuronal phenotype seen in the host tissue occur because of cell fusion between the marrow and host cells or by real transdifferentiation? Replacing patients' BM in the case of blood disorders is well established. However, the clinical application for neurodegenerative diseases such as PD, raises serious questions concerning the safety of the implantation and the competence of the transplanted cell to function as controlled and efficient dopaminergic cells. The use of induced BM-derived neurons for transplantation in animal models of PD is very limited, although several groups reported the improvement in rotational behavior after brain implantation. Thus, although serious basic and clinical studies should be continued, it is not too optimistic to believe that BM-derived stem cells, obviating ethical debate, may provide a therapeutic tool for tissue replacement in PD.

Future Strategies

In establishing stem cells as an alternative graft source, logistical, ethical, and political issues need to be resolved. There is disagreement over the feasibility of "adult" stem cells compared with ES cells. Adult stem cells might be capable of developing only into a limited number of cell types, whereas ES cells can form any fully differentiated cell of the body and exhibit remarkable long-term proliferative potential, offering the possibility of unlimited expansion in culture. However, ES cells retain their mitotic ability after transplantation and this could give rise to tumors. Accordingly, the limited plasticity of adult stem cells might be advantageous in terms of controlling their mitotic ability after transplantation. Furthermore, the use of adult stem cells will not be subject to the ethical concerns that surround the use of fetal tissues, including the ES cells.[145] Thus, safety and efficacy issues on the use of stem cells include the following questions. Do they maintain long-term stable neuronal phenotypes crucial for rescuing the degenerating brain? Are transplanted stem cells functional as a dopaminergic neuron and thus able to provide beneficial effects?

It seems clear that there is an urgent need for more basic research if progress is to be made beyond the level of clinical phenomenology. There are three main challenges. First, it will be necessary to learn much more about neuronal development, in order to define cell types that can be cultured in sufficient quantities and that can adopt appropriate fates when transplanted to different sites in vivo. Second, it will be necessary to establish better animal models – perhaps including genetically modified primates – in order to perform more realistic tests of functional and cognitive recovery after transplantation. Third, it will be important to develop methods for testing whether transplanted neurons can become functionally integrated into brain circuitry; in other words, whether they can actually contribute to the restoration of normal information processing in the damaged brain. It will require the identification and electrophysiological characterization of transplanted neurons in vivo.

The examples we provided in this review serve to demonstrate the numerous issues in cell biology involved in advancing to a functionally valuable therapeutic strategy in PD. However, the most scientific conclusion of all the studies with differentiation and transplantation of rodent, primate, and human stem cells is that cell replacement in neurodegenerative disease in general and PD in particular, can work. However, it is essential to emphasize that clinically helpful cell treatment for PD is not yet available. Dopaminergic cells that are also neurons – dopaminergic neurons – generated from different sorts of stem cells, seem to be the most hopeful option for grafting in PD. The best stem cell source for generating new DA neurons is not yet known. However, we believe that adult stem cells such as

BMSc are the best cells to use in autologous transplantation in the treatment of PD.

References

1. Bjorklund A, Stenevi U. Reconstruction of the nigrostriatal dopamine pathway by intracerebral nigral transplants. Brain Res 1979;177:555–560.
2. Brundin P, Strecker RE, Widner H, et al. Human fetal dopamine neurons grafted in a rat model of Parkinson's disease: immunological aspects, spontaneous and drug-induced behavior, and dopamine release. Exp Brain Res 1988;70:192–208.
3. Lindvall O, Hagell P. Cell replacement therapy in human neurodegenerative disorders. Clin Neurosci Res 2002;2:86–92.
4. Sauer H, Brundin P. Effects of cool storage on survival and function of intrastriatal ventral mesencephalic grafts. Restor Neurol Neurosci 1991;2:123–135.
5. Lindvall O. Neural transplants in Parkinson's disease. In: Dunnett SB, Bjorklund A, eds. Functional Neural Transplantation. New York: Raven; 1994:103–137.
6. Frodl EM, Duan WM, Sauer H, Kupsch A, Brundin P. Human embryonic dopamine neurons xenografted to the rat: effects of cryopreservation and varying regional source of donor cells on transplant survival, morphology, and function. Brain Res 1994;647:286–298.
7. Haque NS, LeBlanc CJ, Isacson O. Differential dissection of the rat E16 ventral mesencephalon and survival and reinnervation of the 6-OHDA-lesioned striatum by a subset of aldehyde dehydrogenase-positive TH neurons. Cell Transplant 1997;6:239–248.
8. Nakao N, Frodl EM, Duan WM, Widner H, Brundin P. Lazaroids improve the survival of grafted rat embryonic dopaminergic neurons. Proc Natl Acad Sci USA 1994;91:12408–12412.
9. Bjorklund A, Lindvall O. Cell replacement therapies for central nervous system disorders. Nat Neurosci 2000;3:537–544.
10. Okano H, Yoshizaki T, Shimazaki T, Sawamotoc K. Isolation and transplantation of dopaminergic neurons and neural stem cells. Parkinsonism Relat Disord 2002;9:23–28.
11. Freed CR, Greene PE, Breeze RE, et al. Transplantation of embryonic dopamine neurons for severe Parkinson's disease. N Engl J Med 2001;344:710–719.
12. Freed CR. Will embryonic stem cells be a useful source of dopamine neurons for transplant into patients with Parkinson's disease? Proc Natl Acad Sci USA 2002;99:1755–1757.
13. Olanow CW, Goetz CG, Kordower JH, et al. A double-blind controlled trial of bilateral fetal nigral transplantation in Parkinson's disease. Ann Neurol 2003;54:403–414.
14. Kopin IJ. The pharmacology of Parkinson's disease therapy: an update. Annu Rev Pharmacol Toxicol 1993;32:467–495.
15. Lang AE, Lozano AM. Parkinson's disease. N Engl J Med 1998;339:1044–1053.
16. Freeman TB, Olanow WC, Hauser RA, et al. Human fetal transplantation. In: Germano IM, ed. Neurosurgical Treatment of Movement Disorders. Park Ridge, IL: American Association of Neurological Surgeons; 1998.
17. Lindvall O. Stem cells for therapy in Parkinson's disease. Pharmacol Res 2003;47:279–287.
18. Chen N, Reith ME. Structure and function of the dopamine transporter. Eur J Pharmacol 2000;405:329–339.
19. Miller GW, Gainetdinov RR, Levey AI, Caron MG. Dopamine transporters and neuronal injury. Trends Pharmacol Sci 1999;20:424–429.
20. Bannon MJ. Dopamine. In: Nature Encyclopedia of Life Sciences. London: Nature Publishing Group; http://www.els.net/ [doi:10.1038/npg.els.0000279], 1998.
21. Sian J, Youdim MBH, Riederer P, Gerlach M. Neurotransmitters and disorders of the basal ganglia. In: Siegel GJ, Agranoff BW, Albers WR, Fisher SK, Uhler MD, eds. Basic Neurochemistry: Molecular, Cellular and Medical Aspects. 6th ed. Philadelphia: Lippincott Williams & Wilkins; 1999. Chapter 45.
22. Perrier AL, Studer L. Making and repairing the mammalian brain: –in vitro production of dopaminergic neurons. Semin Cell Dev Biol 2003;14:181–189.
23. Palkovits M, Brownstein M. Catecholamines in the central nervous system. In: Trendelenberg U, Weiner N, eds. Catecholamines II. Berlin: Springer; 1989:1–26.
24. Arts MP, Groenewegen HJ, Veening JG, Cools AR. Efferent projections of the retrorubral nucleus to the substantia nigra and ventral tegmental area in cats as shown by anterograde tracing. Brain Res Bull 1996;40:219–228.
25. Wurst W, Bally-Cuif L. Neural plate patterning: upstream and downstream of the isthmic organizer. Nat Rev Neurosci 2001;2:99–108.
26. Arenas E. Stem cells in the treatment of Parkinson's disease. Brain Res 2002;57:795–808.
27. Taupin P, Gage FH. Adult neurogenesis and neuronal stem cells of the central nervous system in mammals. J Neurosci Res 2002;69:745–749.
28. Corotto FS, Henegar JA, Maruniak JA. Neurogenesis persists in the subependymal layer of the adult mouse brain. Neurosci Lett 1993;149:111–114.
29. Luskin MB. Restricted proliferation and migration of postnatally generated neurons derived from the forebrain subventricular zone. Neurons 1993;11:173–189.
30. Palmer TD, Schwartz PH, Taupin P, Kaspar B, Stein S, Gage FH. Progenitor cells from human brain after death. Nature 2001;411:42–43.
31. Roy NS, Wang S, Jiang L, et al. In vitro neurogenesis by progenitor cells isolated from the adult human hippocampus. Nat Med 2000;3:271–277.
32. Armstrong RJE, Barker RA. Neurodegeneration: a failure of neuroregeneration? Lancet 2001;358:1174–1176.
33. Okano H. Stem cell biology of the central nervous system. J Neurosci Res 2002;69:698–707.
34. Studer L, Tabar V, McKay RD. Transplantation of expanded mesencephalic precursors leads to recovery in parkinsonian rats. Nat Neurosci 1998;1:290–295.
35. Yan J, Studer L, McKay RD. Ascorbic acid increases the yield of dopaminergic neurons derived from basic fibroblast growth factor expanded mesencephalic precursors. J Neurochem 2001;76:307–311.
36. Studer L, Csete M, Lee SH, et al. Enhanced proliferation survival and dopaminergic differentiation of CNS precursors in lowered oxygen. J Neurosci 2000;20:7377–7383.

37. Carvey PM, Ling ZD, Sortwell CE, et al. A clonal line of mesencephalic progenitor cells converted to dopamine neurons by hematopoietic cytokines: a source of cells for transplantation in Parkinson's disease. Exp Neurol 2001;171:98–108.
38. Storch A, Paul G, Csete M, et al. Long-term proliferation and dopaminergic differentiation of human mesencephalic neural precursor cells. Exp Neurol 2001; 170:317–325.
39. Wagner J, Åkerud P, Castro DS, Holm PC, et al. Induction of midbrain dopaminergic phenotype in Nurr1-overexpressing neural stem cells by type 1 astrocytes. Nat Biotechnol 1999;17:653–659.
40. Takahashi J, Palmer TD, Gage FH. Retinoic acid and neurotrophins collaborate to regulate neurogenesis in adult-derived neural stem cell cultures. J Neurobiol 1999;38:65–81.
41. Sakurada K, Ohshima-Sakurada M, Palmer TD, Gage FH. Nurr1, an orphan nuclear receptor, is a transcriptional activator of endogenous tyrosine hydroxylase in neural progenitor cells derived from the adult brain. Development 1999;126:4017–4026.
42. Daadi MM, Weiss S. Generation of tyrosine hydroxylase-producing neurons from precursors of the embryonic and adult forebrain. J Neurosci 1999; 19:4484–4497.
43. Akerud P, Canals JM, Snyder EY, Arenas E. Neuroprotection through delivery of glial cell line-derived neurotrophic factor by neural stem cells in a mouse model of Parkinson's disease. J Neurosci 2001;21:8108–8118.
44. Lin L, Doherty D, Lile J, Bektesh S, Collins F. GDNF: a glial cell line-derived neurotrophic factor for midbrain dopaminergic neurons. Science 1993;260:1130–1132.
45. Yang M, Stull ND, Berk MA, Snyder EY, Iacovitti L. Neural stem cells spontaneously express dopaminergic traits after transplantation into the intact or 6-hydroxydopamine-lesioned rat. Exp Neurol 2002; 177:50–60.
46. Cameron HA, McKay RD. Adult neurogenesis produces a large pool of new granule cells in the dentate gyrus. J Comp Neurol 2001;435:406–417.
47. Gould E, Reeves AJ, Graziano MS, Gross CG. Neurogenesis in the neocortex of adult primates. Science 1999;286:548–552.
48. Rietze R, Poulin P, Weiss S. Mitotically active cells that generate neurons and astrocytes are present in multiple regions of the adult mouse hippocampus. J Comp Neurol 2000;424:397–408.
49. Kornack DR, Rakic P. Cell proliferation without neurogenesis in adult primate neocortex. Science 2001; 294:2127–2130.
50. Arvidsson A, Collin T, Kirik D, Kokaia Z, Lindvall O. Neuronal replacement from endogenous precursors in the adult brain after stroke. Nat Med 2002;8:963–970.
51. Nakatomi H, Kuriu T, Okabe S, et al. Regeneration of hippocampal pyramidal neurons after ischemic brain injury by recruitment of endogenous neural progenitors. Cell 2002;110:429–441.
52. Lie DC, Dziewczapolski G, Willhoite AR, Kaspar BK, Shults CW, Gage FH. The adult substantia nigra contains progenitor cells with neurogenic potential. J Neurosci 2002;22:6639–6649.
53. Zhao M, Momma S, Delfani K, et al. Evidence for neurogenesis in the adult mammalian substantia nigra. Proc Natl Acad Sci USA 2003;100:7925–7930.
54. Frielingsdorf H, Schwarz K, Brundin P, Mohapel P. No evidence for new dopaminergic neurons in the adult mammalian substantia nigra. Proc Natl Acad Sci USA 2004;101:10177–10182.
55. Levesque MF, Neuman T. Autologous transplantation of adult human neural stem cells and differentiated dopaminergic neurons for Parkinson's disease: a one year post-operative clinical outcome. The 70th annual meeting of the American Association of Neurological Surgeons, Chicago, IL, April 2002.
56. Levesque MF, Neuman T. Autologous transplantation of adult human neural stem cells and differentiated dopaminergic neurons for Parkinson's disease: long term post-operative clinical and functional metabolic results. 8th international conference on neural transplantation and repair, Keystone, CO. Exp Neurol 2002;175:425.
57. Evans MJ, Kaufman MH. Establishment in culture of pluripotent cells from mouse embryos. Nature 1981;5819:154–156.
58. Martin GR. Isolation of a pluripotent cell line from early mouse embryos cultured in medium conditioned by teratocarcinoma stem cells. Proc Natl Acad Sci USA 1981;78:7634–7638.
59. Thomson JA, Kalishman J, Golos TG, et al. Isolation of a primate embryonic stem cell line. Proc Natl Aca Sci USA 1995;92:7844–7848.
60. Thomson JA, Kalishman J, Golos TG, Durning M, Harris CP, Hearn JP. Pluripotent cell lines derived from common marmoset (Callithrix jacchus) blastocysts. Biol Reprod 1996;55:254–259.
61. Thomson JA, Itskovitz-Eldor J, Shapiro SS, et al. Embryonic stem cell lines derived from human blastocysts. Science 1998;282:1145–1147.
62. Suemori H, Tada T, Torii R, et al. Establishment of embryonic stem cell lines from cynomolgus monkey blastocysts produced by IVF or ICSI. Dev Dyn 2001;222:273–279.
63. Reubinoff BE, Pera MF, Fong CY, Trounson A, Bongso A. Embryonic stem cell lines from human blastocysts: somatic differentiation in vitro. Nat Biotechnol 2000;18:399–404.
64. Deacon T, Dinsmore J, Costantini LC, Ratliff J, Isacson O. Blastula-stage stem cells can differentiate into dopaminergic and serotonergic neurons after transplantation. Exp Neurol 1998;149:28–41.
65. Björklund LM, Sánchez-Pernaute R, Chung S, et al. Embryonic stem cells develop into functional dopaminergic neurons after transplantation in a Parkinson rat model. Proc Natl Acad Sci USA 2002; 99:2344–2349.
66. Lee JY, Qu-Petersen Z, Cao B, et al. Clonal isolation of muscle-derived cells capable of enhancing muscle regeneration and bone healing. J Cell Biol 2000;150: 1085–1100.
67. Ye WL, Shimamura K, Rubenstein JL, Hynes MA, Rosenthal A. FGF and Shh signals control dopaminergic and serotonergic cell fate in the anterior neural plate. Cell 1998;93:755–766.
68. Kim JY, Koh HC, Lee JY, et al. Dopaminergic neuronal differentiation from rat embryonic neural precursors by Nurr1 overexpression. J Neurochem 2003; 85:1443–1454.
69. Shim JW, Koh HC, Chang MY, et al. Enhanced in vitro midbrain dopamine neuron differentiation, dopaminergic function, neurite outgrowth, and 1-methyl-4-

phenylpyridium resistance in mouse embryonic stem cells overexpressing Bcl-XL. J Neurosci 2004;24: 843–852.
70. Nishimura F, Yoshikawa M, Kanda S, et al. Potential use of embryonic stem cells for the treatment of mouse parkinsonian models: improved behavior by transplantation of in vitro differentiated dopaminergic neurons from embryonic stem cells. Stem Cells 2003;21:171–180.
71. Kawasaki H, Mizuseki K, Nishikawa S, et al. Induction of midbrain dopaminergic neurons from ES cells by stromal cell-derived inducing activity. Neuron 2000; 28:31–40.
72. Kawasaki H, Suemori H, Mizuseki K, et al. Generation of dopaminergic neurons and pigmented epithelia from primate ES cells by stromal cell-derived inducing activity. Proc Natl Acad Sci USA 2002;99:1580–1585.
73. Morizane A, Takahashi J, Takagi Y, Sasai Y, Hashimoto N. Optimal conditions for in vivo induction of dopaminergic neurons from embryonic stem cells through stromal cell-derived inducing activity. J Neurosci Res 2002;69:934–939.
74. Ying QL, Stavridis M, Griffiths D, Li M, Smith AG. Conversion of embryonic stem cells into neuroectodermal precursors in adherent monoculture. Nat Biotechnol 2003;21:183–186.
75. Barberi T, Klivenyi P, Calingasan NY, et al. Neural subtype specification of fertilization and nuclear transfer embryonic stem cells and application in parkinsonian mice. Nat Biotechnol 2003;21: 1200–1207.
76. Rolletschek A, Chang H, Guan K, Czyz J, Meyer M, Wobus AM. Differentiation of embryonic stem cell-derived dopaminergic neurons is enhanced by survival-promoting factors. Mech Dev 2001;105:93–104.
77. Mizuseki K, Sakamoto T, Watanabe K, et al. Generation of neural crest-derived peripheral neurons and floor plate cells from mouse and primate embryonic stem cells. Proc Natl Acad Sci USA 2003;100:5828–5833.
78. Carpenter MK, Inokuma MS, Denham J, Mujtaba T, Chiu CP, Rao MS Enrichment of neurons and neural precursors from human embryonic stem cells. Exp Neurol 2001;172:383–397.
79. Reubinoff BE, Itsykson P, Turetsky T, et al. Neural progenitors from human embryonic stem cells. Nat Biotechnol 2001;19:1134–1140.
80. Schuldiner M, Yanuka O, Itskovitz-Eldor J, Melton DA, Benvenisty N. Effects of eight growth factors on the differentiation of cells derived from human embryonic stem cells. Proc Natl Acad Sci USA 2000;97:11307–11312.
81. Schuldiner M, Eiges R, Eden A, et al. Induced neuronal differentiation of human embryonic stem cells. Brain Res 2001;913:201–205.
82. Zhang SC, Wernig M, Duncan ID, Brustle O, Thomson JA. In vitro differentiation of transplantable neural precursors from human embryonic stem cells. Nat Biotechnol 2001;19:1129–1133.
83. Kaufman DS, Hanson ET, Lewis RL, Auerbach R, Thomson JA. Hematopoietic colony-forming cells derived from human embryonic stem cells. Proc Natl Acad Sci USA 2001;98:10716–10721.
84. Park S, Lee KS, Lee YJ, et al. Generation of dopaminergic neurons in vitro from human embryonic stem cells treated with neurotrophic factors. Neurosci Lett 2004;359:99–103.
85. Buytaert-Hoefen KA, Alvarez E, Freed CR. Generation of tyrosine hydroxylase positive neurons from human embryonic stem cells after coculture with cellular substrates and exposure to GDNF. Stem Cells 2004;22: 669–674.
86. Perrier AL, Tabar V, Barberi T, et al. Derivation of midbrain dopamine neurons from human embryonic stem cells. Proc Natl Acad Sci USA 2004;101:12543–12548.
87. Khaner H, Singer O, Ben-Hur T, Reubinoff BE. Induction of differentiation of human embryonic stem cells into cultures enriched for dopaminergic neurons. ISSCR 2nd Annual Meeting, Boston, MA, 2004.
88. Reubinoff BE, Idelson M, Khaner H, et al. Human embryonic stem cell-derived neural progenitors correct behavioral deficits in parkinsonian rats. ISSCR 2nd Annual Meeting, Boston, MA, 2004.
89. Wakayama T, Tabar V, Rodriguez I, Perry AC, Studer L, Mombaerts P. Differentiation of embryonic stem cell lines generated from adult somatic cells by nuclear transfer. Science 2001;292:740–743.
90. Lee SH, Lumelsky N, Studer L, Auerbach JM, McKay RD. Efficient generation of midbrain and hindbrain neurons from mouse embryonic stem cells. Nat Biotechnol 2000;18:675–679.
91. Zawada WM, Cibelli JB, Choi PK, et al. Somatic cell cloned transgenic bovine neurons for transplantation in parkinsonian rats. Nat Med 1998;4:569–574.
92. Cibelli JB, Grant KA, Chapman KB, et al. Parthenogenetic stem cells in nonhuman primates. Science 2002;295:819.
93. Vrana KE, Hipp JD, Goss AM, et al. Nonhuman primate parthenogenetic stem cells. Proc Natl Acad Sci USA 2003;100:11911–11916.
94. Lanza RP, Cibelli JB, West MD. Prospects for the use of nuclear transfer in human transplantation. Nat Biotechnol 1999;17:1171–1174.
95. Friedenstein AJ, Gorskaja JF, Kulagina NN. Fibroblast precursors in normal and irradiated mouse hematopoietic organs. Exp Hematol 1976;4:267–274.
96. Friedenstein AJ, Chailakhyan RK, Gerasimov UV. Bone marrow osteogenic stem cells: in vitro cultivation and transplantation in diffusion chambers. Cell Tissue Kinet 1987;20:263–272.
97. Prockop DJ. Marrow stromal cells as stem cells for nonhematopoietic tissues. Science 1997;276:71–74.
98. Pittenger MF, Mackay AM, Beck SC, et al. Multilineage potential of adult human mesenchymal stem cells. Science 1999;284:143–177.
99. Deans RJ, Moseley AB. Mesenchymal stem cells: biology and potential clinical uses. Exp Hematol 2000;28: 875–884.
100. Sanchez-Ramos JR, Song S, Cardozo-Pelaez F, et al. Adult bone marrow stromal cells differentiate into neural cells in vitro. Exp Neurol 2000;164:247–256.
101. Woodbury D, Schwarz EJ, Prockop DJ, Black IB. Adult rat and human bone marrow stromal cells differentiate into neurons. J Neurosci Res 2000;61:364–370.
102. Woodbury D, Reynolds K, Black IB. Adult bone marrow stromal stem cells express germline, ectodermal, endodermal, and mesodermal genes prior to neurogenesis. J Neurosci Res 2002;96:908–917.
103. Black I, Woodbury D. Adult rat and human bone marrow stromal stem cells differentiate into neurons. Blood Cells Mol Dis 2001;27:632–636.

104. Deng W, Obrocka M, Fischer I, Prockop DJ. In vitro differentiation of human marrow stromal cells into early progenitors of neural cells by conditions that increase intracellular cyclic AMP. Biochem Biophys Res Commun 2001;282:148–152.
105. Kohyama J, Abe H, Shimazaki T, et al. Brain from bone: efficient "meta-differentiation" of marrow stroma-derived mature osteoblasts to neurons with Noggin or a demethylating agent. Differentiation 2001;68:235–244.
106. Kabos P, Ehtesham M, Kabosova A, Black KL, Yu JS. Generation of neural progenitor cells from whole adult bone marrow. Exp Neurol 2002;178:288–293.
107. Jin KL, Mao XO, Batteur S, Sun YJ, Greenberg DA. Induction of neuronal markers in bone marrow cells: differential effects of growth factors and patterns of intracellular expression. Exp Neurol 2003;184:78–89.
108. Joannides A, Gaughwin P, Scott M, Watt S, Compston A, Chandran S. Postnatal astrocytes promote neural induction from adult human bone marrow-derived stem cells. J Hematother Stem Cell Res 2003;12:681–688.
109. Levy YS, Merims D, Panet H, Barhum Y, Melamed E, Offen D. Induction of neuron-specific enolase promoter and neuronal markers in differentiated mouse bone marrow stromal cells. J Mol Neurosci 2003;21:121–132.
110. Levy YS, Stroomza M, Melamed E, Offen D. Embryonic and adult stem cells as a source for cell therapy in Parkinson's disease. J Mol Neurosci 2004;24:353–386.
111. Munoz-Elias G, Woodbury D, Black IB. Marrow stromal cells, mitosis, and neuronal differentiation: stem cell and precursor functions. Stem Cells 2003;21:437–448.
112. Padovan CS, Jahn K, Birnbaum T, et al. Expression of neuronal markers in differentiated marrow stromal cells and CD133+ stem-like cells. Cell Transplant 2003;12:839–848.
113. Rismanchi N, Floyd CL, Berman RF, Lyeth BG. Cell death and long-term maintenance of neuron-like state after differentiation of rat bone marrow stromal cells: a comparison of protocols. Brain Res 2003;991:46–55.
114. Dezawa M, Kanno H, Hoshino M, et al. Specific induction of neuronal cells from bone marrow stromal cells and application for autologous transplantation. J Clin Invest 2004;113:1701–1710.
115. Hermann A, Gast R, Liebau S, et al. Efficient generation of neural stem cell-like cells from adult human bone marrow stromal cells. J Cell Sci 2004;117:4411–4422.
116. Qian L, Saltzman WM. Improving the expansion and neuronal differentiation of mesenchymal stem cells through culture surface modification. Biomaterials 2004;25:1331–1337.
117. Schwarz EJ, Alexander GM, Prockop DJ, Azizi SA. Multipotential marrow stromal cells transduced to produce L-DOPA: engraftment in rat model of Parkinson disease. Hum Gene Ther 1999;10:2539–2549.
118. Schwarz EJ, Reger RL, Alexander GM, Class R, Azizi SA, Prockop DJ. Rat marrow stromal cells rapidly transduced with a self-inactivating retrovirus synthesize L-DOPA in vitro. Gene Ther 2001;8:1214–1223.
119. Park KW, Eglitis MA, Mouradian MM. Protection of nigral neurons by GDNF-engineered marrow cell transplantation. Neurosci Res 2001;40:315–323.
120. Cheng FC, Ni DR, Wu MC, Kuo JS, Chia LG. Glial cell line-derived neurotrophic factor protects against 1-methyl-4-phenyl-1,2,3,6-tetrahydropyridine (MPTP)-induced neurotoxicity in C57BL/6 mice. Neurosci Lett 1998;252:87–90.
121. Li Y, Chen J, Wang L, Zhang L, Lu M, Chopp M. Intracerebral transplantation of bone marrow stromal cells in a 1-methyl-4-phenyl-1,2,3,6-tetrahydropyridine mouse model of Parkinson's disease. Neurosci Lett 2001;316:67–70.
122. Jiang Y, Henderson D, Blackstad M, Chen A, Miller RF, Verfaillie CM. Neuroectodermal differentiation from mouse multipotent adult progenitor cells. Proc Natl Acad Sci USA 2003;100(suppl 1):11854–11860.
123. Jiang Y, Jahagirdar BN, Reinhardt RL, et al. Pluripotency of mesenchymal stem cells derived from adult marrow. Nature 2002;418:41–49.
124. Jiang Y, Vaessen B, Lenvik T, Blackstad M, Reyes M, Verfaillie CM. Multipotent progenitor cells can be isolated from postnatal murine bone marrow, muscle, and brain. Exp Hematol 2002;30:896–904.
125. Reyes M, Lund T, Lenvik T, Aguiar D, Koodie L, Verfaillie CM. Purification and ex vivo expansion of postnatal human marrow mesodermal progenitor cells. Blood 2001;98:2615–2625.
126. D'Ippolito G, Diabira S, Howard GA, Menei P, Roos BA, Schiller PC. Marrow-isolated adult multilineage inducible (MIAMI) cells, a unique population of postnatal young and old human cells with extensive expansion and differentiation potential. J Cell Sci 2004;117:2971–2981.
127. Montero-Menei C, Tatard V, Schiller P, Menei P, Benoit Jean-Pierre, D'Ippolito G. Dopaminergic differentiation of human marrow-isolated adult multilineage inducible cells for cell therapy. 2nd Annual Meeting of ISSCR, Boston, MA, 2004.
128. Brazelton TR, Rossi FMV, Keshet GI, Blau HM. From marrow to brain: expression of neuronal phenotypes in adult mice. Science 2000;290:1775–1779.
129. Mezey E, Chandross KJ, Harta G, Maki RA, McKercher SR. Turning blood into brain: cells bearing neuronal antigens generated in vivo from bone marrow. Science 2000;290:1779–1782.
130. Hess DC, Hill WD, Martin-Studdard A, Carroll J, Brailer J, Carothers J. Bone marrow as a source of endothelial cells and NeuN-expressing cells after stroke. Stroke 2002;33:1362–1368.
131. Zhao LR, Duan WM, Reyes M, Keene CD, Verfaillie CM, Low WC. Human bone marrow stem cells exhibit neural phenotypes and ameliorate neurological deficits after grafting into the ischemic brain of rats. Exp Neurol 2002;174:11–20.
132. Mezey E, Key S, Vogelsang G, Szalayova I, Lange GD, Crain B. Transplanted bone marrow generates new neurons in human brain. Proc Natl Acad Sci USA 2003;100:1364–1369.
133. Holden C, Vogel G. Plasticity: time for a reappraisal? Science 2002;296:2126–2129.
134. Lemischka I. A few thoughts about the plasticity of stem cells. Exp Hematol 2002;30:848–852.
135. Wurmser AE, Gage FH. Stem cells: cell fusion causes confusion. Nature 2002;416:485–487.
136. Cogle CR, Yachnis AT, Laywell ED, et al. Bone marrow transdifferentiation in brain after transplantation: a retrospective study. Lancet 2004;363:1432–1437.

137. Pochampally RR, Neville BT, Schwarz EJ, Li MM, Prockop DJ. Rat adult stem cells (marrow stromal cells) engraft and differentiate in chick embryos without evidence of cell fusion. Proc Natl Acad Sci USA 2004;101:9282–9285.
138. Lu D, Li Y, Wang L, Chen J, Mahmood A, Chopp M. Intraarterial administration of marrow stromal cells in a rat model of traumatic brain injury. J Neurotrauma 2001;18:813–819.
139. Lu D, Mahmood A, Wang L, Li Y, Lu M, Chopp M. Adult bone marrow stromal cells administered intravenously to rats after traumatic brain injury migrate into brain and improve neurological outcome. Neuroreport 2001;12:559–563.
140. Lu D, Li Y, Mahmood A, Wang L, Rafiq T, Chopp M. Neural and marrow-derived stromal cell sphere transplantation in a rat model of traumatic brain injury. J Neurosurg 2002;97:935–940.
141. Mahmood A, Lu D, Wang L, Li Y, Lu M, Chopp M. Treatment of traumatic brain injury in female rats with intravenous administration of bone marrow stromal cells. Neurosurgery 2001;49:1196–1204.
142. Chen J, Li Y, Wang L, Lu M, Zhang X, Chopp M. Therapeutic benefit of intracerebral transplantation of bone marrow stromal cells after cerebral ischemia in rats. J Neurol Sci 2001;189:49–57.
143. Chen J, Li Y, Wang L, et al. Therapeutic benefit of intravenous administration of bone marrow stromal cells after cerebral ischemia in rats. Stroke 2001;32:1005–1011.
144. Chopp M, Zhang XH, Li Y, et al. Spinal cord injury in rat: treatment with bone marrow stromal cell transplantation. neuroreport 2000;11:3001–3005.
145. Borlongan CV, Sanberg PR. Neural transplantation for treatment of Parkinson's disease. Drug Discov Today 2002;7:674–682.
146. Kim JH, Auerbach JM, Rodríguez-Gómez JA, et al. Dopamine neurons derived from embryonic stem cells function in an animal model of Parkinson's disease. Nature 2002;418:50–56.
147. Chung S, Sonntag KC, Andersson T, et al. Genetic engineering of mouse embryonic stem cells by Nurr1 enhances differentiation and maturation into dopaminergic neurons. Eur J Neurosci 2002;216:1829–1838.
148. Iacovitti L, Stull ND. Expression of tyrosine hydroxylase in newly differentiated neurons for a human cell line (hNT). Neuroreport 1997;8:1471–1474.
149. Zigova T, Willing AE, Tedesco EM, et al. Lithium chloride induces the expression of tyrosine hydroxylase in hNT neurons. Exp Neurol 1999;157:251–258.
150. Zigova T, Barroso LF, Willing AE, et al. Dopaminergic phenotype of hNT cells in vitro. Dev Brain Res 2000;122:87–90.
151. Iacovitti L, Stull ND, Jin H. Differentiation of human dopamine neurons from an embryonic carcinomal stem cell line. Brain Res 2001;912:99–104.
152. Stull ND, Iacovitti L. Sonic hedgehog and FGF8: inadequate signals for the differentiation of a dopamine phenotype in mouse and human neurons in culture. Exp Neurol 2001;169:36–43.
153. Sodja C, Fang H, Dasgupta T, Ribecco M, Walker PR, Sikorska M. Identification of functional dopamine receptors in human teratocarcinoma NT2 cells. Mol Brain Res 2002;99:83–91.
154. Misiuta IE, Anderson L, McGrogan MP, Sanberg PR, Willing AE, Zigova T. The transcription factor Nurr1 in human NT2 cells and hNT neurons. Dev Brain Res 2003;145:107–115.
155. Baker KA, Hong M, Sadi D, Mendez I. Intrastriatal and intranigral grafting of hNT neurons in the 6-OHDA rat model of Parkinson's disease. Exp Neurol 2000;162:350–360.
156. Yang M, Stull ND, Berk MA, Snyder EY, Iacovitti L. Neural stem cells spontaneously express dopaminergic traits after transplantation into the intact or 6-hydroxydopamine-lesioned rat. Exp Neurol 2002;177:50–60.

8

Cell Replacement Therapy in Acute Stroke: Current State

Yossi Gilgun-Sherki and Jonathan Y. Streifler

Stroke is a leading cause of morbidity in the western world, resulting in chronic disability in many cases. Although huge efforts have been made in the search for effective treatment, so far results have been quite disappointing. Recently, cell replacement therapy has emerged as an experimental approach aiming to restore brain function, which is impaired in several neurodegenerative diseases, as well as in stroke. Porcine fetal cells, neuronal progenitor cells (NPCs), embryonic stem cells (ESCs), immortalized cell lines, bone marrow stromal cells (BMSCs), and umbilical cord blood cells (UCBCs) have been introduced as potential sources for neuronal cells in experimental and clinical stroke trials. However, limited knowledge about their biology (including long-term safety) and insufficient data regarding several issues such as the preferred stroke type and its severity, specific location of the injection, and the preferred cell type restrict their potential clinical use. Therefore, further research on the molecular mechanisms of stroke, the candidate cell lines for transplantation, and bioengineering strategies, is needed before this technique can be implemented safely and effectively in stroke victims.

Acute Stroke

Stroke is defined as an abrupt focal loss of brain function resulting from interference with the blood supply to part of the central nervous system (CNS). Acute stroke comprises two main types: 1) Ischemic stroke (80% of stroke cases), which is mainly caused by extracranial (large artery or cardiac) embolism or intracranial thrombosis, and 2) hemorrhagic stroke (20% of stroke cases), which is further classified to intracerebral hemorrhage, and subarachnoid hemorrhage.

Stroke is a leading cause of mortality and morbidity, particularly in the middle-aged and elderly population, in most developed countries.[1] CNS damage occurs in stroke mainly as a result of hypoxia. In the acute phase of ischemic stroke there is an ischemic gradient comprising the core, which is the central, permanently ischemic zone, and the penumbra, located at the periphery where the ischemic damage is still reversible. In the penumbra, functional alterations occur in the neurons and glial cells. Neurons are most vulnerable to ischemia because of their dependence on the oxidative metabolism and on glucose for energy. The pathophysiological processes in acute CNS injury such as stroke, mechanical trauma, or subarachnoid hemorrhage, are extremely complex and involve pathological permeability of blood-brain barrier, energy failure, loss of cell ion homeostasis, acidosis, increased intracellular calcium, excitotoxicity, and free radical-mediated toxicity.[1] This leads to ischemic necrosis, which occurs in the regions most severely afflicted by ischemia. It can also promote apoptosis, which is more likely to occur in ischemic regions afflicted less severely, evolves at a slower pace, and depends on the activation of a sequence of genes.[2,3]

Although enormous amounts of efforts have been invested throughout the years aiming to provide brain tissue salvage (by using different neuroprotective agents, which were effective in animal models but so far not in humans), currently the effects of acute stroke treatments are modest and chronic disability remains a major medical and economical burden on society. The only approved treatment for acute stroke today is thrombolytic therapy, which is aimed to dissolve the occluding blood clot, thus facilitating early restoration of focal cerebral blood flow. However, because of its short therapeutic time window (delayed administration results in increased risk of hemorrhage), this treatment is not available for most patients. Recently, there has been an increased emphasis on novel treatment for brain function restoration using cell replacement therapies. Indeed, many studies have shown the potential efficacy of neural transplantation in animal models of focal and global cerebral ischemia. However, very few clinical trials have been performed.

In this chapter, we discuss the potential role of cell replacement therapy in stroke, specify several cell lines as potential sources for transplantation, and review the factors and current limitations affecting the safety and efficacy of this method.

Cell Lines as Potential Sources for Transplantation

Various cell lines have been suggested as potential sources for transplantation in stroke; the preferred line, however, has not yet been determined. The molecular complexity of stroke and the involvement of different neuronal phenotypes require that the optimal cell candidate for transplantation is one that can proliferate in high numbers and differentiate into the appropriate neural/glial cell types with maximal efficacy and minimal adverse events. The list of cell lines being investigated is given below.

Porcine Fetal Cells

Fetal (immature) neuronal cells can survive and integrate in the human brain, yet because of the limited availability of human tissue, some investigators have used fetal xenotransplants from pigs, which are considered relatively safe as a donor cell source. These cells, also called lateral ganglionic eminence (LGE) cells, are presumed to be undifferentiated striatal precursor cells and were first used in an animal model of Huntington's disease in the middle of the 1990s. It was shown that transplantation of LGE cells promoted graft integration and improved functional deficits.[4,5] However, the extent of the capability of LGE cells to proliferate or differentiate has not yet been investigated and issues such as the percentage of LGE grafts differentiating into functional neurons versus glial cells, their plasticity, and their differentiation-dependency in the graft site have not yet been clarified.

So far, several studies have shown that transplanted LGE neuroblasts differentiate into striatal neurons after intrastriatal implantation.[6,7] These observations imply that LGE cells seem to be committed to follow a specific lineage pathway, and therefore cast doubts as to their use outside the striatum in the treatment of stroke.

Other concerns include graft rejection and the potential transmission of infectious diseases associated with porcine-to-human neural xenotransplantation [e.g., the porcine endogenous retrovirus (PERV)]. However, no such evidence for clinical in vivo transmission of PERV in the blood of 24 patients with neuronal diseases who underwent transplantation with fetal porcine neurons was found.[8]

Neural Progenitor Cell

During the past few years, it has become clear that the mammalian adult brain contains NPCs that can proliferate, self-renew, and generate all cellular elements in the brain, including neurons. Because of the development of novel technologies, these cells can now be isolated from the subventricular zone (SVZ) and the subgranular zone of the hippocampal dentate gyrus of the developing and the adult CNS tissue. These cells have been shown to proliferate in response to brain damage, including focal ischemia, and therefore are a potential graft source.[9-11] However, these cells cannot be transplanted in every brain region because of their limited growth support and their proliferative/differentiate properties (less in the cortex than in the SVZ).[12]

Embryonic Stem Cells

These cells are derived from pre-embryos at the blastocyst stage and can give rise to all body tissues and cells. Animal models have demonstrated that ESCs, when transplanted into adult hosts, differentiate and develop into cells and tissues and thus may be applicable for treating a variety of conditions, including Parkinson's disease, multiple sclerosis, spinal injuries, stroke, and cancer. Transplanted ESCs are exposed to immune reactions similar to those acting on organ transplants; hence, immunosuppression of the recipient is generally required. It is possible, however, to obtain ESCs that are genetically identical to the patient's own cells using therapeutic cloning techniques.[13]

Several studies showed that these cells are able to migrate in response to damage. Hoehn et al.[14] showed, using magnetic resonance imaging, that ESCs that were implanted into the healthy hemisphere of rat brains 2 weeks after focal cerebral ischemia (FCI), migrated along the corpus callosum to the ventricular walls, and populated en masse at the border zone of the damaged brain tissue (i.e., the hemisphere opposite to the implantation sites).

Another study showed that undifferentiated ESCs – xenotransplanted into the rat brain at the hemisphere opposite to the ischemic injury – migrated along the corpus callosum toward the damaged tissue and differentiated into neurons at the border zone of the lesion. In the homologous mouse brain, the same murine ESCs did not migrate, but produced highly malignant teratocarcinomas at the site of implantation, independent of whether they were predifferentiated in vitro to NPCs.[15]

These results imply that ESCs might migrate to the damaged site. However, the production of teratocarcinoma raises concerns about the safety of ESC transplantation in patients with stroke.

Immortalized Cell Lines

ESC research raises many ethical questions and xenotransplantation limitations. Several laboratories have therefore tracked alternative graft sources including transformed cell lines in vitro. Two major immortalized cell lines have been used: The NTerra-2 cells and the Mandsley hippocampal stem cell line clone 36 (MHP36).

The NTerra-2

This cell line was derived from a human testicular germ cell tumor,[16] and unlike other teratocarcinoma cell lines, it has an exclusive commitment to the neuronal line when exposed to retinoic acid (RA). Several studies have shown that NTerra-2 (NT2) cells resemble NPCs. They express cell surface markers and cytoskeletal proteins unique to neural stem cells, and also yield a complement of daughter cells that retain the original phenotype.[17] In addition, treatment for several weeks with RA and mitotic inhibitors produces postmitotic, neuron-like cells (NT2N), which have asymmetrical morphology with extended axons and dendrites.[17,18] These cells express various neuronal characters, such as neurotransmitters,[19] calcium channels,[20] glutamate receptors,[21] and other proteins, which indicates that they have secretory activity and synaptogenesis.[18,22] However, the major difficulties with these cells are that they cannot develop into completely full-grown neuronal phenotype in vitro, and they show full differentiation only after transplantation.[23]

Apparently, the survival of NT2N cells is dependent on other non-neuronal supportive cells such as glia and oligodendrocytes. Indeed, studies have showed that coculture of NT2N cells with astrocytes substantially prolongs their survival and enhances maturation and synaptogenesis in vitro, compared with NT2N culture alone.[22,24]

The main safety concern with undifferentiated NT2 cells is that their implantation into the rat brain leads to tumor growth and death within 10 weeks, except when they are implanted into the host striatum where grafts cease proliferating and differentiate into neuron-like cells.[25,26]

The Mandsley Hippocampal Stem Cell Line Clone 36

These cells are an immortalized murine stem cell line, derived from the E14 hippocampal proliferative zone of the tsA58 transgenic mouse. The proliferation of this cell line is temperature-dependent, meaning that low temperatures (33°C) result in various neuronal and glial formations, whereas, at high temperatures (37°C), mature neurons and glia are produced.[27]

The survival of these cells after transplantation was speculated to be dependent on immunosuppression treatment; however, Modo et al.[28] showed that in transplanted post-middle cerebral artery occlusion (MCAo) rats no significant differences in cell survival were found between those treated or not treated with cyclosporine A. These results provide evidence for the low immunogenic properties of Mandsley hippocampal stem cell line clone 36 (MHP36) cells during the initial period after implantation, which is known to be associated with an acute host immune response and ensuing graft rejection.

Bone Marrow Stromal Cells

Extraction of bone marrow (BM) gives rise to two cell populations: those that float are hematopoietic cells and those that adhere are referred to as mesenchymal stem cells (MSCs).[29] These cell lines can be obtained readily from BM under local anesthesia, expanded in culture, and potentially could be delivered to injured brain tissue without the need for invasive stereotaxic operations. Using the patient's own BMSCs should prevent host immunity and graft-versus-host disease. These cells are capable of changing their fate and differentiate into a variety of tissues including glia, and neurons.[30–33]

It was shown that when human BMSCs are exposed to neurotrophic factors (NTFs) such as epidermal growth factor (EGF) or brain-derived NTF (BDNF) in vitro or cultured with rat fetal mesencephalic or striatal cells,[32] they differentiate into NPC-like cells, and migrate along paths similar to NPCs.[34]

Several studies found that BMSCs from male C57 BL/6-TgN (ACTbEGFP)1Osb mice expressing GFP that were transplanted into female C57 BL/6J mice that then underwent MCAo, became incorporated into the vasculature of the ischemic zone and expressed an endothelial cell phenotype within 3 days and at 7 and 14 days after MCAo. Some BM-derived cells also expressed the neuronal marker NeuN at 7 and 14 days after ischemia.[35,36] It was also shown that transplantation of nuclear fluorescence-labeled BMSCs into the ipsilateral striatum of mice subjected to MCAo resulted in migration into the corpus callosum and injured cortex. In addition, these cells also expressed neuronal markers, including NeuN, 4 weeks after transplantation.[37]

Another study showed that intravenous injection of human MSC (hMSC) to rats 24 hours after MCAo revealed significant increases in numbers of enlarged and thin walled blood vessels and numbers of newly formed capillaries at the ischemic boundary zone (IBZ). In addition, treatment with hMSCs significantly raised endogenous rat vascular epithelial growth factor (VEGF) levels and endogenous VEGF receptor-immunoreactivity in the IBZ.[38]

Umbilical Cord Blood Cells

This is another potential source of multipotential stem cells that can create neuronal and glial cells in response to NTFs, especially to neuronal growth factor and RA.[39] However, our poor current knowledge regarding the biology of human UCBCs (hUCBCs) restricts their current utilization.

Cell Replacement Therapy in Acute Stroke

Experimental Data

Immortalized Cell Lines

The neuron-like cells (NT2N). Several studies have examined whether grafted NT2N cells to the adult rat brain, after FCI, survive and integrate into the neuronal tissue. One study showed that intrastriatal transplantation of NT2N cells 1 month after MCAo, followed by cyclosporine treatment, led to significant functional improvement at 6 months compared with the control groups receiving either rat fetal cerebellar grafts or growth medium alone or cyclosporine on its own.[40]

No studies have addressed the phenotype of NT2N grafts in the transplanted ischemic brain, nor has it been shown whether they extend processes and integrate into the host brain. Aside from striatal injuries, the effects of NT2N cells in other ischemic infarcts remain to be determined.

MHP36 cells. Veizovic et al.[41] used these cells in an FCI model in rats. Transplantation was followed by immunosuppression with cyclosporine for 2–3 weeks after MCAo. They showed that most of the MHP36 cells transplanted into the intact somatosensory cortex and striatum, remained in the intact hemisphere, whereas some (approximately 30%) migrated to the lesioned cortex and striatum. The MHP36-engrafted animals had significantly reduced infarct volumes and significantly better sensorimotor recovery over the following 18 weeks compared with sham-operated animals, whereas other parameters, such as spatial learning and memory, did not significantly improve.

Several studies have been performed at the Psychology Department in London. The first study investigated whether implantation of 200,000 MHP36 cells in the left (n = 8) or right (n = 9) brain parenchyma or their infusion into the right ventricle (n = 7) 2–3 weeks after right MCAo affected functional recovery. It was found that rats with left and right parenchymal grafts showed reduced bilateral asymmetry (i.e., improved function) but no change in spatial learning. Conversely, spatial learning improved in rats with intraventricular grafts, but a marked asymmetry persisted.[42]

Another recent study showed that intraparenchymal MHP36 grafts either ipsilateral or contralateral to the lesion or intraventricular MHP36 grafts raised apolipoprotein E, a peptide which was associated with plasticity and involved in promoting functional recovery, expression levels in various brain regions 4 months after transplantation.[43] These results imply that both the intact and lesioned hemispheres attract grafted stem cells after stroke, suggesting repair processes that utilize cells both for local repair and to augment plasticity changes in the contralateral motor pathways.

Bone Marrow Stromal Cells

BMSCs may be differentiated into neuron-like and/or glia-like cells, implying that they may have potential use in cell replacement therapy in the CNS. Eglitis et al.[44] (1999) demonstrated that systemically infused BMSCs into irradiated rats, subjected to FCI, migrate to the ischemic cortex and become astrocytes. Another study demonstrated that intrastriatal transplantation of BMSCs in mice 4 days after MCAo, survive, migrate, and differentiate into glial or neuronal-like cells (yet only 1% of the labeled BMSCs expressed neuronal markers[45]). Significant behavioral improvement at 28 days was shown in the transplanted mice compared with controls, although no difference was observed in infarct volume between the groups.[45]

Similar results were obtained by two other studies that administered BMSCs both intravenously and intracarotid and showed improvement in behavioral recovery 14 or 35 days after MCAo, respectively,[46,47] although only 0.02% of the cells stained for neural markers in the ischemic hemisphere.[47]

An additional study showed that transplantation of 3×10^6 BMSCs to MCAo rats improved functional recovery at day 14, compared with the controls.[48] A recent study demonstrated that early intervention with intravenous administration of autologous BM can reduce lesion size in the rat MCAo model and improve functional outcome, as was measured by Morris water maze and treadmill stress test.[49]

Human Mesenchymal Stem Cells

Several studies examined the efficacy of hMSCs in the treatment of experimental stroke. One study reported a significant functional recovery in rats treated with hMSCs at 14 days compared with control rats in a transient MCAo model. Furthermore, few (1%–5%) hMSCs expressed proteins phenotypic of brain parenchymal cells.[50]

An additional study showed that purified hMSCs that were grafted into the cortex surrounding the area of infarction, 1 week after cortical brain ischemia in rats, improved functional performance in several behavior tests. In addition, histologic analyses revealed that transplanted hMSCs expressed markers for astrocytes (GFAP), oligodendrocytes (GalC), and neurons (beta III, NF160, NF200, hNSE, and hNF70). Therefore, it is unlikely that the functional recovery observed in the ischemic rats, which received hMSC grafts, was mediated by the integration of new "neuronal" cells into the circuitry of the host brain. Rather, these results imply that the functional improvement might have been mediated by proteins secreted by the transplanted hMSCs, which could have up-regulated host brain plasticity in response to experimental stroke.[51]

Another recent study showed that intravenous injection of hMSCs to rats that underwent MCAo improved their motor behavior, reduced apoptosis, and promoted endogenous cell proliferation.[52]

According to the preliminary results regarding BMSC transplantation in stroke, it seems likely that these cells might become good candidates for the treatment of stroke. However, because of our limited knowledge on neuronal differentiation, there are many unknown factors such as the capability of these cells to differentiate into mature neurons that are capable of reconstructing the natural neuronal circuitry, and other concerns such as the adequate cell number for transplantation (see Table 8.1) and brain targeting.[46]

Umbilical Cord Blood Cells

UCBCS are the source of hematopoietic stem cells and other stem and progenitor cells. Chen et al.[46] (2001) reported that intravenous infusion of 3×10^6 hUCBCs to rats 24 hours after MCAo, improved behavioral recovery 14 days after implantation compared with control animals subjected to FCI alone or FCI with saline injection. An estimated 2% of these cells expressed neuronal markers, whereas an unknown percentage survived and migrated to the ischemic hemisphere, and also to various other organs.[46]

Another recent study assessed which route of hUCBC administration, intravenously into the femoral vein or directly into the striatum, might produce the greatest behavioral recovery in rats with permanent MCAo. It was found that the spontaneous activity decreased significantly when hUCBCs were transplanted 24 hours after stroke compared with nontransplanted, stroked animals. In addition, in the step test, a significant improvement was found only after femoral delivery of the hUCBCs. This was in contrast to the behavioral recovery that was similar in both striatal and femoral hUCBCs delivery.[53] These results suggest that the intravenous route might be more effective than the striatal route in producing long-term functional benefits to the animals after a stroke.

This source of cells is interesting because of ready availability and it does not raise ethical issues. Although functional improvement has been demonstrated in animal stroke models, much work lies ahead in order to determine unequivocally whether UCBSCs will serve as a potential source for cell transplantation.

Clinical Trials

To date, only one clinical study has been reported, using cultured human neuronal cells (NT2D1, RA treated) in patients with stroke. This was an open, phase I clinical trial that assessed the safety and feasibility of human neuronal cellular transplantation in patients with basal ganglia stroke and fixed motor deficits. It included 12 patients (aged 44–75 years) with an infarct 6 months to 6 years old (and stable for at least 2 months).[54] Four of the 12 subjects were implanted with 2 million cells, divided into three implants, whereas the others received 2 or 6 million cells (at one or three-pass injections), at random. Serial evaluations (12–18 months) showed no adverse cell-related serologic or imaging-defined effects.[54] The European Stroke Scale score was significantly improved in six patients (3 to 10 points), with a mean improvement of 2.9 points in all patients. Motor performance accounted for most of the change, being better in the 6-million cell group. Both the Barthel index and the SF-36 disabilities scales were not consistent as they showed improvement only in the 6-million cell group. In addition, positron emission tomography (PET) scanning at 6 months[54] and 12 months[55] showed greater than 15% relative uptake of 18F-fluorodeoxyglucose (FDG) at the transplant site in six patients. These findings, including the FDG-PET scan, are encouraging; however, because of

Table 8.1. Possible factors that influence the efficacy and safety of transplantation in stroke

- Isolation and expansion techniques
- Number and volume of transplanted cells
- Cell medium (e.g., neurotrophic factors)
- Cell type
- Cell survival (e.g., neurotrophic factors)
- Cell integration (e.g., neurotrophic factors)
- Surgical technique
- Postoperative care
- Place of transplantation and area-specific brain targeting
- Blood supply to the injection site
- Stroke type (ischemic versus hemorrhagic)
- Time of transplantation
- Severity of the damage
- Age and gender of the patient
- Graft rejection and cotherapies such as immunosuppressants
- Appearance of tumors (teratogenicity)
- Co-morbidities and especially other neurological diseases

the small number of patients included in these studies, definitive conclusions cannot be drawn regarding the clinical efficacy.

Factors that Might Affect Efficacy and Safety

Technical Considerations

There are many factors that might influence the efficacy and safety of cell transplantation in stroke (Table 8.1). Among them are the numbers of cells transplanted, which is still relatively unknown. This issue is also important for planning delivery methods given that the different volumes that may be needed for adequate cell numbers may require different methods.

Another important factor is the type of cell to be transplanted. This is of cardinal importance because of the effectiveness and safety properties of each cell type. For example, it is well known that several cell lines (e.g., ESCs) form fatal teratomas at the transplantation site. Tumor formation would be a serious disadvantage to transplantation in humans.

An additional major issue is the site of transplantation as it involves other factors, such as blood supply to the injection site and the stroke type (ischemic versus hemorrhagic). Cells might be implanted intraventricularly or into brain parenchyma. It is reasonable to suggest that the penumbra is the preferred area for cell implantation, because of a reduced content of excitotoxicity and toxic substances such as proinflammatory cytokines and reactive oxygen species and better blood supply through collateral circulation, but this issue requires further examination. In addition, several cell lines cannot be transplanted in every brain region, because of limited growth support (e.g., NPCs are known to be less proliferative in the cortex than in the SVZ).

The timing of the transplantation is also an important factor that might affect the success of transplantation. The optimal timing for a transplant is unknown, yet stroke type, chronicity, and also blood supply (inadequate blood flow would not support graft viability) must be taken into account. The severity of the damage and natural course of recovery from the stroke must also be considered. Many neurologists prefer to transplant at least 1 month after the stroke and preferably when deficits reach a plateau. However, during that delay, the formation of scar tissue may occur, which might adversely affect the implanted grafts. The age of the patient also influences the efficacy of the transplantation, and it is reasonable to presume that younger patients would respond differently than older ones. In addition, the gender and hormonal status of the patient might also have impact on cell survival. Finally, the use of immunosuppressants should also be taken into consideration because they might complicate the interpretation of the therapeutic effect.[56]

Preimplantation Manipulations

These procedures are speculated to be very crucial in the survival of the cells posttransplantation, and might produce better-characterized neuronal donor populations. In addition, they can help to identify the donor glial-neuronal interactions,[57] and can assist in understanding molecular pathways in stroke, such as apoptosis in pre- and posttransplantation.[58] Indeed, apoptosis inhibitors were shown to improve the viability of the grafts when they were administered before or with the implanted cells.[59,60]

One of the most important factors that might contribute to cell survival and integration after transplantation is NTFs, which are naturally secreted peptides from neurons and neuron-supporting cells that act as growth factors for the development, maintenance, repair, and survival of specific neuronal populations[61,62] (see also Table 8.1). These factors stimulate axonal growth and have a key role in the construction of the normal synaptic network during development.[63,64] However, in aging and pathological states, such as head trauma, chronic (e.g., neurodegenerative diseases) or acute (e.g., stroke) diseases, these factors might be deficient, and therefore influence neuronal survival leading to apoptosis.[61,65–67]

Several recent studies support these concepts: A composite graft of fresh BM along with BDNF, transplanted into the IBZ of rat brain, facilitated BM cells to survive and differentiate and improved functional recovery.[68] BDNF and nerve growth factor were also shown to decrease significantly apoptotic cells in the IBZ of the ischemic hemisphere of rats treated with hMSCs.[50]

Another study demonstrated that basic fibroblast growth factor-secreting cell line that was implanted into the right striatum of rats 6 days before MCAo showed a 30% reduction in the infarct volume compared with the controls with encapsulated naive baby hamster kidney cell grafting or those without implantation at all.[69,70]

In a different study, four clones of fetal rat kidney cells producing GDNF at physiological concentrations were transplanted into the ischemic core or penumbra of rats that had undergone MCAo. Three of these four clones showed a reduced volume of infarction and improved behavioral abnormalities as compared with controls.[71]

These results suggest that supplementation of NTFs, either pre-, parallel, or post-transplantation, supports the surviving cells or enhances the local environment to improve function, and therefore might be beneficial in the treatment of stroke.

Conclusions and Future Strategies

A variety of cell types have been used to try to restore brain function after stroke, mainly in rodent models. Some of the findings presented herein imply that cell replacement therapy might indeed ultimately become a novel restorative therapy for stroke. However, because of our limited knowledge on the molecular basis of stroke and cell transplantation, there are many open questions regarding the efficacy (e.g., graft integration, survival, and functionality; see Table 8.1) and safety (e.g., tumor formation) of each cell source. At present, it is also still debatable whether the cells themselves integrate and function as active neurons and glia (i.e., form new neural pathways and connections) or they mainly act through neurohumoral mechanisms (i.e., stimulation of intrinsic host recovery mechanisms). Trophic factors are probably needed and may be even more important than the cell type or vehicles used. It is likely that multiple mechanisms are involved. Therefore, long-term investigations into safety and efficacy, together with comparative studies between cell types, and different trophic factors, are still warranted. They will enhance our understanding of cell replacement therapy in stroke, and facilitate its application in clinical practice.

References

1. Brott T, Bogousslavsky J. Treatment of acute ischemic stroke. N Engl J Med 2000;343:710–722.
2. Pulsinelli WA. Pathophysiology of stroke. Lancet 1992;339:533–536.
3. Dirnagl U, Costantino I, Moskowitz MA. Pathobiology of ischemic stroke: an integrated view. Trends Neurosci 1999;22:391–397.
4. Deacon TW, Pakzaban P, Burns LH, Dinsmore J, Isacson O. Cytoarchitectonic development, axon-glia relationships, and long distance axon growth of porcine striatal xenografts in rats. Exp Neurol 1994;130:151–167.
5. Isacson O, Deacon TW, Pakzaban P, Galpern WR, Dinsmore J, Burns LH. Transplanted xenogeneic neural cells in neurodegenerative disease models exhibit remarkable axonal target specificity and distinct growth patterns of glial and axonal fibres. Nat Med 1995;1:1189–1194.
6. Jacoby DB, Lindberg C, Cunningham MG, Ratliff J, Dinsmore J. Long-term survival of fetal porcine lateral ganglionic eminence cells in the hippocampus of rats. J Neurosci Res 1999;56:581–594.
7. Skogh C, Parmar M, Campbell K. The differentiation potential of precursor cells from the mouse lateral ganglionic eminence is restricted by in vitro expansion. Neuroscience 2003;120:379–385.
8. Dinsmore JH, Manhart C, Raineri R, Jacoby DB, Moore A. No evidence for infection of human cells with porcine endogenous retrovirus (PERV) after exposure to porcine fetal neuronal cells. Transplantation 2000;70:1382–1389.
9. Gu W, Brannstrom T, Wester P. Cortical neurogenesis in adult rats after reversible photothrombotic stroke. J Cereb Blood Flow Metab 2000;20:1166–1173.
10. Jin K, Minami M, Lan JQ, et al. Neurogenesis in dentate subgranular zone and rostral subventricular zone after focal cerebral ischemia in the rat. Proc Natl Acad Sci USA 2001;98:4710–4715.
11. Jiang W, Gu W, Brannstrom T, Rosqvist R, Wester P. Cortical neurogenesis in adult rats after transient middle cerebral artery occlusion. Stroke 2001;32:1201–1207.
12. Svendsen CN, Clarke DJ, Rosser AE, Dunnett SB. Survival and differentiation of rat and human epidermal growth factor-responsive precursor cells following grafting into the lesioned adult central nervous system. Exp Neurol 1996;137:376–388.
13. Sunde A, Eftedal I. Embryonic stem cells and therapeutic cloning. Tidsskr Nor Laegeforen 2001;121:2407–2412.
14. Hoehn M, Kustermann E, Blunk J, et al. Monitoring of implanted stem cell migration in vivo: a highly resolved in vivo magnetic resonance imaging investigation of experimental stroke in rat. Proc Natl Acad Sci USA 2002;99:16267–16272.
15. Erdo F, Buhrle C, Blunk J, et al. Host-dependent tumorigenesis of embryonic stem cell transplantation in experimental stroke. J Cereb Blood Flow Metab 2003;23:780–785.
16. Andrews PW, Damjanov I, Simon D, et al. Pluripotent embryonal carcinoma clones derived from the human teratocarcinoma cell line Tera-2. Differentiation in vivo and in vitro. Lab Invest 1984;50:147–162.
17. Pleasure SJ, Lee VM. NTera 2 cells: a human cell line which displays characteristics expected of a human

committed neuronal progenitor cell. J Neurosci Res 1993;35:585–602.
18. Pleasure SJ, Page C, Lee VM. Pure, postmitotic, polarized human neurons derived from NTera 2 cells provide a system for expressing exogenous proteins in terminally differentiated neurons. J Neurosci 1992;12:1802–1815.
19. Guillemain I, Alonso G, Patey G, Privat A, Chaudieu I. Human NT2 neurons express a large variety of neurotransmission phenotypes in vitro. J Comp Neurol 2000;422:380–395.
20. Neelands TR, King AP, Macdonald RL. Functional expression of L-, N-, P/Q-, and R-type calcium channels in the human NT2-N cell line. J Neurophysiol 2000;84:2933–2944.
21. Younkin DP, Tang CM, Hardy M, et al. Inducible expression of neuronal glutamate receptor channels in the NT2 human cell line. Proc Natl Acad Sci USA 1993;90:2174–2178.
22. Hartley RS, Margulis M, Fishman PS, Lee VM, Tang CM. Functional synapses are formed between human NTera2 (NT2N, hNT) neurons grown on astrocytes. J Comp Neurol 1999;407:1–10.
23. Kleppner SR, Robinson KA, Trojanowski JQ, Lee VM. Transplanted human neurons derived from a teratocarcinoma cell line (NTera-2) mature, integrate, and survive for over 1 year in the nude mouse brain. J Comp Neurol 1995;357:618–632.
24. Bani-Yaghoub M, Felker JM, Naus CC. Human NT2/D1 cells differentiate into functional astrocytes. Neuroreport 1999;10:3843–3846.
25. Miyazono M, Lee VM, Trojanowski JQ. Proliferation, cell death, and neuronal differentiation in transplanted human embryonal carcinoma (NTera2) cells depend on the graft site in nude and severe combined immunodeficient mice. Lab Invest 1995;73:273–283.
26. Miyazono M, Nowell PC, Finan JL, Lee VM, Trojanowski JQ. Long-term integration and neuronal differentiation of human embryonal carcinoma cells (NTera-2) transplanted into the caudoputamen of nude mice. J Comp Neurol 1996;376:603–613.
27. Sinden JD, Rashid-Doubell F, Kershaw TR, et al. Recovery of spatial learning by grafts of a conditionally immortalized hippocampal neuroepithelial cell line into the ischaemia-lesioned hippocampus. Neuroscience 1997;81:599–608.
28. Modo M, Rezaie P, Heuschling P, Patel S, Male DK, Hodges H. Transplantation of neural stem cells in a rat model of stroke: assessment of short-term graft survival and acute host immunological response. Brain Res 2002;958:70–82.
29. Javazon EH, Colter DC, Schwarz EJ, Prockop DJ. Rat marrow stromal cells are more sensitive to plating density and expand more rapidly from single-cell-derived colonies than human marrow stromal cells. Stem Cells 2001;19:219–225.
30. Prockop DJ. Marrow stromal cells as stem cells for nonhematopoietic tissues. Science 1997;276:71–74.
31. Pittenger MF, Mackay AM, Beck SC, et al. Multilineage potential of adult human mesenchymal stem cells. Science 1999;284:143–147.
32. Sanchez-Ramos J, Song S, Cardozo-Pelaez F, et al. Adult bone marrow stromal cells differentiate into neural cells in vitro. Exp Neurol 2000;164:247–256.
33. Woodbury D, Schwarz EJ, Prockop DJ, Black IB. Adult rat and human bone marrow stromal cells differentiate into neurons. J Neurosci Res 2000;61:364–370.
34. Azizi SA, Stokes D, Augelli BJ, DiGirolamo C, Prockop DJ. Engraftment and migration of human bone marrow stromal cells implanted in the brains of albino rats: similarities to astrocyte grafts. Proc Natl Acad Sci USA 1998;95:3908–3913.
35. Hess DC, Hill WD, Martin-Studdard A, Carroll J, Brailer J, Carothers J. Bone marrow as a source of endothelial cells and NeuN-expressing cells after stroke. Stroke 2002;33:1362–1368.
36. Beck H, Voswinckel R, Wagner S, et al. Participation of bone marrow-derived cells in long-term repair processes after experimental stroke. J Cereb Blood Flow Metab 2003;23:709–717.
37. Lee J, Kuroda S, Shichinohe H, et al. Migration and differentiation of nuclear fluorescence-labeled bone marrow stromal cells after transplantation into cerebral infarct and spinal cord injury in mice. Neuropathology 2003;23:169–180.
38. Chen J, Zhang ZG, Li Y, et al. Intravenous administration of human bone marrow stromal cells induces angiogenesis in the ischemic boundary zone after stroke in rats. Circ Res 2003;92:692–699.
39. Sanchez-Ramos JR, Song S, Kamath SG, et al. Expression of neural markers in human umbilical cord blood. Exp Neurol 2001;171:109–115.
40. Borlongan CV, Tajima Y, Trojanowski JQ, Lee VM, Sanberg PR. Transplantation of cryopreserved human embryonal carcinoma-derived neurons (NT2N cells) promotes functional recovery in ischemic rats. Exp Neurol 1998;149:310–321.
41. Veizovic T, Beech JS, Stroemer RP, Watson WP, Hodges H. Resolution of stroke deficits following contralateral grafts of conditionally immortal neuroepithelial stem cells. Stroke 2001;32:1012–1019.
42. Modo M, Stroemer RP, Tang E, Patel S, Hodges H. Effects of implantation site of stem cell grafts on behavioral recovery from stroke damage. Stroke 2002;33:2270–2278.
43. Modo M, Hopkins K, Virley D, Hodges H. Transplantation of neural stem cells modulates apolipoprotein E expression in a rat model of stroke. Exp Neurol 2003;183:320–329.
44. Eglitis MA, Dawson D, Park KW, Mouradian MM. Targeting of marrow-derived astrocytes to the ischemic brain. Neuroreport 1999;10:1289–1292.
45. Li Y, Chopp M, Chen J, et al. Intrastriatal transplantation of bone marrow nonhematopoietic cells improves functional recovery after stroke in adult mice. J Cereb Blood Flow Metab 2000;20:1311–1319.
46. Chen J, Sanberg PR, Li Y, et al. Intravenous administration of human umbilical cord blood reduces behavioral deficits after stroke in rats. Stroke 2001;32:2682–2688.
47. Li Y, Chen J, Chopp M. Adult bone marrow transplantation after stroke in adult rats. Cell Transplant 2001;10:31–40.
48. Lu M, Chen J, Lu D, Yi L, Mahmood A, Chopp M. Global test statistics for treatment effect of stroke and traumatic brain injury in rats with administration of bone marrow stromal cells. J Neurosci Methods 2003;128:183–190.
49. Iihoshi S, Honmou O, Houkin K, Hashi K, Kocsis JD. A therapeutic window for intravenous administration of autologous bone marrow after cerebral ischemia in adult rats. Bain Res 2004;1007:1–9.
50. Li Y, Chen J, Chen XG, et al. Human marrow stromal cell therapy for stroke in rat: neurotrophins and functional recovery. Neurology 2002;59:514–523.

51. Zhao LR, Duan WM, Reyes M, Keene CD, Verfaillie CM, Low WC. Human bone marrow stem cells exhibit neural phenotypes and ameliorate neurological deficits after grafting into the ischemic brain of rats. Exp Neurol 2002;174:11–20.
52. Chen J, Li Y, Katakowski M, et al. Intravenous bone marrow stromal cell therapy reduces apoptosis and promotes endogenous cell proliferation after stroke in female rat. J Neurosci Res 2003;73:778–786.
53. Willing AE, Lixian J, Milliken M, et al. Intravenous versus intrastriatal cord blood administration in a rodent model of stroke. J Neurosci Res 2003;73:296–307.
54. Kondziolka D, Wechsler L, Goldstein S, et al. Transplantation of cultured human neuronal cells for patients with stroke. Neurology 2000;55:565–569.
55. Meltzer CC, Kondziolka D, Villemagne VL, et al. Serial [18F] fluorodeoxyglucose positron emission tomography after human neuronal implantation for stroke. Neurosurgery 2001;49:586–591.
56. Chopp M, Li Y. Treatment of neural injury with marrow stromal cells. Lancet Neurol 2002;1:92–100.
57. Bronstein DM, Perez-Otano I, Sun V, et al. Glia-dependent neurotoxicity and neuroprotection in mesencephalic cultures. Brain Res 1995;704:112–116.
58. Mahalik TJ, Hahn WE, Clayton GH, Owens GP. Programmed cell death in developing grafts of fetal substantia nigra. Exp Neurol 1994;129:27–36.
59. Schierle GS, Hansson O, Leist M, Nicotera P, Widner H, Brundin P. Caspase inhibition reduces apoptosis and increases survival of nigral transplants. Nat Med 1999;5:97–100.
60. Chen J, Li Y, Wang L, Lu M, Chopp M. Caspase inhibition by Z-VAD increases the survival of grafted bone marrow cells and improves functional outcome after MCAo in rats. J Neurol Sci 2002;199:17–24.
61. Hefti F. Neurotrophic factor therapy for nervous system degenerative diseases. J Neurobiol 1994;25:1418–1435.
62. Blesch A, Grill RJ, Tuszynski MH. Neurotrophin gene therapy in CNS models of trauma and degeneration. In: Van Leeuwen FW, Salchi A, Giger RJ, Holtmaat AJGD, Verhaagen J, eds. Progress in Brain Research. Vol. 117. Amsterdam: Elsevier Science BV; 1998:473–484.
63. Grimes ML, Zhou J, Beattie EC, et al. Endocytosis of activated TrkA: evidence that nerve growth factor induces formation of signaling endosomes. J Neurosci 1996;16:7950–7964.
64. Yuen EC, Howe CL, Li Y, Holtzman DM, Mobley WC. Nerve growth factor and the neurotrophic factor hypothesis. Brain Dev 1996;18:362–368.
65. Thoenen H, Barde YA, Davies AM, Johnson JE. Neurotrophic factors and neuronal death. Ciba Found Symp 1987;126:82–95.
66. Connor B, Dragunow M. The role of neuronal growth factors in neurodegenerative disorders of the human brain. Brain Res Rev 1998;27:1–39.
67. Abe K. Therapeutic potential of neurotrophic factors and neural stem cells against ischemic brain injury. J Cereb Blood Flow Metab 2000;20:1393–1408.
68. Chen J, Li Y, Chopp M. Intracerebral transplantation of bone marrow with BDNF after MCAo in rat. Neuropharmacology 2000;39:711–716.
69. Fujiwara K, Date I, Shingo T, et al. Neurotrophic factor-secreting cell grafting for cerebral ischemia: preliminary report. Cell Transplant 2001;10:419–422.
70. Fujiwara K, Date I, Shingo T, et al. Reduction of infarct volume and apoptosis by grafting of encapsulated basic fibroblast growth factor-secreting cells in a model of middle cerebral artery occlusion in rats. J Neurosurg 2003;99:1053–1062.
71. Dillon-Arter O, Johnston RE, Borlongan CV, Truckenmiller ME, Coggiano M, Freed WJ. T155g-immortalized kidney cells produce growth factors and reduce sequelae of cerebral ischemia. Cell Transplant 2002;11:251–259.

9

Gene Therapy to the Nervous System

Hillel Haim and Israel Steiner

Significant advances have been made over the past two decades in our understanding of the basic biology of the nervous system and the molecular basis of neurologic disease. Identification of the complex regulatory mechanisms involved in the maintenance of normal cellular function and the roles assumed by different genes in the pathogenesis of specific diseases have paved the way for a new therapeutic approach based on the alteration of cellular phenotype by genotype manipulation. This new modality, designated gene therapy, has raised high expectations as a potential solution for a large spectrum of currently untreatable conditions. Unfortunately, the rapid transfer from in vitro studies to clinical trials has so far yielded only anecdotal reports of success.

In this chapter, the current status of gene therapy as a regenerative tool for neurologic disease will be reviewed. The principles that underlie the methodology, the main gene delivery vehicle types (vectors), and the different therapeutic approaches adopted for the nervous system will be outlined. This will be followed by a review of several examples of gene therapy use for neurologic diseases. We conclude this chapter by a detailed analysis of those obstacles, technical and conceptual, that still hinder the translation of in vitro efficacy to clinical cure.

Gene Therapy, a Novel Therapeutic Approach

Gene therapy is defined as the introduction of specific nucleic acid sequences into selected target cells for the treatment or prevention of disease. The method was originally contemplated as a potential solution for the wide array of monogenic inherited disorders, such as cystic fibrosis and Duchenne muscular dystrophy, for which conventional pharmacotherapy is unable to provide any adequate response. Restoration of the function of a defective or missing gene product by the introduction of a correct copy of the gene seemed like a simple and feasible concept. It was soon to be appreciated that the approach should not be restricted to single-gene defect replacement therapy. Indeed, alteration of the cellular transcriptional status and in vivo production of a therapeutic protein may be implemented to achieve phenotypic changes in a wide spectrum of disorders. The list of potential applications thus expanded to encompass most neurologic disease states, acute and chronic, inherited and acquired, infectious and neoplastic (see Table 9.1).

Transition into clinical testing was then only a matter of time. Since the initiation of the first gene therapy clinical trial in 1989, nearly 1000 such trials have been approved worldwide.[12] This time period has seen drastic changes in the types of diseases addressed. Most formidable is the slow drift from monogenic inherited disorders to neoplastic disease (in 2003, more than 60% of all gene therapy clinical trials were aimed at neoplastic disease). Two reasons underlie this change. First, the more immediately life-threatening nature of many of these conditions and the lack of efficient alternative therapies have facilitated their transition into clinical testing. Second and perhaps more fundamental, is the current limited ability to achieve efficient gene

Table 9.1. Gene therapy for neurodegenerative disorders: therapeutic approaches

Strategy	Aim of therapy	Targeted pathology	Example disease	Therapeutic gene	References
Introduction of phenotypic changes restricted to the target cell	Replacement of a missing gene function in monogenic disorders	Enzyme deficiency	MPS VII Canavan's disease	β-Glucuronidase Aspartoacylase	1, 2 3
Production of a secreted therapeutic protein to achieve a localized or systemic effect	Alteration of cellular phenotype in non-monogenic disorders	Enzyme deficiency	Parkinson's disease	Tyrosine hydroxylase	4–6
		Decreased neuronal viability	Parkinson's, Alzheimer's, Huntington, ALS, ischemia, traumatic injury	GDNF, NGF, CNTF	7–9
		Neuronal hyperexcitability	Seizures	GAD Potassium channels	10 11

ALS, amyotrophic lateral sclerosis; CNTF, ciliary neurotrophic factor; GAD, glutamic acid decarboxylase; GDNF, glial cell line-derived neurotrophic factor; MPS, mucopolysaccharidosis; NGF, nerve growth factor.

expression in the desired cell population in vivo, to reverse disease phenotypes without causing unwanted side effects.

Thus, while experimentation in the field of gene replacement therapy goes on, the "fast lane" to the clinic has been taken up by cancer gene therapy trials. Accordingly, the number of tumor-destructive approaches increased, to include more cytotoxic genes and replication competent oncolytic viruses.[13–15] Although this class of diseases lies outside the scope of this review, the principles of vector formation and the limitations imposed on the success of in vivo gene transfer similarly apply.

Methods of Gene Delivery

Depending on the application, two modes of delivery may be used to transfer a chosen gene to the target tissue, the ex vivo and in vivo approaches. The ex vivo approach is based on the isolation and in vitro culture of selected cells, where they are manipulated and subsequently returned to the host. Although mainly applied for gene therapy of the immune system where isolation of a specific group of cells is possible,[16] the approach may also be used to generate "mini-factories" that produce and locally secrete desired proteins. The genetically modified cells may thus serve as delivery platforms of neurotrophic factors or neurotransmitter-forming enzymes into the central nervous system (CNS).[17,18]

In contrast, the in vivo approach involves the direct administration of the gene-carrying vector to the host. Delivery may be via simple localized application (such as stereotactic injection into the brain parenchyma), or by the vascular (systemic) route. The main drawback of this approach, and probably the most significant problem currently encountered in gene therapy to the nervous system, is the difficulty in targeting the vector to the selected cell type. To date, this remains the most prominently unsurmounted obstacle.

The Gene-Carrying Vectors

The efficient delivery of the gene to its nuclear target, where it may be expressed, serves as the most basic requirement in gene therapy. Two general types of vectors are used to package and deliver genes: Virus-based and synthetic gene delivery systems. In synthetic systems, the transgene forms part of a plasmid, which is replicated and subsequently purified from bacteria. The only genetic material available for transcription in the target cells is therefore the transgene itself. Plasmid DNA may be delivered (transfected) either alone (naked) or complexed with agents that enhance cellular uptake (such as cationic polymers and liposomes). Although this vector type does not express any toxic or immunogenic foreign protein products, gene transfer is generally inefficient and transient.

In comparison, virus-based systems rely on the natural ability of these infectious agents to package a gene, deliver it to the host cell, and mediate its expression. The gene of interest is incorporated into the modified viral genome, harnessing viral structural and enzymatic components to facilitate delivery and expression. Because the efficiency of gene transfer by viruses exceeds that of the nonviral approach, virus-based vectors currently serve as the most common type of vehicle used in gene therapy at large and for gene transfer to the nervous system in particular.

Viral Vectors

Viral delivery systems are based on modifying the genome of replicative viruses to obtain replication-defective vectors. Such alterations generally include the deletion of coding sequences essential for virus replication and their replacement with the gene of interest. Packaging of the modified genome is performed in specialized cells, which provide in trans those deleted structural and enzymatic components necessary for particle assembly and expression of the carried genome in the target cell. Viral vector infection (designated transduction) results in an abortive cycle, because of the lack of genes necessary for virus replication.

The list of viruses engineered into gene-carrying vectors is continuously growing. From the current arsenal of viral vectors, each retaining several of the properties inherent to the virus from which it was constructed, the vector most appropriate for the specific gene therapy application may be tailored (Table 9.2). Monogenic inherited disorders, such as certain errors of metabolism, require the long-term expression of the transgene, as provided by vectors that achieve stable integration into the host cell chromosomes. In contrast, transient disorders such as acute infections, tissue ischemia, or neoplasms, require shorter time frames of therapeutic gene expression. In the following section, a brief outline of the currently most popular virus-based vectors will be presented, with reference to specific properties, advantages, and disadvantages of each.

Retroviruses

Retroviruses are a large family of enveloped RNA viruses, so named because the genome is reverse transcribed in the infected cell to double-stranded DNA (dsDNA). They are characterized by the establishment of a chronic infection state, generally well tolerated by the host, but slowly progressing diseases such as malignancy and immunodeficiency may ensue. Several members of the retrovirus family have been exploited to serve as vectors: i) C-type retroviruses (also referred to as oncoretroviruses), including the murine leukemia virus (MuLV) group and the avian leukosis virus (ALV), ii) lentiviruses, including the simian, feline, and human immunodeficiency viruses (SIV, FIV, and HIV, respectively), and iii) spumaviruses such as the human foamy virus.

After binding of the viral envelope glycoprotein to the cell-surface receptor, the viral genome enters the host cell and is reverse transcribed in the cytoplasm. Subsequently, the proviral DNA enters the nucleus and integrates into the host cell chromosomes. Viral particles contain two copies of the single-stranded RNA (ssRNA) genome (approximately 9 kb in size), which are incorporated into the assembling virions by the *cis*-acting packaging sequence (ψ). Retrovirus genomes are flanked by long terminal repeat (LTR) sequences, involved *in cis* in reverse transcription, transcriptional control, and chromosomal integration. The LTRs frame the three genes *gag*, *pol*, and *env*, encoding structural proteins, enzymatic components, and the surface glycoprotein, respectively. This structural framework greatly facilitates the construction of retrovirus-based vectors: The *gag*, *pol*, and *env* genes are deleted and replaced by the exogenous transgene of choice. For vector assembly, these missing gene functions are provided *in trans* in specialized cells that express these proteins transiently (packaging cells) or stably (producer cells).

To minimize the chances that replication-competent retroviruses (RCRs) will be generated by homologous recombination, these *trans*-expressed genes are placed on separate constructs, carrying little sequence homology.[19,20] In addition, abolishment of the viral

Table 9.2. Vector properties

	Vector					
	Adenovirus	Retroviruses	Lentivirus	AAV	HSV	Plasmid DNA
Particle size (nm)	70	100	100	20	200	Variable
Genome type and size (kb)	dsDNA (36)	RNA (8.8)	RNA (9.6)	ssDNA (4.7)	dsDNA(152)	—
Packaging capacity (kb)	6–8 (up to 30 kb in gutless vectors)	7	7	5	30 (up to 150 kb in amplicons)	Infinite
Gene transfer to nondividing cells	Yes	No	Yes	Yes	Yes	Minimal
Chromosomal integration	No	Yes	Yes	Yes (random and 19q)	No	No
Preexisting immunity	Yes	No	No	Yes	Yes	No
Immune response	+++	+/−	+/−	+/−	+	None
Typical TU concentration (MI)	10^{13}	10^9	10^9	10^{10}	10^{10}	10^{13}
Major safety concerns	Inflammatory response, cytotoxicity	Insertional mutagenesis, generation of RCRs	Insertional mutagenesis, generation of RCRs	Insertional mutagenesis	Inflammatory response, cytotoxicity	None

dsDNA, double-stranded DNA; ssDNA, single-stranded DNA; TU, transducing units; RCR, replication-competent retroviruses.

LTR promoter prevents the generation of full-length proviral RNA, further increasing vector safety.[21]

Because the retroviral vector genome is chromosomally integrated, the transgene is theoretically expressed for the lifetime of the cell and is passed to daughter cells during mitosis. A potential disadvantage of this retroviral feature is a functional disturbance of the chromosomal material into which it is inserted. This may result in the loss of cell cycle control and malignant transformation (see below).

Lentiviruses. A significant disadvantage of the oncoretrovirus-based vectors is their inability to transduce nondividing cells.[22] In vivo gene delivery to postmitotic cells, most notably in the nervous system, is thus rendered irrelevant. Lentiviruses, however, have evolved the ability to harness the cellular nuclear import machinery to transport the viral genome into the nucleoplasm[23] and are thus able to efficiently transduce postmitotic cells. Although several members of the lentivirus family were developed as gene delivery vehicles, most efforts have focused on the best-characterized lentivirus, the human immunodeficiency virus type 1 (HIV-1).

The genomic structure of lentiviruses closely resembles that of the oncoretroviruses. In addition, they possess two unique regulatory proteins, tat and rev, and several accessory proteins that facilitate viral replication and the persistence of infection.[24–26] Lentiviral vectors deleted of all accessory genes have been constructed, without affecting vector production efficiency.[27,28]

As would be expected of a vector derived from this deadly pathogen, biosafety concerns top the list of aims during vector construction. Splitting the genome into separate constructs, which are cotransfected into the packaging cell line significantly reduced chances of RCR generation.[29,30] As with oncoretrovirus-based vectors, biosafety is further increased by inactivating the LTR promoter, thus abolishing transcription of full-length proviral RNA.[31]

A unique property of retroviruses is the ability to incorporate the envelope glycoprotein of a different virus into their lipid envelope, acquiring its host range for infection in a process designated pseudotyping (see later under "cell-specificity of gene transfer"). HIV-1-based vectors pseudotyped with the vesicular stomatitis virus envelope glycoprotein (VSV-G) have been extensively studied for in vivo transduction of the CNS. Such vectors mediate high-efficiency transduction of both neurons and glial cells of rodent[28,32] and nonhuman primate brains.[33] Transgene expression persists over extended time periods with no associated brain pathology detected.[29] Furthermore, the therapeutic efficacy of this vector to treat neurodegenerative disease in several animal models was demonstrated, including Parkinson's disease,[34] metachromatic leukodystrophy[35] and type VII mucopolysaccharidosis.[2]

Several other lentiviruses have been developed to serve as gene transfer vehicles and recently an FIV-based vector was successfully used to correct cognitive impairments in a mouse model of mucopolysaccharidosis type VII (MPS VII).[36]

Adenoviruses

Adenoviruses are double-stranded nonenveloped DNA viruses, which cause upper respiratory tract infections in humans. They efficiently infect a wide variety of cell types, both dividing and nondividing. More than 50 different human adenoviral serotypes are currently known, of which serotypes 2 and 5 have been most extensively manipulated for gene transfer purposes. Because these two serotypes are also the most common to which humans are exposed, alternative serotypes and nonhuman adenoviruses are currently developed as vectors to surmount potential problems associated with preexisting immunity.[37]

Adenoviral infection is initiated by attachment to the cell surface coxsackie and adenovirus receptor, followed by endocytosis, transport to the nucleus, and translocation into the nucleoplasm where the viral genome remains in the nonintegrated (episomal) state. The replication cycle is then initiated by the sequential transcription of the early (E) genes, DNA replication, and finally the transcription of the late (L) family of genes, which is followed by encapsidation of the newly synthesized genome and viral release by cell lysis.

The first generation of replication-incompetent adenovirus-based vectors was constructed by deleting the E1 gene, the main activator of viral transcription.[38,39] Exogenous sequences of up to 8 kb could thus be introduced in its place. Nevertheless, despite E1 removal, low-level expression of additional genes from these vectors still occurred, eliciting strong cellular and humoral immune responses and resulting in the clearance of transduced cells by cytotoxic T lymphocytes.[40,41] This heralded construction of second- and third-generation vectors containing additional deletions, characterized by decreased expression of viral proteins and improved toxicity profiles.[42] The most extensively deleted adenoviral vector, designated "gutless," is stripped of nearly all viral genes, retaining only the inverted terminal repeats that flank the genome, the packaging signal, and a transgene cassette.[43] Up to 30 kb of exogenous sequences may be accommodated into the vector. *Trans*-complementation of all viral genes is thus necessary for vector assembly and is achieved by coinfection of the packaging cells with a helper virus. "Gutless" vector preparations are minimally contaminated by replication-competent recombinants. They are associated with a significantly reduced inflammatory response,[44,45] produce therapeutic levels of secreted transgene products in experimental animal models,[46] and are currently the vector of choice for adenovirus-mediated gene delivery. Nevertheless, "gutless" vector purification procedures still require improvement in the ability to scale up to concentrations necessary for in vivo delivery.

The episomal status of the adenoviral genome in the transduced cell leads to gradual extinction of transgene expression because of intranuclear degradation and dilution in a dividing cell population. Attempts to overcome the transient expression of the transgene have been made by constructing hybrid adeno/adeno-associated viruses (AAV) and adeno/retrovirus vectors, allowing chromosomal integration of the genome.[47,48] Transduction efficiency by these hybrid vectors is, however, low.

Adeno-Associated Viruses

AAVs are members of the parvovirus family and are not associated with any known disease in humans. A productive replication cycle in the host cell only occurs upon coinfection with a helper virus, such as adenovirus or herpes simplex virus. Six human AAV serotypes are currently known, of which AAV-2 is the most intensively studied for gene therapy purposes.

The tiny AAV virions (20 nm in diameter) carry a ssDNA molecule, of either plus or minus orientation. Inverted terminal repeats flank the genome containing two open reading frames, *rep* and *cap*, each encoding for a number of proteins. *Rep* produces the regulatory proteins required for genome replication and *cap* encodes for the structural proteins of the capsid. After cell entry via the endocytic pathway, the genome is transported to the nucleus and forms dsDNA by either annealing with a complementary strand from a second virus or by de novo formation by the host cell machinery.[49] In the absence of *rep*, the vector will randomly integrate into the host cell chromosomes (as a single provirus or as head-to-tail concatamers by nonhomologous recombination), whereas in its presence, the genome is directed to a specific site in chromosome 19. It should be noted, however, that only a fraction of all intranuclear vector genome copies undergo integration, the rest remain episomal. Following the same principles of vector construction as detailed above, the *rep* and *cap* genes are replaced by a transgene cassette and the missing functions required for vector replication and encapsidation are *trans*-complemented in the packaging cells.[50–52]

AAV-based vectors are extensively used in gene transfer studies to the brain. High transduction efficiency of quiescent cell, minimal toxicity (because of the absence of virus-derived genes), and stable chromosomal integration of the genome render the vector appealing for many applications. In addition, different AAV serotypes selectively transduce different cells in the CNS, enabling cell-type-specific targeting of gene delivery.[53]

A significant disadvantage of AAV-based vectors is the limited size of the transgene sequence that may be inserted (up to 5 kb). This capacity, however, may be doubled by the use of the *trans*-splicing or homologous recombination approaches, taking advantage of the concatamerization of vector genomes that occurs before integration.[54]

Herpes Simplex Virus Type 1

Herpes simplex virus type 1 (HSV-1) is a dsDNA human neurotropic virus. The interest in HSV-1-based vectors is therefore largely concentrated on gene transfer applications to the nervous system. Viral particles (approximately 200 nm in diameter) are composed of a lipid envelope containing 12 different glycoproteins that mediate entry into the host cell, which surrounds the viral capsid that engulfs the 152-kb genome. Between the capsid and envelope, the tegument layer contains several proteins that *trans*-activate viral gene expression and regulate the host cell translation machinery.[55]

The HSV-1 life cycle depends on the type of host cell infected. In epithelial cells, the virus goes through a lytic replication cycle, whereas in neurons it may enter a latent state, persisting episomally in the nucleus. In lytic infection, viral protein expression is conducted in a highly ordered manner, involving the sequential transcription of the immediate-early (IE), early (E), and the late (L) classes of genes. After nuclear entry of the genome, the Vmw65 tegument protein *trans*-activates transcription of the IE genes, leading to E gene expression, whose products enable DNA replication and transcription of the L genes that encode for viral structural components. The encapsidated viral genome then buds through the nucleus, acquires the tegument proteins and envelope within the cytoplasm, and is secreted from the cells in vesicles, culminating in the death of the infected cell.

In neurons, HSV-1 infection may assume a latent form, far less characterized than the lytic cycle.[56] After uptake of the virus by axon terminals, it is retrogradely transported to the cell nucleus where it remains as an episome in a latent state. The events that lead to the establishment of latency and the presence or absence of de novo viral protein synthesis are yet unresolved issues. Latency is, however, known to be associated with the expression of the viral latency associated transcripts (LATs), which are assumed to inhibit the expression of lytic replication cycle genes.[57] From this dormant state, after stimuli such as UV irradiation or stress, the virus may reactivate and go through the lytic infection cycle.

Two major types of gene delivery vectors based on HSV-1 have been constructed: Recombinant and amplicon-based. Recombinant vectors are rendered replication-defective by the deletion of one or more of the five IE genes and the transgene is inserted into the deleted genome by homologous recombination.[58] Such vectors are transcriptionally silent other than expression of the transgene, mimicking the latent infectious state. Propagation of the vector is performed in cell lines that *trans*-complement the missing IE genes. Because nearly half of the HSV-1 genes are not essential for virus replication in cell culture, the recombinant vector genome may accommodate up to 30 kb of foreign DNA.[59,60]

The amplicon vector system is based on bacterially produced plasmids, which contain no viral genes but only the *Escherichia coli* origin of replication, the HSV-1 origin of replication and packaging signal, and the inserted transgene. Packaging of the amplicon in viral particles is enabled by *trans*-complementation using a packaging signal-deleted bacterial artificial chromosome (bac) that expresses the entire HSV-1 genome[61-63] or by multiple cosmids that span the genome.[64] Amplicon-based packaging systems, although producing vector stocks with a decreased content of replication-competent virus, suffer from low titers.

Many animal models of different neurologic diseases have been tested for therapeutic efficiency of gene transfer using HSV-1 vectors, including neuroprotection,[65,66] enzyme replacement therapy for monogenic disorders,[67] and immune modulation for demyelinating disease.[68] Long-term expression from the episomal vector is difficult to achieve. However, in one report, transgene expression in dorsal root ganglia was detected for up to 18 months, from vectors in which the transgene, controlled by the MuLV LTR promoter, was inserted directly upstream of the LAT promoter region.[69] Similarly, using the LAT promoter, continuous systemic release of nerve growth factor (NGF) from an intraarticularly administered vector was observed for at least 6 months in rhesus macaques.[70]

Nonviral Vectors

Whereas the use of viruses as a gene delivery vehicle carries the advantage of mediating high-efficiency gene transfer and the potential to target specific cell types, several significant disadvantages are noted:

a. An immune response is always mounted by the introduction of a foreign protein.
b. Safety risks result from the use of integrating viral vectors.
c. Potential reversion of vectors to replication-competent viruses may ensue.
d. There are limitations on the large-scale production of preparations containing high concentrations of transducing units.
e. The capacity of most viral vector genomes to accommodate large exogenous sequences is limited.

These shortcomings have prompted efforts to produce alternative nonviral systems. The safety and versatility of these latter are, however, traded off by the lack of the functions that viruses have evolved to package, protect, and deliver their genome through the target cell membrane and into the nucleus. A more thorough dissection of the virus infection cycle was thus warranted, to identify and adopt those "ready-made" functions that viruses possess, which render them such efficient gene delivery vehicles. In this respect, the most important functions required are stabilization and protection of the gene in the extra- and intracellular milieu, efficient and selective uptake into the cytoplasm, delivery of the genome into the nucleoplasm, and release from the packaging formulation.

The efficiency of plasmid DNA transfer across the cellular membrane is generally extremely low. To enhance transmembrane transport, both mechanical and chemical approaches are used. Mechanical means, based on increasing membrane permeability to the DNA include: i) Cell bombardment with high-velocity gold or tungsten microparticles complexed to plasmid DNA.[71,72] Routinely used for vaccination protocols that require limited amounts of intramuscular gene expression, application of the methodology for more diffuse and high-level transgene delivery seems unlikely. ii) Increased extracellular pressure was shown to augment uptake of DNA by cells of the cardiovascular system.[73] This method was more recently successfully applied to render vein grafts resistant to hypercholesterolemia-induced atherosclerosis.[74] iii) Transient permeabilization of the plasma membrane by electrical pulses (electroporation). The use of low-voltage, high-frequency pulses significantly reduces the considerable levels of cell mortality previously associated with the treatment and enabled efficient gene expression in mouse skeletal muscle.[75] iv) Ultrasound-mediated gene transfer, based on the same principle as electroporation, has also been shown to increase skeletal muscle transfection efficiency in vivo.[76]

Despite the wide array of membrane permeability-enhancing strategies, mechanical means are generally expected to induce some degree of tissue damage and are therefore currently not considered appropriate for gene transfer to the nervous system. In contrast, chemical agents are constantly gaining momentum as the strategy of choice to increase transfection efficiency. Electrostatically based interactions between the negatively charged DNA and positively charged formulation are used to form complexes that increase cellular deposition, attachment, and uptake of the gene. Among the earliest formulations, most notable are DEAE-dextran and calcium phosphate. Extensively used for in vitro gene transfer, these agents, however, cause significant toxicity and gene expression levels among cells is extremely variable.

A major improvement in nonviral gene transfer technology was introduced by the lipid-based delivery systems. Liposomes are submicron-sized aggregates, composed of amphiphilic lipids that self-assemble to an organized structure surrounding a watery interior. Depending on the composition of the polar head group, liposomes are classified as anionic, cationic, zwitterionic, or nonionic. Cationic liposomes, which associate in aqueous medium with the negatively charged plasmid DNA to form overall positively charged "lipoplexes," are the most widely used. Incorporation of "fusogenic" lipidic elements increases mixing of the lipid phases of the liposome and endosomal membrane, thus enhancing DNA escape from the endosome before fusion with the nuclease-containing lysosomes occurs.[77-79] Although liposomes of different lipid composition are continuously developed to enhance transmembrane delivery, attempts are also made to increase the low efficiency step of plasmid translocation from the cytoplasm into the nucleus.[80] Utilization of virus-derived nuclear localization polypeptide signals, which are conjugated to the vector formulation, has been shown to significantly augment transfection efficiency.[81,82] Moreover, the transfection of nondividing cells, which are more refractory to polynucleotide uptake relative to dividing cells, was significantly enhanced, opening new possibilities for gene transfer to the quiescent cells of the nervous system.

The ability of liposomes to associate with a variety of molecular structures has been further exploited to provide lipoplexes with additional functions. For example, conjugation to polyethylene glycol (PEG) has been shown to protect plasmid DNA from intracellular degradation[83] and increase stability and circulation time upon systemic administration.[84,85] Targeting moieties have also been incorporated into "PEGylated" liposomes, enabling brain-directed delivery of the systemically injected vector,[84,86] as detailed later.

Although liposomal formulations are routinely used in the clinic for the delivery of antifungal and chemotherapeutic drugs, it should be noted that their use for gene transfer applications has been associated with some degree of cytotoxicity.[87] As an alternative, protein-based agents are gaining interest. Cationically charged polypeptides, such as poly-L-lysine, condense DNA and increase transfection efficiency.[88] This formulation allows the chemical conjugation of targeting moieties for specific cell-type targeting.[88,89] Attempts at assembling more complex polypeptide structures, composed of different functional building blocks, have been initiated. One such construct contains the *E. coli* β-galactosidase protein (for DNA protection), an RGD motif (for targeting the cell-surface $\alpha_V\beta_3$ integrin receptor) and a poly-L-lysine tail (for DNA condensation).[90] Intracortical injection of this chimeric protein-gene complex mediated efficient transgene delivery to both the excitotoxically injured and noninjured brain of postnatal rats.[91] Transgene expression was observed in neuronal and nonneuronal cells, with no evidence of inflammation or cytotoxicity 6 days postinjection. Modeling functional polypeptide units with tailor-made characteristics is certain to advance in coming years, replacing those functions provided by viruses with synthetic or human-derived substitutes.

Disease-Targeted Gene Therapy

General Points

There are many neurologic disorders that are amenable to gene therapy.[92,93] In fact, the spectrum may include almost any neurologic condition. Examples abound and include slow and acute viral infections,[94] immune-mediated CNS conditions and multiple sclerosis,[95] traumatic injury to the brain, spinal cord and peripheral nervous system disorders,[96,97] stroke,[98] and epilepsy.[10] At present, however, three conditions receive most of the attention and are at the focus of intensive research: neoplasms, inherited metabolic diseases, and neurodegenerative disorders. Whereas in previous sections of this chapter we focused on the principles underlying vector construction and delivery, here we outline the biological requirements for treatment of neurologic conditions.

The basic requirement to therapy is an understanding of the molecular basis of normal function of the diseased cell and the abnormality that is responsible for the pathological phenotype. Three neurodegenerative conditions will highlight this point. Although much is known about Alzheimer's disease (AD), Parkinson's disease (PD), and amyotrophic lateral sclerosis (ALS), the basic aspects of etiology and pathogenesis are still incompletely understood. The conditions are extremely prevalent and tend specifically to affect the older age groups. They are characterized by dysfunction and early death of selective neuronal subpopulations. In ALS, upper and lower motor neurons in the pyramidal nervous system are affected, leading to paralysis and death. In PD, the pigmented, mainly nigrostriatal dopaminergic, cells are diseased causing severe motor incapacity and in AD the burden seems to rest on a wider range of neuronal subpopulations culminating in dementia. Whereas one approach considers these conditions as the result of an enhanced aging process of selective neuronal cell populations, accumulating data underline either a biochemical basis of cellular dysfunction or the possible involvement of an environmental factor/s.

Gene-based therapy may be attempted in these and other neurodegenerative conditions using two different approaches: Nonspecific delay of cell death and specific disease-tailored strategies.

Delaying Neuronal Cell Death

This may be achieved by the CNS delivery of growth factors and neuroprotective genes, such as NGF,[17] or the antiapoptotic HSV-1 gamma34.5,[99] respectively. The approach is nonspecific and has two major advantages. First, there is no true requirement to fully understand the biochemical basis of the disorder. The therapeutic gene has a general, nonspecific action, and is usually nonselective, namely, it has a broader range of cell populations that it can affect. Second, there is no need to specifically transfer the therapeutic gene to the affected cell type. In many inherited metabolic abnormalities, the intracellular defect calls for intracellular repair (either by providing a normal gene, or by silencing a toxic abnormal gene product), and thus gene therapy has to be targeted to transduce the defective cell from within. With agents such as cytokines or nerve trophic factors, the gene products act from without and, therefore, theoretically, require only that the therapeutic gene product will reach the extracellular compartment. For obvious reasons, this approach has occupied most of the current experimental thrust in ALS,[100,101] PD,[7,102] and AD,[103] using both the "effect from without" and "effect from within" strategies.

Specific Disease-Tailored Strategies

Amyotrophic Lateral Sclerosis

Mutations in the gene coding for Cu/Zn superoxide dismutase enzyme were identified in the familial form of ALS[104] and there is evidence that oxidative stress is involved in motor neuron cell damage in the much more prevalent, sporadic form of ALS.[105] Tissue culture and animal models have been developed to mimic some of the biochemical changes and neuropathology of the disease and antioxidant enzymes (such as superoxide dismutase, catalase, and glutathione peroxidase) have demonstrated therapeutic efficacy in these models (reviewed in Pong[106]).

Parkinson's Disease

Pharmacologic therapy of the disease is based, in part, on supplying the CNS with L-DOPA, the precursor of the neurotransmitter dopamine that is reduced in the disease. Providing the gene that encodes for tyrosine hydroxylase (TH), the enzyme responsible for the synthesis of dopamine, can alleviate extrapyramidal symptomatology in experimental animal models.[4,5]

Alzheimer's Disease

One of the systems severely affected in AD are the cholinergic neurons in the basal forebrain and loss of cholinergic function is closely correlated with the decline in cognitive performance observed in AD patients. Current pharmacotherapy, only partially effective, uses anticholine esterase compounds that reduce neurotransmitter clearance. NGF was previously believed to have a mere neurotrophic role in the survival of cholinergic neurons; however, it is slowly being discovered as a central regulator of both phenotype and function of these cells. Not only does it enhance neurotransmitter synthesis and sprouting in the uninjured cholinergic neurons, but also directly controls cholinergic neurotransmission by mechanisms independent of gene expression or cell signaling.[107] Accordingly, NGF has been shown to improve function in animals bearing cholinergic lesions and has already entered the clinical trial phase for the treatment of AD.

AD is associated with extracellular deposition of the alpha-amyloid protein in senile plaques and the brain microvasculature. It is the product of the alpha-amyloid precursor protein (APP) gene localized on chromosome 21, and is primarily, but not exclusively, expressed in neurons. Interfering with APP expression may reduce the tissue accumulation of the neurotoxic alpha-amyloid protein. For this purpose, antisense oligonucleotides directed at the amyloid beta-peptide region of the APP gene have been used experimentally. Encouraging results from studies with a mouse model of AD that overproduces amyloid beta protein indicate a reversal of cognitive defects after both intracerebroventricular and intravenous administration of such antisense oligonucleotides.[108–110]

Manipulating Postinjury CNS Regeneration

Injury to the adult CNS often results in permanent loss of cells and neuronal function. This is attributed, among others, to the failure of injured axons to regenerate (reviewed in Spencer and Filbin[111] and Fournier and Strittmatter[112]). Extensive work in recent years has uncovered the nature of CNS inhibitory mechanisms that prevent brain tissue regeneration and repair. These include the formation of the glial scar, the participation of several myelin-associated molecules that inhibit axonal regrowth, and the dividing status of neurons. To date, three major myelin-associated inhibitors have been identified: Myelin-associated glycoprotein (MAG[113]), Nogo-A,[114] and oligodendrocyte-myelin glycoprotein (OMgp[115]), all of which exert their effect via the Nogo receptor. Regenerative capacity in the adult CNS may therefore be potentially stimulated by the targeting of one or all of these factors after injury. Such manipulation has so far been attempted only in vitro, and highlighted the potential associated with an approach aimed at inhibiting the inhibition. Suppressing the activity of the Nogo receptor using an AAV vector expressing a dominant-negative form of the Nogo receptor has been shown to increase axon regeneration.[116]

Critical Issues

Targeting Gene Delivery

Whereas much effort is focused on the construction of vectors with increased gene transfer efficiencies and higher safety profiles, the most significant challenge currently faced in gene therapy, prominently exemplified in the CNS, is the achievement of selective transgene expression in a specific cell population within a chosen site. The risks associated with the promiscuous transfer of genetic material mandate the implementation of such selectivity measures.

Conventional pharmacotherapy is based on the systemic administration of a therapeutic drug that is distributed throughout the body via the vascular route. With minimally restricted access to any site or compartment, the specificity of effect is solely determined by the interaction with the target molecule. Gene therapy thus differs from conventional pharmacotherapy in two major respects. First, the biodistribution of a systemically administered vector is strongly biased by the structure and dynamics of the vascular system. Second, the vector itself does not mediate a physiologic effect, but rather serves as a precursor that is processed at the target site to produce the biologically active factor. As a result, the specificity of effect is determined at five different levels: i) Accessibility to the target cells, ii) entry into the target cell, iii) a permissive intracellular environment that enables processing of the vector to a functional gene, iv) expression of the gene by the host cell transcriptional and translational machinery, and v) effect of the transgene protein product.

These levels of specificity were translated into targeting strategies, based on: i) The administration method, ii) selective cellular uptake of the gene-carrying vector, and iii) cell-type-specific transcription.

Modes of Vector Delivery to the CNS

The first consideration in deciding on a mode of vector delivery is the anatomical distribution of afflicted target cells. In PD, for example, the diseased cells are confined to a relatively restricted area, lying deep in the substantia nigra, whereas in AD the afflicted cells are more globally distributed throughout the brain and in lysosomal storage diseases each and every cell in the tissue is involved.

A second consideration is the mode of action of the transgene product. Therapeutic agents that are secreted from the transgene-expressing cells (e.g., growth factors and neurotransmitter precursors) theoretically require gene transfer to a relatively small number of cells. In contrast, for those protein products that induce phenotypic changes restricted to the cell in which they are produced (e.g., ion channels to provide protection from excitotoxic damage), delivery should be conducted so as to achieve maximal gene transfer of the targeted population.

Direct injection. Despite the risks associated with invasive craniotomy-based procedures, as for today, the most common method of vector delivery to the brain used in clinical trials is direct intraparenchymal injection. This approach, however, is associated with local tissue damage by the needle tract, causing secondary damage to the blood-brain barrier (BBB), local inflammation, and hemorrhage. Moreover, standard injection procedures enable vector diffusion over only a few millimeters away from the injection site.[117] The resulting gene transfer is nonhomogenous with a short transduction gradient (i.e., cells proximal to the injection site are significantly more efficiently transduced than those further away).

To increase vector distribution to more distant parts of the injected tissue, convection-enhanced delivery devices have been developed. The pressure gradient-dependent flow current of the vector allows the injection of larger preparation volumes with more homogeneously distributed transduction and minimal tissue damage.[118–120] A setback of this approach is the minimal control over vector flow, which may find its way to unwanted brain regions. Indeed, several studies have shown that diffusion of the injected vector particles throughout the brain is minimally affected by physical tissue barriers, but rather by the interaction between the virus and tissue components (both cellular and extracellular matrix).[118,120,121]

A fundamental shortcoming of the use of reporter genes for in vivo biodistribution studies should be noted. Marker proteins, such as the *E. coli* β-galactosidase, fluorescent proteins, and the firefly luciferase are most often used to determine vector distribution throughout the tissue. Results of such assays reflect the final product of a long sequence of events, starting with arrival at the site and the cell-entry process, through a complex series of intracellular events and culminating in translation and accumulation of the reporter protein. Therefore, differential processing of the gene product may theoretically bias apparent vector distribution. Indeed, intracerebrally injected adenoviral or AAV vectors expressing either the β-galactosidase or the HSV-1 thymidine kinase (TK) gene under identical promoter sequences produced significantly varying results.[120,122,123] HSV-1-TK immunoreactivity was detected over larger areas of the brain and persisted for several months longer. Transgene-specific properties (and assay sensitivity) therefore bias any study of vector distribution, underscoring reservations that should be applied to reporter gene-based studies. A more prudent approach is thus recommended, including both analyses of physical particle distribution (e.g., by fluorescently labeled virions or in situ hybridization for virus-specific sequences) and the use of assays to detect the protein product specific for the application.

The intravascular route. The ability to systemically administer brain-targeted vectors is an appealing alternative to the invasive intraparenchymal procedures. This approach is facilitated by the tremendously high vascularity of the brain, in which every neuron is directly adjacent to a capillary. However, access of vectors from the intravascular compartment and into the brain parenchyma is hindered by the cerebral microvascular endothelium forming the BBB. Transfer across the BBB may be facilitated by temporary disruption of this barrier using an osmotic shock[124] or by drug-induced opening,[125,126] but such methods are associated with chronic neuropathologic changes because of increased access of circulating neurotoxins and potentially pathogens to the brain.[127,128]

An alternative approach, exploiting receptor-mediated transport systems which actively transport large molecules such as insulin and transferrin across the BBB, was recently introduced.[129] By conjugating a monoclonal antibody to the transferrin receptor to a PEGylated liposome, the complexes undergo receptor-mediated transcytosis across the microvascular endothelial cells, followed by receptor-mediated endocytosis into neurons beyond the BBB.[86] Efficient brain delivery of a plasmid expressing the TH gene was shown to result in the normalization of striatal TH levels and reverse motor impairments in a neurotoxin-induced rat model of PD. Similarly, targeting the insulin receptor in primates yielded global brain expression of reporter genes restricted to neurons that express the insulin receptor.[6]

Despite these advances, the most significant disadvantage of systemic vector administration is the biased bodily distribution of these nano-sized particles. Sequestration of the large majority of vectors by organs that have a sinusoidal capillary system (i.e., liver, spleen, bone marrow) requires both higher vector doses and the prevention of transgene expression in these organs.[46] In addition, exposure to circulating components of the immune system is associated with vector inactivation and priming of an immune response (see later).

Intraventricular and intrathecal administration. Intraventricular administration of gene-carrying vectors is generally regarded as a noneffective means to achieve neuronal gene transfer in the brain of adult animals. Transduction is limited to the ependymal cells lining the ventricles, to the choroid plexus, and only a minimal distance into the brain parenchyma itself.[130,131] Nevertheless, this approach can be used to produce transgene products that are secreted into the CSF and may penetrate into the parenchyma.[1,130,132] Unfortunately, not all gene products are able to cross tissue barriers in such a manner.[133]

Transneuronal transfer. The transneuronal portal of entry is used by various neurotropic viruses such as HSV-1, rabies virus, and certain enteroviruses to invade the CNS. Indeed, viruses have been exploited as transneuronal tracers in order to study brain anatomy.[134] Although the efferent transsynaptic transfer of the replication-defective vectors used in gene therapy is not possible, this portal may be used to pass secreted transgene products to higher-order neurons. Thus, vectors administered in the periphery (intramuscularly or subcutaneously) may express the encoded transgenes in the dorsal root ganglia or anterior horn cell bodies and the secreted protein be accessible to second-order neurons in the spinal column.[135] Similarly, import of an adenoviral vector through the olfactory tracts was shown to result in transgene expression in directly related structures in the brain.[136]

Interestingly, brain access of the vector itself is not an absolute necessity for entry of the product. In a study by Hennig et al.,[137] although the intraocularly administered AAV genome remained in the injected eye, efferent transfer of the encoded lysosomal β-glucuronidase enzyme into the CNS occurred, resulting in a reduction of lysosomal storage in brain areas unrelated to the ocular tracts.

Cell Specificity of Gene Transfer

After administration, a fundamental requirement is the ability to direct and restrict gene expression selectively to the cell type of interest. This may be achieved by either selective uptake of the vector by specific cells (targeted entry), or by selective transgene expression through the utilization of cell-specific promoters (transcriptional targeting). These approaches are complementary; whereas targeted entry better addresses the safety issues concerning vector-induced cellular effects, transcriptional targeting provides a secondary line of defense to limit expression to the desired cell type.

Targeted entry. Restriction of vector uptake to selected cell types is based on exploiting surface components unique to the target cell, which serve as receptors to the gene-carrying vector. Because the basic principles of cell entry are derived from the study of viruses, attempts at retargeting viral vectors preceded that of their nonviral counterparts. Cellular tropism of viruses is determined by an interaction between viral glycoproteins and cell-surface expressed receptors. Manipulation of this interaction therefore stands at the basis for all retargeting attempts, which may be categorized into:

1. Selective use of viral glycoproteins that mediate infection of the desired cell type.
2. Genetic engineering of viral glycoproteins to express retargeting moieties.
3. Use of bispecific bridging molecules with specificity to both viral surface and target cell membrane components.

The most basic approach to determine host range is to guide vector choice by the natural tropism of the parental virus from which it is derived. Thus, for example, relying on the variant tropism of the different AAV serotypes, AAV-2 (but not AAV-5) could be used to selectively transduce neuronal cells but not astrocytes.[53] This approach is simplified for retrovirus-derived vectors, which have the unique ability to incorporate envelope glycoproteins of other viruses into their lipid envelope, consequently acquiring their host range for infection. This process of heterologous envelope glycoprotein expression is designated pseudotyping. Initial pseudotypes were in fact aimed to broaden retroviral transduction range to otherwise refractory cells[138–140]; however, several cell-type-specific pseudotypes were also generated. For instance, retrovirus-based vectors, composed of the *gag* gene of the avian reticuloendotheliosis virus (REV-A), the *pol* gene of the spleen necrosis virus (SNV), and the glycoproteins of different rabies virus (RV).[141] These chimeric vectors were able to mediate cell-specific transduction of mouse and human neurons in vitro and demonstrated selective transduction of neurons when injected into the brains of newborn mice.

Retargeting of viral vectors by genetically engineering envelope glycoproteins to express targeting ligands to specific cell-surface receptors was a subject of intensive investigation. A wide variety of proteins and antibody fragments have been inserted into the envelope glycoprotein of virtually all viral vectors.[142–147] Immense differences were observed in the retargeting efficiency among the different vector types. Whereas adenoviral vectors were generally permissive to host range manipulation, retroviruses were more refractory to such alterations. Polypeptide sequences inserted into the retroviral envelope glycoprotein were generally unable to effectively replace the receptor-binding domain of the native protein by activating the complex entry mechanism upon binding to the targeted receptor.[148]

An alternative approach employed is the use of soluble molecules, which function as bridging agents between the viral envelope glycoprotein and a chosen cellular receptor.[149–151] The lack of structure-function disruption of the viral glycoprotein favored the use of this strategy, and such conjugates have been used for in vivo gene transfer with some success[152]. However, the utility of this approach for in vivo administration in humans is still unclear.

By and large, efforts to retarget the entry of viral vectors are progressing at a slower rate than probably expected, are generally disappointing, and may shift attention to their nonviral counterparts. Initial promising results with the brain targeting of PEGylated immunoliposomes[6,86] and the significantly higher degree of flexibility allowed with these vector types, may hopefully mark the way to better accomplishment in this field.

Targeting gene expression (transcriptional targeting). Cell-type-specific promoters serve as an efficient method to restrict transgene expression to selective cell populations within the nervous system. Neuronal and glial cell-specific promoters have long been identified and extensively used to drive the expression of transgenes carried by a variety of vectors.[32,153] Attempts are also conducted to achieve higher levels of differential gene expression, beyond the general neuron-glia delineation, by restricting transcription to specific neuronal cell subtypes. Transgene expression could thus be targeted to noradrenergic neurons by constructing a synthetic promoter based on the multimerization of noradrenergic neuron-specific regulatory sequences from the human dopamine β-hydroxylase (hDBH) promoter.[154] This synthetic promoter was shown to confer cell-type-specific expression in the injected rat brain with higher levels of transgene product than the intact hDBH promoter.

Regulating Gene Expression

Most applications require the ability to control the level of gene expression, because excessive production of the transgene product may cause unwanted side effects. For example, abnormally high levels of the TH enzyme involved in the synthesis of dopamine could induce behavioral and motor dysfunction, as occurs with L-DOPA overdose.

The most basic regulation mechanism is of the "on–off" type, in which transgene transcription can be controlled by the exogenous administration of a drug. In the popular tetracycline-induced regulatory system, *cis*-acting sequences may either up- or down-regulate transcription of a gene after the administration of tetracycline (or its analog doxycycline). This system has been successfully used both in vivo and ex vivo.[155-157] However, it suffers from several shortcomings, the most important one being a retarded effect for induction or repression of transcription, which could last from several days and up to 2 weeks.[155,156] Such systems are therefore only suitable for those applications that do not require a rapid response to an acute state, but rather chronic diseases that can cope with such time frames. A second disadvantage of the "on–off" systems lies in the "all or none" type of therapeutic production. As noted above, the lack of fine-tuning over transgene product levels may not only compromise the efficiency of the therapeutic effect, but also induce toxicity.

A significant advance would be the introduction of inducible genes with a "built-in" regulatory mechanism, driven by sensory input of physiologic status. Such a system, sensing glucocorticoid levels as a marker for acute neurologic insult, was constructed based on a glucocorticoid-responsive promoter.[158] A similar approach was more recently used in a nonviral vector expressing the antiapoptotic bcl-2 gene regulated by the hypoxia-inducible human vascular endothelial growth factor promoter.[159] Gene expression by the inducible construct in vivo was found to be limited to the brain area subjected to experimentally induced hypoxia. Although the infarct volume was not reduced in animals injected with the inducible vector, a significant reduction in the number of apoptotic cells was observed.

A more advanced version of the inducible vectors lies in the realm of biomolecular computers. DNA-based nano-functional units have been constructed, that are able to analyze the levels of distinct mRNA species and release in response a short ssDNA molecule, which regulates gene expression by an antisense mechanism.[160] Although this work has so far been performed only in a cell-free system, the achievement of a molecular "automaton" that is able to sense cellular transcriptional status and respond by the release of a specific therapeutic serves as a huge step forward.

Vector Safety

The turmoils of translating a therapeutic concept into a cure is perhaps none better exemplified than in the course taken by gene transfer technology. With our limited understanding of the "molecular vocabulary" and grammatical rules, difficulties in intervening in the complex conversation conducted within the living organism could have only been foreseen. The potential risks of introducing foreign genetic material and "tamed" pathogens into the human body were soon to be realized during the course of clinical trials. Preclinical calculations of individual risks are therefore modified together with the comprehension gained as to how the tool and system actually work. With the gene transfer systems available today, safety is still the major issue of concern and serves as a primary consideration before translating potential applications into the clinical trial phase (see Table 9.3). The shift of clinical trial attention from monogenic disorders to the more "hopeless" cases of malignant neoplasms may therefore reflect not only the limited efficacy of the methodology, but also the doubts about the safety of this tool. The major hazards and safety concerns associated with gene transfer technology are discussed below.

The Immune Response

In 1999, a young man named Jesse Gelsinger participated in a gene therapy clinical trial at the University of Pennsylvania in Philadelphia for the treatment of ornithine transcarbamylase deficiency. As part of a phase I trial to which he volunteered, he received (via hepatic artery) 3.8×10^{13} particles of the E1/E4-deleted adenoviral vector carrying a correct copy of the gene.

Table 9.3. Risks and hazards of gene therapy

1. Administration method related (e.g., local tissue damage by needle tract).
2. Immune-mediated damage:
   a. Inflammatory reaction.
   b. Cytotoxic T lymphocyte lysis of cells displaying foreign proteins.
3. Vector-induced toxicity:
   a. By non-transgene protein products.
   b. By transgene product.
4. Virus-related:
   a. Insertional mutagenesis.
   b. Reversion to wild-type virus.
   c. Activation of endogenous viruses.
5. Stable gene transfer to germline cells.

Several hours posttreatment he developed a high fever, followed by hepatic failure and disseminated intravascular coagulation. Four days later, he died of multiorgan failure. Results of the postmortem examination revealed that death ensued from an extreme immune response triggered by high vector levels in the systemic circulation.[161,162] It was still unclear, however, why such an immune response was mounted in one patient whereas another, who received the same dose, demonstrated only mild symptoms. The severe depletion of red blood cell precursors in the bone marrow initially suggested a preexisting parvovirus infection or an undetected genetic immune dysfunction.[163] Subsequent studies indicated that the formation of antigen-antibody complexes (caused by preexisting immunity to vector components) caused the inflammatory reaction by activation of the complement system.[164,165] A cytokine-mediated immune response to the systemically disseminated vector (independent of neutralizing antibodies) was also implied.[166] Studies with nonhuman primates indicated that such responses were directed toward viral capsid components rather than to de novo synthesized viral gene products. The dose-dependent reactions triggered by the injected virus cast significant doubt on the utility of this mode of administration for any potentially immunogenic vector.

Direct vector introduction into the brain tissue, previously perceived as shielded from the host immune system, takes on a different form of immune response. After intracerebral injection of a first-generation adenoviral vector to nonprimed animals, an innate inflammatory response, which involves cytokine release, activation of microglial cells, and infiltration by macrophages and lymphocytes, is mounted. This reaction resolves within a month and does not affect transgene expression, persisting for several months. In addition, intracerebral injection does not prime an adaptive immune response. However, if the host is then systemically administered with the vector, an adaptive response is triggered, accompanied by extinction of transgene expression.[167] Both the initial inflammatory response and the priming of the adaptive immune response result from expression of virus-derived genes from first-generation vectors, because these phenomena were not observed with "gutless" adenoviral vectors.[168] Moreover, long-term transgene expression by the "gutless" vector was observed even after peripheral immunization.

Similar to the first generation of adenoviral vectors, both HSV-1 and AAV vectors administered to the brain induce potent immune responses, associated with the abolishment of transgene expression.[169-171] The preimmunization status of the host to the intracerebrally injected AAV determined vector immunogenicity in a serotype specific manner. The inciting factor to the response (i.e., viral capsid or gene expression) is still unclear.

These data emphasize the need to monitor all patients participating in gene therapy clinical trials, both before and after vector administration, for their general immune status, cytokine profile, and, most importantly, for their preimmunization status to the vector.

The most recent unfortunate results of a large nongene therapy clinical trial mandate reference to potential immunogenicity of the therapeutic protein product itself. In a phase II trial for the treatment of PD, recombinant human glial derived neurotrophic factor (GDNF) was infused directly into the striatum of patients.[172] Although initial clinical tests provided encouraging results,[173] the subsequent double-blinded placebo-controlled trial was halted because of both therapeutic inefficacy and safety concerns. Of the 34 patients who received the infusions, four developed antibodies to GDNF, in three of which the antibodies were neutralizing. Whereas the recombinant human GDNF administered in this trial may differ immunogenically from the in vivo produced protein in the gene therapy approach, the concern that such antibodies might also act against endogenous GDNF warrants careful attention.

Viral Vector-Related Risks

Remarkable concern was initially expressed at the idea of using potentially pathogenic viruses as a therapeutic agent. Generation of replication-competent viruses, by recombination with helper constructs or with endogenous silent pathogens, were raised as significant possibilities. Activation of latently residing viruses, such as HSV-1, was similarly proposed to be a potential hazard, but experimental studies have not shown this to occur.[174]

A second risk, associated with the integration of the vector into the host cell genome, proved to be more substantial and occurred in the first and only clinical trial (to date), which has shown a definitive cure provided by gene therapy. X-linked severe combined immunodeficiency XI disease is a fatal condition caused by the lack of a functional γ-c chain cytokine receptor and results in the inability of developing lymphocytes to respond to cytokine signals and mature into functional T and natural-killer cells. In the absence of a full-match bone marrow transplant donor, children usually die during the first years of life from opportunistic infections. In a gene therapy clinical trial conducted by Alain Fischer and colleagues, hematopoietic stem cells were isolated from children with the disease, transduced ex vivo with a retroviral vector expressing a correct copy of the gene, and reinfused to the patients.[16] By 2003, more than 10 patients were treated by this method, the large majority of which reconstituted the function of their immune system. Infants that previously required protective isolation, were thereafter able to conduct a normal lifestyle.

Unfortunately, 3 years after administration of the therapy, two of these patients developed a T cell lymphoproliferative disorder. The proliferating T cells, in both cases, were shown to contain the retroviral vector genome integrated in the proximity of LMO2, a known human T cell protooncogene.[175,176] Cis-activation or disruption of an unidentified silencer could account for the generation of the hyper-proliferative clone. This loss of cell cycle control caused by mutations induced by the chromosomal integration of foreign genetic material is termed insertional mutagenesis. Given the earlier concept of complete randomness in integration, the occurrence of such an adverse event was only considered a theoretical risk. However, vector insertion into the same site in both patients highly suggested that integration is biased toward the more transcriptionally active genes.

In addition, contribution of the transgene product itself to the leukemogenesis was recently noted.[177] Cooperativity between the oncogenic γ-c chain receptor transgene and the overexpression of the LMO2 gene was suggested as the main reason underlying the generation of the leukemic cell clones. These results therefore pinpoint the hazard to this specific case, rather than to the use of integrating viral vectors as a whole. Nevertheless, insertional mutagenesis was shown to be a realistic risk that should be addressed.

Related to the above is the potential of vector transmission to germline cells (i.e., gene transfer to gonadal cells leading to offspring transmission of the transgene). However, studies with several animal species demonstrated no germline transmission after systemic injection of AAV or adenoviral vectors.[178,179]

Conclusions and Future Prospects

The unsatisfactory impact of conventional pharmacotherapy on nervous system pathology is the outcome of a partial understanding of both the regulatory mechanisms that underlie normal system function and the pathophysiology of most neurologic conditions. Naturally, this limits the ability to develop efficient therapeutics by any modality, gene transfer technology inclusive. The mere advantage provided by gene therapy remains the platform it provides for controlled in vivo therapeutic delivery.

Two major obstacles are yet to be surmounted: Achievement of targeted gene delivery to the diseased cell and safety issues associated with gene transfer technology, particularly with the virus-based systems. Although encouraging progress with nonviral vehicles has been achieved, the higher efficiency of virus-based systems still renders them the more common type utilized. Additional required improvements with nonviral vectors include stability, cell-type-specific targeting, and direction to more efficient intracellular routes. With the evolution of molecular modeling and understanding of the sequence-structure-function relationship of proteins, the construction of synthetic functional units that are not based on nature's "ready-made" armamentarium, but merely harness its rules, should facilitate the efficient transfer and expression of genes for the treatment of disease.

References

1. Elliger SS, Elliger CA, Aguilar CP, Raju NR, Watson GL. Elimination of lysosomal storage in brains of MPS VII mice treated by intrathecal administration of an adeno-associated virus vector. Gene Ther 1999;6:1175–1178.
2. Bosch A, Perret E, Desmaris N, Trono D, Heard JM. Reversal of pathology in the entire brain of

mucopolysaccharidosis type VII mice after lentivirus-mediated gene transfer. Hum Gene Ther 2000;11: 1139–1150.
3. Leone P, Janson CG, Bilaniuk L, et al. Aspartoacylase gene transfer to the mammalian central nervous system with therapeutic implications for Canavan disease. Ann Neurol 2000;48:27–38.
4. During MJ, Naegele JR, O'Malley KL, Geller AI. Long-term behavioral recovery in parkinsonian rats by an HSV vector expressing tyrosine hydroxylase. Science 1994;266:1399–1403.
5. Segovia J, Vergara P, Brenner M. Astrocyte-specific expression of tyrosine hydroxylase after intracerebral gene transfer induces behavioral recovery in experimental parkinsonism. Gene Ther 1998;5:1650–1655.
6. Zhang Y, Calon F, Zhu C, Boado RJ, Pardridge WM. Intravenous nonviral gene therapy causes normalization of striatal tyrosine hydroxylase and reversal of motor impairment in experimental parkinsonism. Hum Gene Ther 2003;14:1–12.
7. Do Thi NA, Saillour P, Ferrero L, Dedieu JF, Mallet J, Paunio T. Delivery of GDNF by an E1,E3/E4 deleted adenoviral vector and driven by a GFAP promoter prevents dopaminergic neuron degeneration in a rat model of Parkinson's disease. Gene Ther 2004;11:746–756.
8. Hendriks WT, Ruitenberg MJ, Blits B, Boer GJ, Verhaagen J. Viral vector-mediated gene transfer of neurotrophins to promote regeneration of the injured spinal cord. Prog Brain Res 2004;146:451–476.
9. Regulier E, Pereira de Almeida L, Sommer B, Aebischer P, Deglon N. Dose-dependent neuroprotective effect of ciliary neurotrophic factor delivered via tetracycline-regulated lentiviral vectors in the quinolinic acid rat model of Huntington's disease. Hum Gene Ther 2002;13:1981–1990.
10. Robert JJ, Bouilleret V, Ridoux V, et al. Adenovirus-mediated transfer of a functional GAD gene into nerve cells: potential for the treatment of neurological diseases. Gene Ther 1997;4:1237–1245.
11. Lee AL, Dumas TC, Tarapore PE, et al. Potassium channel gene therapy can prevent neuron death resulting from necrotic and apoptotic insults. J Neurochem 2003;86:1079–1088.
12. The Journal of Gene Medicine (Wiley) clinical trial database: www.wiley.co.uk/genmed/clinical.
13. Hughes RM. Strategies for cancer gene therapy. J Surg Oncol 2004;85:28–35.
14. Scanlon KJ. Cancer gene therapy: challenges and opportunities. Anticancer Res 2004;24:501–504.
15. Vile R, Ando D, Kirn D. The oncolytic virotherapy treatment platform for cancer: unique biological and biosafety points to consider. Cancer Gene Ther 2002;9:1062–1067.
16. Cavazzana-Calvo M, Hacein-Bey S, de Saint Basile G, et al. Gene therapy of human severe combined immunodeficiency (SCID)-X1 disease. Science 2000;288:669–672.
17. Wyman T, Rohrer D, Kirigiti P, et al. Promoter-activated expression of nerve growth factor for treatment of neurodegenerative diseases. Gene Ther 1999;6:1648–1660.
18. Selkirk SM, Greenberg SJ, Plunkett RJ, Barone TA, Lis A, Spence PO. Syngeneic central nervous system transplantation of genetically transduced mature, adult astrocytes. Gene Ther 2002;9:432–443.
19. Otto E, Jones-Trower A, Vanin EF, et al. Characterization of a replication-competent retrovirus resulting from recombination of packaging and vector sequences. Hum Gene Ther 1994;5:567–575.
20. Chong H, Starkey W, Vile RG. A replication-competent retrovirus arising from a split-function packaging cell line was generated by recombination events between the vector, one of the packaging constructs and endogenous retroviral sequences. J Virol 1994;72:2663–2670.
21. Yu SF, von Ruden T, Kantoff PW, et al. Self-inactivating retroviral vectors designed for transfer of whole genes into mammalian cells. Proc Natl Acad Sci USA 1986;83:3194–3198.
22. Miller DG, Adam MA, Miller AD. Gene transfer by retroviral vectors occurs only in cells that are actively replicating at the time of infection. Mol Cell Biol 1990;10:4239–4242.
23. Bukrinsky MI, Haffar OK. HIV-1 nuclear import: in search of a leader. Front Biosci 1999;4:772–781.
24. Sodroski J, Patarca R, Rosen C, Wong-Staal F, Haseltine W. Location of the trans-activating region on the genome of human T-cell lymphotropic virus type III. Science 1985;229:74–77.
25. Fisher AG, Feinberg MB, Josephs SF, et al. The trans-activator gene of HTLV-III is essential for virus replication. Nature 1986;320:367–371.
26. Malim MH, Hauber J, Fenrick R, Cullen BR. Immunodeficiency virus rev trans-activator modulates the expression of the viral regulatory genes. Nature 1988;335:181–183.
27. Naldini L, Blomer U, Gallay P, et al. In vivo gene delivery and stable transduction of nondividing cells by a lentiviral vector. Science 1996;272:263–267.
28. Naldini L, Blomer U, Gage FH, Trono D, Verma IM. Efficient transfer, integration and sustained long-term expression of the transgene in adult rat brains injected with a lentiviral vector. Proc Natl Acad Sci USA 1996;93:11382–11388.
29. Blomer U, Naldini L, Kafri T, Trono D, Verma IM, Gage FH. Highly efficient and sustained gene transfer in adult neurons with a lentivirus vector. J Virol 1997;71:6641–6649.
30. Dull T, Zufferey R, Kelly M, et al. A third-generation lentivirus vector with a conditional packaging system. J Virol 1998;72:8463–8471.
31. Zufferey R, Dull T, Mandel RJ, et al. Self-inactivating lentivirus vector for safe and efficient in vivo gene delivery. J Virol 1998;72:9873–9880.
32. Jakobsson J, Ericson C, Jansson M, Bjork E, Lundberg C. Targeted transgene expression in rat brain using lentiviral vectors. J Neurosci Res 2003;73:876–885.
33. Kordower JH, Bloch J, Ma SY, et al. Lentiviral gene transfer to the nonhuman primate brain. Exp Neurol 1999;160:1–16.
34. Kordower JH, Emborg ME, Bloch J, et al. Parkinson's disease: neurodegeneration prevented by lentiviral vector delivery of GDNF in primate models of Parkinson's disease. Science 2000;290:767–773.
35. Consiglio A, Quattrini A, Martino S, et al. In vivo gene therapy of metachromatic leukodystrophy by lentiviral vectors: correction of neuropathology and protection against learning impairments in affected mice. Nat Med 2001;7:310–316.
36. Brooks AI, Stein CS, Hughes SM, et al. Functional correction of established central nervous system deficits

37. Loser P, Hillgenberg M, Arnold W, Both GW, Hofmann C. Ovine adenovirus vectors mediate efficient gene transfer to skeletal muscle. Gene Ther 2000;7:1491–1498.
38. Berkner KL, Sharp PA. Generation of adenovirus by transfection of plasmids. Nucleic Acids Res 1983;11:6003–6020.
39. Haj-Ahmad Y, Graham FL. Development of a helper-independent human adenovirus vector and its use in the transfer of the herpes simplex virus thymidine kinase gene. J Virol 1986;57:267–274.
40. Yang Y, Li Q, Ertl HC, Wilson JM. Cellular and humoral immune responses to viral antigens create barriers to lung-directed gene therapy with recombinant adenoviruses. J Virol 1995;69:2004–2015.
41. Yang Y, Wilson JM. Clearance of adenovirus-infected hepatocytes by class-I restricted CD4+ CTLs in vivo. J Immunol 1995;155:2564–2570.
42. Lusky M, Christ M, Rittner K, et al. In vitro and in vivo biology of recombinant adenovirus vectors with E1, E1/E2A, or E1/E4 deleted. J Virol 1998;72:2022–2032.
43. Parks RJ, Chen L, Anton M, Sankar U, Rudnicki MA, Graham FL. A helper-dependent adenovirus vector system: removal of helper virus by Cre-mediated excision of the viral packaging signal. Proc Natl Acad Sci USA 1996;93:13565–13570.
44. Kafri T, Morgan D, Krahl T, Sarvetnick N, Sherman L, Verma I. Cellular immune response to adenoviral vector infected cells does not require de novo viral gene expression: implications for gene therapy. Proc Natl Acad Sci USA 1998;95:11377–11382.
45. Morsy MA, Gu M, Motzel S, et al. An adenoviral vector deleted for all viral coding sequences results in enhanced safety and extended expression of a leptin transgene. Proc Natl Acad Sci USA 1998;95:7866–7871.
46. Balague C, Zhou J, Dai Y, et al. Sustained high-level expression of full-length human factor VIII and restoration of clotting activity in hemophilic mice using a minimal adenovirus vector. Blood 2000;95:820–828.
47. Lieber A, Steinwaerder DS, Carlson CA, Kay MA. 1999. Integrating adenovirus-adeno-associated virus hybrid vectors devoid of all viral genes. J Virol 1999;73:9314–9324.
48. Zheng C, Baum BJ, Iadarola MJ, O'Connell BC. Genomic integration and gene expression by a modified adenoviral vector. Nat Biotechnol 2000;18:176–186.
49. Ferrari FK, Samulski T, Shenk T, Samulski RJ. 1996. Second-strand synthesis is a rate-limiting step for efficient transduction by recombinant adeno-associated virus vectors. J Virol 1996;70:3227–3234.
50. Samulski RJ, Chang LS, Shenk T. Helper-free stocks of recombinant adenoassociated viruses: normal integration does not require viral gene expression. J Virol 1989;63:3822–3828.
51. Hermonat PL, Muzyczka N. Use of adeno-associated virus as a mammalian DNA cloning vector: transduction of neomycin resistance into mammalian tissue culture cells. Proc Natl Acad Sci USA 1984;81:6466–6470.
52. Xiao X, Li J, Samulski RJ. Production of high-titer recombinant adeno-associated virus vectors in the absence of helper adenovirus. J Virol 1998;72:2224–2232.
53. Davidson BL, Stein CS, Heth JA, et al. Recombinant adeno-associated virus type 2, 4, and 5 vectors: transduction of variant cell types and regions in the mammalian central nervous system. Proc Natl Acad Sci USA 2000;97:3428–3432.
54. Duan D, Yue Y, Engelhardt JF. Expanding AAV packaging capacity with trans-splicing or overlapping vectors: a quantitative comparison. Mol Ther 2001;4:383–391.
55. Roizman B, Sears A. Herpes simplex viruses and their replication. In: Fields BN, Knipe DM, Howley PM, et al., eds. Fields Virology. 3rd ed. Philadelphia: Lippincott–Raven; 1996:2231–2295.
56. Kent JR, Kang W, Miller CG, Fraser NW. Herpes simplex virus latency-associated transcript gene function. J Neurovirol 2003;9:285–290.
57. Mador N, Goldenberg D, Cohen O, Panet A, Steiner I. Herpes simplex virus type 1 latency-associated transcripts suppress viral replication and reduce immediate-early gene mRNA levels in a neuronal cell line. J Virol 1998;72:5067–5075.
58. Krisky DM, Wolfe D, Goins WF, et al. Deletion of multiple immediate-early genes from herpes simplex virus reduces cytotoxicity and permits long-term gene expression in neurons. Gene Ther 1998;5:1593–1603.
59. Marconi P, Krisky D, Oligino T, et al. Replication-defective herpes simplex virus vectors for gene transfer in vivo. Proc Natl Acad Sci USA 1996;93:11319–11320.
60. Samaniego LA, Neiderhiser L, DeLuca NA. Persistence and expression of the herpes simplex virus genome in the absence of immediate-early proteins. J Virol 1998;72:3307–3320.
61. Saeki Y, Ichikawa T, Saeki A, et al. Herpes simplex virus type 1 DNA amplified as bacterial artificial chromosome in Escherichia coli: rescue of replication-competent virus progeny and packaging of amplicon vectors. Hum Gene Ther 1998;9:2787–2794.
62. Geller AI, Yu L, Wang Y, Fraefel C. Helper virus-free herpes simplex virus-1 plasmid vectors for gene therapy of Parkinson's disease and other neurological disorders. Exp Neurol 1997;144:98–102.
63. Stavropoulos TA, Strathdee CA. An enhanced packaging system for helper-dependent herpes simplex virus vectors. J Virol 1998;72:7137–7143.
64. Cunningham C, Davison AJ. A cosmid-based system for constructing mutants of herpes simplex virus type 1. Virology 1993;197:116–124.
65. Yenari MA, Fink SL, Sun GH, et al. Gene therapy with HSP72 is neuroprotective in rat models of stroke and epilepsy. Ann Neurol 1998;44:584–591.
66. Yamada M, Oligino T, Mata M, Goss JR, Glorioso JC, Fink DJ. Herpes simplex virus vector-mediated expression of Bcl-2 prevents 6-hydroxydopamine-induced degeneration of neurons in the substantia nigra in vivo. Proc Natl Acad Sci USA 1999;96:4078–4083.
67. Zhu J, Kang W, Wolfe J, Fraser N. Significantly increased expression of beta-glucuronidase in the central nervous system of mucopolysaccharidosis type VII mice from the latency-associated transcript promoter in a nonpathogenic herpes simplex virus type 1 vector. Mol Ther 2000;2:82–94.
68. Martino G, Poliani PL, Marconi PC, Comi G, Furlan R. Cytokine gene therapy of autoimmune demyelination revisited using herpes simplex virus type-1-derived vectors. Gene Ther 2000;7:1087–1093.

69. Carpenter DE, Stevens JG. Long-term expression of a foreign gene from a unique position in the latent herpes simplex virus genome. Hum Gene Ther 1996;7:1447–1454.
70. Wolfe D, Goins WF, Kaplan TJ, et al. Herpesvirus-mediated systemic delivery of nerve growth factor. Mol Ther 2001;3:61–69.
71. Yang NS, Burkholder J, Roberts B, Martinell B, McCabe D. In vivo and in vitro gene transfer to mammalian somatic cells by particle bombardment. Proc Natl Acad Sci USA 1990;87:9568–9572.
72. Yang NS, Sun WH. Gene gun and other non-viral approaches for cancer gene therapy. Nat Med 1995;1:481–483.
73. Mann MJ, Gibbons GH, Hutchinson H, et al. Pressure-mediated oligonucleotide transfection of rat and human cardiovascular tissues. Proc Natl Acad Sci USA 1999;96:6411–6416.
74. Ehsan A, Mann MJ, Dell'Acqua G, Dzau VJ. Long-term stabilization of vein graft wall architecture and prolonged resistance to experimental atherosclerosis after E2F decoy oligonucleotide gene therapy. J Thorac Cardiovasc Surg 2001;121:714–722.
75. Rizzuto G, Cappelletti M, Maione D, et al. Efficient and regulated erythropoietin production by naked DNA injection and muscle electroporation. Proc Natl Acad Sci USA 1999;96:6417–6422.
76. Taniyama Y, Tachibana K, Hiraoka K, et al. Development of safe and efficient novel nonviral gene transfer using ultrasound: enhancement of transfection efficiency of naked plasmid DNA in skeletal muscle. Gene Ther 2002;9:372–380.
77. El Ouahabi A, Thiry M, Pector V, Fuks R, Ruysschaert JM, Vandenbranden M. The role of endosome destabilizing activity in the gene transfer process mediated by cationic lipids. FEBS Lett 1997;414:187–192.
78. Monkkonen J, Urtti A. Lipid fusion in oligonucleotide and gene delivery with cationic lipids. Adv Drug Delivery Rev 1998;34:37–49.
79. Farhood H, Serbina N, Huang L. The role of dioleyl phosphatidyl-ethanolamine in cationic liposomes mediated gene transfer. Biochim Biophys Acta 1995;1235:289–295.
80. Holmes AR, Dohrman AF, Ellison AR, Goncz KK, Gruenert DC. Intracellular compartmentalization of DNA fragments in cultured airway epithelial cells mediated by cationic lipids. Pharm Res 1999;16:1020–1025.
81. Sebestyen MG, Ludtke JJ, Bassik MC, et al. DNA vector chemistry: the covalent attachment of signal peptides to plasmid DNA. Nat Biotechnol 1998;16:80–85.
82. Subramanian A, Ranganathan P, Diamond SL. Nuclear targeting peptide scaffolds for lipofection of nondividing mammalian cells. Nat Biotechnol 1999;17:873–877.
83. Lee RJ, Huang L. Lipidic vector systems for gene transfer. Crit Rev Ther Drug Carrier Syst 1997;14:173–206.
84. Shi N, Pardridge WM. Noninvasive gene targeting to the brain. Proc Natl Acad Sci USA 2000;97:7567–7572.
85. Shi N, Boado RJ, Pardridge WM. Receptor-mediated gene targeting to tissues in vivo following intravenous administration of pegylated immunoliposomes. Pharm Res 2001;18:1091–1095.
86. Zhang Y, Schlachetzki F, Pardridge WM. Global nonviral gene transfer to the primate brain following intravenous administration. Mol Ther 2003;7:11–18.
87. Filion MC, Phillips NC. Major limitations in the use of cationic liposomes for DNA delivery. Int J Pharm 1998;162:159–170.
88. Zauner W, Ogris M, Wagner E. Polylysine-based transfection systems utilizing receptor-mediated delivery. Adv Drug Delivery Rev 1998;30:97–113.
89. Schaffer DV, Lauffenburger DA. Optimization of cell surface binding enhances efficiency and specificity of molecular conjugate gene delivery. J Biol Chem 1998;273:28004–28009.
90. Aris A, Feliu JX, Knight A, Coutelle C, Villaverde A. Exploiting viral cell-targeting abilities in a single polypeptide, non-infectious, recombinant vehicle for integrin-mediated DNA delivery and gene expression. Biotechnol Bioeng 2000;68:689–696.
91. Peluffo H, Aris A, Acarin L, Gonzalez B, Villaverde A, Castellano B. Nonviral gene delivery to the central nervous system based on a novel integrin-targeting multifunctional protein. Hum Gene Ther 2003;14:1215–1223.
92. Kennedy PG, Steiner I. The potential use of viral vectors for gene therapy in neurological diseases. In: Lightman S, ed. Horizons in Medicine. London: Blackwell Science; 1996:406–417.
93. Costantini LC, Bakowska JC, Breakefield XO, Isacson O. Gene therapy in the CNS. Gene Ther 2000;7:93–109.
94. Mester JC, Pitha PM, Glorioso JC. Antiviral activity of herpes simplex virus vectors expressing murine alpha 1-interferon. Gene Ther 1995;2:187–196.
95. Broberg E, Setala N, Roytta M, et al. Expression of interleukin-4 but not of interleukin-10 from a replicative herpes simplex virus type 1 viral vector precludes experimental allergic encephalomyelitis. Gene Ther 2001;8:769–777.
96. Natsume A, Wolfe D, Hu J, et al. Enhanced functional recovery after proximal nerve root injury by vector-mediated gene transfer. Exp Neurol 2003;184:878–886.
97. Eaton MJ, Blits B, Ruitenberg MJ, Verhaagen J, Oudega M. Amelioration of chronic neuropathic pain after partial nerve injury by adeno-associated viral (AAV) vector-mediated over-expression of BDNF in the rat spinal cord. Gene Ther 2002;9:1387–1395.
98. Shirakura M, Inoue M, Fujikawa S, et al. Postischemic administration of Sendai virus vector carrying neurotrophic factor genes prevents delayed neuronal death in gerbils. Gene Ther 2004;11:784–790.
99. Roy M, Hom JJ, Sapolsky RM. HSV-mediated delivery of virally derived anti-apoptotic genes protects the rat hippocampus from damage following excitotoxicity, but not metabolic disruption. Gene Ther 2002;9:214–219.
100. Yamashita S, Mita S, Arima T, et al. Bcl-2 expression by retrograde transport of adenoviral vectors with Cre-loxP recombination system in motor neurons of mutant SOD1 transgenic mice. Gene Ther 2001;8:977–986.
101. Boillee S, Cleveland DW. Gene therapy for ALS delivers. Trends Neurosci 2004;27:235–238.
102. Wang L, Muramatsu S, Lu Y, et al. Delayed delivery of AAV-GDNF prevents nigral neurodegeneration and promotes functional recovery in a rat model of Parkinson's disease. Gene Ther 2002;9:381–389.
103. Tuszynski MH, Smith DE, Roberts J, McKay H, Mufson E. Targeted intraparenchymal delivery of human NGF by gene transfer to the primate basal forebrain for 3 months does not accelerate beta-amyloid plaque deposition. Exp Neurol 1998;154:573–582.

104. Rosen DR, Siddique T, Patterson D, et al. Mutations in Cu/Zn superoxide dismutase gene are associated with familial amyotrophic lateral sclerosis. Nature 1993;362:59–62.
105. Carri MT, Ferri A, Cozzolino M, Calabrese L, Rotilio G. Neurodegeneration in amyotrophic lateral sclerosis: the role of oxidative stress and altered homeostasis of metals. Brain Res Bull 2003;61:365–374.
106. Pong K. Oxidative stress in neurodegenerative diseases: therapeutic implications for superoxide dismutase mimetics. Expert Opin Biol Ther 2003;3:127–139.
107. Rattray M. Is there nicotinic modulation of nerve growth factor? Implications for cholinergic therapies in Alzheimer's disease. Biol Psychiatry 2001;49:185–193.
108. Kumar VB, Farr SA, Flood JF, et al. Site-directed antisense oligonucleotide decreases the expression of amyloid precursor protein and reverses deficits in learning and memory in aged SAMP8 mice. Peptides 2000;21:1769–1775.
109. Banks WA, Farr SA, Butt W, Kumar VB, Franko MW, Morley JE. Delivery across the blood-brain barrier of antisense directed against amyloid beta: reversal of learning and memory deficits in mice overexpressing amyloid precursor protein. J Pharmacol Exp Ther 2001;297:1113–1121.
110. Poon HF, Joshi G, Sultana R, et al. Antisense directed at the Abeta region of APP decreases brain oxidative markers in aged senescence accelerated mice. Brain Res 2004;1018:86–96.
111. Spencer T, Filbin MT. A role for cAMP in regeneration of the adult mammalian CNS. J Anat 2004;204:49–55.
112. Fournier AE, Strittmatter SM. Regenerating nerves follow the road more traveled. Nat Neurosci 2002;5:821–822.
113. McKerracher L, David S, Jackson DL, Kottis V, Dunn RJ, Braun PE. Identification of myelin-associated glycoprotein as a major myelin-derived inhibitor of neurite growth. Neuron 1994;13:805–811.
114. GrandPre T, Nakamura F, Vartanian T, Strittmatter SM. Identification of the Nogo inhibitor of axon regeneration as a Reticulon protein. Nature 2000;403:439–444.
115. Kottis V, Thibault P, Mikol D, et al. Oligodendrocyte-myelin glycoprotein (OMgp) is an inhibitor of neurite outgrowth. J Neurochem 2002;82:1566–1569.
116. Fischer D, He Z, Benowitz LI. Counteracting the Nogo receptor enhances optic nerve regeneration if retinal ganglion cells are in an active growth state. J Neurosci 2004;24:1646–1651.
117. Boviatsis EJ, Scharf JM, Chase M, et al. Antitumor activity and reporter gene transfer into rat brain tumors inoculated with herpes simplex virus vectors defective in thymidine kinase or ribonucleotide reductase. Gene Ther 1994;1:323–331.
118. Hamilton JF, Morrison PF, Chen MY, et al. Heparin coinfusion during convection-enhanced delivery (CED) increases the distribution of the glial-derived neurotrophic factor (GDNF) ligand family in rat striatum and enhances the pharmacological activity of neurturin. Exp Neurol 2001;168:155–161.
119. Bankiewicz KS, Eberling JL, Kohutnicka M, et al. Convection-enhanced delivery of AAV vector in parkinsonian monkeys: in vivo detection of gene expression and restoration of dopaminergic function using pro-drug approach. Exp Neurol 2000;164:2–14.
120. Nguyen JB, Sanchez-Pernaute R, Cunningham J, Bankiewicz KS. Convection-enhanced delivery of AAV-2 combined with heparin increases TK gene transfer in the rat brain. Neuroreport 2001;12:1961–1964.
121. Thomas CE, Edwards P, Wickham TJ, Castro MG, Lowenstein PR. Adenovirus binding to the coxsackievirus and adenovirus receptor or integrins is not required to elicit brain inflammation but is necessary to transduce specific neural cell types. J Virol 2002;76:3452–3460.
122. Zermansky AJ, Bolognani F, Stone D, et al. Towards global and long-term neurological gene therapy: unexpected transgene dependent, high-level, and widespread distribution of HSV-1 thymidine kinase throughout the CNS. Mol Ther 2001;4:490–498.
123. Dewey RA, Morrissey G, Cowsill CM, et al. Chronic brain inflammation and persistent herpes simplex virus 1 thymidine kinase expression in survivors of syngeneic glioma treated by adenovirus-mediated gene therapy: implications for clinical trials. Nat Med 1999;5:1256–1263.
124. Doran SE, Ren XD, Betz AL, et al. Gene expression from recombinant viral vectors in the central nervous system after blood-brain barrier disruption. Neurosurgery 1995;36:965–970.
125. Muldoon LL, Nilaver G, Kroll RA, et al. Comparison of intracerebral inoculation and osmotic blood-brain barrier disruption for delivery of adenovirus, herpesvirus, and iron oxide particles to normal rat brain. Am J Pathol 1995;147:1840–1851.
126. Kroll RA, Neuwelt EA. Outwitting the blood-brain barrier for therapeutic purposes: osmotic opening and other means. Neurosurgery 1998;42:1083–1099.
127. Salahuddin TS, Johansson BB, Kalimo H, Olsson Y. Structural changes in the rat brain after carotid infusions of hyperosmolar solutions: a light microscopic and immunohistochemical study. Neuropathol Appl Neurobiol 1988;14:467–482.
128. Nadal A, Fuentes E, Pastor J, McNaughton PA. Plasma albumin is a potent trigger of calcium signals and DNA synthesis in astrocytes. Proc Natl Acad Sci USA 1995;92:1426–1430.
129. Pardridge WM. Drug and gene delivery to the brain: the vascular route. Neuron 2002;36:555–558.
130. Betz AL, Yang GY, Davidson BL. Attenuation of stroke size in rats using an adenoviral vector to induce overexpression of interleukin-1 receptor antagonist in brain. J Cereb Blood Flow Metab 1995;15:547–551.
131. Ooboshi H, Welsh MJ, Rios CD, Davidson BL, Heistad DD. Adenovirus-mediated gene transfer in vivo to cerebral blood vessels and perivascular tissue. Circ Res 1995;77:7–13.
132. Bajocchi G, Feldman SH, Crystal RG, Mastrangeli A. Direct in vivo gene transfer to ependymal cells in the central nervous system using recombinant adenovirus. Nat Genet 1993;3:229–234.
133. Yan Q, Matheson C, Sun J, Radeke MJ, Feinstein SC, Miller JA. Distribution of intracerebral ventricularly administered neurotrophins in rat brain and its correlation with trk receptor expression. Exp Neurol 1994;127:23–36.

134. Card JP. Pseudorabies virus neuroinvasiveness: a window into the functional organization of the brain. Adv Virus Res 2001;56:39–71.
135. Ghadge GD, Roos RP, Kang UJ, et al. CNS gene delivery by retrograde transport of recombinant replication-defective adenoviruses. Gene Ther 1995;2:132–137.
136. Draghia R, Caillaud C, Manicom R, Pavirani A, Kahn A, Poenaru L. Gene delivery into the central nervous system by nasal instillation in rats. Gene Ther 1995;2:418–423.
137. Hennig AK, Levy B, Ogilvie JM, et al. Intravitreal gene therapy reduces lysosomal storage in specific areas of the CNS in mucopolysaccharidosis VII mice. J Neurosci 2003;23:3302–3307.
138. Spector DH, Wade E, Wright DA, et al. Human immunodeficiency virus pseudotypes with expanded cellular and species tropism. J Virol 1990;64:2298–2308.
139. Emi N, Friedmann T, Yee JK. Pseudotype formation of murine leukemia virus with the G protein of vesicular stomatitis virus. J Virol 1991;65:1202–1207.
140. Burns JC, Friedmann T, Driever W, Burrascano M, Yee JK. Vesicular stomatitis virus G glycoprotein pseudotyped retroviral vectors: concentration to very high titer and efficient gene transfer into mammalian and nonmammalian cells. Proc Natl Acad Sci USA 1993;90:8033–8037.
141. Parveen Z, Mukhtar M, Rafi M, et al. Cell-type-specific gene delivery into neuronal cells in vitro and in vivo. Virology 2003;314:74–83.
142. Russell SJ, Hawkins RE, Winter G. Retroviral vectors displaying functional antibody fragments. Nucleic Acids Res 1993;21:1081–1085.
143. Cosset FL, Morling FJ, Takeuchi Y, Weiss RA, Collins MK, Russell SJ. Retroviral retargeting by envelopes expressing an N-terminal binding domain. J Virol 1995;69:6314–6322.
144. Hall FL, Gordon EM, Wu L, et al. Targeting retroviral vectors to vascular lesions by genetic engineering of the MoMLV gp70 envelope protein. Hum Gene Ther 1997;8:2183–2192.
145. Peng KW, Morling FJ, Cosset FL, Murphy G, Russell SJ. A gene delivery system activatable by disease-associated matrix metalloproteinases. Hum Gene Ther 1997;8:729–738.
146. Yang Q, Mamounas M, Yu G, et al. Development of novel cell surface CD34-targeted recombinant adenoassociated virus vectors for gene therapy. Hum Gene Ther 1998;9:1929–1937.
147. Laquerre S, Anderson DB, Stolz DB, Glorioso JC. Recombinant herpes simplex virus type 1 engineered for targeted binding to erythropoietin receptor-bearing cells. J Virol 1998;72:9683–9697.
148. Peng KW, Russell SJ. Viral vector targeting. Curr Opin Biotechnol 1999;10:454–457.
149. Trepel M, Grifman M, Weitzman MD, Pasqualini R. Molecular adaptors for vascular-targeted adenoviral gene delivery. Hum Gene Ther 2000;11:1971–1981.
150. Etienne-Julan M, Roux P, Carillo S, Jeanteur P, Piechaczyk M. The efficiency of cell targeting by recombinant retroviruses depends on the nature of the receptor and the composition of the artificial cell-virus linker. J Gen Virol 1992;73:3251–3255.
151. Snitkovsky S, Young JA. Cell-specific viral targeting mediated by a soluble retroviral receptor-ligand fusion protein. Proc Natl Acad Sci USA 1998;95: 7063–7068.
152. Reynolds PN, Nicklin SA, Kaliberova L, et al. Combined transductional and transcriptional targeting improves the specificity of transgene expression in vivo. Nat Biotechnol 2001;19:838–842.
153. Cucchiarini M, Ren XL, Perides G, Terwilliger EF. Selective gene expression in brain microglia mediated via adeno-associated virus type 2 and type 5 vectors. Gene Ther 2003;10:657–667.
154. Hwang DY, Carlezon WA Jr, Isacson O, Kim KS. A high-efficiency synthetic promoter that drives transgene expression selectively in noradrenergic neurons. Hum Gene Ther 2001;12:1731–1740.
155. Chtarto A, Bender HU, Hanemann CO, et al. Tetracycline-inducible transgene expression mediated by a single AAV vector. Gene Ther 2003;10:84–94.
156. Kafri T, van Praag H, Gage FH, Verma IM. Lentiviral vectors: regulated gene expression. Mol Ther 2000;1: 516–521.
157. Johansen J, Rosenblad C, Andsberg K, et al. Evaluation of Tet-on system to avoid transgene down-regulation in ex vivo gene transfer to the CNS. Gene Ther 2002;9:1291–1301.
158. Ozawa CR, Ho JJ, Tsai DJ, Ho DY, Sapolsky RM. Neuroprotective potential of a viral vector system induced by a neurological insult. Proc Natl Acad Sci USA 2000;97:9270–9275.
159. Cao YJ, Shibata T, Rainov NG. Liposome-mediated transfer of the bcl-2 gene results in neuroprotection after in vivo transient focal cerebral ischemia in an animal model. Gene Ther 2002;9:415–419.
160. Benenson Y, Gil B, Ben-Dor U, Adar R, Shapiro E. An autonomous molecular computer for logical control of gene expression. Nature 2004;429:423–429.
161. Marshall E. Gene therapy death prompts review of adenovirus vector. Science 1999;286:2244–2245.
162. Assessment of adenoviral vector safety and toxicity: report of the National Institutes of Health Recombinant DNA Advisory Committee. Hum Gene Ther 2002;13:3–13.
163. Marshall E. Gene therapy on trial. Science 2000;288:951–957.
164. Cichon G, Boeckh-Herwig S, Schmidt HH, et al. Complement activation by recombinant adenoviruses. Gene Ther 2001;8:1794–1800.
165. Bostanci A. Blood test flags agent in death of Penn subject. Science 2002;295:604–605.
166. Schnell MA, Zhang Y, Tazelaar J, et al. Activation of innate immunity in nonhuman primates following intraportal administration of adenoviral vectors. Mol Ther 2001;3:708–722.
167. Lowenstein PR, Castro MG. Progress and challenges in viral vector-mediated gene transfer to the brain. Curr Opin Mol Ther 2002;4:359–371.
168. Thomas CE, Schiedner G, Kochanek S, Castro MG, Lowenstein PR. Peripheral infection with adenovirus causes unexpected long-term brain inflammation in animals injected intracranially with first-generation, but not with high-capacity, adenovirus vectors: toward realistic long-term neurological gene therapy for chronic diseases. Proc Natl Acad Sci USA 2000;97:7482–7487.

169. Wood MJ, Byrnes AP, Pfaff DW, Rabkin SD, Charlton HM. Inflammatory effects of gene transfer into the CNS with defective HSV-1 vectors. Gene Ther 1994;1:283–291.
170. McMenamin MM, Byrnes AP, Charlton HM, Coffin RS, Latchman DS, Wood MJ. A gamma34.5 mutant of herpes simplex 1 causes severe inflammation in the brain. Neuroscience 1998;83:1225–1237.
171. Peden CS, Burger C, Muzyczka N, Mandel RJ. Circulating anti-wild-type adeno-associated virus type 2 (AAV2) antibodies inhibit recombinant AAV2 (rAAV2)-mediated, but not rAAV5-mediated, gene transfer in the brain. J Virol 2004;78:6344–6359.
172. Lang A. The 129th annual meeting of the American Neurological Association, October 2004, Toronto, Canada.
173. Gill SS, Patel NK, Hotton GR, et al. Direct brain infusion of glial cell line-derived neurotrophic factor in Parkinson disease. Nat Med 2003;9:589–595.
174. Sundaresan P, Hunter WD, Martuza RL, Rabkin SD. Attenuated, replication-competent herpes simplex virus type 1 mutant G207: safety evaluation in mice. J Virol 2000;74:3832–3841.
175. Royer-Pokora B, Loos U, Ludwig WD. TTG-2, a new gene encoding a cysteine-rich protein with the LIM motif, is overexpressed in acute T-cell leukaemia with the t(11;14)(p13;q11). Oncogene 1991;6:1887–1893.
176. Hacein-Bey-Abina S, von Kalle C, Schmidt M, et al. A serious adverse event after successful gene therapy for X-linked severe combined immunodeficiency. N Engl J Med 2003;348:255–256.
177. Dave UP, Jenkins NA, Copeland NG. Gene therapy insertional mutagenesis insights. Science 2004;303:333.
178. Arruda VR, Fields PA, Milner R, et al. Lack of germline transmission of vector sequences following systemic administration of recombinant AAV-2 vector in males. Mol Ther 2001;4:586–592.
179. Peters AH, Drumm J, Ferrell C, et al. Absence of germline infection in male mice following intraventricular injection of adenovirus. Mol Ther 2001;4:603–613.

Section 3

Musculoskeletal

Section 3
Musculoskeletal

Zvi Nevo and Mark M. Levy

The skeletal tissues, cartilage and bone, are coined expressions in biology (twin idioms) considered to have common progenitor-ancestor cells. Deducing from the evolutionary history, the appearance of cartilage structures in marine creatures preceded the appearance of hard-bony tissues in creatures of the universe. This phylogenic order is supported as well by the autogenesis profile and in the wound-healing saga of bone fractures, where the events recapitulate the events of the embryonic development, where a cartilaginous callus is preceding the final bony callus of the reparative tissue. Understanding the phylogenic order and the individual developmental-sequential events, repair, and regeneration sequel at the molecular and cellular levels, might help to develop innovative clinical approaches for long-term solutions in skeletal pathological issues.

However, a major difference exists between the two tissues, cartilage and bone. Whereas cartilage loses its self-wound healing (repair and regeneration) already early in life, the bone and bone marrow regeneration vigor is outstanding among the body tissues to old age. As emerging from nowaday's hottest cell source, the stem cells in general and mesenchymal stem cell progenitors in particular, are enriched in bone marrow serving as a major vital fountain for progenitor cells of both tissues, cartilage and bone. The "vital" power for bone induction and regeneration of devitalized bone pieces – demineralized bone matrix – was learned in the scientific period by Urist, Reddi, and Huggins during experiments in the sixties and early seventies of the last century.

However, the vigor of bone marrow stem cells in supporting renewal of tissues and organs to a compete individual was already reported in the biblical story on the creation of Adam's wife – Eve (Genesis, Chapter II, verses 21 and 22: *"The Lord God caused a deep sleep to fall upon Adam, and he slept, and the Lord took one of his ribs, and closed up the flesh instead there of; and the rib, which the Lord God had taken from man, made be a women, and brought her unto the man"*). Hence, the first product from bone marrow stem cells was Eve.

Furthermore, we are told that Eve used to stand at the entrance of her tent in the afternoons waiting for Adam to come back home from the field. Upon his arrival, she fell into his arms and hugged him strongly. Biblical interpreters disputed in their explanations to this ritual of Eve. The most logic explanation claimed by one of them was that during the hugging she was counting Adam's ribs, to make sure that no competitor might have been created somewhere else.

Discussing already the Old Testament, we might bring another point in case to our matter, that bone-derived substances can serve for regeneration and renewal, as outlined in the following phrases of the "Dry Bones Prophesy" in Ezekiel Chapter XXXVII, verses 1–14: *"The hand of the Lord was upon me, and carried me out in the spirit of the Lord, and set me down in the midst of the valley which was full of bones ... they were very dry ... can these bones live? ... I will lay sinews upon you, and will bring flesh upon you, and cover you with skin, and put breath in you."*

Irregular developmental processes of skeletal tissues, small to massive losses in the structures of cartilages, bones, and/or joints caused by either traumatic, accidental events or diseases leading to pathological damage (tumors and genetic abnormalities) are tackled and discussed in all the various chapters of the current section.

The scope of regenerative medicine is to recreate an efficient natural tissue to function in the original place of the missing or defective one. In a sense, it is to play the role of nature by human wisdom, where disciplines such as tissue engineering, cell, and gene therapy fueled by molecular biology are operating to treat the diseased organ.

The study of the lineages of the musculoskeletal stem cells, the mesenchymal cells, and the differentiation patterns, as well as the interactions among them, provides the pillars of the tissue constituents. The way in which those stem cells are directed to certain paths is governed by factors and cytokines well synchronized in time, place, and in accordance with the surrounding environment, physical conditions, genetic legacy, and age. Not less important is the supporting infrastructure or intercellular matrix molecules making the difference of yielding a mere pulp or a real fruit. The vascularization aspect adds another factor to the equation that obliges an in vivo phase for certain tissues to get their mature and functional expression.

In the first chapter, "Mesenchymal Stem Cells: Where Can You Find Them? How Can You Use Them," the trinity of the elements composing the composite implant for the repair of losses and injuries of cartilage and bone are discussed: (a) The optimal cellular source(s)-cell types, (b) the adhesive milieu-gels containing the growth factors/signaling molecules, and (c) the structural template and matrix, the so-called ideal scaffold, platform of technologies building the innovative niche of biomaterials and tissue engineering for the sake of inducing repair and regeneration in cartilages and bones.

The chapter "Cartilage" is divided into two subsections. The first subsection discusses cartilage as a biological entity, the basics of the molecular and cellular structure, and growth factors involved in its formation and maintenance, from embryogenesis to old age. The second subsection emphasizes cartilage as a clinical entity and the dynamic changes of the medical strategic solutions in the past, present, and future.

Detailed descriptions regarding the structures, components, and functions of articular cartilage are outlined in the first subsection – starting from limb morphogenesis, limb organogenesis, cartilage homeostasis and its dependence on growth factors, hormones, cytokines, proteases, and proteases inhibitors. Furthermore, approaches to cartilage repair, mesenchymal stem cells, and cartilage regeneration, and the latest tissue engineering and biomaterials recruited to help achieve the optimal renewal goals by in vitro reconstructed cartilage replacement grafts are described as well.

The second half of the cartilage chapter is devoted to the practical, clinical, and scientific steps and protocols of the cell therapeutic procedure for cartilage repair in the new era, started in the middle of the nineties of the last century. The so-called Autologous Chondrocyte Transplantation procedure is reported here by members of the original pioneering team. The details include: Cell harvest from a biopsy, cultured cell expansion, tips for directing the dedifferentiated cells to undergo redifferentiation, and cell implantation ensuring their integration with the surrounding tissues. Attempts for improvement of the reparative outcomes by introducing new information of molecular biology, meaning gene therapy and the expression of essential growth factors, were gained recently, in animal experimentation. The latest biomaterials and scaffolds involved in the composite implants are described as well.

The chapter "Bone Regeneration" describes the family of the morphogenetic protein signals – the BMPs, more than 15 members including cartilage-derived morphogenetic protein. Bone morphogens operate in the frame of gene therapy via BMPs' receptors that are distributed on cells and on extracellular matrix molecules. This accumulated knowledge and know-how help to direct stromal stem cells with morphogens for bone cell therapy. The intensive powers for regeneration of bone and bone marrow make them a good prototype model for creating tissue engineered products for bone repair. Future perspectives are discussed, as challenges for optimal delivery systems of BMPs and growth factors to serve as osteoinductive and osteoconductive substances.

Impressive advances were achieved with the inclusion of an appropriate matrix seeded with cells grown under determined physical conditions including mechanical stimuli, nutrients, and factors, obtaining vital tissues suitable for human treatment. Although integration of engineered tissue with the normal surrounding tissues is still considered a barrier in cartilage repair of big defects and whole articular surfaces, that should be overcome with further research. Bones, in contrast, integrate easily when new vascularization is assured, giving more options to engineered compounds with multilayered tissue implants, to be readily integrated into the bone region.

Osteoarthritis involves pathologies of cartilage, bone, tendon, muscles, and synovial membrane tissues. Osteoarthritis is considered the major clinical entity of joint disorders. This clinical entity serves as the ultimate target of most studies conducted in connective tissue research, including the very latest developed niches of stem cells, regenerative medicine, biomaterials, and tissue engineering. Obesity, lowered physical activities, increased mechanical loading, characteristic gait patterns, stem cell dysfunction, especially toward recruitment for the chondrogenic differentiation, and on the other hand, at osteophyte formation, have been related to osteoarthritic development. It appears that in vitro manipulation of stem cells to strengthen their chondrogenic phenotype at the expense of osteogenic phenotype might be beneficial upon in vivo transplantation of the constructs into regions with initial signs of osteoarthrosis.

10

Mesenchymal Stem Cells: Where Can You Find Them? How Can You Use Them?

Anna Derubeis, Giuseppina Pennesi, and Ranieri Cancedda

In the last decade, the definition of stem cell has been widely and inappropriately used because of the lack of specific markers that could allow for the isolation of the true stem cell. A stem cell, by a universally accepted definition, is a cell able to proliferate indefinitely and to maintain the multipotentiality throughout its lifetime. Embryonic stem cells are true stem cells, but because of the ethical concerns they raise, they have been lately overtaken by research on stem cells isolated from adult tissues.

Several laboratories have successfully isolated stem cells from many tissues: the brain, the blood, the skin, the skeletal muscle, the cord blood, and the bone marrow and many have also attempted to translate their discoveries on stem cells into clinical practice.

Nevertheless, as of today, several plugs are still missing:

- Is there a single stem cell pool from which all other tissue-specific stem cells originate?
- Are the isolated stem cell populations real stem cells?
- Does in vitro culture alter cell biology and/or cell potential and can we use it as an evaluation technology?

This chapter will give a brief general introduction on what is known about stem cells, in particular mesenchymal stem cells (MSCs), then it will concentrate on an overview of different sources of stem cells and highlight the most up-to-date disputes in the field. Finally, it will report the most promising clinical applications of MSCs, and provide a summary of the successes and failures of the technology.

Mesenchymal Stem Cells

Embryonic stem cells represent the true expression of stemness: they are able to proliferate indefinitely, to self-renew, and to differentiate toward all tissues of the adult organism. Embryonic stem cells injected in adult mice develop into benign tumors called teratomas containing cell types deriving from all three germ layers, further demonstrating their extensive differentiation potential.[1,2] Ethical considerations and a still limited understanding of the molecular mechanisms controlling the differentiation pathways, however, has greatly limited research in this field and consequently the use of this very promising cell population.

Following these considerations, the attention of the scientific community has turned to adult tissues and research in the past decade has focused on the isolation, characterization, and possible use of adult stem cells. Friedenstein and coworkers[3,4] were among the first to isolate mesenchymal cells from the bone marrow and to discover the multipotentiality of the population. They harvested bone marrow samples from the iliac crest, plated the suspension in plastic culture dishes, and observed that, after a few days, by progressive removal of the hematopoietic counterpart, adhering fibroblasts started to appear attached to the bottom of the culture plate.[4] Their observations led to the discovery that these cells had a fibroblastic morphology, formed distinct colonies, and when implanted in vivo were able to develop into a mature bone tissue.[5] Since then, studies have followed that further characterized the bone marrow-derived MSCs (BMSCs).[6-10]

BMSCs have been shown to represent 0.001% of the whole marrow, they can be isolated primarily by adhesion to plastic, but could also be concentrated by Percoll gradient centrifugation.[11] BMSCs are clonogenic and multipotent and are able to differentiate into bone, cartilage, hematopoiesis supportive stroma, and adipocytes[6,12-14] [Figure 10.1 (see color section)]. So far, nothing surprising: They reside in the bone marrow and appear to contribute to the replenishment or formation of most tissues of the skeleton. Are they true stem cells? The turning point arrived when Ferrari et al.[15] reported that bone marrow-derived cells engrafted in injured skeletal muscle, indicating that a population in the bone marrow could colonize and possibly undertake a myogenic commitment. Similar conclusions were reached when Gussoni et al.[16] transplanted beta-gal bone marrow cells in a murine model of Duchenne's muscular dystrophy.

Interestingly, few reports have shown that bone marrow cells, transplanted in mice where liver damage was induced, integrated in the parenchyma.[17,18] In one case, the integration of bone marrow cells reached such a high level that a restoration of liver function was observed.[18] In humans, Alison et al.[19] were the first to show that cells within the liver had an extrahepatic origin.

These findings changed dramatically the otherwise generally accepted concept that the multipotentiality of a MSC was restricted to lineages derived from the same germ layer and that only stem cells residing in the tissues could be activated by environmental cues, possibly when injury occurred.

BMSCs are easy to harvest from the iliac crest of healthy donors and could be expanded many-fold in vitro to increase the amount of transplantable cells but, most importantly, they are multipotential, therefore allowing their use in a variety of clinical situations. The possibility of using BMSCs in the treatment of disease and in particular in the reconstruction of bone defects requires that they maintain their proliferation capability after transplantation and throughout the lifetime of the individual and that this potential is not lost after in vitro passaging.

Here is the first problem:

- Can MSCs be expanded in vitro indefinitely? Do cultured cells express telomerase, an enzyme having a major role in cell immortalization, as embryonic cells do?
- Is the multipotentiality maintained after in vitro expansion?

Several studies have been undertaken in this respect. Bruder et al.[9] showed that BMSCs extensively expanded in vitro undergo senescence after about 38 population doublings, although maintaining the ability to differentiate toward the osteogenic phenotype. Banfi et al.[20] found that BMSCs in culture undergo a drastic decrease in proliferation capacity at the 23rd population doubling. Parallel to a decrease in proliferation appears a decrease in multipotentiality where bone formation in vivo in the nude mouse model is dramatically impaired.

Evaluation of human Telomerase Reverse Transcriptase (hTERT) expression in cultured cells and telomere length reduction during time in culture confirmed that MSCs isolated from the bone marrow age in culture and fail to respect one of the fundamental criteria of a stem cell, the presence of telomerase and the maintenance of telomere length[21,22] [Figure 10.2 (see color section)].

Attempts have been undertaken to optimize the culture environment and growth factor requirements needed to implement culture expansion and maintenance of the phenotype.[8,23-26] In particular, Bianchi et al.[21] and Martin et al.[25] have reported that the addition of fibroblast growth factor-2 (FGF2) to the culture promotes a reduction in the colony number and an increase in the colony size of plated BMSCs. Furthermore, the amount of cells needed to stimulate bone formation in vivo is much lower than if the cells were cultured without the factor. Bianchi et al. have gone further and postulated that FGF2 acts as a selective agent that selects a more primitive subpopulation within the whole cells plated.[27]

A great contribution to the field has come from Reyes et al.[28] They were able to isolate from the bone marrow mesenchymal cells with stem cell characteristics by depleting the bone marrow suspension of glycophorin A+ CD45+ cells and subsequently by plating the cells on fibronectin in low serum and at low density. Mesodermal progenitor cells in the above-mentioned culture conditions proliferate up to 50 cell doublings without obvious senescence, maintaining their differentiation potential. The maintenance of the telomere length despite subsequent in vitro passaging further reinforced the stem cell nature of the isolated population.[28]

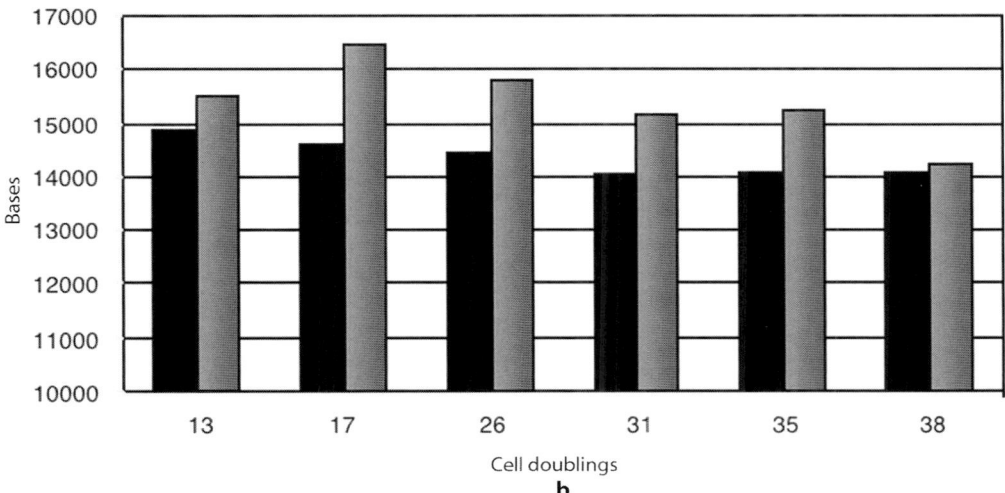

Figure 10.2.b The diagram shows telomere length reduction in BMSCs during time in culture (black bars). The addition of FGF2 to the culture selects for a more primitive cell population whose telomere length is higher (gray bars). The progressive shortening of telomeres in both conditions confirms the lack of hTERT expression. (Redrawn from Bianchi et al., 2003[27].)

The above article suggests that more sophisticated isolation procedures and possibly the identification of specific markers could greatly contribute to the selection and subsequent isolation of the true stem cell from adult tissues.

Every Tissue Has Its Own Stem Cell Pool

Since Friedenstein first discovered the existence of an MSC reservoir in the bone marrow, studies have accumulated that identified stem/progenitor cells in tissues other than the bone marrow.

Recently, Lee et al. and others[29] have identified and isolated stem/progenitor cells from umbilical cord blood (UCB).[30,31] It is well accepted that UCB is a source for hematopoietic stem cells and concentration of hematopoietic stem cells in cord blood has been shown to be greatly higher than in the bone marrow. In addition, the hematopoietic stem cells isolated from the UCB have a higher proliferative potential associated with an extended lifespan.[32] Lee et al. were able to isolate from UCB a population of MSCs, lineage negative and glycophorin A+ that were fibroblastic in shape and size, adhered to the culture dish, and were able to proliferate extensively in vitro. Furthermore, they induced UCB-derived cells toward the osteoblastic, chondroblastic, and adipogenic phenotype in vitro by culturing the cells in specific inducing media presenting a behavior similar to BMSCs.[29]

Lee et al. attempted also to investigate a neuroglial-like and hepatocyte-like phenotype of the isolated population and succeeded in demonstrating that UCB-derived cells changed morphology assuming a glial-like phenotype and did indeed express neuroglial markers such as glial fibrillary acidic protein and microtubule-associated protein 2. In addition, after culturing the cells in hepatogenic medium for 6 weeks, the cells expressed albumin and exhibited the ability to take up low-density lipoprotein.[29]

More compelling evidence was given in 2004 by Kogler et al., who isolated a CD45−, adherent cell population from the cord blood called USSCs (unrestricted somatic stem cells) that "without spontaneous differentiation, had the intrinsic and directable potential to develop into mesodermal, endodermal, and ectodermal cell fates."[33] Kogler et al. showed for the first time the ability of cord blood-derived MSCs to extensively proliferate in vitro up to at least 10^{15} cells maintaining the telomere length for at least up to 36 population doublings. USSCs formed bone when implanted on a bioceramic scaffold in critical-size defects in rats and cartilage when associated to gel foams and implanted subcutaneously into immunocompromised mice. Furthermore, transplantation of USSCs in the preimmune fetal sheep model resulted in a substantial number of human cardiomyocytes in both atria and ventriculi of the sheep.[33] In this respect, MSCs from the cord blood appear slightly different from MSCs from the bone marrow, which engrafted predominantly in the Purkinje fiber system.[34] This suggests that MSCs from the UCB could be more primitive than those from the bone marrow.

MSCs with extensive multipotentiality have also been isolated from the skeletal muscle of different animal models, and still controversy exists on how many types of progenitors are in the skeletal muscle and whether the cell populations isolated by different laboratories are the same or exist according to a hierarchy. The general consensus is that satellite cells are the progenitor cells for myocytes and myotubes of the skeletal muscle and reside quiescently within the tissue.[35,36] Nevertheless, Asakura et al.[37] and Wada et al.[38] isolated satellite cells and were able to differentiate them toward the osteogenic phenotype in vitro, after induction with bone morphogenetic proteins (BMPs).

Levy et al.[39] were the first to show that a cell population isolated from the human skeletal muscle was alkaline phosphatase positive, and up-regulated osteocalcin expression in vitro after a 24-hour induction with 1,25-dihydroxyvitamin D3. To this respect, the theory proposed by Minasi et al.[40] (2002) is interesting, suggesting that progenitors of the mesodermal tissues are associated with the vasculature and delivered in most tissues of the body through fetal angiogenesis. Subsequently local events of the microenvironment would trigger the exit of these stem cell pools from the quiescent phase and into active proliferation.

A possible candidate for this role is the pericyte. Pericytes encircle capillaries in the microvasculature of the connective tissues, the nervous tissue including the cerebral cortex, peripheral nerves, and the retina, the muscle tissue, and the lungs.[41–46] Doherty et al.,[45] for example, isolated pericytes from the bovine retina and implanted them in diffusion chambers in vivo. Harvest of the implants showed formation of both bone and cartilage, suggesting an extensive multipotential capability of the cell population.

After these initial findings, the search for stem/progenitor cells in adult tissues has dramatically spread and several stem cell pools have been identified from a variety of tissues that possess at least the potential to undergo differentiation toward the mesenchymal lineages of the skeleton. Lee et al.[47] and Suva et al.[48] have isolated MSCs from the femoral head of patients undergoing hip replacement surgery and were able to induce differentiation of these cells into at least bone, cartilage, and fat.

Osteogenic potential of cells isolated from the periosteum has been documented since 1932 when Fell[49] succeeded in culturing periosteal cells and appropriately induced them to form a mineralized matrix in vitro. In 1990, Nakahara et al.[50] were the first to demonstrate that cells isolated from the periosteum of young chicks could undergo osteochondrogenic differentiation in vivo when transplanted into athymic mice. Since then, extensive research has been done on periosteal-derived stem cells until 2001 when Vacanti et al.[51] reported the successful replacement of a distal phalanx with tissue-engineered bone. They isolated cells from the periosteum and cultured them in vitro. After the cells reached 20E6, they were loaded on a coral-based scaffold reproducing the shape of the missing phalanx and under general anesthesia delivered to the site.[51]

To this respect, it is interesting to remember that Brittberg et al.[52] have developed a protocol for the reconstruction/repair of cartilage damage: The site of the lesion is cleaned and covered with a periosteal flap sutured to the cartilage; ex vivo expanded chondrocytes are injected in the pocket and, after a variable amount of time, the lesion gets repaired. Discussions are underway to establish whether the repair is only the result of engraftment of the chondrocytes or progenitor cells from the periosteum contribute to the healing.[52] Nevertheless, as of today, to our knowledge, no proof has been shown of the ability of the cells isolated from the periosteum to undergo differentiation pathways other than the osteogenic and chondrogenic ones.[53]

Worth mentioning is the work by De Bari et al.[54] (2001) who isolated stem cells from the synovial membrane. They demonstrated that MSCs isolated from the synovial membrane (hSM-MSC) under appropriate cell culture conditions differentiate toward the chondrogenic, adipogenic, and osteogenic lineage. hSM-MSCs proliferate extensively in culture without marked signs of senescence up to 10 passages and injected into regenerating mouse muscle restore the muscle fibers. In addition, hSM-MSCs administered to dystrophic muscle succeed in restoring the sarcolemmal expression of dystrophin.[54]

Far more appealing for tissue engineering purposes is the possibility to isolate MSCs from adipose tissues. Several reports have been published that show the existence of MSCs in fat.[55] In particular, Zuk et al.[56] were among the first to show that MSCs isolated from lipoaspiration could differentiate into bone, cartilage, and adipose tissue in vitro. They extended their study by inducing the processed lipoaspirate toward the neurogenic and the myogenic phenotype and showed that the cells they had isolated were indeed able to express markers characteristic of the two lineages.[56] Cowan et al.[57] have gone further by showing how cells isolated from the adipose tissue, ADAS (adipose-derived adult stromal) cells, can be used in a tissue engineering approach and can be considered a valid alternative to bone marrow stromal cells. In their publication, Cowan and coworkers presented healing of a critical-size calvarial defect in rats by the implant of polylactide-co-glycolide-coated hydroxyapatite cubes loaded with ADAS cells.

What is greatly appealing about this population is that ADAS cells present several advantages over BMSCs: The yield of cells is much higher from fat than from bone marrow, the proliferation rate of ADAS cells is substantially higher than in BMSCs during expansion in vitro, and they are relatively easy to harvest.[55,57]

Stem Cell Therapy of Skeletal Tissues

Bone Reconstruction

The ability of BMSCs to form bone has been among the first properties to be exploited. Bone formation and repair has been evaluated first in small animal models, then in larger ones, and the successful results obtained led to the first clinical trial.

Goshima et al.[57a] for the first time developed a protocol in which cells loaded on a bioceramic scaffold and implanted subcutaneously into immunocompromised mice allowed for the evaluation of the osteogenic potential of the transplanted cell population. Bruder et al.[58] and Kon et al.[59] have gone further and evaluated the potential of BMSCs to repair bone defects in vivo in larger animal models. Bruder et al. in dogs and Kon et al. in sheep created a bone critical-size defect in the long bones and reconstructed the missing segment by implant of appropriately designed scaffolds with and without adsorbed BMSCs. Two months after surgery, the filled defect was examined and evaluated and bone formation was observed. In particular, even though bone formation was evidenced in both experimental and control implants, the rate of bone formation was markedly increased in implants loaded with cells. Furthermore, the bone formed had much higher stiffness when compared with the bone formed without cells.[59]

Similar observations were conducted by Petite et al.[60] who repaired critical-size segmental defects with in vitro-expanded BMSCs loaded on a coral-based scaffold. Efficient repair of segmental defects in both small and large animal models has encouraged the initiation of clinical trials. Quarto et al.[61] were the first to report the repair of large segmental defects in humans using a tissue engineering approach. BMSCs from the patients were harvested from the iliac crest and expanded many-fold in vitro. The shape of the defect gave appropriate information for the design of the hydroxyapatite scaffold and, at the time of surgery, cells were detached from the culture dish and loaded on the bioceramic. After variable time frames, all three patients presented a repair of the defect where abundant callus formation was evident.[61] This approach, although highly successful, still needs optimization. For example, studies are underway to establish if total, unfractioned bone marrow could prime bone repair and how fast the repair develops when compared with in vitro-expanded BMSCs.

In addition, much research is conducted on biomaterials to increase the resorbability of the implant without losing resistance. Bioceramics composed of 100% hydroxyapatite provide high strength to loading but are not resorbed and reside in the defect for several years after callus formation. On the contrary, scaffolds mainly composed of tricalcium phosphate have a greater capacity to resorption but are too fragile to sustain the weight load. Scaffolds in which different ratios of the two biomaterials are formed are currently under investigation. Nevertheless, research on stem cells has been lately paralleled by research on scaffolds, both as delivery vehicles and also as active inducers of the goal that one wants to achieve.

Cartilage Repair

The ability of BMSCs to differentiate into cartilage in pellet culture in vitro prompted several research laboratories to investigate the possibility of using these cells to repair cartilage defects.[13,62] Lesions in cartilage tissue, particularly articular cartilage of the knee, are subjected to the development of osteoarthritis.[63,64] In adults, when the cartilaginous tissue is damaged, it undergoes a repair process that involves mostly the development of fibrocartilage where the amount of collagen type I/III greatly encompasses the physiologic amounts of collagen type II.[65,66] The substitution of hyaline cartilage with fibrocartilage impairs the viscoelastic properties of the joint. In addition, chondrocytes are relatively quiescent cells mostly committed toward a mature phenotype and their proliferation potential is very limited.[67] Therefore, lesions in the articular cartilage rarely undergo spontaneous healing.

In 1994, Brittberg et al.[51] developed a very successful protocol in which they harvest a cartilage sample from a healthy area, dissect it, and amplify chondrocytes in vitro. The lesion, sutured with a periosteal flap is filled with the chondrocyte suspension. Although healing occurs and the repaired cartilage appears hyaline cartilage, a great limitation of the protocol is the limited proliferative capacity of the cell population. Therefore, MSCs have been evaluated as a valid alternative as a tissue engineering tool that could substitute chondrocytes in cartilage repair processes.[68] BMSCs present several advantages over chondrocytes: They proliferate extensively in culture and are relatively easy to harvest. In addition, being multipotential, they can be considered a repair tool for full-thickness cartilage defects in which both the subchondral bone and the thin cartilaginous layer are damaged.

Wakitani et al.[69] in 1994 implanted BMSCs previously in vitro expanded in a large full-thickness defect in a weight-bearing rabbit knee. Twenty-four weeks after transplantation, both cartilage and subchondral bone repaired and the defect was completely filled. Gao et al.,[70] in 2002, have gone further and investigated the possibility of using different scaffolds to promote differentiation of BMSCs toward the two lineages: They proposed a two-phase composite material composed of an injectable calcium phosphate and a hyaluronan derivative. In this case, BMSCs loaded on the scaffold will be prompted by the calcium phosphate to go toward bone differentiation and by the hyaluronic acid to differentiate into cartilage tissue. They concluded that by playing on the scaffold composition, BMSCs can be redirected toward the lineage of choice and efficiently repair the full-thickness defect in the rabbit knee.[70] Possible disadvantages of the technology that are still under investigation are the type of cartilage that forms, and possibly the inability of BMSCs to control the differentiation stage perhaps progressing toward hypertrophy.

Ligaments and Tendon: The New Era

Soft tissue injuries account for half of all the musculoskeletal injuries in the United States each year. Normal healing frequently occurs through the development of scar tissue whose elastic properties are far inferior than the original tissue.[71] Because tendon and ligaments have a major role in the movement of the joint, their rupture or lesion could dramatically influence the stability of the joint leading to subsequent degenerative diseases.

All of this considered, investigation has begun in the use of MSCs to engineer ligaments and tendon.[72,73] A first attempt to redirect Achille's tendon repair was conducted by Young et al.[74] in 1998 where a defect was created in the rabbit Achille's tendon. BMSCs were harvested, cultured in vitro, and subsequently loaded on a collagen gel sutured to the defect. A similar protocol was used to repair a surgically induced defect in the patellar tendon.[75] In both studies, healing of the defect was evident but, most importantly, when compared with the control in which the scaffold was implanted without cells, greater improvement of the mechanical stability and the elastic modulus was measured.

Awad et al.[75] (1999) showed that BMSC-loaded implants increased to up to 15%–40% their structural properties, keeping in mind that the maximum force of the tendon dramatically decreases when the medial segment is removed to host the implant. After Awad et al.'s investigations, many have attempted to reconstruct tendons and ligaments in vivo, whereas others have begun to engineer tendon and/or ligaments in vitro via the establishment of bioreactors and the use of BMSCs subjected to cyclic strength.[76] Altman et al.[77] have developed a bioreactor system in which BMSCs are seeded on a silk matrix scaffold and placed in a bioreactor able to apply independent and well-controlled mechanical strains. The bioreactor is able to provide nutriment to the construct at a controlled rate and to reproduce a multidimensional strength to the developing tendon that reminds the forces applied in development. In particular, resolution of less than 0.1 mm for translational and less than 0.1 for rotational strain could be applied to the developing tissue.[77]

Immunomodulatory Role of BMSCs

In the past few years, several laboratories have begun to investigate the immunomodulatory role of BMSCs. Different independent in vitro studies performed with human or mouse cells agree that autologous or allogeneic BMSCs strongly suppress T lymphocyte proliferation, triggered by cellular, nonspecific mitogenic stimuli, or antigenic peptide, in a dose-dependent way.[78,79] Immunologic restriction appears not to be involved, indicating that third-party nonhistocompatible cells can be used to suppress the lymphocyte activation.[80,81]

Studies in animal models showed that BMSCs could have a critical role in the regulation of the immune response also in an in vivo setting. Mechanisms by which this phenomenon occurs are not yet known. Autoimmune-prone mice, who have undergone allogeneic transplant with cotransplantation of donor bone as a source of stromal cells, survived 48 weeks after transplantation without recurrence of any autoimmune phenomenon, suggesting that stromal cells prevented the occurrence of graft failure, regulating T and B cell reactions.[82] Adult bone marrow stromal cells administered intravenously to rats after traumatic brain injury migrate into brain and improve neurologic outcome.[83]

BMSCs were also found in other organs and primarily localized to the vascular structures, without any obvious adverse effects. In humans, allogeneic transplantation in osteogenesis imperfecta patients resulted in 1.5%–2.0% engraftment of donor osteoblasts, suggesting that mesenchymal precursors present in the marrow may have a potential therapeutic role.[84] An immunomodulatory activity could be a characteristic also of stem/progenitors cells of other lineages.[83,85–88]

Experimental evidences supporting the hypothesis that BMSCs are able to regulate the immune response have been reported, indicating that BMSCs suppress the activation of the immune response by mechanisms that are still unknown. The perspective of using BMSCs in preventing or curing graft rejection is intriguing, especially in the case of transplant of engineered tissues.

Acknowledgment. Supported by funds from the Italian Ministry of Instruction, University and Research (MIUR) and from the European and the Italian Space Agencies (ESA and ASI).

References

1. Pera MF, Reubinoff B, Trounson A. Human embryonic stem cells. J Cell Sci 2000;113(pt 1):5–10.
2. Odorico JS, Kaufman DS, Thomson JA. Multilineage differentiation from human embryonic stem cell lines. Stem Cells 2001;19(3):193–204.
3. Friedenstein AJ. Precursor cells of mechanocytes. Int Rev Cytol 1976;47:327–359.
4. Friedenstein AJ. Marrow stromal fibroblasts. Calcif Tissue Int 1995;56(suppl 1):S17.
5. Friedenstein AJ, Chailakhyan RK, Gerasimov UV. Bone marrow osteogenic stem cells: in vitro cultivation and transplantation in diffusion chambers. Cell Tissue Kinet 1987;20(3):263–272.
6. Owen M, Friedenstein AJ. Stromal stem cells: marrow-derived osteogenic precursors. Ciba Found Symp 1988;136:42–60.
7. Caplan AI. Mesenchymal stem cells. J Orthop Res 1991;9(5):641–650.
8. Kuznetsov SA, Friedenstein AJ, Robey PG. Factors required for bone marrow stromal fibroblast colony formation in vitro. Br J Haematol 1997;97(3):561–570.
9. Bruder SP, Jaiswal N, Haynesworth SE. Growth kinetics, self-renewal, and the osteogenic potential of purified human mesenchymal stem cells during extensive subcultivation and following cryopreservation. J Cell Biochem 1997;64(2):278–294.
10. Bianco P, Riminucci M, Gronthos S, Robey PG. Bone marrow stromal stem cells: nature, biology, and potential applications. Stem Cells 2001;19(3):180–192.
11. Barry FP, Murphy JM. Mesenchymal stem cells: clinical applications and biological characterization. Int J Biochem Cell Biol 2004;36(4):568–584.
12. Beresford JN, Bennett JH, Devlin C, Leboy PS, Owen ME. Evidence for an inverse relationship between the differentiation of adipocytic and osteogenic cells in rat marrow stromal cell cultures. J Cell Sci 1992;102(pt 2):341–351.
13. Muraglia A, Cancedda R, Quarto R. Clonal mesenchymal progenitors from human bone marrow differentiate in vitro according to a hierarchical model. J Cell Sci 2000;113(pt 7):1161–1166.
14. Ahdjoudj S, Lasmoles F, Oyajobi BO, Lomri A, Delannoy P, Marie PJ. Reciprocal control of osteoblast/chondroblast and osteoblast/adipocyte differentiation

14. of multipotential clonal human marrow stromal F/STRO-1(+) cells. J Cell Biochem 2001;81(1):23–38.
15. Ferrari G, Cusella-De Angelis G, Coletta M, et al. Muscle regeneration by bone marrow-derived myogenic progenitors [see comments]. Science 1998;279 (5356):1528–1530.
16. Gussoni E, Soneoka Y, Strickland CD, et al. Dystrophin expression in the mdx mouse restored by stem cell transplantation. Nature 1999;401(6751):390–394.
17. Petersen BE, Bowen WC, Patrene KD, et al. Bone marrow as a potential source of hepatic oval cells. Science 1999;284(5417):1168–1170.
18. Lagasse E, Connors H, Al-Dhalimy M, et al. Purified hematopoietic stem cells can differentiate into hepatocytes in vivo. Nat Med 2000;6(11):1229–1234.
19. Alison MR, Poulsom R, Jeffery R, et al. Hepatocytes from non-hepatic adult stem cells. Nature 2000;406 (6793):257.
20. Banfi A, Muraglia A, Dozin B, Mastrogiacomo M, Cancedda R, Quarto R. Proliferation kinetics and differentiation potential of ex vivo expanded human bone marrow stromal cells: implications for their use in cell therapy. Exp Hematol 2000;28(6):707–715.
21. Bianchi G, Muraglia A, Daga A, Corte G, Cancedda R, Quarto R. Microenvironment and stem properties of bone marrow-derived mesenchymal cells. Wound Repair Regen 2001;9(6):460–466.
22. Banfi A, Bianchi G, Notaro R, Luzzatto L, Cancedda R, Quarto R. Replicative aging and gene expression in long-term cultures of human bone marrow stromal cells. Tissue Eng 2002;8(6):901–910.
23. Pitaru S, Kotev-Emeth S, Noff D, Kaffuler S, Savion N. Effect of basic fibroblast growth factor on the growth and differentiation of adult stromal bone marrow cells: enhanced development of mineralized bone-like tissue in culture. J Bone Miner Res 1993;8(8):919–929.
24. Gronthos S, Simmons PJ. The growth factor requirements of STRO-1-positive human bone marrow stromal precursors under serum-deprived conditions in vitro. Blood 1995;85(4):929–940.
25. Martin I, Muraglia A, Campanile G, Cancedda R, Quarto R. Fibroblast growth factor-2 supports ex vivo expansion and maintenance of osteogenic precursors from human bone marrow. Endocrinology 1997; 138(10):4456–4462.
26. Locklin RM, Oreffo RO, Triffitt JT. Effects of TGFbeta and bFGF on the differentiation of human bone marrow stromal fibroblasts. Cell Biol Int 1999;23(3): 185–194.
27. Bianchi G, Banfi A, Mastrogiacomo M, Notaro R, Luzzatto L, Cancedda R, et al. Ex vivo enrichment of mesenchymal cell progenitors by fibroblast growth factor 2. EXP Cell Res 2003;287(1):98–105.
28. Reyes M, Lund T, Lenvik T, Aguiar D, Koodie L, Verfaillie CM. Purification and ex vivo expansion of postnatal human marrow mesodermal progenitor cells. Blood 2001;98(9):2615–2625.
29. Lee OK, Kuo TK, Chen WM, Lee KD, Hsieh SL, Chen TH. Isolation of multipotent mesenchymal stem cells from umbilical cord blood. Blood 2004;103(5): 1669–1675.
30. Erices A, Conget P, Minguell JJ. Mesenchymal progenitor cells in human umbilical cord blood. Br J Haematol 2000;109(1):235–242.
31. Goodwin HS, Bicknese AR, Chien SN, Bogucki BD, Quinn CO, Wall DA. Multilineage differentiation activity by cells isolated from umbilical cord blood: expression of bone, fat, and neural markers. Biol Blood Marrow Transplant 2001;7(11):581–588.
32. Szilvassy SJ, Meyerrose TE, Ragland PL, Grimes B. Differential homing and engraftment properties of hematopoietic progenitor cells from murine bone marrow, mobilized peripheral blood, and fetal liver. Blood 2001;98(7):2108–2115.
33. Kogler G, Sensken S, Airey JA, et al. A new human somatic stem cell from placental cord blood with intrinsic pluripotent differentiation potential. J Exp Med 2004;200(2):123–135.
34. Airey JA, Almeida-Porada G, Colletti EJ, et al. Human mesenchymal stem cells form Purkinje fibers in fetal sheep heart. Circulation 2004;109(11):1401–1407.
35. Le Moigne A, Martelly I, Barlovatz-Meimon G, et al. Characterization of myogenesis from adult satellite cells cultured in vitro. Int J Dev Biol 1990;34(1):171–180.
36. Seale P, Asakura A, Rudnicki MA. The potential of muscle stem cells. Dev Cell 2001;1(3):333–342.
37. Asakura A, Komaki M, Rudnicki M. Muscle satellite cells are multipotential stem cells that exhibit myogenic, osteogenic, and adipogenic differentiation. Differentiation 2001;68(4–5):245–253.
38. Wada MR, Inagawa-Ogashiwa M, Shimizu S, Yasumoto S, Hashimoto N. Generation of different fates from multipotent muscle stem cells. Development 2002; 129(12):2987–2995.
39. Levy MM, Joyner CJ, Virdi AS, et al. Osteoprogenitor cells of mature human skeletal muscle tissue: an in vitro study. Bone 2001;29(4):317–322.
40. Minasi MG, Riminucci M, De Angelis L, et al. The meso-angioblast: a multipotent, self-renewing cell that originates from the dorsal aorta and differentiates into most mesodermal tissues. Development 2002;129(11): 2773–2783.
41. Diaz-Flores L, Gutierrez R, Varela H, Rancel N, Valladares F. Microvascular pericytes: a review of their morphological and functional characteristics. Histol Histopathol 1991;6(2):269–286.
42. Diaz-Flores L, Gutierrez R, Lopez-Alonso A, Gonzalez R, Varela H. Pericytes as a supplementary source of osteoblasts in periosteal osteogenesis. Clin Orthop 1992(275):280–286.
43. Decker B, Bartels H, Decker S. Relationships between endothelial cells, pericytes, and osteoblasts during bone formation in the sheep femur following implantation of tricalcium phosphate-ceramic. Anat Rec 1995;242(3):310–320.
44. Hirschi KK, D'Amore PA. Pericytes in the microvasculature. Cardiovasc Res 1996;32(4):687–698.
45. Doherty MJ, Ashton BA, Walsh S, Beresford JN, Grant ME, Canfield AE. Vascular pericytes express osteogenic potential in vitro and in vivo. J Bone Miner Res 1998;13(5):828–838.
46. Doherty MJ, Canfield AE. Gene expression during vascular pericyte differentiation. Crit Rev Eukaryot Gene Expr 1999;9(1):1–17.
47. Lee HS, Huang GT, Chiang H, et al. Multipotential mesenchymal stem cells from femoral bone marrow near the site of osteonecrosis. Stem Cells 2003; 21(2):190–199.
48. Suva D, Garavaglia G, Menetrey J, et al. Non-hematopoietic human bone marrow contains long-lasting, pluripotential mesenchymal stem cells. J Cell Physiol 2004;198(1):110–118.

49. Fell HB. The osteogenic capacity in vivo of periosteum and endosteum isolated from the limb skeleton of fowl embryos and young chicks. J Anat 1932;66:157.
50. Nakahara H, Bruder SP, Haynesworth SE, et al. Bone and cartilage formation in diffusion chambers by subcultured cells derived from the periosteum. Bone 1990;11(3):181–188.
51. Vacanti CA, Bonassar LJ, Vacanti MP, Shufflebarger J. Replacement of an avulsed phalanx with tissue-engineered bone. N Engl J Med 2001;344(20):1511–1514.
52. Brittberg M, Lindahl A, Nilsson A, Ohlsson C, Isaksson O, Peterson L. Treatment of deep cartilage defects in the knee with autologous chondrocyte transplantation. N Engl J Med 1994;331(14):889–895.
53. Hutmacher DW, Sittinger M. Periosteal cells in bone tissue engineering. Tissue Eng 2003;9(suppl 1):S45–64.
54. De Bari C, Dell'Accio F, Vandenabeele F, Vermeesch JR, Raymackers JM, Luyten FP. Skeletal muscle repair by adult human mesenchymal stem cells from synovial membrane. J Cell Biol 2003;160(6):909–918.
55. Halvorsen YD, Franklin D, Bond AL, et al. Extracellular matrix mineralization and osteoblast gene expression by human adipose tissue-derived stromal cells. Tissue Eng 2001;7(6):729–741.
56. Zuk PA, Zhu M, Ashjian P, et al. Human adipose tissue is a source of multipotent stem cells. Mol Biol Cell 2002;13(12):4279–4295.
57. Cowan CM, Shi YY, Aalami OO, et al. Adipose-derived adult stromal cells heal critical-size mouse calvarial defects. Nat Biotechnol 2004;22(5):560–567.
57a. Goshima J, Goldberg VM, Caplan AI. The osteogenic potential of culture-expanded rat marrow mesenchymal cells assayed in vivo in calcium phosphate ceramic blocks. Clin Orthop 1991;262:298–311.
58. Bruder SP, Kraus KH, Goldberg VM, Kadiyala S. The effect of implants loaded with autologous mesenchymal stem cells on the healing of canine segmental bone defects. J Bone Joint Surg Am 1998;80(7):985–996.
59. Kon E, Muraglia A, Corsi A, et al. Autologous bone marrow stromal cells loaded onto porous hydroxyapatite ceramic accelerate bone repair in critical-size defects of sheep long bones. J Biomed Mater Res 2000;49(3):328–337.
60. Petite H, Viateau V, Bensaid W, et al. Tissue-engineered bone regeneration. Nat Biotechnol 2000;18(9):959–963.
61. Quarto R, Mastrogiacomo M, Cancedda R, et al. Repair of large bone defects with the use of autologous bone marrow stromal cells. N Engl J Med 2001;344(5):385–386.
62. Muraglia A, Corsi A, Riminucci M, et al. Formation of a chondro-osseous rudiment in micromass cultures of human bone-marrow stromal cells. J Cell Sci 2003;116(pt 14):2949–2955.
63. Sandell LJ, Aigner T. Articular cartilage and changes in arthritis. An introduction: cell biology of osteoarthritis. Arthritis Res 2001;3(2):107–113.
64. Dozin B, Malpeli M, Camardella L, Cancedda R, Pietrangelo A. Response of young, aged and osteoarthritic human articular chondrocytes to inflammatory cytokines: molecular and cellular aspects. Matrix Biol 2002;21(5):449–459.
65. Benya PD, Padilla SR, Nimni ME. Independent regulation of collagen types by chondrocytes during the loss of differentiated function in culture. Cell 1978;15(4):1313–1321.
66. Hunziker EB. Articular cartilage repair: basic science and clinical progress. A review of the current status and prospects. Osteoarthritis Cartilage 2002;10(6):432–463.
67. Malpeli M, Randazzo N, Cancedda R, Dozin B. Serum-free growth medium sustains commitment of human articular chondrocyte through maintenance of Sox9 expression. Tissue Eng 2004;10(1–2):145–155.
68. Solchaga LA, Yoo JU, Lundberg M, et al. Hyaluronan-based polymers in the treatment of osteochondral defects. J Orthop Res 2000;18(5):773–780.
69. Wakitani S, Goto T, Pineda SJ, et al. Mesenchymal cell-based repair of large, full-thickness defects of articular cartilage. J Bone Joint Surg Am 1994;76(4):579–592.
70. Gao J, Dennis JE, Solchaga LA, Goldberg VM, Caplan AI. Repair of osteochondral defect with tissue-engineered two-phase composite material of injectable calcium phosphate and hyaluronan sponge. Tissue Eng 2002;8(5):827–837.
71. Beredjiklian PK, Favata M, Cartmell JS, Flanagan CL, Crombleholme TM, Soslowsky LJ. Regenerative versus reparative healing in tendon: a study of biomechanical and histological properties in fetal sheep. Ann Biomed Eng 2003;31(10):1143–1152.
72. Sato M, Maeda M, Kurosawa H, Inoue Y, Yamauchi Y, Iwase H. Reconstruction of rabbit Achilles tendon with three bioabsorbable materials: histological and biomechanical studies. J Orthop Sci 2000;5(3):256–267.
73. Ouyang HW, Goh JC, Thambyah A, Teoh SH, Lee EH. Knitted poly-lactide-co-glycolide scaffold loaded with bone marrow stromal cells in repair and regeneration of rabbit Achilles tendon. Tissue Eng 2003;9(3):431–439.
74. Young RG, Butler DL, Weber W, Caplan AI, Gordon SL, Fink DJ. Use of mesenchymal stem cells in a collagen matrix for Achilles tendon repair. J Orthop Res 1998;16(4):406–413.
75. Awad HA, Butler DL, Boivin GP, et al. Autologous mesenchymal stem cell-mediated repair of tendon. Tissue Eng 1999;5(3):267–277.
76. Altman GH, Lu HH, Horan RL, et al. Advanced bioreactor with controlled application of multi-dimensional strain for tissue engineering. J Biomech Eng 2002;124(6):742–749.
77. Altman GH, Horan RL, Martin I, et al. Cell differentiation by mechanical stress. FASEB J 2002;16(2):270–272.
78. Di Nicola M, Carlo-Stella C, Magni M, et al. Human bone marrow stromal cells suppress T-lymphocyte proliferation induced by cellular or nonspecific mitogenic stimuli. Blood 2002;99(10):3838–3843.
79. Krampera M, Glennie S, Dyson J, et al. Bone marrow mesenchymal stem cells inhibit the response of naive and memory antigen-specific T cells to their cognate peptide. Blood 2003;101(9):3722–3729.
80. Le Blanc K, Rasmusson I, Sundberg B, et al. Treatment of severe acute graft-versus-host disease with third party haploidentical mesenchymal stem cells. Lancet 2004;363(9419):1439–1441.
81. Frank M, Sayegh M. Immunomodulatory functions of mesenchymal stem cells. Lancet 2004;363:1411–1412.
82. Ishida T, Inaba M, Hisha H, et al. Requirement of donor-derived stromal cells in the bone marrow for successful allogeneic bone marrow transplantation. Complete prevention of recurrence of autoimmune diseases in MRL/MP-Ipr/Ipr mice by transplantation of bone marrow plus bones (stromal cells) from the same donor. J Immunol 1994;152(6):3119–3127.

83. Lu D, Mahmood A, Wang L, Li Y, Lu M, Chopp M. Adult bone marrow stromal cells administered intravenously to rats after traumatic brain injury migrate into brain and improve neurological outcome. Neuroreport 2001; 12(3):559–563.
84. Horwitz E, Prockop D, Fitzpatrick L, et al. Transplantability and therapeutic effects of bone marrow-derived mesenchymal cells in children with osteogenesis imperfecta. Nat Med 1999;5(3):309–313.
85. Li Y, Hisha H, Inaba M, et al. Evidence for migration of donor bone marrow stromal cells into recipient thymus after bone marrow transplantation plus bone grafts: a role of stromal cells in positive selection. Exp Hematol 2000;28(8):950–960.
86. Li Q, Ashraf F, Rana T, et al. Long-term survival of allogeneic donor cell-derived corneal epithelium in limbal deficient rabbits. Curr Eye Res 2001;23(5):336–345.
87. Modo M, Rezaie P, Heuschling F, Patel S, Male D, Hodges H. Transplantation of neural stem cells in a rat model of stroke: assessment of short-term graft survival and acute host immunological response. Brain Res 2002;958(1):70–82.
88. Sugita S, Streilein J. Iris pigment epithelium expressing CD86 (B7-2) directly suppresses T cell activation in vitro via binding to cytotoxic T lymphocyte-associated antigen 4. J Exp Med 2003;198(1):161–171.

11

Basic to Clinical Cartilage Engineering: Past, Present, and Future Discussions

Mats Brittberg, Tommi Tallheden, and Anders H. Lindahl

Articular cartilage has limited capacity for self-repair and this inability may be the reason for the development of the end stage of cartilage loss, osteoarthritis (OA). OA is today a disability producer in many millions of people all over the world, and to find reliable methods of early repair of cartilage injuries and thereby prevent the development of OA seems of utmost importance. To learn more about how cartilage functions and how cartilage develops, studies on skeletal development during embryonic life could be helpful, especially as cartilage serves multiple functions in the developing embryo and those functions and events could tell us more about cartilage produced for postnatal life.

When a cartilage surface is injured, there are few chondrocytes that can start the repair partly because of the avascularity of cartilage and because of the low cell-to-matrix quota. But important knowledge that can be useful is that the embryonic cartilage development involves a mesenchymal high-density cell aggregation.[1–3] Subsequently, to imitate embryonic cartilage development, the goal for the orthopedic surgeon is to try to deliver as many of the chondrogenic cells as possible into the cartilage lesion to achieve some sort of repair.

In Gothenburg, Sweden, the experience with biological articular resurfacing dates back to the early 1980s and the research has been focused on using the autologous articular chondrocytes[4–6] for local cartilage defect repair even though other chondrogenic cells such as allergenic chondrocytes, auricular chondrocytes, nasal chondrocytes, autologous rib perichondrial cells, periosteal cells, or mesenchymal bone marrow stromal cells could have been possible alternatives. However, the articular chondrocytes are responsible for the unique features of articular cartilage; therefore, it seems rational to use true committed chondrocytes to repair a cartilaginous defect.

Autologous Chondrocyte Transplantation

Cell Harvest

Biopsies of articular cartilage can be harvested by arthroscopy from a minor load-bearing area in the affected joint and at the same time 10 × 10 mL of autologous venous blood can be collected for preparation of serum additive to the culture medium.[7,8] To get an idea of the amount of cartilage needed to be harvested, biopsies from 1000 patients were studied. The mean value of biopsy weight was 280 mg (4–1700 mg). Furthermore, the mean value for cells/mg studied on 500 patients was 2600 cells/mg.[9]

Normally, the biopsies are taken as full thickness, through all layers down to the subchondral bone.[4,5] However, recent studies by Dowthwaite et al.[10] tell us of the existence of a progenitor cell from the surface zone of articular cartilage. That population of cells exhibits high affinity for fibronectin, possesses a high colony-forming efficiency, expresses the cell fate selector gene Notch 1, and also exhibits phenotypic plasticity. There seems to be a chondrocyte subpopulation with progenitor-like characteristics in the surface layer of cartilage indicating that it might be enough to harvest the superficial layers for chondrocyte isolation and expansion.[10]

In Vitro Cell Expansion

From such a piece of harvested cartilage, chondrocytes can be isolated by enzymatic digestion and the primary goal of in vitro chondrocyte expansion is to increase the cell number without loosening the redifferentiation ability of the cells. Individual chondrocytes are isolated by collagenase digestion overnight and cultured in Dulbecco's modified Eagle medium/F12 with 10% autologous serum supplement. Primary cultures are performed in 25-cm^2 culture flasks and after 1 week the cells are subcultured by trypsin to 75-cm^2 culture flasks at a cell density of 8000 cells/cm^2 and the cells are cultured for another 1–2 weeks. During this period, the initial cells are expanded to 20–50 times the initial amount of cells.[4,5]

The culture environment favors fast proliferating cells and therefore it is possible that certain subpopulations could be concentrated. Whether this is an explanation to why chondrocytes during in vitro culture lose their phenotype if the cells actually revert to a fetal stage, needs to be further elucidated.

Condensation

During the initial 12-week period of embryonic life, the formation of the skeleton begins. The beginning process involves a mesenchymal cell aggregation, which is the fundamental feature of cartilage differentiation in the developing limb with the formation of the prechondrogenic cell condensation, a blastema.[1] In vitro studies, it has been shown that mesenchymal cell aggregates must achieve a threshold size before chondrogenesis can proceed.[2] Subsequently, to start chondrogenesis in order to repair a cartilaginous tissue, a large number of chondrogenic cells for implantation in high densities are needed.

The dedifferentiated chondrocytes have a similarity to primitive mesenchymal cells and an implantation of a high density of those in vitro-expanded primitive immature chondrocytes could imitate the prechondrogenic cell condensation and cartilage formation.[6] The repair process initiated by implantation of the cells into the defect initiates cell condensation and cartilage formation similar to the mesenchymal condensation in limb formation discussed above. To evaluate that similarity, special primers for limited key genes expressed during limb and cartilage development have been studied by Lindahl et al.[8]: collagen type IIA and IIB, osteocalcin, SRY-related HMG box gene (Sox9), cartilage-derived morphogenetic protein 1, wingless type MMTV integration site family member 14 (Wnr-14), and core-binding factor alpha 1. All the described genes were expressed by the cultured cells and especially Sox9 and Wnt-14 expression were of interest because of their importance in embryonal cartilage cell condensation and joint development.[8]

Redifferentiation

Doubts have been expressed that the dedifferentiated cells would not revert enough to contribute to a repair after implantation. However, several researchers have shown that dedifferentiated chondrocytes are able to reexpress phenotypic markers of the articular chondrocyte.[11–13] The tests include three-dimensional cultures in gels of agarose, collagen, and alginate. The redifferentiation can also be obtained after treatment of chondrocytes in monolayer by dihydrocytochalasin B or staurosporine.[11,12] Tallheden et al.[13] studied monolayer culture-expanded chondrocytes that redifferentiated in a pellet model as seen by an increase in collagen type II immunoreactivity between days 7 and 14. The late phase consisted of a strong down-regulation of extracellular signal-regulated protein kinase (ERK-1) and an up-regulation of p38 kinase and Sox9, suggesting that the late phase mimicked parts of the signaling processes involved in the early chondrogenesis in limb bud cells. Other genes, which indicated a transition from proliferation to tissue formation, were the down-regulated cell cycle genes GSPT1 and the up-regulated growth-arrest-specific protein (gas)[13] [Figure 11.1 (see color section)].

Although the mechanisms involved in restoration of the differentiated phenotype have not been elucidated yet, it has been shown that the synthesis of specific proteoglycans and type II collagen can be related to a modification of actin architecture.

Cell Implantation

The culture-expanded cells normally arrive to the operating room in syringes at a density of 30 million cells/mL.[7,8] The damaged joint is opened and the cartilage injury is debrided to healthy cartilage. A flap of periosteum or a collagen membrane is sutured over the defect and finally the cells are implanted into the defect with a treatment dose of 1×10^6 cells/cm^2 of defect area [Figure 11.2 (see color section)].

The ability of the culture-expanded chondrocytes to adhere to the debrided surface has been questioned but several studies in vivo and in vitro have shown that the chondrocytes are able to adhere and redifferentiate within the joint. Chen et al.[14] used radiolabeled chondrocytes for quantification and showed that the efficiency of transplantation onto a cartilage substrate was 93% ± 4% for seeding densities of as much as 650,000 cells per cm^2 after a seeding duration of 1 hour. During the 16 hours after seeding onto a cartilage substrate, the transplanted cells synthesized sulfated proteoglycan in direct proportion to the number of cells seeded. Most (83%) of the newly synthesized proteoglycan was released into the medium rather than retained within the layer of transplanted cells and the recipient cartilage substrate, thus suggesting that at least early on, an overlying membrane is important.[14]

These results implicate that, at least in experiments with chondrocytes directly seeded to cartilage explants, a linear relationship between biosynthetic activity and the number of seeded chondrocytes could be seen, which means that the number of seeded cells seems important.[14] However, the number of cells clinically needed for the implantation either as a suspension or in a scaffold has not been studied enough. LeBaron and Athanasiou[15] noted that polylactide-polyglycolide scaffolds seeded with a density of less than 10 million cells per milliliter, resulted in very little cartilaginous material. They stated that seeding at high cell densities seemed advisable.[15] Puelacher et al.[16] presented a study that revealed that seeding scaffolds at a density ranging from 20 to 100 million cells per milliliter resulted in formation of clinically appropriate cartilage when implanted into nude mice subcutaneously.

In another study,[17] histologic analysis indicated that chondrocytes grown on devitalized cartilage discs produced new matrix that bonded and integrated individual cartilage elements with mechanically functional tissue. Biomechanical testing demonstrated a time-dependent increase in tensile strength, failure strain, failure energy, and tensile modulus to values 5%–30% of normal articular cartilage by 8 months in vivo. The values recorded at 4 months were not statistically different from those collected at the latest time point, indicating that the limits of the biomechanical property values were reached after 4 months from implantation.

Sohn et al.[18] used an ex vivo bovine model to study the implanted chondrocytes' behavior and orientation relative to gravity of a repaired full-thickness articular cartilage defect and found that the gravity affected the initial distribution of transplanted chondrocytes, prelabeled with 3H-thymidine. Those results indicate that injected chondrocytes localize under the influence of gravity within the initial few hours after injection. Therefore, the defect orientation during this time can be an important factor in the uniformity of cell distribution in the autologous chondrocyte implantation procedure and may be an important determinant of the ultimate clinical outcome.

To monitor the persistence and the phenotype of injected chondrocytes in repair tissue, Dell'Accio et al.[19] used a fluorescence labeling protocol for articular chondrocytes, which allowed cell tracking in vivo using the fluorescence dye PKH26. Their data indicate that the implanted cells can persist for at least 14 weeks in the defects, can participate in integration with the surrounding tissues, and become a structural part of the repair tissue rich in collagen type II and sulfated proteoglycans.

Cell-to-Cell Contact and Integration to the Surrounding Tissue

The initial attachment of transplanted chondrocytes to the surface of a cartilage defect is crucial for the success of chondrocyte transplantation. The attachment is important regarding the start of chondrogenesis, induction of the differentiation program, and integration of neocartilage produced into surrounding native cartilage.

Wang and Kandel[20] used freshly isolated primary or passaged chondrocytes that were seeded on the top of bone plugs having a surface composed of mid-deep zone hyaline cartilage or calcified cartilage or onto bone only. Both primary and passaged chondrocytes attached efficiently to all three surfaces (>88% of seeded cells). As a sign of start of a chondrogenesis, there was expression of type II collagen and aggrecan core protein mRNA by 2 hours postimplantation.

Kurtis and coworkers[21] studied the time influence on cell attachment. After culture in monolayer, adhesion of chondrocytes to cartilage increased with time, from 6%–16% at 10 minutes to a maximum of 59%–82% at 80–320 minutes. They also found that $\beta1$, $\alpha5\ \beta1$, and $\alpha v \beta 5$ integrins seem to be involved in human chondrocyte initial adhesion and retention to cartilage. Enzymatic treatment of a cartilage surface can further enhance the chondrocyte adhesion to surrounding native cartilage.

Tacchetti et al.[22] have shown that with chick embryo-derived undifferentiated cells, a reduced rate of cell clustering and cell-to-cell contact parallels a reduction of cell recruitment into the cartilage differentiation program. They suggested that there was a cascade of events important in the early stages of chondrocyte differentiation consisting of the acquisition of the ability to establish cell-to-cell contacts, the formation of a permissive environment capable of activating the differentiation program, and finally the expression of differentiation markers.

Gene Therapy

To alter or improve the cells before implantation or by directly changing the function of the chondrocytes in situ, gene therapy is a possible option. Different cDNAs have been cloned, which may be used to stimulate biological processes that could improve cartilage healing by (1) inducing mitosis and the synthesis and deposition of cartilage extracellular matrix components by chondrocytes, (2) induction of chondrogenesis by mesenchymal progenitor cells, or (3) inhibiting cellular responses to inflammatory stimuli. It is possible that the chondrogenic cells transfer genes encoded for cartilage repair promoting factors directly to the lesion site. The transferred genes must enter the cell's nucleus where it can be transcribed followed by a transportation of the generated mRNA out from the nucleus to serve as matrix for protein production in the ribosomes.

Viral gene vectors are regarded as more efficient than nonviral vectors such as liposomes. Milbrandt et al.[23] explored the feasibility of using transduced cells for gene therapy to induce healing of osteochondral defects. Both a mouse mesenchymal cell line and mixed rabbit adherent stromal cells were transduced with either liposomal transfection or retroviral transduction using a traceable gene. Transduction efficiency was more than 95% with the retroviral construct and expression was maintained for more than 6 months of passage. The liposomal transfection led to a transient expression with an efficiency of 50%. The expression of osteochondral genes was diminished but preserved after transduction in vitro. Transduced rabbit cells were transplanted into osteochondral defects in rabbit femoral condyles. Cells transplanted in vivo could be detected for 4 weeks in the repair tissue. Milbrandt et al.[23] demonstrated that mesenchymal cells from bone marrow, stably transduced with a traceable gene product, retain the bone and cartilage phenotype and can be followed in vivo after transplantation into cartilage defects. Similar animal experiments clearly demonstrate the utility of tissue engineering strategies in which gene therapy is used to locally influence the repair environment.

One drawback with gene therapy is the relatively short half-lives in vivo of the gene expression, which often require high doses and repeated injection, and still much research remains until a safe clinical procedure can be used.

Growth Factors

Relatively little is known about the intracellular signaling pathways involved with growth factors and cartilage repair processes but one important group of growth factors that have raised special interest are the peptide growth factors. Of these factors, there are three growth factor classes that are especially interesting, the fibroblast growth factor family, the insulin-like growth factors including insulin, and transforming growth factor β (TGFβ) and related molecules.[24,25] All these factors have been implicated in three aspects of cartilage growth and metabolism: The induction of mesoderm and differentiation of a cartilaginous skeleton in the early embryo, the growth and differentiation of chondrocytes within the epiphyseal growth plates leading to endochondral calcification, and the processes of articular cartilage damage and repair.[24] Repair of defects in tissues normally requires regeneration of injured cells via control of the cell cycle, differentiation, and cell death (apoptosis). The peptide growth factors usually work through paracrine effects and are able to initiate cell replication through cell surface receptors and thereby initiate cascades that amplify the cell's response.

Because of the poor in situ capacity of cartilage repair, it would be ideal if growth factors could be loaded into a device designed to stimulate the cells already present in the joint to repair the injury. Potential candidates are TGFβ and related bone morphometric proteins, which can induce the differentiation of cartilage from primitive mesenchyme, and together with basic fibroblast growth factor and insulin-like growth factors promote cartilage growth.[26–28] Of interest also are other members of the TGFβ superfamily that are thought to have key roles in chondrocyte growth and differentiation. Notably, bone morphogenetic protein-2 (BMP-2) may be a useful cytokine to improve healing of cartilaginous defects.[28–30] The problem, however, is that the control of chondrocytic differentiation of primitive stem cells is affected by interplay and expression of several factors such as Brachyury, BMP-4 (BMP-2B), TGFβ3. Important for the phenotypic expression is also the Smads 1, 4, and 5.[31] The situation is therefore rather complex and, instead of a single growth factor at one occasion, several factors in a cascade are needed.

Animal Experiments

In 1984 and 1989 Peterson et al.[32] and Grande et al.,[33] respectively, presented their results in rabbit models with autologous chondrocytes grown in vitro on the healing rate of chondral defects not penetrating the subchondral bone plate. In defects that had received transplants 8 weeks' postimplantation, a significant amount of cartilage was reconstituted (82%) compared with engrafted controls (18%). Autoradiography on reconstituted cartilage showed that there was labeled cells incorporated into the repair matrix.[33] Goldberg and Caplan[3] compared implantation of mature chondrocytes, so-called committed, with mesenchymal stem cells for the repair of full-thickness defects in the femoral condyles of adult rabbits. Both cell types repaired the defect with hyaline-like neocartilage. However, the mesenchymal stem cell repair had a more hyaline-like morphology and cartilage zonal characteristics than the repair from the committed chondrocytes. Mesenchymal cells as chondrogenic progenitors have also been studied by Nevo et al.,[34] who found problems such as a delayed pace of endochondral ossification in the deep zones of the subchondral region of the study defects, or ossification above the tide mark, within the superficial cartilaginous articular regions. They found that autogenetic, chondrocytic-enriched bone marrow-derived mesenchymal cells were superior to other cell sources for articular cartilage regeneration.

Brittberg et al.[5] compared periosteal grafts with and without chondrocytes in rabbit patellar chondral defects. One year after implantation, periosteum and chondrocytes demonstrated an average repair area of 87% compared with the 30% repair area observed in the periosteum-alone graft. A histologic grading system also demonstrated a statistically significant difference between the two graft types, with the tissue produced by chondrocytes in combination with a periosteal flap resulting in much higher histologic scoring compared with defects treated with only a periosteal flap.

Rahfoth et al.[35] transplanted allograft chondrocytes embedded in agarose gel into rabbit articular cartilage defects and followed up the repair for 6–18 months. At 18 months, in 47% of the grafts, a morphologically stable hyaline-like cartilage was noted to develop, and extent of recovery was never observed in controls.

Using a dog model to study autologous chondrocyte repair on chondral repair, Breinan et al.[36] found that, at 12–18 months postsurgery, there were no differences in the repair with autologous chondrocytes and periosteum versus periosteum alone, but a substantial number of animals had a break through to the subchondral bone.

Recently, using the previously established canine model for repair of articular cartilage defects, Lee et al.[37] evaluated the 15-week healing of chondral defects (e.g., to the tidemark) implanted with an autologous articular chondrocyte-seeded type II collagen scaffold that had been cultured in vitro for 4 weeks before implantation. The amount and composition of the reparative tissue were compared with results from the Breinan study using the same animal model in which the following groups were analyzed: Defects implanted with autologous chondrocyte-seeded collagen scaffolds that had been cultured in vitro for approximately 12 hours before implantation, defects implanted with autologous chondrocytes alone, and untreated defects. Chondrocytes, isolated from articular cartilage harvested from the left knee joint of six adult canines, were expanded in number in a monolayer for 3 weeks, seeded into porous type II collagen scaffolds, cultured for another 4 weeks in vitro, and implanted into chondral defects in the trochlear groove of the right knee joints. The percentages of specific tissue types filling the defects were evaluated histomorphometrically and certain mechanical properties of the repair tissue were determined. The reparative tissue filled 88% ± 6% of the cross-sectional area of the original defect, with hyaline cartilage accounting for 42% ± 10% (range 7%–67%) of defect area. These values were greater than those reported previously for untreated defects and defects implanted with a type II collagen scaffold seeded with autologous chondrocytes within 12 hours before implantation. Most interesting was the decreased amount of fibrous tissue filling the defects in the current study, 5% ± 5% as compared with previous treatments. Despite this improvement, indentation testing of the repair tissue formed revealed that the compressive stiffness of the repair tissue was well below (20-fold lower stiffness) that of native articular cartilage.

Still, long follow-ups with a reliable and maybe larger animal are lacking. However, it appears that the above different animal models with allogenous or autologous chondrocytes used in the treatment of cartilage defects show benefit over cartilage defects treated without cells or not treated at all, at least in reports of little more than 1 year's follow-up.

The Clinical Research

Clinically, the first patients with articular cartilage defects were treated by implanting autologous cells expanded in vitro in combination with a biomechanical membrane – the periosteum in 1987.[4] This, the first generation of chondrocyte transplantation, was initially termed autologous chondrocyte transplantation (ACT). Because the periosteum itself has chondrogenic potential,[38] a dual chondrogenic response when using the chondrocytes in combination with the periosteum may be expected. Today, the technique is called either ACT or ACI (autologous chondrocyte implantation). In Sweden, autologous chondrocyte transplantation in combination with a periosteal graft has been used in approximately 1200 patients since October 1987 and, worldwide now, variants of ACT/ACI have been tried in approximately 12,000 patients. The use of ACT is always considered alongside other techniques.

In patients with small, acute defects, ACT is mostly used after failure of other techniques after 6 months. In large, acute defects, ACT and osteochondral grafting (up to 4 cm^2) may be used immediately because such large defects are difficult to resurface with bone marrow stimulation techniques.

In a clinical evaluation of 244 patients with 2–10 years' follow-up,[9] subjective and objective improvements were seen in high numbers of patients with femoral condyle lesions and osteochondritis dissecans. There was a high percentage of clinical good to excellent results (84%–90%) in patients with different types of single femoral condyle lesions whereas other types of lesions had a lower degree of success (mean 74%). Biopsies of repair tissue showed mostly a mixed repair tissue with a fibrous top layer and more hyaline-like middle and bottom layer [Figure 11.3 (see color section)].

To study the long-term durability of ACT-treated patients, 61 patients that had passed 2 years postsurgery were followed for at least 5 years up to 11 years postsurgery (mean 7.4 years). After 2 years, 50 of 61 patients were graded good–excellent.

At the 5- to 11-year follow-up, 51 of the 61 were graded good–excellent. The total failure rate was 16% (10/61) at mean 7.4 years. All ACT failures occurred in the first 2 years, so patients showing good to excellent improvement at 2 years had a high percentage of good results at long-term follow-up.

Most reports on the use of autologous chondrocyte transplantation from other centers show similar figures with a high degree of success in regard to the total number of improved patients but the criticism has been that ACT needs to be evaluated versus other cartilage repair techniques in randomized trials.[39] A very comprehensive analysis of the ACT technology was recently presented.[40] The authors stated that, on the basis of literature, no definite conclusions can be drawn about the clinical effectiveness of ACT, which should be regarded as an experimental procedure. However, on these grounds, almost all other techniques used for treating disabling cartilage defects, could be regarded as experimental. The cost of ACT is substantial in comparison to the other techniques, and surgeons have reported similar good results with those techniques as have been reported with ACT. Most of those other cartilage repair techniques have still quite short follow-ups (2–4 years) and the authors speculate that it is possible that, by extending the time horizon and assuming that better outcomes are sustained with ACT, but not with other therapies, financial and human costs might in the long run be less with ACT. Such speculations, according to the authors, are not justified until data from randomized studies become available. It is easy to agree with that statement, but you may emphasize the importance of long-term follow-ups in such studies with the definitions of a short-term study being a minimum of 2 years, mid-term 5 years, and a long-term study at least 10 years.

To date, three such clinical randomized trials have been reported on. Those studies as described below could be seen as short-term studies. Knutsen et al.[41] studied 80 patients who needed local cartilage repair because of symptomatic lesions on the femoral condyles measuring 2–10 cm^2. The patients came from four hospitals and were randomized into ACT or microfracture treatment and followed at 12 and 24 months. At 2 years, both groups had significant clinical improvement. According to the SF-36 physical component score at 2 years postoperatively, the improvement in the microfracture group was significantly better than that in the autologous chondrocyte implantation group. Both methods had acceptable short-term clinical results. There was no significant difference in macroscopic or histologic results between the two treatment groups.

Horas et al.[42] performed a prospective clinical study to investigate the 2-year outcomes in 40 patients with an articular cartilage lesion of the femoral condyle who had been randomly treated with either transplantation of an autologous osteochondral cylinder or implantation of autologous chondrocytes. Both treatments resulted in a decrease in symptoms. However, the improvement provided by the autologous chondrocyte implantation lagged behind that provided by the osteochondral cylinder transplantation. Histologically, the defects treated with autologous chondrocyte implantation were primarily filled with fibrocartilage, whereas the osteochondral cylinder transplants retained their hyaline character, although there was a persistent interface between the transplant and the surrounding original cartilage. The authors mentioned the limitations of their study because it included a small number of patients, the relatively short (2-year) follow-up, and the absence of a control group.

Bentley and associates[43] studied 100 patients with a mean age of 31.3 years (16–49) with symptomatic chondral and osteochondral lesions of the knee, which were suitable for cartilage repair, and were randomized to undergo either ACT or mosaicplasty: 58 patients had ACI and 42 mosaicplasty. Most lesions were posttraumatic and the mean size of the defect was 4.66 cm^2. The mean duration of symptoms was 7.2 years and the mean number of previous operations, excluding arthroscopy, was 1.5. The mean follow-up was 19 months (12–26). Functional assessment using the modified Cincinnati and Stanmore scores and objective clinical assessment showed that 88% had excellent or good results after ACT compared with 69% after mosaicplasty. Arthroscopy at 1 year demonstrated excellent or good repairs in 82% after ACI and in 34% after mosaicplasty. All five patellar mosaicplasties failed. This prospective, randomized, clinical trial showed significant superiority of ACT over mosaicplasty for the repair of articular defects in the knee.

The ankle joint, shoulder, elbow, hip, and wrist[44–48] are other locations that have been tried in smaller numbers of patients. With the development of arthroscopic techniques,[49,50] the use of ACI will be increased also in those smaller joint compartments. Specially, the use of resorbable membranes instead of the periosteum will be important for those joints by which one may avoid the risk of hypertrophy. The periosteal hypertrophy may become a problem in the smaller joints.

The first generation of ACT is a combination treatment with two chondrogenic factors involved: The implanted suspension of chondrocytes and the cambium cells from the periosteum. The disadvantages include the potential leakage of cells from defects, dedifferentiation of cellular phenotype as the cells have been grown in monolayer just before implantation, and uneven distribution of cells as well as substantial risk of periosteal hypertrophy. Resorbable membranes, such as Chondro-Gide (a type I/type III collagen membrane, Geistlich, Pharma AG, CH-6110 Wolhausen, Switzerland), are a possible alternative to the periosteum[51,52] and the clinical results with that membrane seem promising. Similar good short-term results have also been presented with the hyaluronan-based biodegradable polymer scaffold HYAFF-11(Fidia Advanced Biopolymers, Abano Terme, Italy).[53,54]

The Future

We will see more and more different cell-containing resorbable scaffolds to be used for arthroscopic implantation; some scaffolds with cells cultured for several weeks(mature grafts) whereas others just seeded with cells 1–2 days before surgery(immature grafts) or even just at implantation time. However, the repair is also dependent on a fast integration of the implant and immature constructs have poorer mechanical properties but integrate better than either more mature constructs or cartilage explants. Integration of immature constructs involves cell proliferation and the progressive formation of cartilaginous tissue, in contrast to the integration of more mature constructs or native cartilage, which involves only the secretion of extracellular matrix components. Trypsin and chondroitinase ABC treatments of the adjacent cartilage further enhance the integration of immature constructs.[55]

The ACT technology needs to be further improved and there is a search for new biomaterials, which are aimed to secure the cells in the defect area and permit their proliferation and differentiation. The maintenance of the original phenotype by isolated chondrocytes grown in vitro is an important requisite for their use and handling in a future transarthroscopic technique in articular cartilage resurfacing.

Conclusion

An analysis of the literature provides no evidence so far for regular regeneration of hyaline cartilage in animal experiments and still today's treatments for cartilage resurfacing are less than satisfactory, and rarely restore full function or return the tissue to its native normal state. The rapidly growing field of tissue engineering holds great promise for the generation of functional cartilage tissue substitutes. Cell biologists, engineers, and surgeons work closely together with combined knowledge of using biocompatible, biomimetic, biomechanical suitable scaffolds seeded with chondrogenic cells and loaded with bioactive molecules that promote time-relapsed cellular differentiation and/or maturation.

References

1. Caplan AI, Elyaderani M, Mochizuki Y, Wakitani S, Goldberg VM. Principles of cartilage repair and regeneration. Clin Orthop Relat Res 1997(342):254–269.
2. Cottrill CP, Archer CW, Wolpert L. Cell sorting and chondrogenic aggregate formation in micromass culture. Dev Biol 1987;122(2):503–515.
3. Goldberg VM, Caplan AI. Cellular repair of articular cartilage. In: Kuettner KE, Goldberg V, eds. Osteoarthritic Disorders. Rosemont, IL: American Academy of Orthopaedic Surgeons; 1994:357–364.
4. Brittberg M, Lindahl A, Nilsson A, Ohlsson C, Isaksson O, Peterson L. Treatment of deep cartilage defects in the knee with autologous chondrocyte transplantation. N Engl J Med 1994;331(14):889–895.
5. Brittberg M, Nilsson A, Lindahl A, Ohlsson C, Peterson L. Rabbit articular cartilage defects treated with autologous cultured chondrocytes. Clin Orthop Relat Res 1996(May):270–283.
6. Brittberg M. Cartilage Repair. MD Thesis, Göteborg University; 1996.
7. Sjögren-Jansson ET, Tallheden T, Lindahl A. Growing the cells. In: Ashton IK, Brittberg M, Richardson JB, eds. The Eurocell Experience of Autologous Chondrocyte Implantation. Oswestry: The Institute of Orthopaedics (Oswestry) Publishing Group; 2004 47–51.
8. Lindahl A, Brittberg M, Peterson L. Cartilage repair with chondrocytes: clinical and cellular aspects. Novartis Found Symp 2003;249:175–186; discussion 86–89, 234–238, 9–41.
9. Brittberg M, Peterson L, Sjogren-Jansson E, Tallheden T, Lindahl A. Articular cartilage engineering with autologous chondrocyte transplantation. A review of recent developments. J Bone Joint Surg Am 2003;85-A(suppl 3):109–115.
10. Dowthwaite GP, Bishop JC, Redman SN, et al. The surface of articular cartilage contains a progenitor cell population. J Cell Sci 2004;117(pt 6):889–897.
11. Borge L, Lemare F, Demignot S, Adolphe M. Restoration of the differentiated functions of serially passaged chondrocytes using staurosporine. In Vitro Cell Dev Biol Anim 1997;33(9):703–709.
12. Adolphe M, Demignot S. Versatility of differentiated functions of cultured joint chondrocytes. Eventual usefulness in treatment. Bull Acad Natl Med 2000;184(3):593–600; discussion 1–4.
13. Tallheden T, Karlsson C, Brunner A, et al. Gene expression during redifferentiation of human articular chondrocytes. Osteoarthritis Cartilage 2004;12(7):525–535.

14. Chen AC, Nagrampa JP, Schinagl RM, Lottman LM, Sah RL. Chondrocyte transplantation to articular cartilage explants in vitro. J Orthop Res 1997;15(6): 791–802.
15. LeBaron RG, Athanasiou KA. Ex vivo synthesis of articular cartilage. Biomaterials 2000;21(24):2575–2587.
16. Puelacher WC, Kim SW, Vacanti JP, Schloo B, Mooney D, Vacanti CA. Tissue-engineered growth of cartilage: the effect of varying the concentration of chondrocytes seeded onto synthetic polymer matrices. Int J Oral Maxillofac Surg 1994;23(1):49–53.
17. Peretti GM, Zaporojan V, Spangenberg KM, Randolph MA, Fellers J, Bonassar LJ. Cell-based bonding of articular cartilage: an extended study. J Biomed Mater Res 2003;64A(3):517–524.
18. Sohn DH, Lottman LM, Lum LY, et al. Effect of gravity on localization of chondrocytes implanted in cartilage defects. Clin Orthop 2002;(394):254–262.
19. Dell'Accio F, Vanlauwe J, Bellemans J, Neys J, De Bari C, Luyten FP. Expanded phenotypically stable chondrocytes persist in the repair of tissue and contribute to cartilage matrix formation and structural integration in a goat model of autologous chondrocyte implantation. J Orthop Res 2003;21(1):123–131.
20. Wang H, Kandel RA. Chondrocytes attach to hyaline or calcified cartilage and bone. Osteoarthritis Cartilage 2004;12(1):56–64.
21. Kurtis MS, Schmidt TA, Bugbee WD, Loeser RF, Sah RL. Integrin-mediated adhesion of human articular chondrocytes to cartilage. Arthritis Rheum 2003; 48(1):110–118.
22. Tacchetti C, Tavella S, Dozin B, Quarto R, Robino G, Cancedda R. Cell condensation in chondrogenic differentiation. Exp Cell Res 1992;200(1):26–33.
23. Milbrandt T, Berthoux L, Christenson J, et al. Tracing transduced cells in osteochondral defects. J Pediatr Orthop 2003;23(4):430–436.
24. Hill DJ, Logan A. Peptide growth factors and their interactions during chondrogenesis. Prog Growth Factor Res 1992;4(1):45–68.
25. Fortier LA, Mohammed HO, Lust G, Nixon AJ. Insulin-like growth factor-I enhances cell-based repair of articular cartilage. J Bone Joint Surg Br 2002;84(2):276–288.
26. Weisser J, Rahfoth B, Timmermann A, Aigner T, Brauer R, von der Mark K. Role of growth factors in rabbit articular cartilage repair by chondrocytes in agarose. Osteoarthritis Cartilage 2001;9(suppl A):S48–54.
27. Tanaka H, Mizokami H, Shiigi E, et al. Effects of basic fibroblast growth factor on the repair of large osteochondral defects of articular cartilage in rabbits: dose-response effects and long-term outcomes. Tissue Eng 2004;10(3–4):633–641.
28. Frenkel SR, Saadeh PB, Mehrara BJ, et al. Transforming growth factor beta superfamily members: role in cartilage modeling. Plast Reconstr Surg 2000;105(3): 980–990.
29. van den Berg WB, van der Kraan PM, Scharstuhl A, van Beuningen HM. Growth factors and cartilage repair. Clin Orthop 2001;(391 suppl):S244–250.
30. Sellers RS, Zhang R, Glasson SS, et al. Repair of articular cartilage defects one year after treatment with recombinant human bone morphogenetic protein-2 (rhBMP-2). J Bone Joint Surg Am 2000;82(2): 151–160.
31. Otto WR, Rao J. Tomorrow's skeleton staff: mesenchymal stem cells and the repair of bone and cartilage. Cell Prolif 2004;37(1):97–110.
32. Peterson L, Menche D, Grande D, Pitman M. Chondrocyte transplantation: an experimental model in the rabbit. Trans Orthop Res Soc 1984;9:218.
33. Grande DA, Pitman MI, Peterson L, Menche D, Klein M. The repair of experimentally produced defects in rabbit articular cartilage by autologous chondrocyte transplantation. J Orthop Res 1989;7(2):208–218.
34. Nevo Z, Robinson D, Horowitz S, Hasharoni A, Yayon A. The manipulated mesenchymal stem cells in regenerated skeletal tissues. Cell Transplant 1998;7(1):63–70.
35. Rahfoth B, Weisser J, Sternkopf F, Aigner T, von der Mark K, Brauer R. Transplantation of allograft chondrocytes embedded in agarose gel into cartilage defects of rabbits. Osteoarthritis Cartilage 1998;6(1):50–65.
36. Breinan HA, Minas T, Hsu HP, Nehrer S, Sledge CB, Spector M. Effect of cultured autologous chondrocytes on repair of chondral defects in a canine model. J Bone Joint Surg Am 1997;79(10):1439–1451.
37. Lee CR, Grodzinsky AJ, Hsu HP, Spector M. Effects of a cultured autologous chondrocyte-seeded type II collagen scaffold on the healing of a chondral defect in a canine model. J Orthop Res 2003;21(2):272–281.
38. O'Driscoll SW, Salter RB. The induction of neochondrogenesis in free intra-articular periosteal autografts under the influence of continuous passive motion. An experimental investigation in the rabbit. J Bone Joint Surg Am 1984;66(8):1248–1257.
39. Lohmander LS. Tissue engineering of cartilage: do we need it, can we do it, is it good and can we prove it? Novartis Found Symp 2003;249:2–10; discussion 6, 170–174, 239–241.
40. Jobanputra P, Parry D, Fry-Smith A, Burls A. Effectiveness of autologous chondrocyte transplantation for hyaline cartilage defects in knees: a rapid and systematic review. Health Technol Assess 2001;5(11):1–57.
41. Knutsen G, Engebretsen L, Ludvigsen TC, et al. Autologous chondrocyte implantation compared with microfracture in the knee. A randomized trial. J Bone Joint Surg Am 2004;86-A(3):455–464.
42. Horas U, Pelinkovic D, Herr G, Aigner T, Schnettler R. Autologous chondrocyte implantation and osteochondral cylinder transplantation in cartilage repair of the knee joint. A prospective, comparative trial. J Bone Joint Surg Am 2003;85-A(2):185–192.
43. Bentley G, Biant LC, Carrington RW, et al. A prospective, randomised comparison of autologous chondrocyte implantation versus mosaicplasty for osteochondral defects in the knee. J Bone Joint Surg Br 2003;85(2):223–230.
44. Petersen L, Brittberg M, Lindahl A. Autologous chondrocyte transplantation of the ankle. Foot Ankle Clin 2003;8(2):291–303.
45. Giannini S, Buda R, Grigolo B, Vannini F. Autologous chondrocyte transplantation in osteochondral lesions of the ankle joint. Foot Ankle Int 2001;22(6):513–517.
46. Johansen O, Lindahl A, Peterson L, Olsen B, JF W, Knutsen G. Hip osteochondritis-treated by debridement, suture of periosteal flap and chondrocyte implantation. A case report. In: Hunziker E, Mainil-Varlet, eds.Updates in Cartilage Repair. A multimedia production on cartilage repair on 6 CD ROMS. Philadelphia: Lippincott, Williams & Wilkins; CD 6.
47. Nilsson A, Lindahl A, Peterson L, Brittberg M, C. S. Autologous chondrocyte transplantation of the human wrist. In: Hunziker E, Mainil-Varlet, eds.Updates in

48. Romeo AA, Cole BJ, Mazzocca AD, Fox JA, Freeman KB, Joy E. Autologous chondrocyte repair of an articular defect in the humeral head. Arthroscopy 2002;18(8):925–929.
49. Marcacci M, Zaffagnini S, Kon E, Visani A, Iacono F, Loreti I. Arthroscopic autologous chondrocyte transplantation: technical note. Knee Surg Sports Traumatol Arthrosc 2002;10(3):154–159.
50. Erggelet C, Sittinger M, Lahm A. The arthroscopic implantation of autologous chondrocytes for the treatment of full-thickness cartilage defects of the knee joint. Arthroscopy 2003;19(1):108–110.
51. Behrens P, Ehlers EM, Kochermann KU, Rohwedel J, Russlies M, Plotz W. New therapy procedure for localized cartilage defects. Encouraging results with autologous chondrocyte implantation. MMW Fortschr Med 1999;141(45):49–51.
52. Russlies M, Behrens P, Wunsch L, Gille J, Ehlers EM. A cell-seeded biocomposite for cartilage repair. Ann Anat 2002;184(4):317–323.
53. Grigolo B, Roseti L, Fiorini M, et al. Transplantation of chondrocytes seeded on a hyaluronan derivative (hyaff-11) into cartilage defects in rabbits. Biomaterials 2001;22(17):2417–2424.
54. Grigolo B, Lisignoli G, Piacentini A, et al. Evidence for redifferentiation of human chondrocytes grown on a hyaluronan-based biomaterial (HYAff 11): molecular, immunohistochemical and ultrastructural analysis. Biomaterials 2002;23(4):1187–1195.
55. Obradovic B, Martin I, Padera RF, Treppo S, Freed LE, Vunjak-Novakovic G. Integration of engineered cartilage. J Orthop Res 2001;19(6):1089–1097.

Above references 47 (Cartilage Repair. A multimedia production on cartilage repair on 6 CD ROMS. Philadelphia: Lippincott, Williams & Wilkins; CD 6.) completes the list from previous page.

12

Cartilage

Rocky S. Tuan and Faye H. Chen

Articular cartilage is the load-bearing material of the joint, and it is vital for normal joint motion. Because of its poor healing capacity, the increasing prevalence of osteoarthritis, and the aging, yet active, population, there is an increasing clinical need for improved treatment options for cartilage degeneration. This has motivated developments in cartilage tissue engineering to produce in vitro cartilage replacement grafts that can meet the functional demand in vivo. Although significant progress has been made, an implantable cartilage tissue substitute that eventually reproduces the structural and functional properties of the native tissue has not been developed. In this chapter, we will first discuss the normal structure and function of mature articular cartilage, its structural components and their organization, which are important for the function of this tissue. Next, we will review the factors that are critical for maintenance of its homeostasis. In addition, we will also discuss the key events during embryonic limb development. This information should serve as the foundation to guide the rational design of cartilage constructs for cartilage tissue repair and functional tissue engineering. In the following sections, we will survey the current effort and state of art of cartilage repair and tissue engineering, and will discuss the potential use of mesenchymal stem cells (MSCs) in these processes.

General Structure and Function of Articular Cartilage

Cartilage is a connective tissue that serves multiple functions throughout development. It provides structural support for the early embryo, and forms a template for bone formation through endochondral ossification. Postnatally, upon completion of endochondral growth, cartilage covers the surfaces of the joints to cushion and lubricate the joints during movement. It also participates in the repair of bone fracture through endochondral ossification.

Mature cartilage is a soft connective tissue that is composed of a single cell type, chondrocyte, and a highly specialized extracellular matrix (ECM). Three major types of cartilaginous tissues are present in the body: Hyaline cartilage, fibrocartilage, and elastic cartilage. The biochemical composition and molecular structure of the matrix give rise to distinct biomechanical properties of different types of cartilage, and their functions.

Hyaline cartilage is the most common type of cartilage. The most common hyaline cartilage, and the most studied, is articular cartilage.[1,2] This tissue covers the articulating surfaces of long bones and sesamoid bones within synovial joints. Articular cartilage in freely movable joints, such as hip and knee, can withstand very large loads, up to 20 mPa during normal joint movement,[3-6] while providing a smooth, lubricating bearing material with minimal wear. Another example of hyaline cartilage is the growth plate, which develops to form bones of the axial skeleton and long bones of the appendicular skeleton via condensation of mesenchymal cells and their subsequent differentiation into chondrocytes that proceed along the endochondral ossification pathway. Fibrocartilage contains thick layers of larger collagen fibers in the ECM that contribute to its fibrous appearance. Two major fibrocartilage tissues are the meniscus, and the annulus fibrosus of the intervertebral disc. Articular cartilage and meniscus are vital to the maintenance of normal joint motion, and both are involved in degenerative diseases such as osteoarthritis.

Structural Component and Organization of Articular Cartilage

One of the most important functions of articular cartilage is to support large loads during joint movement. To achieve this function is a primary goal of current cartilage repair and cartilage tissue engineering efforts, and has yet to be accomplished. The load-bearing property of cartilage depends on the structural composition and organization of its ECM, which is synthesized and maintained by chondrocytes. Cartilage ECM contains three classes of proteins: Collagens, proteoglycans, and other noncollagenous proteins.

The ability of articular cartilage to resist compression is primarily attributed to the presence of proteoglycan aggregates. The high density of fixed negative charge of the glycosaminoglycan chains draws water into the tissue, resulting in a large osmotic pressure.[7–10] The balance between the osmotic pressure of the proteoglycans and the tension in the collagen fibers results in a highly specialized connective tissue well suited for bearing compressive loads.[11,12] Cartilage tensile stiffness and strength, however, is determined primarily by the collagen network.[13,14] In addition, collagen can also contribute to the compressive behavior of cartilage.[15] Thus, the biomechanical properties of articular cartilage are dependent on the integrity of the collagen network and on the maintenance of high proteoglycan content within the matrix.

The third class of cartilage ECM proteins, the noncollagenous proteins, includes hyaluronan, link protein, the smaller proteoglycans, fibronectin, matrilins, and cartilage oligomeric matrix protein (COMP) (Table 12.1). Although these are not major components in terms of the absolute cartilage solid mass, some of them may approach the molar concentrations of collagen and aggrecan and serve important regulating functions. For example, small proteoglycans such as decorin, lumican, and fibromodulin, may be important for collagen fibril formation and assembly.[16–18] Much research effort has focused on collagens and proteoglycans for their critical role in maintaining cartilage ECM structure. Now it has become clear that the minor noncollagenous components are also important regulators of cartilage matrix integrity through interacting with the cells and the other matrix proteins.

Articular cartilage displays considerable heterogeneity in its composition and structure throughout its depth. Along with the differences in collagen fiber and proteoglycan network, chondrocyte cell shape and size also vary with depth[11,19,20] (Figure 12.1). This gives the tissue a layered appearance under electron microscopy and probably gives rise to different mechanical characteristics of the different zones. The superficial zone represents 10%–20% of articular cartilage thickness, and has the highest collagen content and the lowest level of aggrecan.[7,21,22] Fine collagen fibrils densely organized in parallel to the articular surface in this zone[23–25] may help to resist shear forces generated during joint use, and may be the reason why tensile strength has been shown to be the highest in this zone.[26,27] The cells in this zone are elongated and oriented in parallel to the articular surface. Whereas the number of cells per unit volume is maximal beneath the surface and decreases toward the tidemark, cell size increases with the distance from the articular surface. The next zone, which comprises 40%–60% of the total thickness, is the middle zone. Collagen content decreases from the superficial zone to the middle zone, and

Table 12.1. Extracellular matrix molecules of articular cartilage

% Wet Weight	Molecule
60–85	Water
15–22	Collagen type II
4–7	Aggrecan
	Hyaluronan
	Link protein
	Type VI collagen
	Type IX collagen
	Type XI collagen
	COMP
	Matrilins
	Decorin
	Biglycan
	Fibromodulin
	Fibronectin
	Thrombospondins

Source: Adapted from Mow et al.[11]

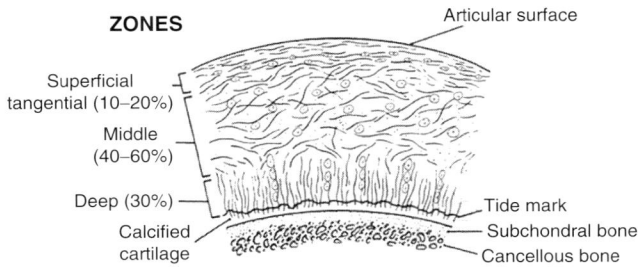

Figure 12.1. Zonal organization of collagen fibers and chondrocytes in articular cartilage. Three zones of articular cartilage are illustrated. The superficial tangential zone contains collagen fibers and chondrocytes oriented in parallel to the articular surface. In the middle zone, collagen fibers have larger diameters with random orientation. In the deep zone, the fibers appear to be organized perpendicular to the surface and cross the "tidemark" to insert into the calcified cartilage and subchondral bone. The cells are spherical in the middle zone, and oblong in vertical columns in the deep zone. (Adapted from Mow et al.[11])

remains relatively constant in the deeper zones, whereas aggrecan content increases to the greatest in the middle zone.[7,21,28] The collagen fibrils in the middle zone have a larger diameter that is less tightly packed with random orientation. In the deep zone (about 30% of the total thickness), the fibers appear to be woven together to form large fiber bundles organized perpendicular to the surface.[23,29,30] These bundles cross the "tidemark" to insert into the calcified cartilage and subchondral bone, thus function to securely anchor the uncalcified tissue onto the bone ends. The cells are spherical in the middle zone, and oblong in vertical columns in the deep zone. It is possible that the combination of collagen fiber organization, proteoglycan matrix, and shape of chondrocytes are intimately related and are likely adapted to optimize the mechanical stability and load-bearing capacity of the articular cartilage.[31]

Cartilage Homeostasis

Under normal circumstances, healthy articular cartilage is expected to maintain its function throughout life. Balanced anabolic and catabolic processes result in the homeostasis and maintenance of cartilage ECM and its biological function. Matrix turnover is an integral and ongoing process during growth and development and in mature cartilage. It is normally under the tight control of growth factors, cytokines, and proteases that can regulate the synthesis of matrix proteins and various proteases and inhibitors. However, this balance can be disturbed during disease processes, traumatic injury, or normal aging, resulting in remodeling, and degradation of the ECM, as observed in articular cartilage during osteoarthritis. When degradation of healthy cartilage is induced, aggrecan is lost rapidly followed by collagen type II, which leads to the eventual loss of cartilage ECM and chondrocyte cell death. Degradation enzymes that are primarily responsible for the degradation of these cartilage matrix proteins include aggrecanases and matrix metalloproteinases (Table 12.2).

Chondrocytes are metabolically active in response to changes in their environment, which include soluble mediators, e.g., cytokines, growth factors, hormones, proteases, pharmaceutical agents (Table 12.2), and mechanical environment, e.g., loading-induced stresses, strains, osmotic and hydraulic pressures, and electric currents and potentials. These factors

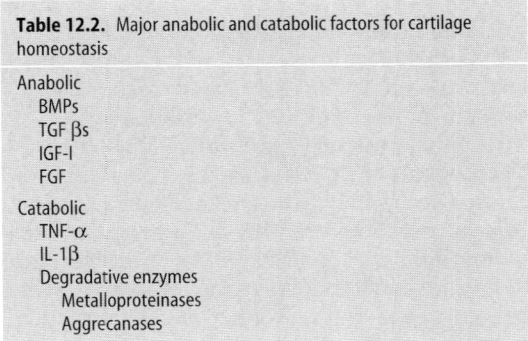

Table 12.2. Major anabolic and catabolic factors for cartilage homeostasis

Anabolic
  BMPs
  TGF βs
  IGF-I
  FGF

Catabolic
  TNF-α
  IL-1β
  Degradative enzymes
    Metalloproteinases
    Aggrecanases

control chondrocyte metabolism and affect cartilage homeostasis in either autocrine or paracrine manner with either anabolic or catabolic effects on the chondrocytes. Of the cytokines with predominantly anabolic activities, members of the transforming growth factor β (TGFβ)/bone morphogenetic protein (BMP) family maintain cartilage homeostasis by stimulating chondrocyte mitogenesis and increasing cartilage matrix synthesis as well as decreasing proteoglycan degradation. They can stimulate chondrocyte differentiation and cartilage formation during development. TGFβ1 has also been shown to protect cartilage against interleukin-1 (IL-1)-induced degradation process. Other important anabolic growth factors for articular cartilage include insulin-like growth factor-I (IGF-I)[32] and fibroblast growth factor (FGF). The cytokines that have catabolic activities include IL-1, tumor necrosis factor-α (TNF-α), IL-17, IL-18, and leukemia inhibitory factor. Cytokines such as IL-6 can have dual effect on chondrocytes.

Mechanical force is another important factor affecting the health of articular cartilage and consequently the function of the joint. That cartilage requires normal mechanical loading to maintain its normal balance of ECM is obvious in in vivo immobilization experiments. In animal models, when limbs are immobilized, the weight-bearing limbs often see increase in cartilage matrix synthesis and content, whereas the immobilized limb incurs decreased matrix synthesis and content, which often leads to cartilage thinning.[33–35] Using a variety of techniques (e.g., X-ray, ultrasound, magnetic resonance imaging), changes in cartilage thickness from 6% to 20% have been observed for physiological load levels of 1–5 body weight.[36–38] The effect of loading also depends on loading magnitude as well as frequency. Many physical and chemical stimuli with potential effects on chondrocytes and its ECM can be generated by loading. These include direct deformational loading on the cell and ECM, hydrostatic pressure, fluid flow and shear stress, osmolarity gradient, streaming potential, and convection of nutrients. Mechanical loading has been demonstrated both in vivo and in vitro to be important for the normal maintenance of articular cartilage and the metabolic response of the chondrocyte, whether the cell is within the native tissue or an artificial three-dimensional construct.[39] However, the mechanism of loading on chondrocyte metabolism, despite intensive investigation, remains largely elusive.

Limb Morphogenesis

There is a current school of thought that adult reparative or regenerative skeletogenesis recapitulates the events of embryonic skeletal development. Therefore, it is important to understand the mechanisms controlling limb morphogenesis and related dysmorphogenesis. Embryonic skeletal development is controlled exquisitely at the levels of gene transcription, cellular signaling, cell–cell and cell–matrix interactions, as well as systemic modulation. Mediators include transcription factors, growth factors, cytokines, metabolites, hormones, as well as environmentally derived influences, and involve the recruitment, commitment, differentiation, and maturation of mesenchymal cells into those in the skeletal tissue lineage, specifically cartilage and bone, along the intramembranous and endochondral ossification pathways.

The limbs develop from paired primordia, referred to as limb fields, along its anterior-posterior body axis. At the early stages of limb development, the buds exhibit a paddle shape consisting of undifferentiated mesenchymal cells derived from the lateral plate and somitic mesoderm, covered by ectoderm. Through the gradual recruitment of cells, precartilage condensation (Figure 12.2) results in closely packed mesenchymal cells in the chondrogenic regions surrounded by the nonchondrogenic mesenchyme. Both in vivo and in vitro observations have demonstrated a high cell density requirement for chondrogenesis to occur.[40–42] Positional information is determined in part by the expression of Hox genes. The process of mesenchymal cell condensation is directed by cell–cell and cell–matrix interactions as well as secreted factors interacting with their cognate receptors. This is correlated with restricted temporal and spatial patterns of ECM expression[43] (Figure 12.2). Before condensation, mesenchymal cells present in the limb secrete an ECM rich in hyaluronan and collagen type I that prevents intimate cell–cell interaction. As condensation begins, an increase in hyaluronidase activity is observed with a decrease in hyaluronan in the ECM. Hyaluronan is thought to facilitate cell

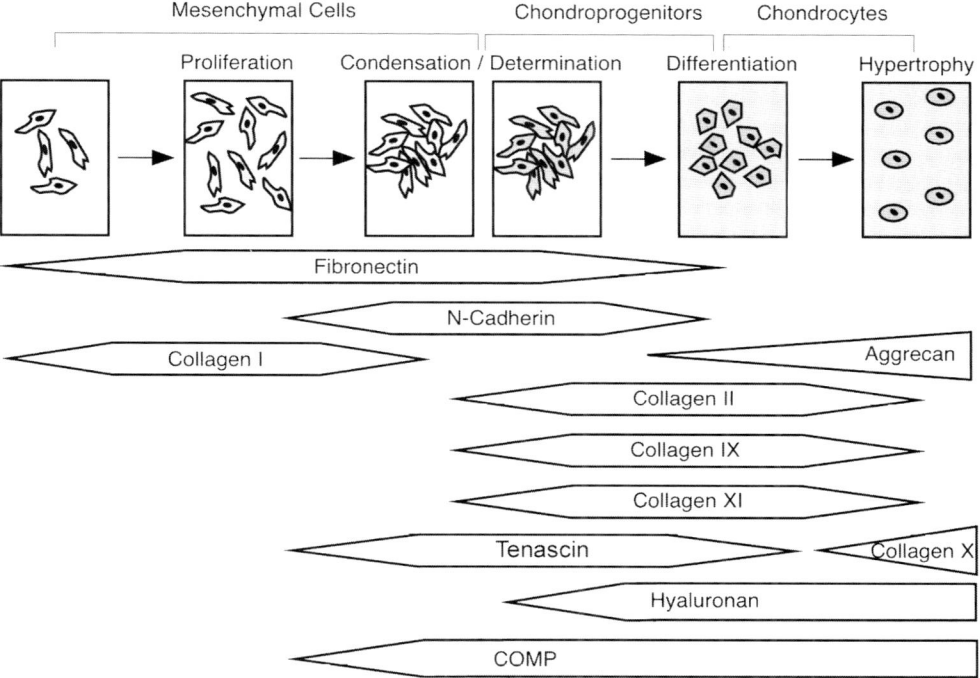

Figure 12.2. Schematic diagram of mesenchymal cell differentiation into chondrocytes and the accompanying alterations in ECM. Loosely arranged mesenchymal cells proliferate and condense, a process regulated by cell–cell adhesion molecules such as N-cadherin. N-cadherin protein production increases specifically during mesenchymal cell condensation/determination and decreases as these chondroprogenitor cells differentiate. The condensing mesenchymal cells undergo cellular determination to become chondroprogenitor cells, differentiate into chondrocytes, and eventually become hypertrophic chondrocytes. Chondroprogenitor determination and chondrocyte differentiation are accompanied by dynamic ECM remodeling. Fibronectin production increases during the proliferation phase of chondrogenesis, but decreases as chondroprogenitor cells differentiate into chondrocytes. Aggrecan expression in the ECM increases as chondrocytes differentiate and become hypertrophic. Collagen type I is present specifically in the matrix of undifferentiated mesenchymal cells, and is replaced by collagen type II as the chondroprogenitors differentiate into chondrocytes. Expression of collagen types IX and XI mirrors the expression pattern of collagen type II. Collagen type X is present in the ECM of only hypertrophic chondrocytes. The presence of tenascin in the ECM increases during mesenchymal cell condensation, is maintained through chondroprogenitor cell differentiation and is reduced as these cells differentiate. Hyaluronan is found in the ECM of chondroprogenitor cells and is maintained through chondrocyte hypertrophy. COMP expression localizes to the ECM of condensing mesenchymal cells and remains through cellular hypertrophy. (*Source:* Shum et al.[43])

movement and the increase in hyaluronidase and subsequent decrease in hyaluronan allows for close cell–cell interactions.[44–47] The establishment of cell–cell interactions is presumably involved in triggering one or more signal transduction pathways that initiate chondrogenic differentiation. Two cell adhesion molecules implicated in this process are N-cadherin and N-CAM. Both of these molecules are expressed in condensing mesenchyme and then disappear in differentiating cartilage.[48,49] Perturbing the function(s) of N-cadherin[50] or N-CAM[51] causes reduction or alterations in chondrogenesis both in vitro and in vivo, further supporting a role for these cell adhesion molecules in mediating the mesenchymal condensation step.

In addition to cell–cell interactions, cell–matrix interactions also seem to have an important role in mesenchymal cell condensation. The involvement of fibronectins, syndecans, tenascins, thrombospondins, focal adhesion kinase, and paxillin in this process have been reported.[52–55] Cell–cell and cell–matrix interactions activate cytoplasmic kinases, phosphatases, and GTPases that can, in turn, be modulated by signaling from growth and differentiation factors, such as the BMPs and Wnts.[56–58]

After condensation, osteoprogenitor and chondroprogenitor cells initiate their differentiation while neighboring cells undergo apoptosis, thus defining the boundaries of the developing skeletal elements. Mesenchymal condensations followed by chondrocyte differentiation and maturation occur in digital zones, whereas mesenchymal cells undergo apoptotic elimination in interdigital web zones to give rise to the delineation of the digits.[59] BMP, GDF5, and Wnt-14 signaling are key regulators of interdigital apoptosis and digit patterning,[60,61] and FGF2 has been shown to antagonize BMP-4 apoptotic effect.[62] Cellular differentiation into chondrocytes includes an increase in proteoglycan and collagen type II secretion into the ECM.[63,64] In the growth plate, during endochondral ossification, proliferating chondrocytes exit the cell cycle, become rounded, and undergo hypertrophy. The hypertrophic chondrocyte secretes a new ECM rich in collagen type X and increased levels of alkaline phosphatase whereas the secretion of collagen types II and IX is reduced[65,66] (Figure 12.2). Chondrocyte proliferation and maturation in the growth plate is regulated by a negative feedback loop of intercellular communication mediated by the secreted signaling molecules, parathyroid hormone-related protein (PTHrP) and Indian hedgehog (Ihh).[67–69] Regulation and coordination of the rates of chondrocyte proliferation, hypertrophic maturation, apoptosis, and bone collar formation are essential to normal bone morphogenesis.

It is obvious that skeletal morphogenesis requires the intricate interaction and coordination of various signaling molecules and structural molecules. Mutations that cause disruption to both the structural proteins and signaling molecules of growth factors, their receptors, and the ensuing intracellular signaling pathways have been found to lead to congenital skeletal and limb defects (see review by Shum et al.[43]).

Current Approaches to Cartilage Repair

Age-related degenerative diseases such as osteoarthritis, trauma-induced injury, bone tumors, and genetic and developmental abnormalities are the principal causes of cartilage tissue damage or loss. In clinical settings, the consequences of these damages manifest as joint stiffness or locking, swelling, pain, and ultimately immobility. In the United States, osteoarthritis affects approximately 20 million people, and its incidence increases with age, with most people older than 60 years of age having varying degree of osteoarthritis in at least one joint. Because of its acellular and avascular nature, damaged cartilage lacks the ability to repair and regenerate, and degeneration is generally irreversible. Chondral defects are challenging in terms of achieving adequate tissue healing. Naturally occurring repair processes after cartilage damage often give rise to fibrocartilage tissues, which are mechanically inferior and may ultimately lead to tissue necrosis and loss.

Various surgical interventions and procedures have been in use for patients to relieve pain and regain joint function. Relatively simple procedures include lavage, shaving, and laser abrasion; drilling, including microfracture of the subchondral bone for focal chondral defects, aim at eliciting help from subchondral bone and marrow space to induce spontaneous cartilage repair; more extensive surgical procedures include autogenic or allogeneic osteochondral transplantation, and autologous perichondral and periosteal graft; and recently, autologous chondrocyte implantation technique has shown promises with short-term patient satisfaction.[70] Drastic measures of total joint replacement remains the choice today for large area lesion or joint destruction, although this procedure itself is a risky procedure, especially for elderly patients who are mostly affected. The above procedures have been successful to varying degrees in treating articular defects; however, short of total joint replacement, they are effective only for treating chondral defects of limited sizes. Availability of tissue graft material and donor site morbidity remain problematic.[70] Therefore, there is a need for tissue engineered constructs that closely mimic the native tissue in both structure and functionality, that preferably do not utilize cells from cartilage. Because of the ease of isolation and expansion, and the multiple differentiation potential, the MSCs are gaining acceptance as the cell type of choice for future cartilage repair and functional tissue engineering.

Cartilage Tissue Engineering

The clinical need for improved treatment options for the numerous patients with cartilage injuries has motivated tissue engineering aimed at the generation of cartilage replacement tissues in vitro that can meet the functional demands in vivo. Two types of tissue engineering approaches are used, one being constructed entirely in vitro with full functionality before transplantation, the second being constructed partially in vitro followed by transplantation for full in vivo differentiation. In either case, three fundamental components determine the success of a tissue engineered construct: Scaffold, responsive cells, and an environment that promotes the differentiation of cells and regeneration of the tissue structure.

The three-dimensional properties of tissues, particularly those of the skeleton including the cartilage, require that tissue engineered replacement be produced with the appropriate shape and form that can be achieved by the use of appropriate scaffolds. The desired characteristics of a tissue engineered scaffold would include biocompatibility, bioresorbability, and biodegradability upon tissue healing. In addition, the scaffold should be highly porous to permit cell penetration and tissue impregnation, permeable enough to facilitate nutrient delivery and gas exchange, and adaptable to and strong enough to withstand the mechanical environment. Moreover, the scaffold should have a surface that is conducive to cell attachment and migration to permit appropriate extracellular assembly and the transmittal of signaling molecules. Additional modification of the scaffold may involve bioactivation, in that the cells are not merely lodged in the matrix but are exposed to an environment that is conducive to tissue generation. Various types of matrices for cartilage tissue engineering are under investigation, and have been tested either in vitro, or in vivo. These matrices include the protein-based matrices of collagen, fibrin, gelatin, carbohydrate-based scaffolds including agarose, alginate, hyaluronan, chitosan, polylactic/polyglycolic acids, and synthetic polymers of carbon fiber and Teflon-based meshes (for review, see Hunziker[70]). These matrices show varying degrees of success, although none has fulfilled the requirement of an ideal matrix for human implantation.

The cells are important for the production of new replacement tissue through synthesis and assembly of the ECM, and are important for the long-term stability and the success of the tissue engineered constructs. Although naked matrices have been used for cartilage repair, studies have shown that in most cases cartilage repair is improved with cell-seeded scaffolds than with acellular scaffolds alone (e.g., see Kawamura et al.[71] and Rahfoth et al.[72]). Until now, one of the major limitations of tissue engineering has been the successful isolation, expansion, and maintenance of tissue-specific cells. For example, chondrocytes, when isolated and expanded in vitro, will dedifferentiate into fibroblast-like cells that cease to make cartilage-specific matrix proteins. Although these dedifferentiated cells can be redifferentiated into chondrocytes using various techniques, the degree of cell differentiation is uncertain.[73,74] Therefore, the alternative use of multipotential and almost unlimited MSCs instead of committed and limited tissue-specific cells represents an attractive and powerful alternative approach.

Tissue engineering is dependent on the local environment to initiate and maintain the functional cell/tissue type and, therefore, the successful outcome of the engineered constructs. In general, the environment consists of bioactive factors, including signaling molecules, appropriate ECM, and mechanical stimulation. Different anabolic growth factors that are shown to be important for cartilage differentiation and anabolic activity, including IGF-I and members of the TGFβ and the BMP family, including BMP-2, BMP-7, BMP-9, BMP-12, and BMP-13, have been shown to expand the cell population, to increase the production of the appropriate ECM, and to influence the differentiation state of the cells during in vitro culture, which ultimately improves the outcome of cartilage tissue engineering.[75-82] In addition, various forms of physical stimuli have been successfully used to stimulate cartilage matrix production and improve mechanical strength.[83-86] Under in vivo physiological conditions, the loading of diarthrodial joints is generally cyclical and/or intermittent.[87,88] Engineered cartilage constructs subjected to cyclical deformational loading have been found to respond with biosynthetic and gene expression changes similar to articular cartilage explants.[85,86,89-91] In contrast, long-term (up to 12 months) free swelling cultures are unable to achieve material properties similar to either dynamically loaded constructs or the native tissue. Using combinations of growth factors and various mechanical stimulation, in vitro cartilage tissue engineering has generated cartilage tissues with proteoglycan and collagen contents as well as mechanical strength approaching, yet never as high as, the native articular cartilage tissue.[85,92] So far, the experimental challenges in cartilage tissue engineering remain to be the identification of an appropriate source of chondrogenic cells, stimulation and maintenance of chondrocyte cell phenotype, and the development of an adequate three-dimensional matrix.

MSCs and Cartilage Regeneration

Since the groundbreaking work of Friedenstein et al.,[93] who isolated bone-forming progenitor cells from rat marrow, it has been widely accepted that there exists in bone marrow nonhematopoietic progenitor cells with the potential to develop into a variety of mesenchymal as well as nonmesenchymal cells. These are called the mesenchymal stem cells – MSCs.[94] Derived from adult tissues, MSCs can differentiate into various cell types of mesenchymal tissues, including cartilage,[95-98] bone,[99-101] fat,[97] muscle,[102-104] tendon,[105,106] and hematopoietic supporting marrow stroma[107] (Figure 12.3). In addition, MSCs have been shown to be able to differentiate into neural tissues.[108] Although MSCs represent a very small fraction (0.001%–0.01%) of the total population of nucleated cells in marrow,[97] they can be easily isolated from bone marrow and can be extensively expanded by in vitro cultivation without obvious spontaneous differentiation whereas retaining the potential of differentiation upon appropriate stimulation (Figure 12.3).[97,109-111] Techniques for isolation of the bone marrow-derived MSCs range from simple direct plating, to density gradient centrifugation, and magnetic bead sorting based on cell surface markers. The isolated MSCs can be grown in the presence of selective batches of fetal bovine serum, and can remain in a stable undifferentiated state upon long-term culture up to 30–40 passages.[97]

Although bone marrow stroma remains the most accessible and enriched source for MSCs, multipotential cells have been isolated from almost all tissues, including adipose,[112] periosteum,[113,114] synovial membrane,[115,116] muscle,[117,118] dermis,[117] deciduous teeth,[119] pericytes,[120] blood,[121] bone marrow,[97] trabecular bone,[122,123] infrapatellar fat pad,[124] and articular cartilage[125-127] (Table 12.3). The origin of these tissue stem cells remains unclear at present. They can be derived from local tissue-specific cells or recruited remotely, e.g., from bone marrow. Furthermore, what role or advantage, if any, these cells contribute to disease progression or tissue regeneration, in comparison with bone marrow-derived MSCs, needs further investigation.

There has been evidence indicating the decreasing proliferation and differentiation activities of MSCs with age and/or with diseases, e.g., osteoporosis and osteoarthritis.[128-130] For example, bone marrow MSCs isolated from patients with advanced osteoarthritis exhibit significantly lower proliferative capacity and significant reduction in in vitro chondrogenic and adipogenic activities compared with MSCs from normal controls. It remains to be determined whether or not the characteristics of MSCs from these diseases are different from those of healthy individuals, and the underlying reasons for the differences. This might affect the usefulness of autologous MSCs for tissue repair in eventual clinical settings.

Experimentally, MSCs are identified by the expression of Thy-1 (CD90), endoglin (CD105), hyaluronic acid receptor CD44, integrin $\alpha 1$ subunit CD29, and activated leukocyte cell-adhesion molecules, as well as SH3 and SH4 antigen, and are negative for the hematopoietic markers (CD34, CD45, CD14) (for review, see Minguell[131]). Inconsistency in the literature on the growth characteristics and differentiation potential of MSCs underscores the need for a functional definition of MSCs. At present, there is lack of a unifying definition as well as information on specific markers that define the cell types characterized as MSCs, with the sole definition being their ability to (1) differentiate along specific mesenchymal lineages when induced to do so, (2) remain in an undifferentiated state until provided the signal to divide asymmetrically, and, finally, (3) undergo many more replicative cycles than normal, fully differentiated cells.

Although there have been numerous data describing the lineage induction and associated lineage-specific molecular expression in MSCs (see Figure 12.3), the biological mechanisms responsible for the broad developmental potential of adult MSCs remain largely unclear. Extensive knowledge regarding MSC lineage development, especially regarding MSC differentiation control by various growth factors and their underlying signaling pathways, and factors regulating the complete differentiation capacity, will be essential for future development of MSCs

Cartilage

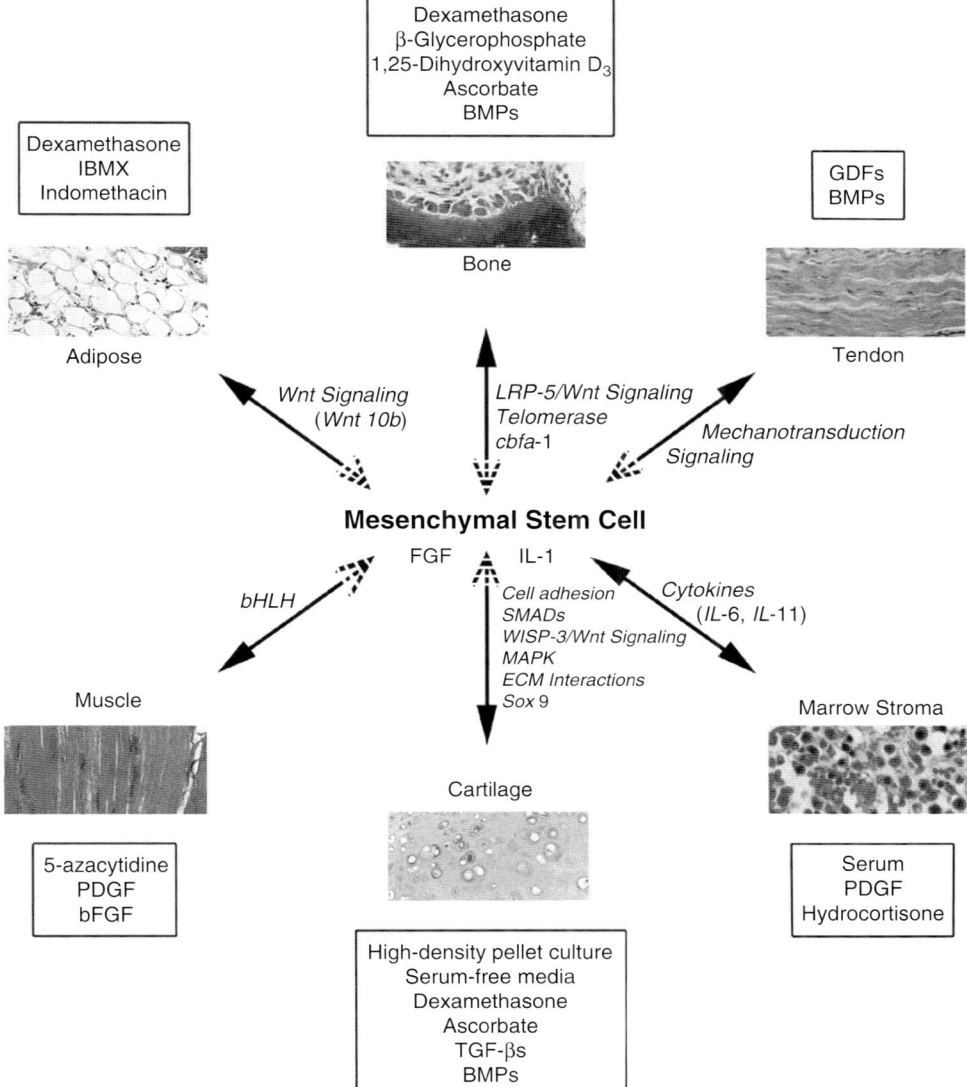

Figure 12.3. Lineage potential of adult human mesenchymal stem cells (MSCs). MSCs are characterized by their multilineage differentiation potentials, including bone, cartilage, adipose, muscle, tendon, and stroma. This figure depicts some of the in vitro culture conditions (boxed) that promote the respective differentiation process into a specific lineage. Known signaling pathways and/or components or events shown to be involved in lineage-specific differentiation are in italics. Dotted arrowheads denote potential "reverse" differentiation events. (Adapted from Tuan et al.[147])

for the purpose of tissue engineering and clinical application. Molecules involved in the Wnt signaling pathways, including the various Wnts, their receptor Frizzleds, and inhibitors Dickkopf-1 (Dkk1) and secreted frizzled-related proteins (sFRP1), are critical factors involved in the differentiation of MSCs along the chondrogenic pathways.[132,133] In recapitulation of limb chondrogenesis in which cell–cell contacts have pivotal roles in initiating chondrogenic differentiation, pellet or micromass culture of MSCs have been used in vitro to initiate chondrogenic differentiation in chemically defined serum-free medium supplemented with TGFβ1, TGFβ2, or

Table 12.3. Sources of multipotential adult mesenchymal stem cells

Source tissue	Multilineage differentiation potential
Bone marrow	Adipocyte
	Astrocyte
	Neuron
	Cardiomyocyte
	Hepatocyte
	Mesangial cell
	Muscle
	Chondrocyte
	Osteoblast
	Stromal cell
	Various embryonic tissue lineages
Muscle	Endothelial cell, neuron
	Adipocyte, myotubes, osteocyte
	Chondrocyte
	Osteoblast
Trabecular bone	Adipocyte, chondrocyte, osteoblast
Dermis	Adipocyte, chondrocyte, muscle, osteoblast
Adipose	Chondrocyte, muscle, osteoblast
	Stromal cell
Periosteum	Chondrocyte, osteoblast
Pericyte	Chondrocyte
	Osteoblast
Blood	Adipocyte, fibroblast, osteoblast, osteoclast
Synovial membrane	Adipocyte, chondrocyte, muscle, osteoblast
Articular cartilage	Osteoblast, chondrocyte, adipocyte
Placenta	Chondrocyte, osteoblast, adipocyte
Cord blood	Chondrocyte, osteoblast, adipocyte

Source: Adapted from Tuan et al.[147]

TGFβ3.[96,98,134] It has been shown that TGFβ1 activated TGFβ as well as Wnt signaling pathways in promoting MSC differentiation into chondrocytes.[135] TGFβ-mediated chondrogenesis of human mesenchymal progenitor cells also involves N-cadherin and mitogen-activated protein kinase and Wnt signaling crosstalk.[136] In addition, IGF-I, BMP-2, BMP-6, BMP-7, and BMP-9 may also enhance chondrogenic differentiation.

There are increasing numbers of reports concerning the hypoimmunogenic nature of the MSCs. Undifferentiated MSCs and differentiated MSCs do not elicit alloreactive lymphocyte proliferative responses and modulate immune responses. In animal models, MSCs delay graft rejection,[137,138] and in children with osteogenesis imperfecta, allogeneic bone marrow transplantation resulted in engraftment of donor-derived MSCs and new bone formation.[139] The immuno-privilege of MSCs suggests that MSCs can be potentially transplantable between human leukocyte antigen-incompatible individuals. However, MSCs have also been shown to inhibit T cell proliferation through an immunosuppressive effect mediated by CD8 regulatory T cells and permit tumor growth in allogeneic recipients.[140]

The usefulness of MSCs for cartilage repair has been demonstrated in studies with animal models. In a New Zealand white rabbit model in which full-thickness lesions were mechanically induced and filled with collagen sponges loaded with MSCs, MSCs were shown to differentiate into chondrocytes that secreted a cartilaginous matrix, which was then replaced by bone in the subchondral zone to reconstitute the different layers in the femoral condyle.[141] In a goat model in which osteoarthritis was induced by medial meniscectomy and anterior cruciate ligament resection, intraarticular injection of MSCs labeled with green fluorescent protein showed cartilage healing, with increased proteoglycan content and reduced fibrillar lesions. Along with marked regeneration of the medial meniscus, there is engraftment of the labeled cells in the regenerated meniscus, fat pad, and synovium. However, there is no apparent incorporation of the MSCs into the damaged articular cartilage. Despite this, degeneration of the articular cartilage, osteophytic remodeling, and subchondral sclerosis were reduced in cell-treated joints compared with joints treated with vehicle alone without cells.[142]

In view of their use in tissue engineering of articular cartilage, it has been shown in various culture systems that MSCs are able to differentiate into chondrocyte lineage in three-dimensional matrices.[143-147] For example, when MSCs from skeletally mature goats were encapsulated in a photopolymerizing poly(ethylene glycol)-based hydrogel and cultured with TGFβ1, the encapsulated MSCs form cartilage-like tissue in vitro, expressing aggrecan, link protein, and type II collagen.[144] In our own laboratory, a three-dimensional amalgam scaffold consisting of the biodegradable polymer poly-L-lactic acid (PLA) and alginate was used to study the chondrogenic potential of adult human MSCs. The alginate was used to improve cell loading and retention within the construct, and PLA scaffold to provide adequate mechanical strength and structural stability. With TGFβ1 as stimulant, by day 21, expression of cartilage-specific ECM proteins were detected in the constructs, including collagen types II and IX, and aggrecan.[145] In another system, human adult MSCs readily attached to electron spun nanofibrous scaffold made of a synthetic biodegradable polymer, poly(ε-caprolactone). In the presence of TGFβ1, the MSCs differentiated to a chondrocytic phenotype, as evidenced by chondrocyte-specific gene expression and synthesis of cartilage-associated ECM proteins. The levels of chondrogenesis observed in MSCs seeded within the nanofibrous scaffold were comparable to that observed for MSCs maintained as cell aggregates or pellets.[146] These studies demonstrate the feasibility of using human adult MSCs for in vitro cartilage tissue engineering. Future investigations need to better define bioactive factors and suitable scaffolds that can promote complete and specific articular cartilage phenotypic differentiation, that support the in vitro fabrication of tissue engineered constructs with ECM composites, and mechanical properties that closely approximate the native mature articular cartilage.

Summary and Future Perspectives

Articular cartilage is the major load-bearing tissue of the body, and is vital for the mobility and health of humans. Because of its limited potential to self-repair and regenerate, and the increasing incidence of cartilage degeneration in the aging, yet active, population, there is an increasing demand for cartilage tissue engineering to produce a cartilage tissue construct that can replace the damaged tissue and meet the functional demands in vivo. The success of cartilage tissue engineering depends on three interacting components: Scaffold, cells, and bioactive factors. Because of their ease of isolation and expansion as well as multipotential differentiation, MSCs undoubtedly are most desirable as the cell source for cartilage tissue engineering. Numerous studies, based on the notion that MSC differentiation recapitulates events of embryonic limb development, have identified factors that are important for MSC chondrogenic differentiation. However, the microenvironment within the mature cartilage tissue, and the unclear origin and characterization of the various sources of MSCs, call for rigorous and systematic investigations into the mechanisms of adult MSC phenotypic differentiation modulation. The feasibility of using adult MSCs for cartilage repair and cartilage tissue engineering promises great potential for eventual clinical use, and demands rational design and strategies that combine optimal scaffold and bioactive factors that will ultimately push the MSCs along complete and true articular chondrogenic differentiation pathway, and regenerate a tissue either in vitro, or in vivo, that reproduces the structural and functional properties of the native, healthy tissue. Along the line of functional cartilage tissue engineering using adult MSCs, a few issues warrant further investigation. There remain to be formulated rigorous standards for tissue engineered construct, be it cartilage ECM composition, or mechanical strength, that can best predict the functional success of the construct in vivo. This entails studies on the long-term behavior of MSCs associated with the biomaterials and implanted in pathological joints that present an inflammatory and catabolic environment that is also biomechanically demanding. Integration of the grafts into host tissues remains problematic and requires further investigation. In addition, more studies are needed to generate fully functional tissue constructs with zonal distribution of cells and organization of ECM that is characteristic of articular cartilage, with distinct architecture of the superficial, middle, and deep zones.

Acknowledgment

This work was supported by NIH Z01 41131.

References

1. Mankin HJ, Mow VC, Buckwalter JA, Ianotti JP, Ratcliffe A. Articular cartilage structure, composition and function. In: Buckwalter JA, Einhorn TA, Simon SR, eds. Orthopaedic Basic Science: Biology and Biomechanics of the Musculoskeletal System. Rosemont, IL: American Academy of Orthopaedic Surgeon; 2000:443–470.
2. Mow VC, Ratcliffe A, Poole AR. Cartilage and diarthrodial joints as paradigms for hierarchical materials and structures. Biomaterials 1992;13:67–97.
3. Ahmed AM, Burke DL. In-vitro measurement of static pressure distribution in synovial joints. Part I. Tibial surface of the knee. J Biomech Eng 1983;105:216–225.
4. Ahmed AM, Burke DL, Yu A. In-vitro measurement of static pressure distribution in synovial joints. Part II. Retropatellar surface. J Biomech Eng 1983;105:226–236.

5. Greenwald AS, O'Connor JJ. The transmission of load through the human hip joint. J Biomech 1971;4:507–528.
6. Hodge WA, Fijan RS, Carlson KL, et al. Contact pressures in the human hip joint measured in vivo. Proc Natl Acad Sci USA 1986;83:2879–2883.
7. Maroudas A. Physicochemical properties of articular cartilage. In: Freeman MAR, ed. Adult Articular Cartilage. Kent, UK: Pitman Medical Publishing; 1979:215–290.
8. Buschmann MD, Grodzinsky AJ. A molecular model of proteoglycan-associated electrostatic forces in cartilage mechanics. J Biomech Eng 1995;117:170–192.
9. Lai WM, Hou JS, Mow VC. A triphasic theory for the swelling and deformation behaviors of articular cartilage. J Biomech Eng 1991;113:245–258.
10. Hardingham TE, Fosang AJ, Dudhia J. Aggrecan, the chondroitin sulfate/keratan sulfate proteoglycan from cartilage. In: Kuettner KE, Schleyerbach R, Peyron JG, Hascall VC, eds. Articular Cartilage and Osteoarthritis. New York: Raven Press; 1992:5–20.
11. Mow VC, Gu WY, Chen FH. Structure and function of articular cartilage and meniscus. In: Mow VC, Huiskes R, eds. Basic Orthopaedic Biomechanics and Mechanobiology. Philadelphia: Lippincott-Raven; 2005:183–258.
12. Kempson GE. Mechanical properties of articular cartilage. In: Freeman MAR, ed. Adult Articular Cartilage. Kent, UK: Pitman Medical; 1979:333–414.
13. Kempson GE, Tuke MA, Dingle JT, Barrett AJ, Horsfield PH. The effects of proteolytic enzymes on the mechanical properties of adult human articular cartilage. Biochim Biophys Acta 1976;428:741–760.
14. Kempson GE, Muir H, Swanson SA, Freeman MA. Correlations between stiffness and the chemical constituents of cartilage on the human femoral head. Biochim Biophys Acta 1970;215:70–77.
15. Williamson AK, Chen AC, Sah RL. Compressive properties and function-composition relationships of developing bovine articular cartilage. J Orthop Res 2001;19:1113–1121.
16. Ameye L, Aria D, Jepsen K, et al. Abnormal collagen fibrils in tendons of biglycan/fibromodulin-deficient mice lead to gait impairment, ectopic ossification, and osteoarthritis. FASEB J 2002;16:673–680.
17. Neame PJ, Kay CJ, McQuillan DJ, Beales MP, Hassell JR. Independent modulation of collagen fibrillogenesis by decorin and lumican. Cell Mol Life Sci 2000;57:859–863.
18. Danielson KG, Baribault H, Holmes DF, et al. Targeted disruption of decorin leads to abnormal collagen fibril morphology and skin fragility. J Cell Biol 1997;136:729–743.
19. Eggli PS, Hunziker EB, Schenk RK. Quantitation of structural features characterizing weight- and less-weight-bearing regions in articular cartilage: a stereological analysis of medial femoral condyles in young adult rabbits. Anat Rec 1988;222:217–227.
20. Wong M, Wuethrich P, Eggli P, Hunziker EB. Zone-specific cell biosynthetic activity in mature bovine articular cartilage: a new method using confocal microscopic stereology and quantitative autoradiography. J Orthop Res 1996;14:424–432.
21. Lipshitz H, Etheredge R 3rd, Glimcher MJ. Changes in the hexosamine content and swelling ratio of articular cartilage as functions of depth from the surface. J Bone Joint Surg 1976;58:1149–1153.
22. Muir H, Bullough P, Maroudas A. The distribution of collagen in human articular cartilage with some of its physiological implications. J Bone Joint Surg 1970;52:554–563.
23. Clark JM. The organization of collagen in cryofractured rabbit articular cartilage: a scanning electron microscopic study. J Orthop Res 1985;3:17–29.
24. Mow VC, Lai WM. Some surface characteristics of articular cartilage. I. A scanning electron microscopy study and a theoretical model for the dynamic interaction of synovial fluid and articular cartilage. J Biomech 1974;7:449–456.
25. Weiss C, Rosenberg L, Helfet AJ. An ultrastructural study of normal young adult human articular cartilage. J Bone Joint Surg 1968;50:663–674.
26. Roth V, Mow VC. The intrinsic tensile behavior of the matrix of bovine articular cartilage and its variation with age. J Bone Joint Surg 1980;62:1102–1117.
27. Kempson GE, Muir H, Pollard C, Tuke M. The tensile properties of the cartilage of human femoral condyles related to the content of collagen and glycosaminoglycans. Biochim Biophys Acta 1973;297:456–472.
28. Franzen A, Inerot S, Hejderup SO, Heinegard D. Variations in the composition of bovine hip articular cartilage with distance from the articular surface. Biochem J 1981;195:535–543.
29. Broom ND. The collagen framework of articular cartilage: its profound influence on normal and abnormal load-bearing function. In: Nimni ME, ed. Collagen: Chemistry, Biology and Biotechnology. Boca Raton, FL: CRC Press; 1988:243–265.
30. Redler I, Mow VC, Zimny ML, Mansell J. The ultrastructure and biomechanical significance of the tidemark of articular cartilage. Clin Orthop Relat Res 1975;112:357–362.
31. Wu JZ, Herzog W. Elastic anisotropy of articular cartilage is associated with the microstructures of collagen fibers and chondrocytes. J Biomech 2002;35:931–942.
32. Trippel SB. Growth factor actions on articular cartilage. J Rheumatol Suppl 1995;43:129–132.
33. Jortikka MO, Inkinen RI, Tammi MI, et al. Immobilisation causes longlasting matrix changes both in the immobilised and contralateral joint cartilage. Ann Rheum Dis 1997;56:255–261.
34. Palmoski M, Perricone E, Brandt KD. Development and reversal of a proteoglycan aggregation defect in normal canine knee cartilage after immobilization. Arthritis Rheum 1979;22:508–517.
35. Kiviranta I, Jurvelin J, Tammi M, Saamanen AM, Helminen HJ. Weight bearing controls glycosaminoglycan concentration and articular cartilage thickness in the knee joints of young beagle dogs. Arthritis Rheum 1987;30:801–809.
36. Armstrong CG, Bahrani AS, Gardner DL. In vitro measurement of articular cartilage deformations in the intact human hip joint under load. J Bone Joint Surg Am 1979;61:744–755.
37. Macirowski T, Tepic S, Mann RW. Cartilage stresses in the human hip joint. J Biomech Eng 1994;116:10–18.
38. Eckstein F, Tieschky M, Faber SC, et al. Effect of physical exercise on cartilage volume and thickness in vivo: MR imaging study. Radiology 1998;207:243–248.
39. Guilak F, Hung CT. Physical regulation of cartilage metabolism. In: Mow VC, Huiskies R, eds. Basic Orthopaedic Biomechanics. Philadelphia: Lippincott-Raven; 2005:259–300.

40. Ahrens PB, Solursh M, Reiter RS. Stage-related capacity for limb chondrogenesis in cell culture. Dev Biol 1977;60:69–82.
41. DeLise AM, Stringa E, Woodward WA, Mello MA, Tuan RS. Embryonic limb mesenchyme micromass culture as an in vitro model for chondrogenesis and cartilage maturation. Methods Mol Biol 2000;137:359–375.
42. San Antonio JD, Tuan RS. Chondrogenesis of limb bud mesenchyme in vitro: stimulation by cations. Dev Biol 1986;115:313–324.
43. Shum L, Coleman CM, Hatakeyama Y, Tuan RS. Morphogenesis and dysmorphogenesis of the appendicular skeleton. Birth Defects Res C Embryo Today 2003;69:102–122.
44. Knudson CB, Toole BP. Hyaluronate-cell interactions during differentiation of chick embryo limb mesoderm. Dev Biol 1987;124:82–90.
45. Knudson CB. Hyaluronan and CD44: strategic players for cell-matrix interactions during chondrogenesis and matrix assembly. Birth Defects Res C Embryo Today 2003;69:174–196.
46. Toole BP, Jackson G, Gross J. Hyaluronate in morphogenesis: inhibition of chondrogenesis in vitro. Proc Natl Acad Sci USA 1972;69:1384–1386.
47. Toole BP, Linsenmayer TF. Newer knowledge of skeletogenesis: macromolecular transitions in the extracellular matrix. Clin Orthop Relat Res 1977;129:258–278.
48. Oberlender SA, Tuan RS. Spatiotemporal profile of N-cadherin expression in the developing limb mesenchyme. Cell Adhes Commun 1994;2:521–537.
49. Tavella S, Raffo P, Tacchetti C, Cancedda R, Castagnola P. N-CAM and N-cadherin expression during in vitro chondrogenesis. Exp Cell Res 1994;215:354–362.
50. Oberlender SA, Tuan RS. Expression and functional involvement of N-cadherin in embryonic limb chondrogenesis. Development 1994;120:177–187.
51. Widelitz RB, Jiang TX, Murray BA, Chuong CM. Adhesion molecules in skeletogenesis. II. Neural cell adhesion molecules mediate precartilaginous mesenchymal condensations and enhance chondrogenesis. J Cell Physiol 1993;156:399–411.
52. Gehris AL, Stringa E, Spina J, et al. The region encoded by the alternatively spliced exon IIIA in mesenchymal fibronectin appears essential for chondrogenesis at the level of cellular condensation. Dev Biol 1997;190:191–205.
53. Bang OS, Kim EJ, Chung JG, et al. Association of focal adhesion kinase with fibronectin and paxillin is required for precartilage condensation of chick mesenchymal cells. Biochem Biophys Res Commun 2000;278:522–529.
54. Seghatoleslami MR, Kosher RA. Inhibition of in vitro limb cartilage differentiation by syndecan-3 antibodies. Dev Dyn 1996;207:114–119.
55. Mackie EJ, Thesleff I, Chiquet-Ehrismann R. Tenascin is associated with chondrogenic and osteogenic differentiation in vivo and promotes chondrogenesis in vitro. J Cell Biol 1987;105:2569–2579.
56. Haas AR, Tuan RS. Chondrogenic differentiation of murine C3H10T1/2 multipotential mesenchymal cells. II. Stimulation by bone morphogenetic protein-2 requires modulation of N-cadherin expression and function. Differentiation 1999;64:77–89.
57. Stott NS, Jiang TX, Chuong CM. Successive formative stages of precartilaginous mesenchymal condensations in vitro: modulation of cell adhesion by Wnt-7A and BMP-2. J Cell Physiol 1999;180:314–324.
58. Oh CD, Chang SH, Yoon YM, et al. Opposing role of mitogen-activated protein kinase subtypes, erk-1/2 and p38, in the regulation of chondrogenesis of mesenchymes. J Biol Chem 2000;275:5613–5619.
59. Pizette S, Niswander L. Early steps in limb patterning and chondrogenesis. Novartis Found Symp 2001;232:23–36.
60. Hogan BL. Bone morphogenetic proteins: multifunctional regulators of vertebrate development. Genes Dev 1996;10:1580–1594.
61. Macias D, Ganan Y, Sampath TK, et al. Role of BMP-2 and OP-1 (BMP-7) in programmed cell death and skeletogenesis during chick limb development. Development 1997;124:1109–1117.
62. Merino R, Ganan Y, Macias D, et al. Morphogenesis of digits in the avian limb is controlled by FGFs, TGFbetas, and noggin through BMP signaling. Dev Biol 1998;200:35–45.
63. Archer CW, Rooney P, Wolpert L. Cell shape and cartilage differentiation of early chick limb bud cells in culture. Cell Differ 1982;11:245–251.
64. Shinomura T, Kimata K, Oike Y, et al. Appearance of distinct types of proteoglycan in a well-defined temporal and spatial pattern during early cartilage formation in the chick limb. Dev Biol 1984;103:211–220.
65. Schmid TM, Linsenmayer TF. Immunohistochemical localization of short chain cartilage collagen (type X) in avian tissues. J Cell Biol 1985;100:598–605.
66. Osdoby P, Caplan AI. Characterization of a bone-specific alkaline phosphatase in chick limb mesenchymal cell cultures. Dev Biol 1981;86:136–146.
67. Kronenberg HM, Karaplis AC, Lanske B. Role of parathyroid hormone-related protein in skeletal development. Ann NY Acad Sci 1996;785:119–123.
68. Lanske B, Karaplis AC, Lee K, et al. PTH/PTHrP receptor in early development and Indian hedgehog-regulated bone growth. Science 1996;273:663–666.
69. Vortkamp A, Lee K, Lanske B, et al. Regulation of rate of cartilage differentiation by Indian hedgehog and PTH-related protein. Science 1996;273:613–622.
70. Hunziker EB. Articular cartilage repair: basic science and clinical progress. A review of the current status and prospects. Osteoarthritis Cartilage 2002;10:432–463.
71. Kawamura S, Wakitani S, Kimura T, et al. Articular cartilage repair. Rabbit experiments with a collagen gel-biomatrix and chondrocytes cultured in it. Acta Orthop Scand 1998;69:56–62.
72. Rahfoth B, Weisser J, Sternkopf F, et al. Transplantation of allograft chondrocytes embedded in agarose gel into cartilage defects of rabbits. Osteoarthritis Cartilage 1998;6:50–65.
73. Benya PD, Shaffer JD. Dedifferentiated chondrocytes reexpress the differentiated collagen phenotype when cultured in agarose gels. Cell 1982;30:215–224.
74. Zaucke F, Dinser R, Maurer P, Paulsson M. Cartilage oligomeric matrix protein (COMP) and collagen IX are sensitive markers for the differentiation state of articular primary chondrocytes. Biochem J 2001;358:17–24.
75. Hunziker EB. Growth-factor-induced healing of partial-thickness defects in adult articular cartilage. Osteoarthritis Cartilage 2001;9:22–32.
76. Flechtenmacher J, Huch K, Thonar EJ, et al. Recombinant human osteogenic protein 1 is a potent stimulator of the synthesis of cartilage proteoglycans and collagens by human articular chondrocytes. Arthritis Rheum 1996;39:1896–1904.

77. Jelic M, Pecina M, Haspl M, et al. Regeneration of articular cartilage chondral defects by osteogenic protein-1 (bone morphogenetic protein-7) in sheep. Growth Factors 2001;19:101–113.
78. Blunk T, Sieminski AL, Appel B, et al. Bone morphogenetic protein 9: a potent modulator of cartilage development in vitro. Growth Factors 2003;21:71–77.
79. Fortier LA, Mohammed HO, Lust G, Nixon AJ. Insulin-like growth factor-I enhances cell-based repair of articular cartilage. J Bone Joint Surg Br 2002;84:276–288.
80. Elisseeff J, McIntosh W, Fu K, Blunk T, Langer R. Controlled-release of IGF-I and TGFβ1 in a photopolymerizing hydrogel for cartilage tissue engineering. J Orthop Res 2001;19:1098–1104.
81. Blunk T, Sieminski AL, Gooch KJ, et al. Differential effects of growth factors on tissue-engineered cartilage. Tissue Eng 2002;8:73–84.
82. Loeser RF, Pacione CA, Chubinskaya S. The combination of insulin-like growth factor 1 and osteogenic protein 1 promotes increased survival of and matrix synthesis by normal and osteoarthritic human articular chondrocytes. Arthritis Rheum 2003;48:2188–2196.
83. Vunjak-Novakovic G, Martin I, Obradovic B, et al. Bioreactor cultivation conditions modulate the composition and mechanical properties of tissue-engineered cartilage. J Orthop Res 1999;17:130–138.
84. Freed LE, Langer R, Martin I, Pellis NR, Vunjak-Novakovic G. Tissue engineering of cartilage in space. Proc Natl Acad Sci USA 1997;94:13885–13890.
85. Mauck RL, Nicoll SB, Seyhan SL, Ateshian GA, Hung CT. Synergistic effects of growth factors and dynamic loading for cartilage tissue engineering. Tissue Eng 2003;9:697–611.
86. Mauck RL, Soltz MA, Wang CC, et al. Functional tissue engineering of articular cartilage through dynamic loading of chondrocyte-seeded agarose gels. J Biomech Eng 2000;122:252–260.
87. Paul JP. Forces transmitted by joints in the human body. Proc Inst Mech Eng 1967;181:8.
88. Dillman CJ. Kinematic analysis of running. In: Wimore JH, ed. Exercise and Sport Sciences Review. New York: Academic Press; 1975:193–218.
89. Buschmann MD, Gluzband YA, Grodzinsky AJ, Hunziker EB. Mechanical compression modulates matrix biosynthesis in chondrocyte/agarose culture. J Cell Sci 1995;108:1497–1508.
90. Lee DA, Bader DL. Compressive strains at physiological frequencies influence the metabolism of chondrocytes seeded in agarose. J Orthop Res 1997;15:181–188.
91. Davisson T, Kunig S, Chen A, Sah R, Ratcliffe A. Static and dynamic compression modulate matrix metabolism in tissue engineered cartilage. J Orthop Res 2002;20:842–848.
92. Seidel JO, Pei M, Gray ML, et al. Long-term culture of tissue engineered cartilage in a perfused chamber with mechanical stimulation. Biorheology 2004;41:445–458.
93. Friedenstein AJ, Piatetzky-Shapiro II, Petrakova KV. Osteogenesis in transplants of bone marrow cells. J Embryol Exp Morphol 1966;16:381–390.
94. Caplan AI. Mesenchymal stem cells. J Orthop Res 1991;9:641–650.
95. Mackay AM, Beck SC, Murphy JM, et al. Chondrogenic differentiation of cultured human mesenchymal stem cells from marrow. Tissue Eng 1998;4:415–428.
96. Johnstone B, Hering TM, Caplan AI, Goldberg VM, Yoo JU. In vitro chondrogenesis of bone marrow-derived mesenchymal progenitor cells. Exp Cell Res 1998;238:265–272.
97. Pittenger MF, Mackay AM, Beck SC, et al. Multilineage potential of adult human mesenchymal stem cells. Science 1999;284:143–147.
98. Barry F, Boynton RE, Liu B, Murphy JM. Chondrogenic differentiation of mesenchymal stem cells from bone marrow: differentiation-dependent gene expression of matrix components. Exp Cell Res 2001;268:189–200.
99. Aubin JE, Liu F, Malaval L, Gupta AK. Osteoblast and chondroblast differentiation. Bone 1995;17:77S–83S.
100. Jaiswal N, Haynesworth SE, Caplan AI, Bruder SP. Osteogenic differentiation of purified, culture-expanded human mesenchymal stem cells in vitro. J Cell Biochem 1997;64:295–312.
101. Long MW. Osteogenesis and bone-marrow-derived cells. Blood Cells Mol Dis 2001;27:677–690.
102. Galmiche MC, Koteliansky VE, Briere J, Herve P, Charbord P. Stromal cells from human long-term marrow cultures are mesenchymal cells that differentiate following a vascular smooth muscle differentiation pathway. Blood 1993;82:66–76.
103. Ferrari G, Cusella-De Angelis G, Coletta M, et al. Muscle regeneration by bone marrow-derived myogenic progenitors. Science 1998;279:1528–1530.
104. Wakitani S, Saito T, Caplan AI. Myogenic cells derived from rat bone marrow mesenchymal stem cells exposed to 5-azacytidine. Muscle Nerve 1995;18:1417–1426.
105. Young RG, Butler DL, Weber W, et al. Use of mesenchymal stem cells in a collagen matrix for Achilles tendon repair. J Orthop Res 1998;16:406–413.
106. Awad HA, Butler DL, Boivin GP, et al. Autologous mesenchymal stem cell-mediated repair of tendon. Tissue Eng 1999;5:267–277.
107. Cheng L, Qasba P, Vanguri P, Thiede MA. Human mesenchymal stem cells support megakaryocyte and pro-platelet formation from CD34(+) hematopoietic progenitor cells. J Cell Physiol 2000;184:58–69.
108. Kopen GC, Prockop DJ, Phinney DG. Marrow stromal cells migrate throughout forebrain and cerebellum, and they differentiate into astrocytes after injection into neonatal mouse brains. Proc Natl Acad Sci USA 1999;96:10711–10716.
109. Pereira RF, Halford KW, O'Hara MD, et al. Cultured adherent cells from marrow can serve as long-lasting precursor cells for bone, cartilage, and lung in irradiated mice. Proc Natl Acad Sci USA 1995;92:4857–4861.
110. Colter DC, Class R, DiGirolamo CM, Prockop DJ. Rapid expansion of recycling stem cells in cultures of plastic-adherent cells from human bone marrow. Proc Natl Acad Sci USA 2000;97:3213–3218.
111. Reyes M, Lund T, Lenvik T, et al. Purification and ex vivo expansion of postnatal human marrow mesodermal progenitor cells. Blood 2001;98:2615–2625.
112. Zuk PA, Zhu M, Mizuno H, et al. Multilineage cells from human adipose tissue: implications for cell-based therapies. Tissue Eng 2001;7:211–228.
113. De Bari C, Dell'Accio F, Luyten FP. Human periosteum-derived cells maintain phenotypic stability and chondrogenic potential throughout expansion regardless of donor age. Arthritis Rheum 2001;44:85–95.
114. Nakahara H, Goldberg VM, Caplan AI. Culture-expanded human periosteal-derived cells exhibit osteochondral potential in vivo. J Orthop Res 1991;9:465–476.

115. De Bari C, Dell'Accio F, Tylzanowski P, Luyten FP. Multipotent mesenchymal stem cells from adult human synovial membrane. Arthritis Rheum 2001;44:1928–1942.
116. Hunziker EB, Rosenberg LC. Repair of partial-thickness defects in articular cartilage: cell recruitment from the synovial membrane. J Bone Joint Surg Am 1996;78:721–733.
117. Young HE, Steele TA, Bray RA, et al. Human reserve pluripotent mesenchymal stem cells are present in the connective tissues of skeletal muscle and dermis derived from fetal, adult, and geriatric donors. Anat Rec 2001;264:51–62.
118. Bosch P, Musgrave DS, Lee JY, et al. Osteoprogenitor cells within skeletal muscle. J Orthop Res 2000;18:933–944.
119. Miura M, Gronthos S, Zhao M, et al. SHED: stem cells from human exfoliated deciduous teeth. Proc Natl Acad Sci USA 2003;100:5807–5812.
120. Brighton CT, Lorich DG, Kupcha R, et al. The pericyte as a possible osteoblast progenitor cell. Clin Orthop Relat Res 1992;(257):287–299.
121. Zvaifler NJ, Marinova-Mutafchieva L, Adams G, et al. Mesenchymal precursor cells in the blood of normal individuals. Arthritis Res 2000;2:477–488.
122. Noth U, Osyczka AM, Tuli R, et al. Multilineage mesenchymal differentiation potential of human trabecular bone-derived cells. J Orthop Res 2002;20:1060–1069.
123. Osyczka AM, Noth U, Danielson KG, Tuan RS. Different osteochondral potential of clonal cell lines derived from adult human trabecular bone. Ann NY Acad Sci 2002;961:73–77.
124. Wickham MQ, Erickson GR, Gimble JM, Vail TP, Guilak F. Multipotent stromal cells derived from the infrapatellar fat pad of the knee. Clin Orthop Relat Res 2003;(412):196–212.
125. Dell'Accio F, De Bari C, Luyten FP. Microenvironment and phenotypic stability specify tissue formation by human articular cartilage-derived cells in vivo. Exp Cell Res 2003;287:16–27.
126. Dowthwaite GP, Bishop JC, Redman SN, et al. The surface of articular cartilage contains a progenitor cell population. J Cell Sci 2004;117:889–897.
127. Alsalameh S, Amin R, Gemba T, Lotz M. Identification of mesenchymal progenitor cells in normal and osteoarthritic human articular cartilage. Arthritis Rheum 2004;50:1522–1532.
128. Murphy JM, Dixon K, Beck S, et al. Reduced chondrogenic and adipogenic activity of mesenchymal stem cells from patients with advanced osteoarthritis. Arthritis Rheum 2002;46:704–713.
129. Quarto R, Thomas D, Liang CT. Bone progenitor cell deficits and the age-associated decline in bone repair capacity. Calcif Tissue Int 1995;56:123–129.
130. Rodriguez JP, Garat S, Gajardo H, Pino AM, Seitz G. Abnormal osteogenesis in osteoporotic patients is reflected by altered mesenchymal stem cells dynamics. J Cell Biochem 1999;75:414–423.
131. Minguell JJ, Erices A, Conget P. Mesenchymal stem cells. Exp Biol Med (Maywood) 2001;226:507–520.
132. Sato N, Meijer L, Skaltsounis L, Greengard P, Brivanlou AH. Maintenance of pluripotency in human and mouse embryonic stem cells through activation of Wnt signaling by a pharmacological GSK-3-specific inhibitor. Nat Med 2004;10:55–63.
133. Gregory CA, Singh H, Perry AS, Prockop DJ. The Wnt signaling inhibitor dickkopf-1 is required for reentry into the cell cycle of human adult stem cells from bone marrow. J Biol Chem 2003;278:28067–28078.
134. Awad HA, Halvorsen YD, Gimble JM, Guilak F. Effects of transforming growth factor beta1 and dexamethasone on the growth and chondrogenic differentiation of adipose-derived stromal cells. Tissue Eng 2003;9:1301–1312.
135. Zhou S, Eid K, Glowacki J. Cooperation between TGF-beta and Wnt pathways during chondrocyte and adipocyte differentiation of human marrow stromal cells. J Bone Miner Res 2004;19:463–470.
136. Tuli R, Tuli S, Nandi S, et al. Transforming growth factor-beta-mediated chondrogenesis of human mesenchymal progenitor cells involves N-cadherin and mitogen-activated protein kinase and Wnt signaling cross-talk. J Biol Chem 2003;278:41227–41236.
137. Bartholomew A, Sturgeon C, Siatskas M, et al. Mesenchymal stem cells suppress lymphocyte proliferation in vitro and prolong skin graft survival in vivo. Exp Hematol 2002;30:42–48.
138. Le Blanc K, Tammik C, Rosendahl K, Zetterberg E, Ringden O. HLA expression and immunologic properties of differentiated and undifferentiated mesenchymal stem cells. Exp Hematol 2003;31:890–896.
139. Horwitz EM, Prockop DJ, Gordon PL, et al. Clinical responses to bone marrow transplantation in children with severe osteogenesis imperfecta. Blood 2001;97:1227–1231.
140. Djouad F, Plence P, Bony C, et al. Immunosuppressive effect of mesenchymal stem cells favors tumor growth in allogeneic animals. Blood 2003;102:3837–3844.
141. Wakitani S, Goto T, Pineda SJ, et al. Mesenchymal cell-based repair of large, full-thickness defects of articular cartilage. J Bone Joint Surg 1994;76:579–592.
142. Murphy JM, Fink DJ, Hunziker EB, Barry FP. Stem cell therapy in a caprine model of osteoarthritis. Arthritis Rheum 2003;48:3464–3474.
143. Awad HA, Wickham MQ, Leddy HA, Gimble JM, Guilak F. Chondrogenic differentiation of adipose-derived adult stem cells in agarose, alginate, and gelatin scaffolds. Biomaterials 2004;25:3211–3222.
144. Williams CG, Kim TK, Taboas A, et al. In vitro chondrogenesis of bone marrow-derived mesenchymal stem cells in a photopolymerizing hydrogel. Tissue Eng 2003;9:679–688.
145. Caterson EJ, Li WJ, Nesti LJ, et al. Polymer/alginate amalgam for cartilage-tissue engineering. Ann NY Acad Sci 2002;961:134–138.
146. Li WJ, Tuli R, Okafor C, et al. A three-dimensional nanofibrous scaffold for cartilage tissue engineering using human mesenchymal stem cells. Biomaterials 2005;26:599–609.
147. Tuan RS, Boland G, Tuli R. Adult mesenchymal stem cells and cell-based tissue engineering. Arthritis Res Ther 2003;5:32–45.

13

Bone Regeneration

A.H. Reddi

Morphogenesis is the developmental cascade of pattern formation, establishment of body plan, and the architecture of mirror-image bilateral symmetry of musculoskeletal structures culminating in the adult form. Regenerative medicine is the emerging discipline of the fabrication of spare parts for the human body including the skeleton to restore function of lost parts caused by disease cancer and trauma. It is based on rational principles of developmental biology and morphogenesis. The three key ingredients for regenerative medicine and tissue engineering are inductive morphogenetic signals, responding stem cells, and extracellular matrix scaffolding.[1] Recent advances in molecular cell biology of morphogenesis will aid in the design principles and architecture for tissue engineering and regeneration. Regeneration recapitulates embryonic development and morphogenesis. Among the many tissues in the human body, bone has considerable powers for regeneration; therefore, it is a prototype model for tissue engineering. Implantation of demineralized bone matrix into subcutaneous sites results in local bone induction. The sequential cascade of bone morphogenesis mimics sequential skeletal morphogenesis in limbs and permits the isolation of bone morphogens. Although it is traditional to study morphogenetic signals in embryos and bone morphogenetic proteins (BMPs), the primordial inductive signals for bone are isolated from demineralized bone matrix from adults. BMPs initiate, promote, and maintain chondrogenesis and osteogenesis and have actions beyond bone. The recently identified cartilage-derived morphogenetic proteins (CDMPs) are critical for cartilage and joint morphogenesis. The symbiosis of bone inductive and conductive strategies is critical for regeneration of bone, and is in turn governed by the context and biomechanics. The context is the microenvironment, consisting of extracellular matrix scaffolding, and can be duplicated by biomimetic biomaterials such as collagens, hydroxyapatite, proteoglycans, and cell adhesion proteins including fibronectins and laminins. The rules of architecture for tissue engineering are an imitation and adoption of the laws of developmental biology and morphogenesis, thus they may be universal for all tissues, including bones, joints, and associated musculoskeletal tissues.

Bone Morphogenetic Proteins

Bone grafts have been used by orthopedic surgeons for nearly a century to aid in recalcitrant bone repair. Decalcified bone implants have been used to treat patients with osteomyelitis.[2] It was hypothesized that bone might contain a substance, osteogenin, that initiates bone growth.[3] Urist[4] made the key discovery that demineralized, lyophilized segments of rabbit bone induced new bone formation when implanted intramuscularly. Bone induction is a sequential multistep cascade.[5-7] The key steps in this cascade are chemotaxis, mitosis, and differentiation. Chemotaxis is the directed migration of cells in response to a chemical gradient of signals released from the insoluble demineralized bone matrix. The demineralized bone matrix is predominantly composed of type I insoluble collagen and it binds plasma fibronectin.[8] Fibronectin has domains for binding to collagen, fibrin, and heparin. The responding mesenchymal cells attached to the collagenous matrix and proliferated as indicated by [^{3}H]thymidine autoradiography and incorporation into acid-precipitable DNA on day 3.[9] Chondroblast differentiation was evident on day 5, chondrocytes on days 7–8, and cartilage hypertrophy on day 9. There was concomitant vascular invasion on day 9 with osteoblast differentiation. On days 10–12, alkaline phosphatase was maximal. Osteocalcin, bone γ-carboxyglutamic acid containing gla protein (BGP), increased on day 28. Hematopoietic marrow differentiated in the ossicle and was maximal by day 21. This entire sequential bone development cascade is reminiscent of bone and cartilage morphogenesis in the limb bud.[7,10] Hence, it has immense implications for isolation of inductive signals initiating cartilage and bone morphogenesis. In fact, a systematic investigation of the chemical components responsible for bone induction was undertaken.

A prerequisite for any quest for novel morphogens is the establishment of a battery of bioassays for new bone formation. A panel of in vitro assays was established for chemotaxis, mitogenesis, and chondrogenesis, and an in vivo bioassay for bone formation. Although the in vitro assays were expedient, we routinely monitored a labor-intensive in vivo bioassay as it was the only bona fide bone induction assay. A major limitation in the approach was that the demineralized bone matrix is insoluble and in the solid state. In view of this, dissociative extractants such as 4 M guanidine HCl or 8 M urea as 1% sodium dodecyl sulfate at pH 7.4 were used[11] to solubilize proteins. Approximately 3% of the proteins were solubilized from demineralized bone matrix, and the remaining residue was mainly insoluble type I bone collagen. The extract alone, or the residue alone, was incapable of new bone induction. However, addition of the extract to the residue (insoluble collagen) and then implantation in a subcutaneous site resulted in bone induction. Thus, it would appear that for optimal osteogenic activity there was collaboration between a soluble signal in the extract and insoluble substratum.[12] This bioassay was a useful advance in the final purification of BMPs and led to the determination of limited tryptic peptide sequences, which led to the eventual cloning of BMPs.[13–15]

The cloning of BMP-2, BMP-2B (now called BMP-4) and BMP-3 (also called osteogenin) by Wozney and colleagues[13] was important. Osteogenic protein-1 and −2 (OP-1 and OP-2) were cloned by Ozkaynak and colleagues.[15] There are more than 15 members of the BMP family (Table 13.1). The other members of the extended transforming growth factor β (TGFβ)/BMP superfamily include inhibins and activins (implicated in follicle-stimulating hormone release from pituitary) Müllerian duct inhibitory substance, growth/differentiation factors (GDFs), nodal, and lefty, a gene implicated in establishing right/left asymmetry.[16,17] BMPs are also implicated in embryonic induction.[1,18–20]

BMPs are dimeric molecules and the conformation is critical for biological actions. Reduction of the single interchain disulfide bond resulted in the loss of biological activity. The mature monomer molecule consists of about 120 amino acids, with seven canonical cysteine residues. There are three intrachain disulfides per monomer and one interchain disulfide bond in the dimer. The cysteine knot is in the critical core of the BMP monomer. The crystal structure of BMP-7 has been determined.[21] It is a good possibility in the near future that the crystal structure of the BMP-

Table 13.1. Bone morphogenetic proteins

BMP	Other names	Function
BMP-2	BMP-2A	Bone and cartilage morphogenesis
BMP-3	Osteogenin	Bone morphogenesis
BMP-3B	GDF-10	Intramembranous bone formation
BMP-4	BMP-2B	Bone formation
BMP-5		Bone morphogenesis
BMP-6		Cartilage hypertrophy
BMP-7	Osteogenic protein-1	Bone formation
BMP-8	Osteogenic protein-2	Bone formation
BMP-8B		Spermatogenesis
BMP-9		Liver differentiation
BMP-10		?
BMP-11	GDF-11	?
CDMP-1	GDF-5	Chondrogenesis, joint formation
CDMP-2	GDF-6	Chondrogenesis
CDMP-3	GDF-7	Tendon/ligament formation

BMPs Bind to Extracellular Matrix

It is well known that extracellular matrix components have a critical role in morphogenesis. The structural macromolecules and their supramolecular assembly in the matrix do not explain their role in epithelial–mesenchymal interaction and morphogenesis. This riddle can now be explained by the binding of BMPs to heparan sulfate heparin, and type IV collagen[22-24] of the basement membranes. In fact, this might explain in part the necessity for angiogenesis before osteogenesis during development. In addition, the actions of activin in the development of the frog, in terms of dorsal mesoderm induction, are modified to neuralization by follistatin.[25] Similarly, Chordin and Noggin from the Spemann organizer induce neuralization by binding and inactivation of BMP-4. Neural induction is likely to be a default pathway when BMP-4 is nonfunctional.[26,27] Thus, this is an emerging principle in development and morphogenesis that binding proteins can terminate a dominant morphogen's action and initiate a default pathway. Finally, the binding of a soluble morphogen to extracellular matrix converts it into an insoluble matrix-bound morphogen to act locally in the solid state.[22]

BMP Receptors

Recombinant human BMP-4 and BMP-7 bind to BMP receptor IA (BMPR-IA) and BMP receptor IB (BMPR-IB).[28] CDMP-1 also binds to both type I BMP receptors. There is a collaboration between type I and type II BMP receptors.[29] The type I receptor serine/threonine kinase phosphorylates a signal-transducing protein substrate called Smad 1 or 5.[30] Smad is a term derived from fusion of Drosophila Mad gene and *Caenorhabtitis elegans* (nematode) Sma gene. Smads 1 and 5 signal in partnership with a common co-Smad, Smad 4. The transcription of BMP response genes are initiated by Smad 1/Smad 4 heterodimers. Smads are trimeric molecules as gleaned by X-ray crystallography. The phosphorylation of Smads 1 and 5 by type I BMP receptor kinase is inhibited by inhibitory Smads 6 and 7.[31] Smad interacting protein may interact with Smad 1 and modulate BMP response gene expression.[15,32] The downstream targets of BMP signaling are likely to be homeobox genes, the cardinal genes for morphogenesis and transcription. BMPs, in turn, may be regulated by members of the hedgehog family of genes such as Sonic and Indian hedgehog[33] including receptors patched and smoothened and transcription factors such as Gli 1, 2, and 3. The actions of BMPs can be terminated by specific binding proteins such as noggin.[26]

Responding Stem Cells

It is well known that the embryonic mesoderm-derived mesenchymal cells are progenitors for bone, cartilage, tendons, ligaments, and muscle. However, certain stem cells in adult bone marrow, muscle, and fascia can form bone and cartilage. The identification of stem cells readily sourced from bone marrow may lead to banks of stem cells for cell therapy and perhaps gene therapy with appropriate "homing" characteristics to bone marrow and hence to the skeleton. The pioneering work of Friedenstein et al.[34] and Owen and Friedenstein[35] identified bone marrow stromal stem cells. These stromal cells are distinct from the hematopoietic stem cell lineage. The bone marrow stromal stem cells consist of inducible and determined osteoprogenitors committed to osteogenesis. Determined osteogenic precursor cells have the propensity to form bone cells without any external cues or signals. However, inducible osteogenic precursors require an inductive signal such as BMP or demineralized bone matrix. The stromal stem cells of Friedenstein and Owen are also called mesenchymal stem cells,[36] with potential to form bone, cartilage, adipocytes, and myoblasts in response to cues from environment and/or intrinsic factors. There is very recently considerable hope and anticipation that these bone marrow stromal cells may be excellent vehicles for cell and gene therapy.[37]

From a practical standpoint, these stromal stem cells can be obtained by bone marrow biopsies and expanded rapidly for use in cell therapy after pretreatment with BMPs. The potential uses in both cell and gene therapy are very promising. There are continuous improvements in the viral vectors and efficiency of gene therapy.[38,39] It is possible to use BMP genes transfected in stromal stem cells to target to the bone marrow to induce bone.[40]

Morphogens and Gene Therapy

The recent advances in morphogens are ripe for techniques of regional gene therapy for orthopedic tissue engineering. The availability of cloned genes for BMPs and CDMPs and the requisite platform technology of gene therapy may have immediate applications. Whereas protein therapy provides an immediate bolus of morphogen, gene therapy achieves a sustained prolonged secretion of gene products. Furthermore, recent improvements in regulated gene expression allow the turning on and off of gene expression. The progress in vectors for delivering genes also bodes well. The use of adenoviruses, adeno-associated viruses, and tetroviruses is poised for applications in bone and joint repair.[38,39,41,42] Although gene therapy has some advantages for orthopedic tissue engineering, an optimal delivery system for protein and gene therapy is needed, especially in replacement of large segmented defects and in fibrous non-unions and malunions.

Challenges

The earlier discussion of inductive signals (BMPs), responding stem cells (stromal cells) leads us to the scaffolding (the microenvironment/extracellular matrix) for optimal tissue engineering. The natural biomaterials in the composite tissue of bones and joints are collagens, proteoglycans, and glycoproteins of cell adhesion such as fibronectin and the mineral phase. The mineral phase in bone is predominantly hydroxyapatite. In native state, the associated citrate, fluoride, carbonate, and trace elements constitute the physiological hydroxyapatite. The high protein binding capacity makes hydroxyapatite a natural delivery system. Comparison of insoluble collagen, hydroxyapatite, tricalcium phosphate, glass beads, polymethylmethacrylate as carriers, revealed collagen to be an optimal delivery system for BMPs.[43] It is well known that collagen is an ideal delivery system for growth factors in soft and hard tissue wound repair.[44]

During the course of systematic work on hydroxyapatite of two pore sizes (200 or 500 µm) in two geometrical forms (beads or discs), an unexpected observation was made. The geometry of the delivery system is critical for optimal bone induction. The discs were consistently osteoinductive with BMPs in rats, but the beads were inactive.[45] The chemical composition of the two hydroxyapatite configurations was identical. In certain species, the hydroxyapatite alone appears to be "osteoinductive."[46] In subhuman primates, the hydroxyapatite induces bone, albeit at a much slower rate. One interpretation is that osteoinductive endogenous BMPs in circulation progressively bind to implanted discs of hydroxyapatite. When an optimal threshold concentration of native BMPs is achieved, the hydroxyapatite becomes osteoinductive. Strictly speaking, most hydroxyapatite substrata are ideal osteoconductive materials. This example in certain species also serves to illustrate how an osteoconductive biomimetic biomaterial may progressively function as an osteoinductive substance by binding to endogenous BMPs. Thus, there is a physiological–physicochemical continuum between the hydroxyapatite alone and a progressive composite with endogenous BMPs. Recognition of this experimental nuance will save unnecessary arguments among biomaterials scientists about the osteoinductive action of a conductive substratum such as hydroxyapatite.

Complete regeneration of a baboon craniotomy defect was accomplished by recombinant human osteogenic protein (rhOP-1; human BMP-7).[47] Recombinant BMP-2 was delivered by poly(α-hydroxy acid) carrier for calvarial regeneration.[48] Copolymer of polylactic and polyglycolic acid in a non-union model in the rabbit ulna was used and the results were satisfactory.[49]

An important problem in the clinical application of biomimetic biomaterials with BMPs and/or other morphogens is the sterilization. Although gas (ethylene oxide) is used, one should always be concerned about reactive free radicals. Using allogeneic demineralized bone matrix with endogenous native BMPs, as long as low temperature (4°C or less) was maintained, the samples tolerated up to 5–7 M Rads of irradiation.[50,51] The standard dose acceptable to the Food and Drug Administration is 2.5 M Rads. This information would be useful to the biotechnology companies preparing to market recombinant BMP-based osteogenic devices. Perhaps the tissue banking industry with an interest in bone grafts[52] could also use this critical information. The various freeze-dried and demineralized allogeneic bone may be used in the interim as satisfactory carriers for BMPs. The moral of this experiment is it is not the irradiation dose, but the ambient sample temperature during irradiation that is absolutely critical.

Unlike bone with its considerable prowess for repair and even regeneration, cartilage is recalcitrant. But why? It may be attributable in part to relative avascularity of hyaline cartilage, high concentration of protease inhibitors, and perhaps even growth inhibitors. The wound debridement phase is not optimal to prepare the cartilage wound bed for the optimal milieu interieur for repair. Although cartilage has been successfully engineered to predetermined shapes,[53] true repair of the tissue continues to be a real challenge in part because of hierarchical organization and geometry.[54] However, considerable excitement in the field has been generated by a group of Swedish workers in Göteborg, using autologous culture-expanded human chondrocytes.[55] A continuous challenge in chondrocyte cell therapy is progressive dedifferentiation and loss of characteristic cartilage phenotype. The redifferentiation and maintenance of the chondrocytes for cell therapy can be aided by BMPs, CDMPs, TGFβ isoforms, and insulin-like growth factors. It is also possible to repair cartilage using muscle-derived mesenchymal stem cells.[56] The potential possibility of the problems posed by cartilage proteoglycans in preventing cell immigration for repair was investigated by chondroitinase ABC and trypsin pretreatment in partial-thickness defects,[57] with and without TGFβ. Pretreatment with chondroitinase ABC followed by TGFβ revealed a contiguous layer of cells from the synovial membrane hinting at the potential source of "repair" cells from synovium. Multiple avenues of cartilage morphogens, cell therapy with chondrocytes and stem cells from marrow and muscle, and biomaterial scaffolding may lead to an optimal tissue engineered articular cartilage.

It is inevitable during the aging of humans that one will confront impaired locomotion caused by wear and tear in bones and joints. Therefore, the repair and possibly complete regeneration of the musculoskeletal system and other vital organs such as skin, liver, and kidney may potentially need optimal repair or a spare part for replacement. Can we create spare parts for the human body? There is much reason for optimism that tissue engineering can help patients. We are living at an extraordinary time in the biology, medicine, surgery, and computational and related technology. The confluence of advances in molecular developmental biology and attendant advances in inductive signals for morphogenesis, stem cells, biomimetic biomaterials, and extracellular matrix biology augers well for imminent breakthroughs.

The symbiosis of biotechnology and biomaterials has set the stage for systematic advances in tissue engineering.[58-60] The recent advances in enabling platform technology include molecular imprinting.[61] In principle, specific recognition and catalytic sites are imprinted using templates. The applications range from biosensors, catalytic applications to antibody, and receptor recognition sites. For example, the cell binding RGD site in fibronectin[62] or YIGSR domain in laminin can be imprinted in complementary sites.[63]

The rapidly advancing frontiers in morphogenesis with BMPs, hedgehogs, homeobox genes, and a veritable cornucopia of general and specific transcription factors, coactivators, and repressors will lead to cocrystallization of ligand–receptor complexes, protein–DNA complexes, and other macromolecular interactions. Let us imagine a head of the femur and a mold is fabricated with computer-assisted design and manufacture. It faithfully reproduces the structural features and may be imprinted with morphogens, inductive signals, and cell adhesion sites. This assembly can be loaded with stem cells and BMPs and other inductive signals with a nutrient medium optimized for optimal number of cell cycles, and then predictably exit into the differentiation phase to reproduce a totally new bone femoral head. In fact, such a biological approach with vascularized muscle flap and BMPs yielded new bone with a defined shape and has demonstrated the proof of principle for further development and validation.[64] We indeed are entering a brave new world of prefabricated biological spare parts for the regeneration of bone for the human body based on sound architectural rules of inductive signals for morphogenesis, responding stem cells with lineage control, and with growth factors immobilized on a template of biomimetic biomaterial based on extracellular matrix. The BMPs are now approved by the Food and Drug Administration for clinical uses in spine fusion and fracture healing.

Acknowledgment

This work was supported by the Lawrence Ellison Chair in Musculoskeletal Molecular Biology. I thank Ms. Danielle Neff for outstanding help and enthusiastic bibliographic assistance.

References

1. Reddi AH. Role of morphogenetic proteins in skeletal tissue engineering and regeneration. Nat Biotechnol 1998;16:247–252.
2. Senn N. On the healing of aseptic bone cavities by implantation of antiseptic decalcified bone. Am J Med Sci 1989;98:219–240.
3. Lacroix P. Recent investigations on the growth of bone. Nature 1945;156:576.
4. Urist MR. Bone: formation by autoinduction. Science 1965;150:893–899.
5. Reddi AH, Huggins CB. Biochemical sequences in the transformation of normal fibroblasts in adolescent rat. Proc Natl Acad Sci USA 1972;69:1601–1605.
6. Reddi AH, Anderson WA. Collagenous bone matrix-induced endochondral ossification and hemopoiesis. J Cell Biol 1976;69:557–572.
7. Reddi AH. Cell biology and biochemistry of endochondral bone development. Coll Relat Res 1981;1:209–226.
8. Weiss RE, Reddi AH. Synthesis and localization of fibronectin during collagenous matrix mesenchymal cell interaction and differentiation of cartilage and bone in vivo. Proc Natl Acad Sci USA 1980;77:2074–2078.
9. Rath NC, Reddi AH. Collagenous bone matrix is a local mitogen. Nature 1979;278:855–857.
10. Reddi AH. Extracellular matrix and development. In: Piez KA, Reddi AH, eds. Extracellular Matrix Biochemistry. New York: Elsevier; 1984:375–412.
11. Sampath TK, Reddi AH. Homology of bone inductive proteins from human, monkey, bovine, and rat extracellular matrix. Proc Natl Acad Sci USA 1983;80:6591–6595.
12. Sampath TK, Reddi AH. Dissociative extraction and reconstitution of bone matrix components involved in local bone differentiation. Proc Natl Acad Sci USA 1981;78:7599–7603.
13. Wozney JM, Rosen V, Celeste AJ, et al. Novel regulators of bone formation: molecular clones and activities. Science 1988;242:1528–1534.
14. Luyten F, Cunningham NS, Ma S, et al. Purification and partial amino acid sequence of osteogenin, a protein initiating bone differentiation. J Biol Chem 1989;265:13377–13380.
15. Ozkaynak E, Rueger DC, Drier EA, et al. OP-1 cDNA encodes an osteogenic protein in the TGF-β family. EMBO J 1990;9:2085–2093.
16. Reddi AH. Bone morphogenetic proteins: an unconventional approach to isolation of first mammalian morphogens. Cytokine Growth Factor Rev 1997;8:11–20.
17. Cunningham NS, Jenkins NA, Gilbert DJ, Copeland NG, Reddi AH, Lee S-J. Growth/differentiation factor-10: a new member of the transforming growth factor-beta[Page No. 13-10] superfamily related to bone morphogenetic protein-3. Growth Factors 1995;12:99–109.
18. Lemaire P, Gurdon JB. Vertebrate embryonic inductions. Bioessays 1994;16(9):617–620.
19. Melton DA. Pattern formation during animal development. Science 1991;252:234–241.
20. Lyons KM, Hogan BLM, Robertson EJ. Colocalization of BMP-2 and BMP-7 RNA suggest that these factors cooperatively act in tissue interactions during murine development. Mech Dev 1995;50:71–83.
21. Griffith DL, Keck PC, Sampath TK, Rueger DC, Carlson WD. Three-dimensional structure of recombinant human osteogenic protein-1: structural paradigm for the transforming growth factor-β superfamily. Proc Natl Acad Sci USA 1996;93:878–883.
22. Paralkar VM, Nandedkar AKN, Pointers RH, Kleinman HK, Reddi AH. Interaction of osteogenin, a heparin binding bone morphogenetic protein, with type IV collagen. J Biol Chem 1990;265:17281–17284.
23. Paralkar VM, Vukicevic S, Reddi AH. Transforming growth factor-β type I binds to collagen IV of basement membrane matrix: Implications for development. Dev Biol 1991;143:303–308.
24. Paralkar VM, Weeks BS, Yu YM, Kleinman HK, Reddi AH. Recombinant human bone morphogenetic protein 2B stimulates PC12 cell differentiation: potentiation and binding to type IV collagen. J Cell Biol 1992;119:1721–1728.
25. Hemmati-Brivanlou A, Kelly OG, Melton DA. Follistatin, an antagonist of activin, is expressed in the Spemann organizer and displays direct neuralizing activity. Cell 1994;77:283–295.
26. Piccolo S, Sasai Y, Lu B, De Robertis EM. Dorsoventral patterning in Xenopus: inhibition of ventral signals by direct binding of chordin to BMP-4. Cell 1996;86:589–598.
27. Zimmerman LB, Jesus-Escobar JM, Harland RM. The Spemann organizer signal Noggin binds and inactivates bone morphogenetic protein-4. Cell 1996;86:599–606.
28. ten Dijke P, Yamashita H, Sampath TK, et al. Identification of type I receptors for OP-1 and BMP-4. J Biol Chem 1994;269:16986–16988.
29. Nishitoh H, Ichijo H, Kimura M, et al. Identification of type I and type II serine/threonine kinase receptors for growth and differentiation factor-5. J Biol Chem 1996;271:21345–21352.
30. Chen X, Rubock MJ, Whitman M. A transcriptional partner for Mad proteins in TGF-β signalling. Nature 1996;383:691–696.
31. Hayashi H, Abdollah S, Qui Y, et al. The MAD-related protein Smad 7 associates with the TGFβ receptor and functions as an antagonist of TGFβ signalling. Cell 1997;89:1165–1173.
32. Heldin CH, Miyazono K, ten Dijke P. TGFβ signaling from cell membrane to nucleus through Smad proteins. Nature 1997;390:465–471.
33. Johnson RL, Tabin CJ. Molecular models for vertebrate limb development. Cell 1997;90:979–990.
34. Friedenstein AJ, Petrakova KV, Kurolesova AI, Frolora GP. Heterotopic transplants of bone marrow: analysis

of precursor cell for osteogenic and hemopoietic tissues. Transplantation 1968;6:230–247.
35. Owen ME, Friedenstein AJ. Stromal stem cells: marrow derived osteogenic precursors. CIBA Found Symp 1988;136:42–60.
36. Caplan AI. Mesenchymal stem cell. J Orthop Res 1991;9:641–650.
37. Prockop DJ. Marrow stromal cells and stem cells for non hematopoietic tissues. Science 1997;276:71–74.
38. Bank A. Human somatic cell gene therapy. Bioessays 1996;18:999–1007.
39. Mulligan RC. The basic science of gene therapy. Science 1993;260:926–932.
40. Peng H, Wright V, Vsas A, et al. Synergistic enhancement of bone formation and healing by stem cell expressed VEGF and BMP-4. J Clin Ivest 2002;110:751–759.
41. Kozarsky KF, Wilson JM. Gene therapy: adenovirus vectors. Curr Opin Genet Dev 1993;3:499–503.
42. Morsy MA, Mitani K Clemens P, Caskey T. Progress toward human gene therapy. JAMA 1993;270(19): 2338–2345.
43. Ma S, Chen G, Reddi AH. Collaboration between collagenous matrix and osteogenin is required for bone induction. Ann NY Acad Sci 1990;580:524–525.
44. McPherson JM. The utility of collagen-based vehicles in delivery of growth factors for hard and soft tissue wound repair. Clin Mater 1992;9:225–234.
45. Ripamonti U, Ma S, Reddi AH. The critical role of geometry of porus hydroxyapatite delivery system induction of bone by osteogenin, a bone morphogenetic protein. Matrix 1992;12:202–212.
46. Ripamonti U. Osteoinduction in porous hydroxyapatite implanted in heterotopic sites of different animal models. Biomaterials 1996;17:31–35.
47. Ripamonti U, Van den Heever B, Sampath TK, Tucker MM, Rueger DC, Reddi AH. Complete regeneration of bone in the baboon by recombinant human osteogenic protein-1 (hOP-1, bone morphogenetic protein-7). Growth Factors 1996;123:273–289.
48. Hollinger J, Mayer M, Buck D, et al. Poly(alpha-hydroxy acid) carrier for delivering recombinant human bone morphogenetic protein-2 for bone regeneration. J Controlled Release 1996;39:287–304.
49. Bostrom M, Lane JM, Tomin E, et al. Use of bone morphogenetic protein-2 in the rabbit ulnar nonunion model. Clin Orthop Relat Res 1996;327:272–282.
50. Weintroub S, Reddi AH. Influence of irradiation on the osteoinductive potential of demineralized bone matrix. Calcif Tissue Int 1988;42:255–260.
51. Weintroub S, Weiss JF, Catravas GN, Reddi AH. Influence of whole body irradiation and local shielding on matrix-induced endochondral bone differentiation. Calcif Tissue Int 1990;46:38–45.
52. Damien CJ, Parson JR. Bone graft and bone graft substitutes: a review of current technology and applications. J Appl Biomater 1991;2:187–208.
53. Kim WS, Vacanti JP, Cima L, et al. Cartilage engineered in predetermined shapes employing cell transplantation on synthetic biodegradable polymers. Plast Reconstr Surg 1994;94:233–237.
54. Mow VC, Ratcliffe A, Poole AR. Cartilage and diarthrodial joints as paradigms for hierarchical materials and structures. Biomaterials 1992;13:67–97.
55. Brittberg M, Lindahl A, Nilsson A, Ohlsson C, Isaksson O, Peterson L. Treatment of deep cartilage defects in the knee with autologous chondrocyte transplantation. N Engl J Med 1994;331:889–895.
56. Grande DA, Southerland SS, Manji R, Pate DW, Schwartz RE, Lucas PA. Repair of articular cartilage defects using mesenchymal stem cells. Tissue Eng 1995;1:345–353.
57. Hunzinker EB, Rosenberg LC. Repair of partial-thickness defects in articular cartilage: cell recruitment from the synovial membrane. J Bone Joint Surg 1996;78-A:721–733.
58. Reddi AH. Bone and cartilage differentiation. Curr Opin Genet Dev 1994;4:937–944.
59. Langer R, Vacanti JP. Tissue engineering. Science 1993;260:930–932.
60. Hubbell JA. Biomaterials in tissue engineering. Biotechnology 1995;13:565–575.
61. Mosbach K, Ramstrom O. The emerging technique of molecular imprinting and its future impact on biotechnology. Biotechnology 1996;14:163–170.
62. Ruoslahti E, Pierschbacher MD. New perspectives in cell adhesion: RGD and integrins. Science 1987;238: 491–497.
63. Vukicevic S, Luyten FP, Kleinman HK, Reddi AH. Differentiation of canalicular cell processes in bone cells by basement membrane matrix component: regulation by discrete domains of laminin. Cell 1990;64:437–445.
64. Khouri RK, Koudsi B, Reddi AH. Tissue transformation into bone in vivo. JAMA 1991;266:1953–1955.

14

Osteoarthritis and Mesenchymal Cells – The Prospects for Repair of the Disease by Cell Transplantation and Tissue Engineering

Dror Robinson

Current Understanding of Osteoarthritis

Understanding of osteoarthritis has greatly evolved in recent years. The disease was once described as a "wear and tear" disorder affecting articular cartilage. This is a gross underestimation of the affectation. Evidence now exists showing that osteoarthritis in fact involves many tissues including subchondral bone, muscles, and tendons. It is debatable whether the bone involvement is primary or secondary in osteoarthritis.[1] In addition, the synoviocytes lining the joint capsule appear to be involved in the joint destruction by issuing various cytokines. Another clear association exists between obesity and osteoarthritis. Obviously, obesity itself might lead to increased mechanical loading of joint surfaces because of both total body weight and alterations in gait patterns. However, obese people tend to be less physically active and, thus, although peak joint forces might be increased, repeated cumulative loads might actually be decreased in obese people as compared with athletic ones. Thus, although it is true that a mechanical relation might be responsible for the cartilage destruction, other factors might also be involved. However, the relationship between osteoarthritis and obesity seems more complex. Increased levels of fatty acids are found in osteoarthritic cartilage.[2] Fatty acids and other metabolites related to obesity could presumably be related to the progression of polyarticular osteoarthritis, i.e., the generalized form of the disorder as suggested by Aspden et al.[3]

Furthermore, several studies have documented abnormal bone metabolism in osteoarthritic individuals including altered bone metabolism in remote sites (iliac bone) in patients with hand osteoarthritis.[4] The disorder in osteoarthritis seems to affect not only bone and cartilage but muscle as well. Although it is debatable whether muscle weakness precedes or follows the joint dysfunction, some authors suggest that muscle dysfunction is a primary disorder in these individuals eventually leading to joint destruction.[5]

If the above observations are correct, a possible explanation for the affectation of different cell types in these disorders might be a stem cell dysfunction. It is well known that the chondrocytic, osteoblastic, fibroblastic, and adipocytic lineages share a common stem cell – i.e., the mesenchymal stem cell (MSC). If osteoarthritis is a manifestation of stem cell dysfunction, then manipulated stem cells might be a possible solution to this disorder.

MSCs in Osteoarthritis

What is the role of MSCs in osteoarthritis? Bone marrow contains a subpopulation of cells demonstrating a mesenchymal progenitor cell behavior.[6] These cells are capable in vitro of forming both bone and cartilage under the appropriate environmental conditions. Such cells exist as well in osteoarthritis joints. The frequency of the subpopulation of stromal cells that are CD9/CD90/CD166 positive seems to be around 5% in osteoarthritic synovial membrane.[7] These mesenchymal cells appear to be attracted to repair sites of partial-thickness injuries of articular cartilage by transforming growth factor β.[8] Although even end-stage osteoarthritis joints contain MSCs,[7] their activity, both adipogenic and chondrogenic, seems to be reduced as compared with normal joints.[9] This conforms to the known increase in osteoblastic activity in osteoarthritic bones, both adjacent to affected joints and in remote sites. It has been shown that osteoblasts from patients with osteoarthritis proliferate in vitro more rapidly than those from healthy individuals and express different concentrations of markers.[10] Implantation of MSCs into osteoarthritic defects in humans during high tibial osteotomy led to improvement in the quality of repair tissue formed in the defects. However, clinical improvement could not be demonstrated as compared with the group undergoing high tibial osteotomy alone.[11] The conclusion from these two studies seems to be that although mesenchymal cells exist in osteoarthritic joints, they appear to be of reduced quality especially with regard to chondrogenic differentiation. Thus, improvement of clinical results might require an induction of differentiation toward a more typical chondrogenic phenotype. In addition, it seems to be desirable to deliver large numbers of MSCs into osteoarthritic joints. Culture in vitro appears to enrich the culture with cells capable of chondroosseous differentiation by approximately an order of magnitude.[7] In osteoarthritic joints in contrast with rheumatoid arthritis, the number of MSCs in the synovium seems to be reduced.[12] The difference may be related to the lack of MSC recruitment in osteoarthritis. In contrast, in an experimental arthritis model mimicking rheumatoid arthritis, stem cells were recruited by tumor necrosis factor-α.[13] An interesting work by Murphy et al.[14] has demonstrated that even a scaffold-free approach of delivering bone marrow-derived stem cells can lead to regeneration of joint's injured tissues. In this landmark study, repair of a caprine model of osteoarthritis had been enhanced by the use of intraarticular injections of a suspension of bone marrow mesenchymal cells and hyaluronic acid.

Osteoarthritis has been induced surgically by resection of both the medial meniscus and the anterior cruciate ligament. In this model, osteophyte formation and articular cartilage degeneration rapidly ensues. The animals were treated by either injection of bone marrow-derived MSCs in hyaluronic acid or hyaluronic acid alone. It is particularly noteworthy that not only was cartilage quality maintained better in the former group, but evidence of medial meniscus regeneration was seen in the MSC-augmented group indicating that also meniscus repair might be improved by MSC addition. It is important to note that this study did not utilize a scaffold for immobilizing the cells in the articular cartilage defect. It is probably not feasible in most clinical situations to fill defects with scaffolds. In contrast to most experimental situations, clinically encountered focal cartilage defects are large, shallow, and often uncontained. An uncontained defect is a defect that is not totally surrounded by articular cartilage. Such a defect is very difficult to fill with a stable scaffold, because the scaffold has a tendency to displace toward the uncontained side. Furthermore, most articular cartilage defects in the osteoarthritis joint are so-called "kissing lesions," i.e., the cartilage is damaged on both sides of the joint at areas that make contact with each other during joint motion. Thus, it is likely that any scaffold placed in "kissing lesions" will tend to be eroded and displaced by joint motion. This study describes the use of hyaluronan as a cell-delivery vehicle. Hyaluronan is not an inert substance but rather is necessary for granulation-tissue production and cell proliferation. The substance also encourages migration and proliferation of MSCs.[14] Thus, it seems that repair of articular cartilage might not require scaffolds to carry the cells but rather addition of stem cells.

Source of Mesenchymal Progenitor Cells

Another question to be answered refers to the source of mesenchymal progenitor cells needed to regain joint homeostasis. The currently accepted technique of autologous chondrocyte implantation seems to involve MSCs. The chondrocytes undergo dedifferentiation in vitro during cell culture. Some of the cells in these cultures appear to be mesenchymal progenitors.[15] The success of this technique depends on implantation of the cells into a cartilage defect and locally mediated signals that induce cartilage repair and lead to chondrogenic redifferentiation of these cells. Recently, it has been shown that synovial fluid contains MSCs.[16] These seem to be more common in osteoarthritis than in rheumatoid arthritis. The role of these cells in the osteoarthritic process is not clear. It is possible that the cells are just debris released from the injured articular surfaces. However, it is possible that the cells represent a repair attempt gone awry. The latter theory is supported by the clinical observation of secondary synovial chondromatosis, i.e., bone and cartilage formation inside the synovial membrane that might derive from these floating mesenchymal cells. Recently, the sequence of osteophyte formation has been characterized on the histologic and immunohistochemical level.[17] Osteophyte formation begins with mesenchymal condensation, passes through a stage similar to growth plate formation, and ends with a mature osteophyte covered by hyaline-like cartilage. Thus, it seems plausible that MSCs present locally within the diseased joint, are capable of forming synovial chondroosseous bodies[18] as well as forming osteophytes,[17] but are not capable of repairing the joint surfaces. The locally present MSCs have been termed "niche" stem cells, which are inherently more suitable for repair of local tissues. Unfortunately, it seems that in osteoarthritis these cells malfunction.[34] It is possible that cells recruited from autologous bone marrow and cultured in vitro could be selected to express a more chondrogenic phenotype and to attach into cartilage defects to allow better repair of joint surfaces without osteophyte formation. Recently, an exciting new technique of targeting repair cells into damaged joint surfaces has been termed cell painting.[20] In this technique, cells are coated by noncytotoxic antibodies that allow site-specific attachment to damaged cartilaginous surfaces. The solution to the osteoarthritic enigma might be related to selective proliferation of stem cells in culture, selecting for the chondrogenic phenotype at the expense of the osteogenic phenotype and later delivering the cells locally into the joint allowing matrix-specific binding of the cells so that they will concentrate at damaged areas instead of the joint periphery. There is some evidence that articular cartilage in osteoarthritis contains MSCs, possibly derived from bone marrow. The cells in bone marrow capable of chondrocytic differentiation coexpress CD105 and CD166.[21] CD105 is endoglin, a type of transforming growth factor β receptor (III). CD166 is activated leukocyte cell adhesion molecule. Cells expressing CD166 in the perichondrium are capable of generating MSCs.[22] Coexpression of these two antigens appears to indicate a subpopulation of mesenchymal stem cells capable of generating cartilage-like tissue. A recent study has shown that osteoarthritic cartilage contains more MSCs than normal cartilage.[21] It is possible that curing osteoarthritis could involve addition of mesenchymal progenitors and encouragement of the cells to undergo differentiation into cartilage.

References

1. Radin EL, Rose RM. The role of subchondral bone in the initiation and progression of cartilage damage. Clin Orthop 1986;213:34–40.
2. Lippiello L, Walsh T, Fienhold M. The association of lipid abnormalities with tissue pathology in human osteoarthritic articular cartilage. Metabolism 1991;40:571–576.
3. Aspden RM, Scheven BAA, Hutchison JD. Osteoarthritis as a systemic disorder including stromal cell differentiation and lipid metabolism. Lancet 2001;357:1118–1121.
4. Dequeker J, Mokassa L, Aerssens J. Bone density and osteoarthritis. J Rheumatol 1995;22:98–100.
5. Hurley MV. The role of muscle weakness in the pathogenesis of osteoarthritis. Rheum Dis Clin North Am 1999;25:283–298.
6. Conget PA, Minguell JJ. Phenotypical and functional properties of human bone marrow mesenchymal progenitor cells. J Cell Physiol 1999;181(1):67–73.
7. Fickert S, Fiedler J, Brenner RE. Identification, quantification and isolation of mesenchymal progenitor cells from osteoarthritic synovium by fluorescence automated cell sorting. Osteoarthritis Cartilage 2003;11:790–800.
8. Hunziker EB, Rosenberg LC. Repair of partial thickness defects in articular cartilage: cell recruitment from the synovial membrane. J Bone Joint Surg Am 1996;78(5):721–733.
9. Murphy JM, Dixon K, Beck S, Fabian D, Feldman A, Barry F. Reduced chondrogenic and adipogenic activity of mesenchymal stem cells from patients with advanced osteoarthritis. Arthritis Rheum 2002;46(3):704–713.
10. Hilal G, Martel-Pelletier J, Pelletier J-P, Ranger P, Lajeunesse D. Osteoblast-like cells from human subchondral osteoarthritic bone demonstrate an altered phenotype in vitro: possible role in subchondral bone sclerosis. Arthritis Rheum 1998;41:891–899.
11. Wakitani S, Imoto K, Yamamoto T, Saito M, Murata N, Yoneda M. Human autologous culture expanded bone

marrow mesenchymal cell transplantation for repair of cartilage defects in osteoarthritic knees. Osteoarthritis Cartilage 2002;10:199–206.
12. Marinova-Mutafchieva L, Taylor P, Funa K, et al. Mesenchymal cells expressing bone morphogenetic protein receptors are present in the rheumatoid arthritis joint. Arthritis Rheum 2000;43:2046–2055.
13. Marinova-Mutafchieva L, Williams RO, Funa K, et al. Inflammation is preceded by tumor necrosis factor-dependent infiltration of mesenchymal cells in experimental arthritis. Arthritis Rheum 2002;46:507–513.
14. Murphy JM, Fink DJ, Hunziker EB, Barry FP. Stem cell therapy in a caprine model of osteoarthritis. Arthritis Rheum 2003;48:(12):3464–3474.
15. Tallheden T, Dennis JE, Lennon DP, et al. Phenotypic plasticity of human articular chondrocytes. J Bone Joint Surg Am 2003;85A(suppl 2):93–100.
16. Jones EA, English A, Henshaw K, et al. Enumeration and phenotypic characterization of synovial fluid multipotential mesenchymal progenitor cells in inflammatory and degenerative arthritis. Arthritis Rheum 2004;50:(3)817–827.
17. Gelse K, Eger W, Diemtar T, Aigner T. Osteophyte development: molecular characterization of differentiation stages. Osteoarthritis Cartilage 2003;11: 141–148.
18. Robinson D, Hasharoni A, Evron Z, Segal M, Nevo Z. Synovial chondromatosis: the possible role of FGF 9 and FGF receptor 3 in its pathology. Int J Exp Pathol 2000;81(3):183–189.
19. Luyten FP. Mesenchymal stem cells in osteoarthritis. Curr Opin Rheumatol 2004;16(5):599–603.
20. Dennis JE, Cohen N, Goldberg VM, Caplan AI. Targeted delivery of progenitor cells for cartilage repair. J Orthop Res 2004;22(4):735–741.
21. Alsalameh S, Amin R, Gemba T, Lotz M. Identification of mesenchymal progenitor cells in normal and osteoarthritic human articular cartilage. Arthritis Rheum 2004;50(5):1522–1532.
22. Arai F, Ohneda O, Miyamoto T, Zhang XQ, Suda T. Mesenchymal stem cells in perichondrium express activated leukocyte cell adhesion molecule and participate in bone marrow formation. J Exp Med 2002;195: 1549–1563.

Colorplates

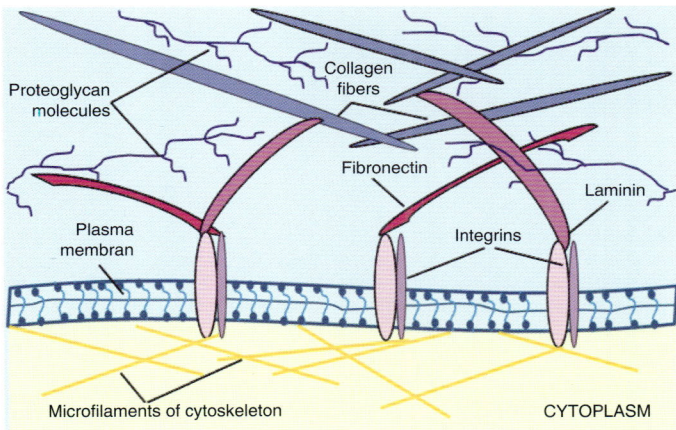

Figure 1.2. Cardiomyocytes are tethered in an extensive extracellular network of collagen and other structural proteins, including fibronectins and proteoglycans.

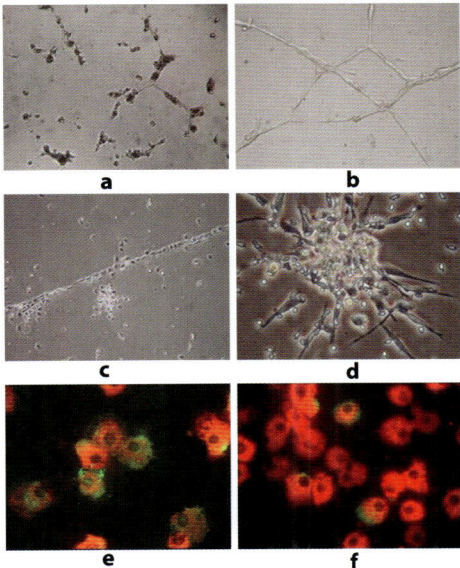

Figure 2.3. Endothelial phenotype and function. **a** Vascular-like network formation of cultured MSCs from adult human BM in 12-hour three-dimensional Matrigel culture. **b** Vascular network formation of human umbilical vein endothelial cells in 12-hour three-dimensional Matrigel culture. **c** Formation of cord-like structures by primary MSCs from adult BM in suspension culture. **d** Endothelial colony (CFU-EC) from nonmobilized adult human PB. **e** Putative EPCs from nonmobilized adult human PB as characterized by Dil-Ac-LDL uptake (red) and BS-1 lectin binding (green). **f** Putative EPCs from PB characterized by Dil-Ac-LDL uptake (red) and UEA lectin binding (green). (Courtesy of Daniela Thaler and Eva Rohde, MD.)

COLOR PLATE II

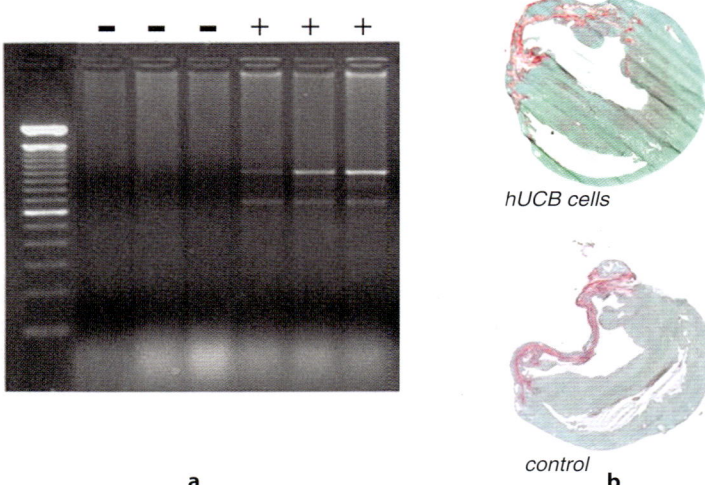

Figure 2.4. **a** Human stem cells selectively home to the infarcted myocardium in mice. Here, this is demonstrated by detection of human-specific DNA in the hearts of immunoincompetent SCID mice that had undergone intravenous injection of human umbilical cord blood (hUCB) cells after myocardial infarction by coronary artery occlusion (+). The first three lanes (−) have been obtained from mouse hearts that underwent human umbilical cord blood cell injection without prior myocardial infarction. There is no cell migration to the normal myocardium. **b** Cross-section through infarcted hearts of mice that had (top) or had not (bottom) undergone intravenous injection of human umbilical cord blood cells. The infarct area appears smaller in cell-treated hearts.

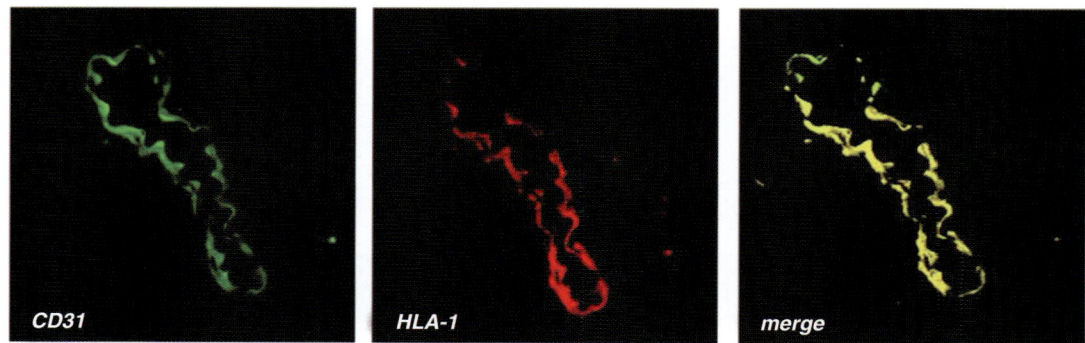

Figure 2.5. A capillary blood vessel in a mouse heart after myocardial infarction and intravenous delivery of human umbilical cord blood cells. The CD31 staining (right) determines the endothelial phenotype. The HLA-1 expression indicates that the cells are indeed of human origin (center). The merged image gives the impression that the vessels consist of both human (yellow) and mouse (green) endothelial cells. (Reprinted from Ma N, Stamm C, Kaminski A, et al. Human cord blood cells induce angiogenesis following myocardial infarction in NOD/SCID-mice. Cardiovasc Res 2005;66:45–54, © 2005, with permission from European Society of Cardiology.)

COLOR PLATE III

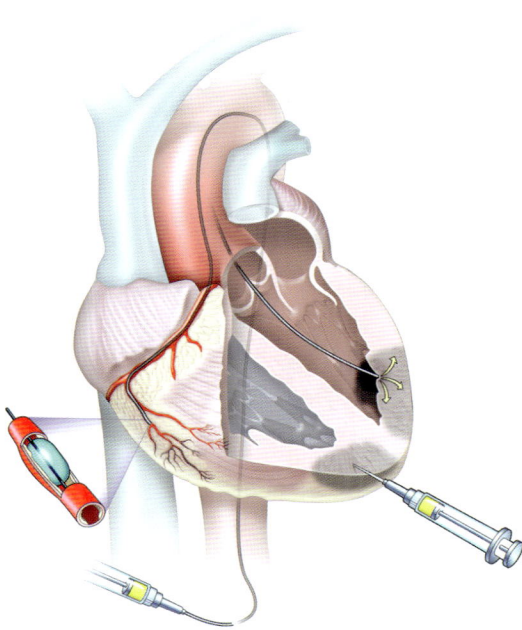

Figure 2.7. The principal strategies for delivery of stem/progenitor cells to the ischemic myocardium are shown. In patients who have to undergo heart surgery, cells can easily be injected directly into the myocardium. An alternative way of cell injection into chronically ischemic myocardium is transventricular catheter approach with transendocardial puncture. To locate the target area, complex electrophysiology and imaging techniques are used. The intracoronary cell injection is currently the preferred mode of cell delivery in acute myocardial infarction. Here, interaction between stem cells and endothelial cells is required to mediate adhesion of cells to the vascular wall as well as penetration of the endothelial layer and basement membrane. (With permission from Wort & Bild Verlag/Apotheken Umschau, 2005.)

COLOR PLATE IV

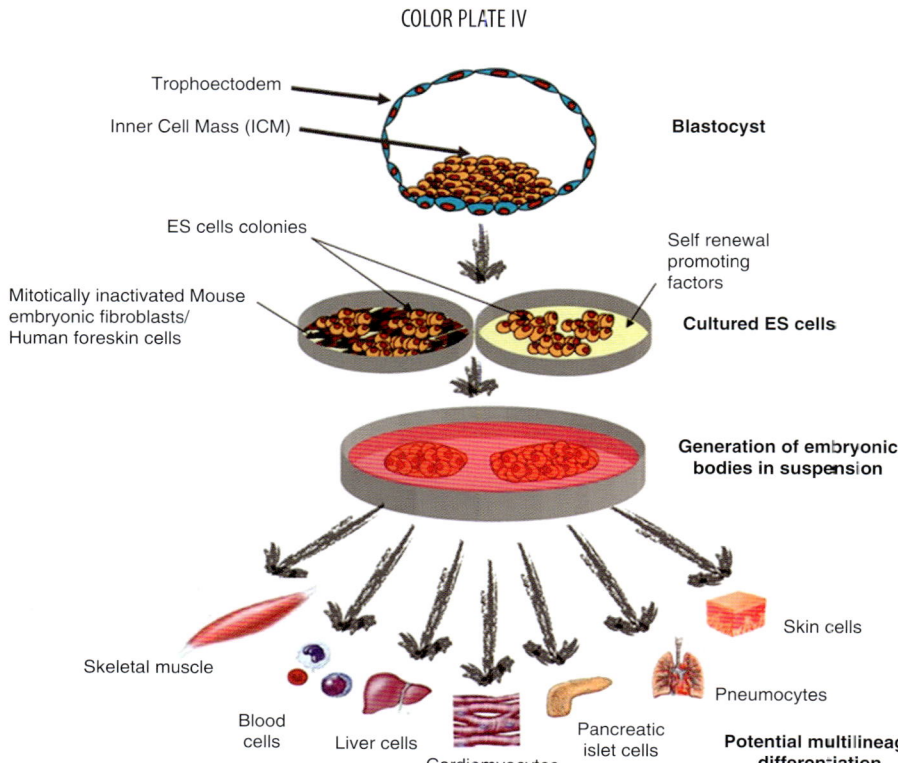

Figure 3.1. Early embryonic development and hESC isolation, propagation, and in vitro differentiation. The hESC lines can be generated from human blastocysts. At this stage, the embryo comprises the trophectoderm and the inner cell mass (ICM), which eventually will give rise to all tissue types in the embryo. hESC lines can be isolated from the ICM by immunosurgery and plated on the MEF feeder layer, human foreskin cells, or self-renewal promoting factors. hESCs can be propagated continuously in the undifferentiated state when grown with feeder layers or the factor supplements. When removed from these conditions and grown in suspension, they begin to generate three-dimensional differentiating cell aggregates that are termed embryoid bodies (EBs). This in vitro differentiating system may be used to generate a plurality of tissue types, including skeletal muscles, hematopoietic cells, liver cells, cardiomyocytes, pancreatic islet cells, lung cells, and keratinocytes.

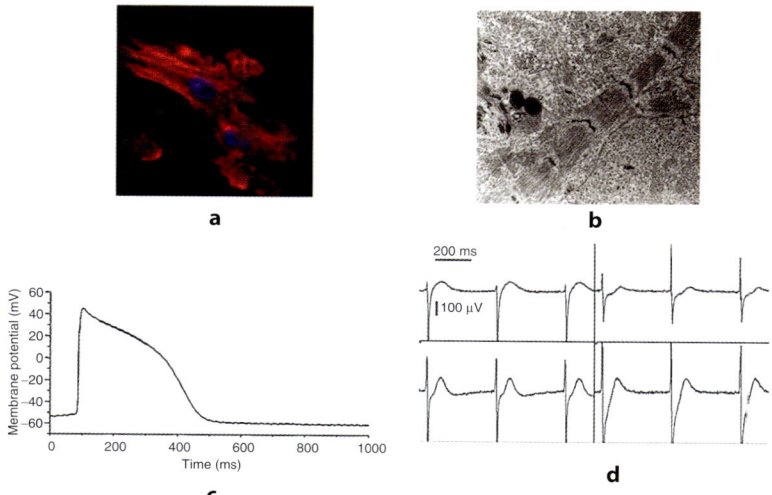

Figure 3.2. Structural and electrophysiological prosperities of hESDCMs. **a** Immunofluorescence staining demonstrating the cardiac phenotype of the hESDCMs [cardiac troponin I (red) nuclei (TO-PRO)]. **b** Transmission electron micrograph of sectioned beating EB demonstrating the presence of organized sarcomeres and Z bands. Intracellular **c** and extracellular **d** electrophysiological recording from hESDCMs.

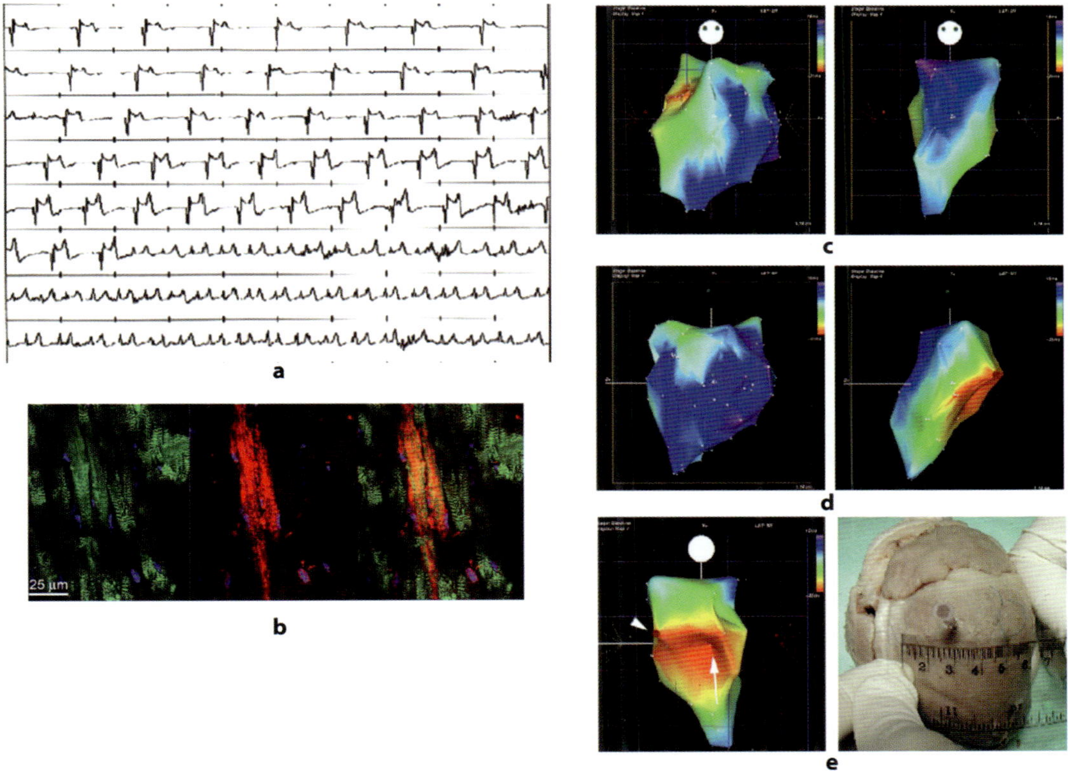

COLOR PLATE V

Figure 3.4. Electromechanical integration of human ES cell derived cardiomyocytes. **a** ECG strip containing part of the sustained ventricular ectopic activity (top) interspersed with a period of junctional escape rhythm (bottom). **b** Histologic assessment of the area of earliest activation. The left and middle panel shows the results of immunostaining with antisarcomeric alpha-cardiac actinin (green) and anti-human mitochondria (red) antibodies, respectively, whereas the right panel shows the superposition of both images. **c-e** Electroanatomical mapping and pathological correlation of the swine after His bundle ablation and cell transplantation. Mapping of the junctional (left) and ectopic ventricular (right) rhythms. Maps are shown from anteroposterior (c) and left lateral views (d). The junctional rhythm originated from the superior septum (left) whereas the new ectopic rhythm originated from the posterolateral wall (right) (earliest activation – red, latest activation – purple). **d** Spatial correlation between the electroanatomical map (left) and the sight of cell transplantation (right). During mapping, a focal ablation (arrowhead, left) was generated 2 cm away from the earliest area of activation (arrow, left). The pathological findings demonstrated correlation between the ablation site (pink needle) and the area of cell transplantation (blue suture).

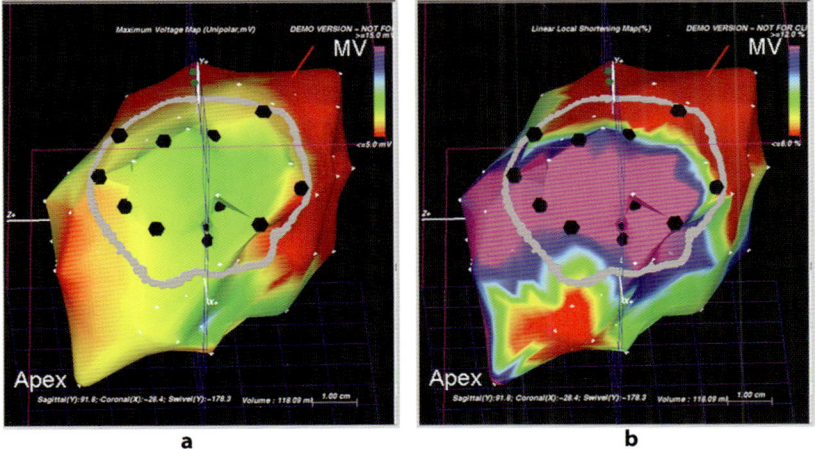

Figure 4.1. Bottom view of color-coded electromechanical maps. **a** Local shortening map. **b** Unipolar voltage map. Twelve injections (black dots) were delivered into predefined inferoposterior area. The marked zone also allows avoiding injection into the mitral valve area.

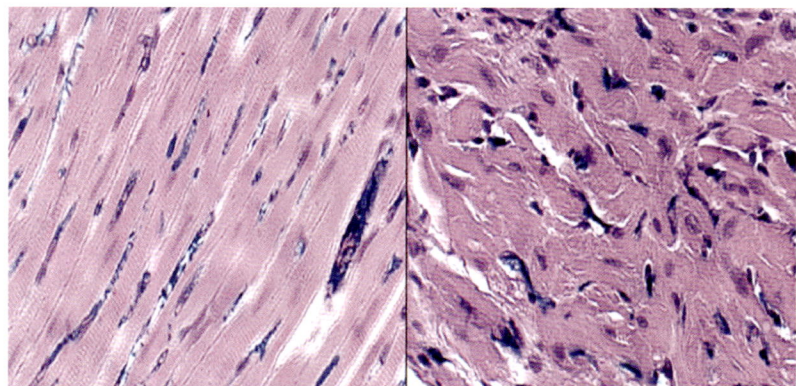

Figure 5.2. Left, Normal myocardium, hematoxylin-eosin, 40-fold magnification (after in vivo perfusion staining with Uniperse blue, a suspension of blue particles, capillaries within the myocardium appear blue). Right, Grafted tissue 3 weeks after intramyocardial injection of neonatal cells into infarcted tissue created by permanent coronary artery ligation, hematoxylin-eosin, 40-fold magnification.

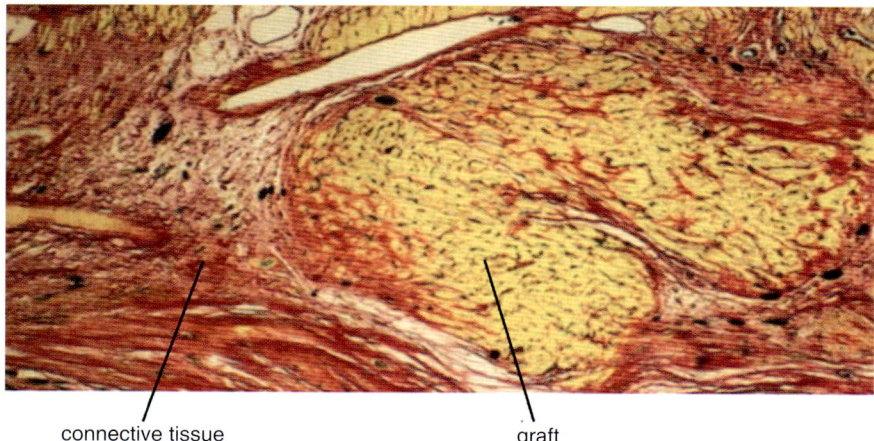

Figure 5.3. Graft 4 weeks after transplantation of neonatal cardiomyocytes in the scar, created by permanent coronary artery occlusion. The graft is largely surrounded by connective tissue and collagen, separating it from the host. Yellow, cardiomyocytes; red, collagen; Picrosirius red staining, 40-fold magnification.

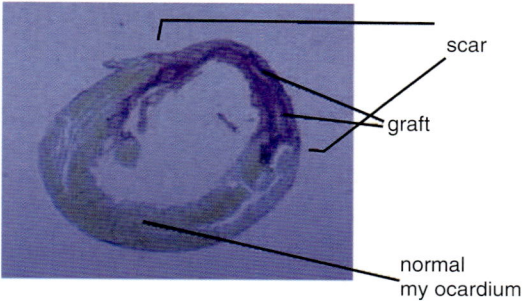

Figure 5.4. Cross-section of an infarcted heart (permanent coronary artery occlusion) 4 weeks after transplantation of neonatal cardiomyocytes. Clusters of grafted cells have developed, leading to thickening of the infarcted wall. On macroscopic assessment, the scar (collagen) appears red (Picrosirius red staining), the graft and normal myocardium yellow (Picrosirius red).

COLOR PLATE VII

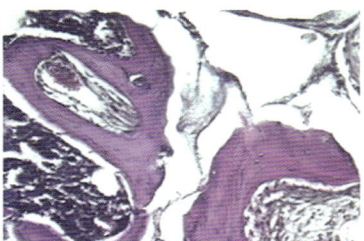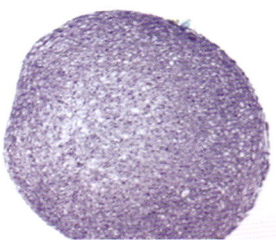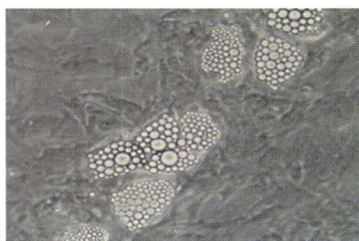

Figure 10.1. Differentiation of BMSCs toward three mesenchymal lineages: BMSCs loaded on a hydroxyapatite scaffold and implanted subcutaneously into immunocompromised mice form bone (left panel). BMSCs cultured in vitro in the presence of transforming growth factor differentiate into cartilage as evidenced by deposition of proteoglycans and formation of lacunae around the cells (center panel). In low serum and in the presence of insulin, BMSCs develop into preadipocytes filled with lipid droplets as evidenced in the right panel.

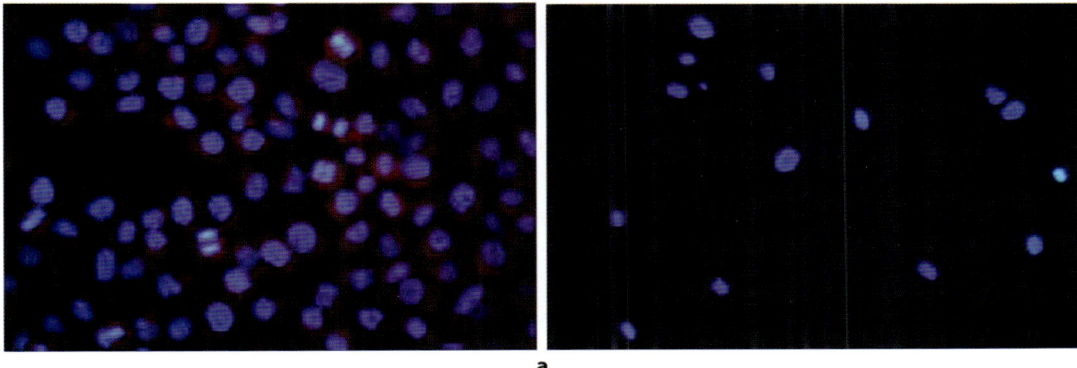

a

Figure 10.2. a Telomerase expression as evidenced in immunofluorescence experiments in BMSCs. BMSCs appear negative (right) for the presence of hTERT. The right panel presents Hela cells as a positive control (DAPI staining evidences cell nuclei).

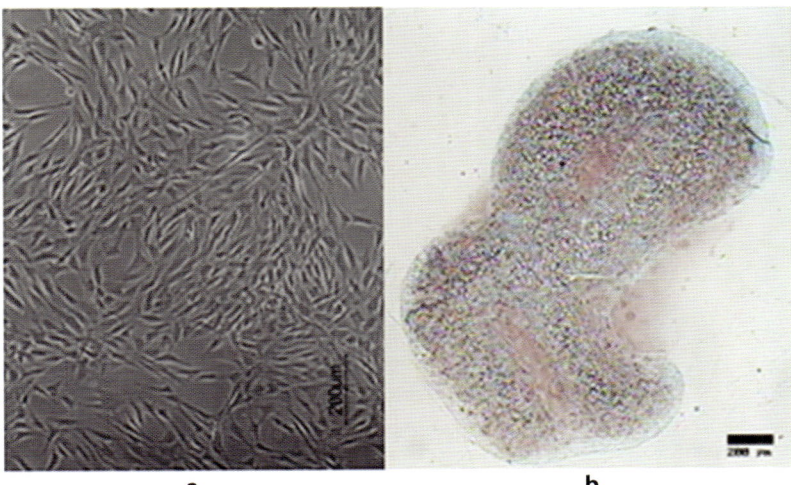

a b

Figure 11.1. Redifferentiation of human articular chondrocytes. **a** Monolayer culture of dedifferentiated human articular chondrocytes (passage one). **b** Redifferentiated articular chondrocytes in high-density pellet culture. Type II collagen is shown by red immunohistochemical staining (Vector VIP).

COLOR PLATE VIII

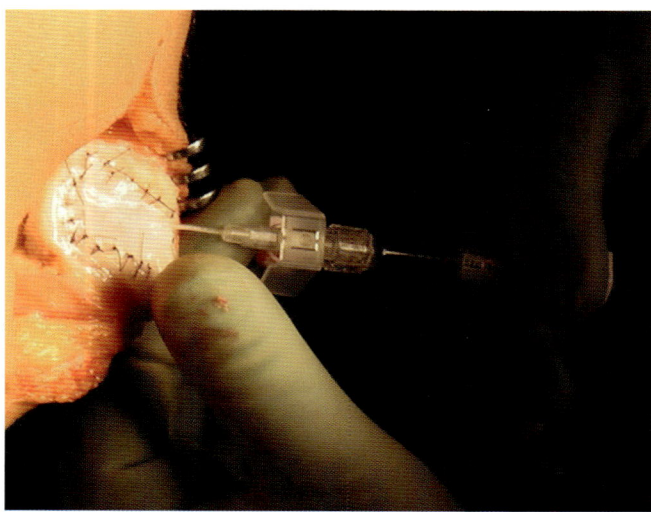

Figure 11.2. A cartilage defect on a human patella has been covered by a resorbable collagen I/III membrane. In vitro-expanded choncrocytes are implanted from a syringe into the defect.

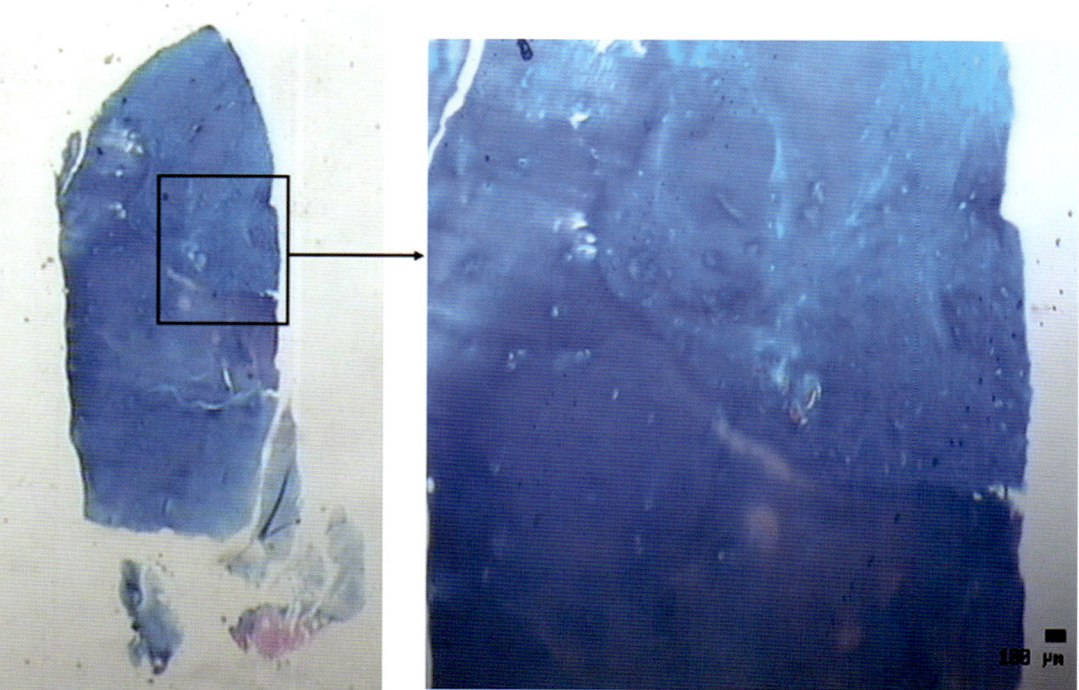

Figure 11.3. A full-thickness osteochondral biopsy from a cartilage defect that has been treated by autologous chondrocyte implantation 2 years earlier. Note fibrous top layer with remnants from periosteal top membrane and the underlying more cartilaginous repair tissue. Alcian blue – van Gieson staining.

COLOR PLATE IX

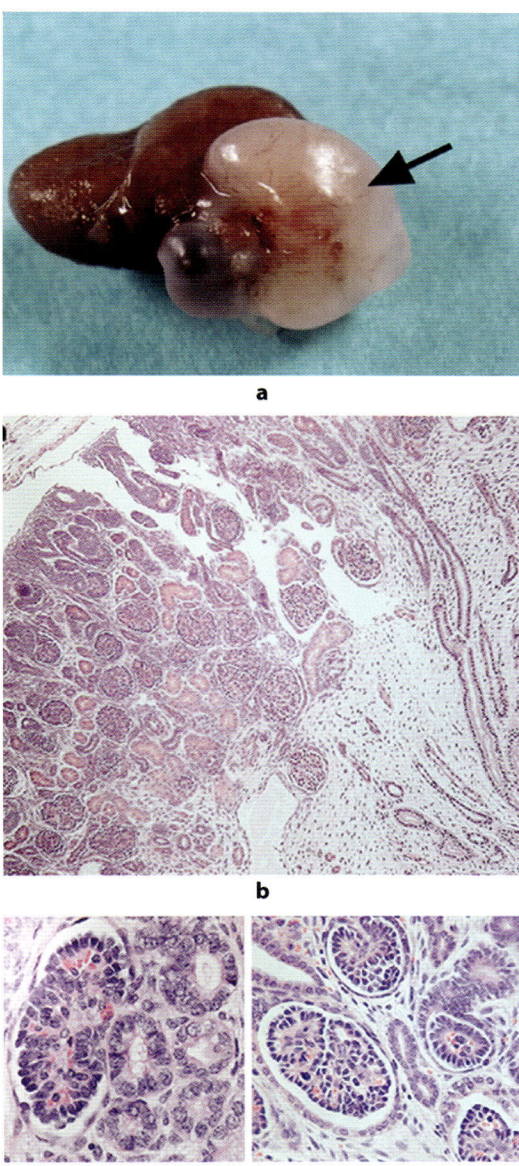

Figure 15.2. Growth and differentiation of an early human kidney precursor after transplantation into mice (8 weeks' posttransplant). **a** Macroscopic view; note massive growth and the formed shape of a kidney (arrow). **b** Histology (hematoxylin and eosin) (original magnification ×10); note preserved architecture and differentiation into layers of glomeruli and tubules. **c** Higher magnification (original magnification ×40) showing developed glomeruli and tubules.

COLOR PLATE X

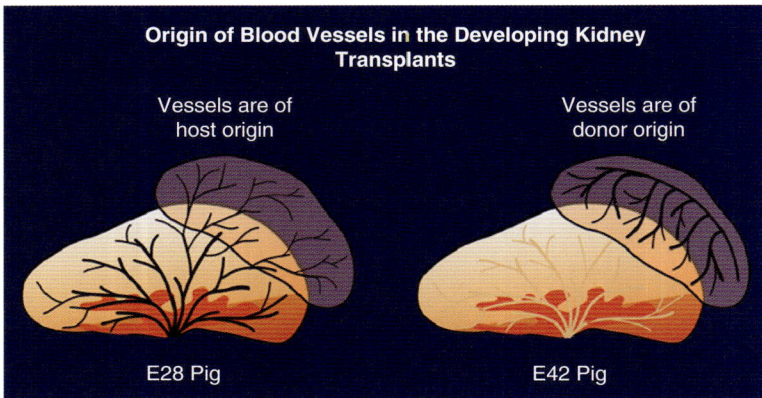

Figure 15.3. A scheme demonstrating the origin of blood vessels in the developing kidney transplants. Upon transplantation of early embryonic kidney precursors, a predominance of host-derived vessels are observed (left). On the contrary, when later-gestation kidneys are transplanted, a predominance of donor-derived vessels is found (right).

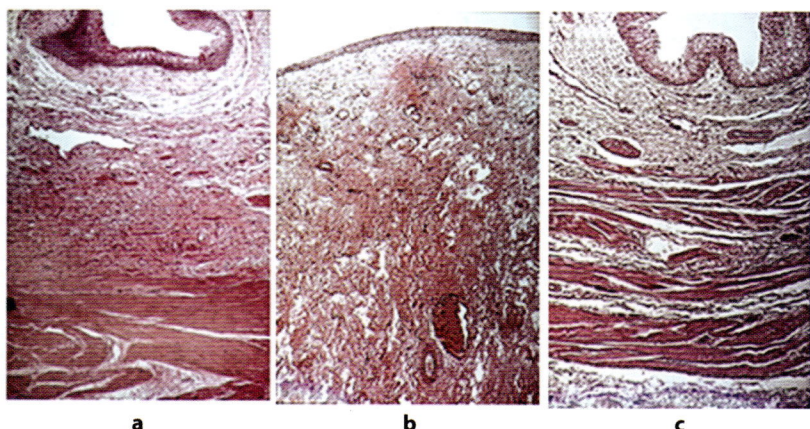

Figure 16.1. Hematoxylin and eosin histologic results 6 months after surgery (original magnification: ×250). **a** Normal canine bladder. **b** The bladder dome of the cell-free polymer reconstructed bladder consists of a thickened layer of collagen and fibrotic tissue. **c** The tissue engineered neo-organ shows a histomorphologically normal appearance. A trilayered architecture consisting of urothelium, submucosa, and smooth muscle is evident.

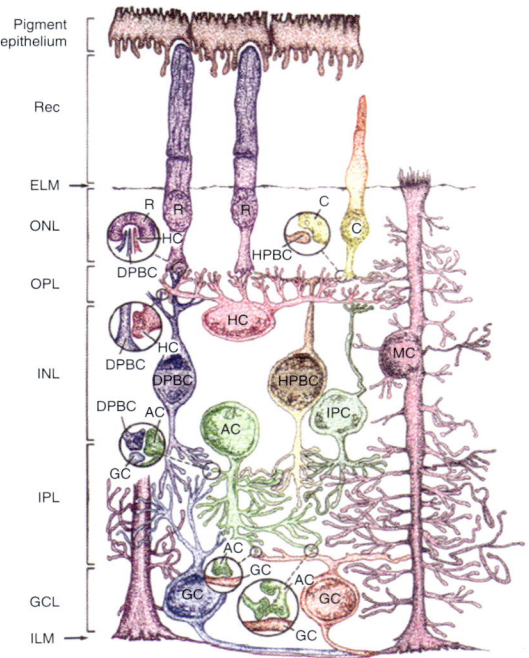

Figure 19.1. Schematic wiring diagram of the retina.

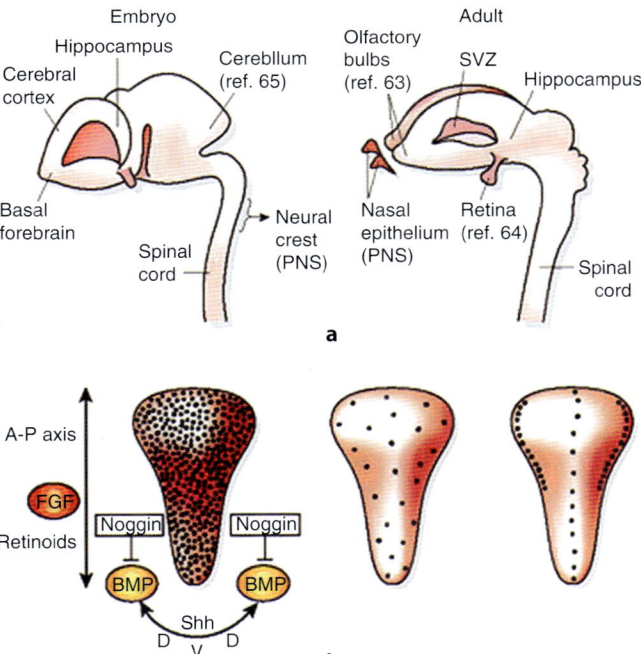

Figure 19.2. The location of neural stem cells. **a** The principal regions of the embryonic and adult nervous system from which neural stem cells have been isolated. **b** Three models describing stem cells in the vertebrate neural plate. All neural plate cells are stem cells (left), or stem cells are a minor population that is evenly distributed (middle) or located in particular regions such as the midline and lateral edges (right). Factors such as bone morphogenetic proteins (BMPs), Noggin, retinoids, sonic hedgehog (Shh), and fibroblast growth factors (FGFs), which provide anterior–posterior (A–P) and dorsal–ventral (D–V) patterning information, may regionalize stem cells. (Reproduced from Temple, 2001, Nature, with permission.)

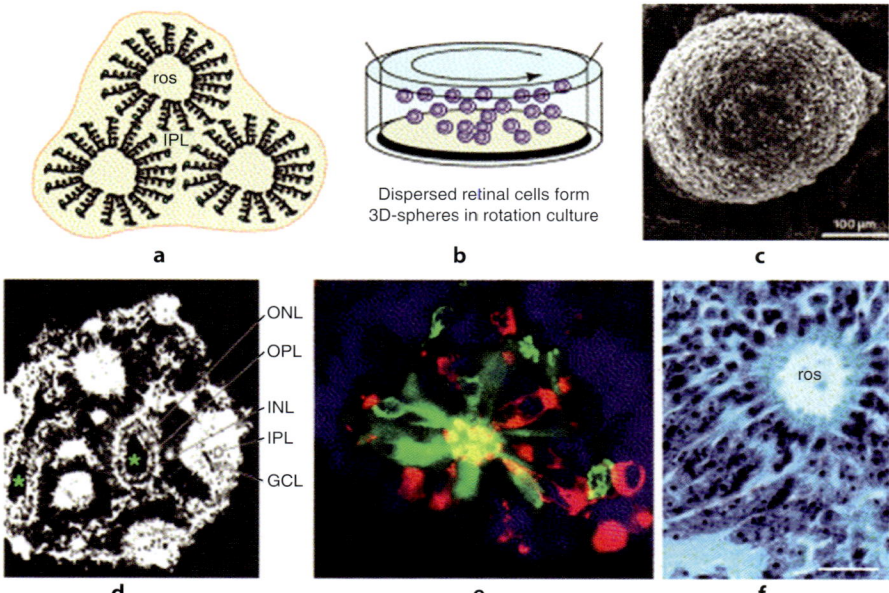

Figure 19.4. Production of histotypical retinal spheres by reaggregation of dispersed embryonic chick retinal cells. Schemes of **a** the internal structure, and **b** the reaggregate culture, are shown. **c** A scanning electron micrograph of a rosetted retinosphere. **d** F11-stained cryosection of a rosetted sphere after 9 days in vitro. All retinal layers are represented, including large internal photoreceptor rosettes [green stars; "ros" in a and f] and laminar areas corresponding to an OPL, INL, and IPL matrix, and ganglion cells. d–f, Rosettes hold rods and cones [red and green, respectively in e]. Note that the laminar structure is inverted compared with that of a normal retina. GCL, ganglion cell layer; INL, inner nuclear layer; IPL, inner plexiform layer; ONL, outer nuclear layer; OPL, outer plexiform layer. Scale bar in **f** corresponds to 120 μm in **d** 23 μm in **e** and 17 μm in **f**. (Reproduced from Layer et al.,[130] 2002, Trends in Neuroscience, with permission.)

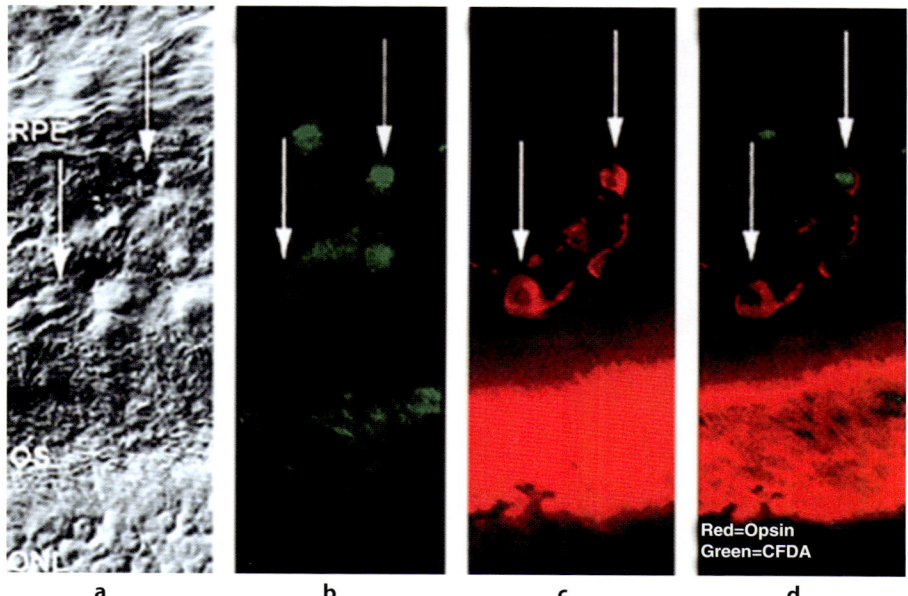

Figure 19.5. Differentiation of cultured retinal stem cells-progenitors in the subretinal space. Retinal stem cells-progenitors isolated from embryonic retina were cultured for a week in the presence of EGF. Proliferating cells were stained with vital dye, CFDA, and transplanted into the subretinal space of PN10 rats. Two weeks after transplantation, grafted cells **a**, **b** expressed photoreceptor-specific markers, opsin **c**. **d** Merged images. Arrows, grafted cells; RPE, retinal pigment epithelium; OS, outer segment; ONL, outer nuclear layer. (Reproduced from Ahmad, 2001, Investigative Ophthalmology and Visual Science, with permission.)

COLOR PLATE XIII

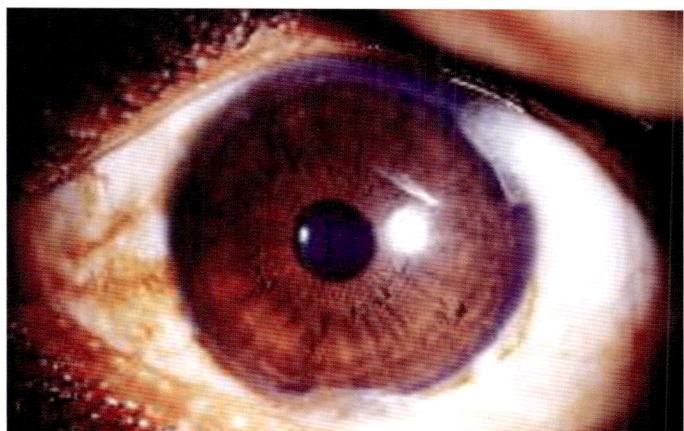

Figure 20.2. Ocular surface reconstruction after a severe chemical burn. [From Basti S, Rao SK. Current status of limbal conjunctival autograft. Curr Opin Ophthalmol 2000;11:224–232.]

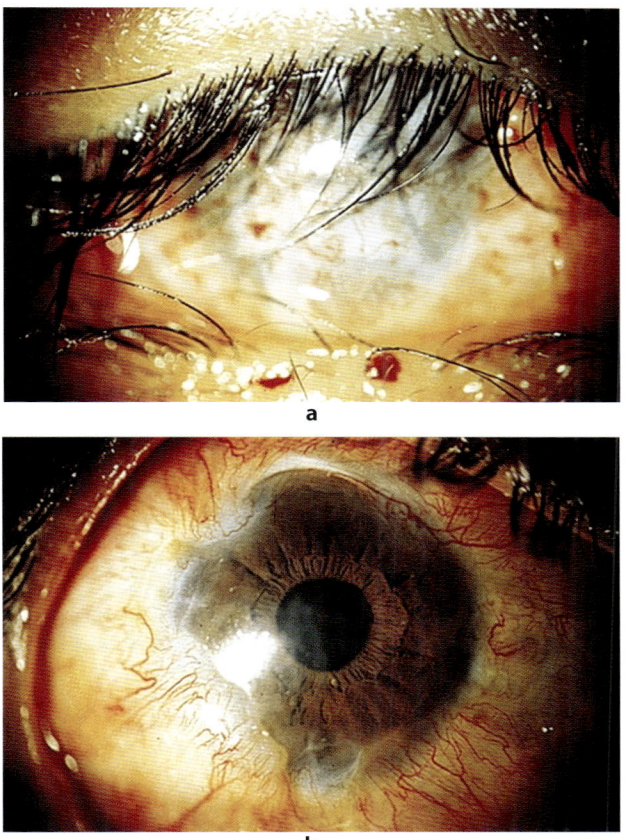

Figure 20.3. Limbal autografts, early postoperative and the donor eye. [Reprinted from Basti S, Rao SK. Current status of limbal conjunctival autograft. Curr Opin Ophthalmol 2000;11:224–232, Figures 1 and 2.]

COLOR PLATE XIV

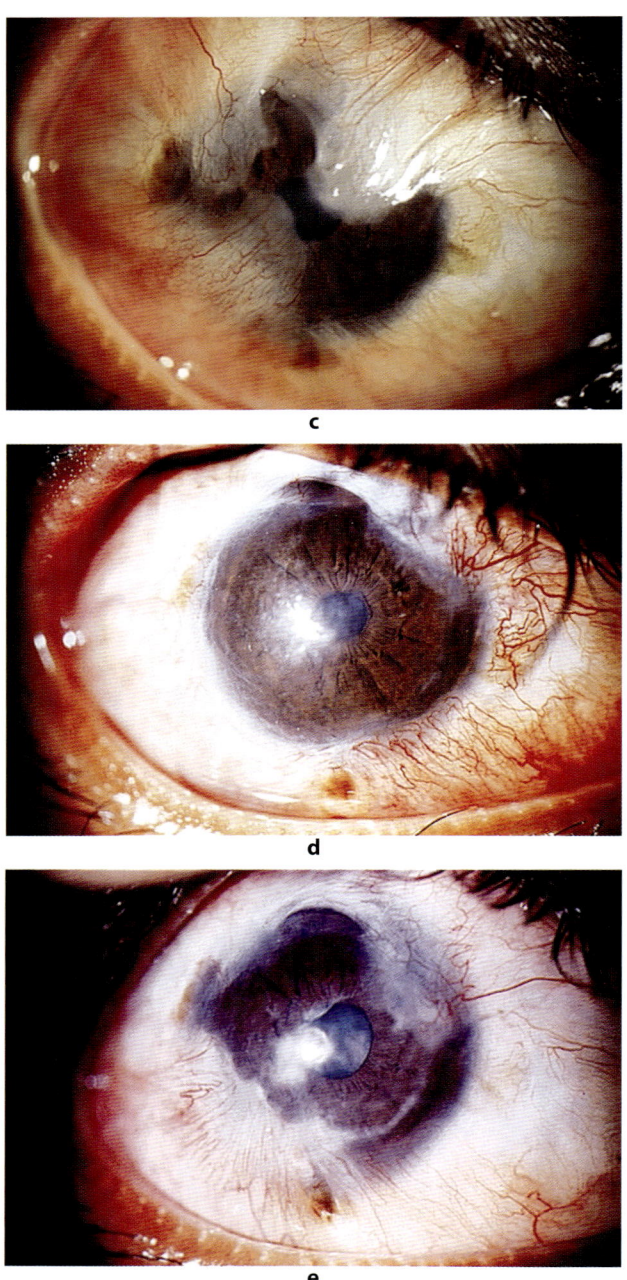

Figure 20.3. (*Continued*)

COLOR PLATE XV

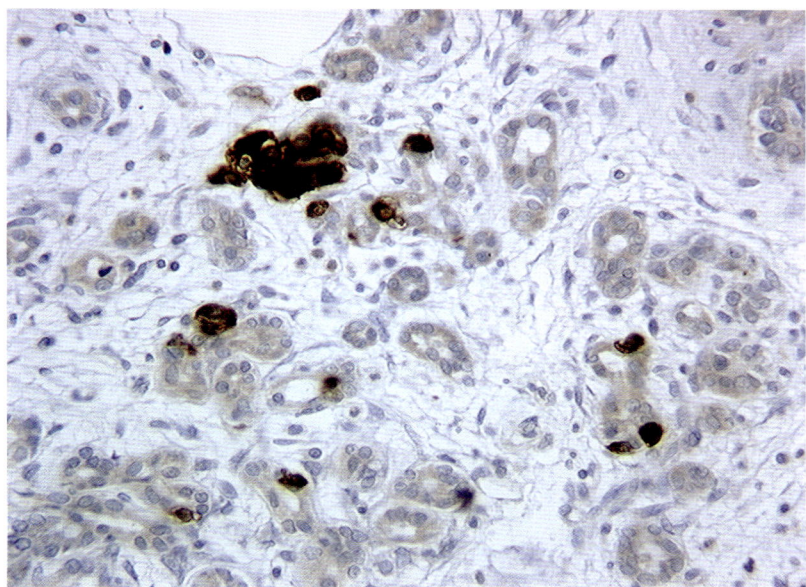

Figure 22.2. Neogenesis in human pancreas. The budding of islet tissue (here immunostained for insulin) from ducts is interpreted as neogenesis or new islet formation. This pancreas was from a 57-year-old female organ donor.

COLOR PLATE XVI

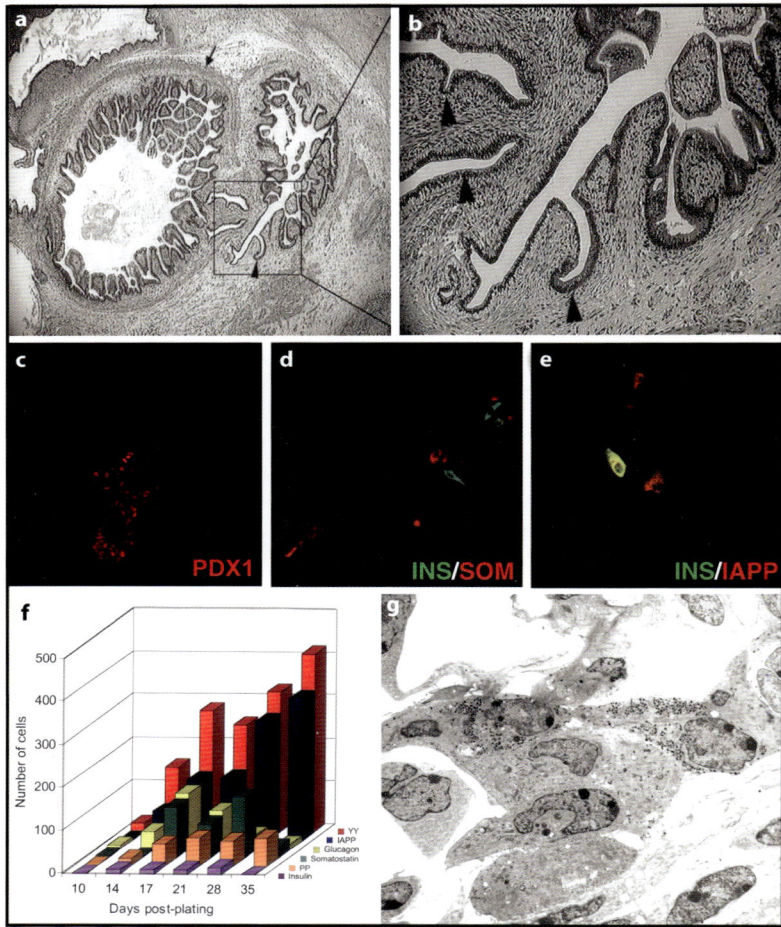

Figure 23.2. Endoderm and pancreas-like differentiation in murine and human ES cells. **a** Hematoxylin and eosin-stained tissue section of a teratoma generated after intramuscular injection of human ES cells into an immunodeficient mouse. A gut-like structure is clearly present. Original magnification 200×. **b** Enlargement of area shown in **a**. Original magnification 400×. Arrowheads in **a** and **b** mark cuboidal epithelium and areas of duct-like branching morphogenesis. Small arrow indicates layer of circular smooth muscle surrounding the gut-like structure. **c–e** Murine ES cells were differentiated into embryoid bodies (EBs) for 7 days, and then EBs were plated intact onto gelatinized coverslips and grown in the presence of serum for an additional period of time X (denoted as EB7+X). **c** EB7+7 stained with antisera to PDX1. Original magnification 40×. **d** EB7+28 stained with antisera to insulin (green) and somatostatin (red). Original magnification 40×. **e** EB7+21 stained with antisera to insulin (green) and IAPP (red). Costaining cells appear yellow. Original magnification 60×. **f** Bar graph depicting numbers of differentiated murine ES cells stained for insulin, pancreatic polypeptide (PP), somatostatin, glucagon, IAPP, or peptide YY (YY) after a 7-day EB formation and additional time in culture, shown on the x axis. Numbers graphed are averages of counts from 4–7 coverslips for each time point. **g** Electron micrograph of murine ES cells differentiated for 17 days after plating EBs. Adjacent cells with multiple electron-dense neurosecretory granules are visible. Magnification 6000×.

Section 4

Kidney

Section 4

Kidney

Benjamin Dekel and Yair Reisner

End-stage renal disease is a deadly disease unless supportive treatment is administered in the form of hemodialysis, peritoneal dialysis, or kidney transplantation. The morbidity, poor quality of life, and extensive burden on the health service of patients on chronic dialysis are major factors that prompt the development of alternatives for patients with kidney disease. However, there is a severe shortage of donor organs that is worsening yearly given the aging population.

Scientists in the field of regenerative medicine and tissue engineering apply the principles of cell transplantation, material science, and bioengineering to construct biological substitutes that will restore and maintain normal function in diseased and injured tissues. This approach could be also applicable to the kidney and urogenital tract. Induction of appropriate kidney differentiation and growth out of stem or progenitor cell populations, with or without the aid of growth factors and permissive scaffolds, represents an attractive option to combat renal disease and chronic kidney donor shortage.

Will we be able to grow or regenerate kidneys and bladders for use as graft materials in the future? Are we about to embark on a revolution in renal medicine? How does one sort through the hype of regenerative medicine to judge the true promise?

In this section, we and Atala outline the realms of investigation that are capturing the most attention in the field of kidney and bladder tissue regeneration. Our objective is to provide a framework for appreciating the promise while at the same time understanding the challenges behind translating fundamental tissue engineering and stem cell biology into novel clinical therapies.

15

Progenitor Cell Therapy for Kidney Regeneration

Benjamin Dekel and Yair Reisner

End-stage renal disease (ESRD) is a deadly disease unless supportive treatment is administered in the form of hemodialysis, peritoneal dialysis, or kidney transplantation. The morbidity, poor quality of life, and extensive burden on the health service of patients on chronic dialysis and the shortage of kidney donors for renal transplantation are major factors that prompt the development of alternative therapies for patients with ESRD.[1]

Regenerative medicine is focused on the development of cells, tissues, and organs for the purpose of restoring function through transplantation. The general thought is that replacement, repair, and restoration of function is best accomplished by cells, tissues, or organs that can perform the appropriate physiologic/metabolic duties better than any mechanical device, recombinant protein therapeutic, or chemical compound.[2]

Because of the kidney's is complex structure and function, its reconstruction represents a major challenge. Thus, during the past few years, sophisticated bioengineering methods of renal cell replacement have combined biologic and synthetic components. For instance, a renal tubule assist device engineered of porcine renal proximal tubule cells and connected in series to a hemofiltration device within an extracorporeal blood circuit was shown to be beneficial in acutely uremic animals and might therefore prove to be valuable in the treatment of acute renal failure.[3,4]

Induction of appropriate kidney differentiation and growth out of stem or progenitor cell populations represents an attractive option to combat kidney disease and possibly chronic kidney donor shortage. In that regard, the use of embryonic and adult stem cells as starting material offers new and powerful strategies for future kidney tissue development and engineering.

Growing Demands for Kidney Allograft Transplantation

Organ transplantation has been one of the major medical advances of the past 30 years. A growing number of patients can be transplanted successfully because of the continuing progress in surgery and medical treatments, and the development of new immunosuppressive drugs.[5] About 1 million people have received an organ, 73 kidneys from cadaver donors have survived more than 25 years, 17 heart and 27 liver transplant recipients more than 15 years.[6,7] Although the transplant community attempts to keep up with the increasing demand for transplantable organs, the supply continues to decrease far short of the need. This also applies to kidney transplant programs. It has been estimated that the number of patients with ESRD – for most of whom renal transplantation is the treatment of choice – is increasing at the rate of 7%–8% per year in the United States.[8] The United Network for Organ Sharing (UNOS) database shows that between 1988 and April 2002, the number of patients on a waiting list for renal transplantation increased from

13,943 to 51,753 patients.[9] From 1988 to 2000, the patients' waiting time has almost tripled from a median of 400 days to more than 1100 days,[9] and the number of patients who have died every year awaiting a cadaveric renal transplantation has increased from 736 to 2875, a 290% increase.[9] Moreover, in 2000, only 26% of the patients on the waiting list for a kidney transplant actually underwent renal transplantation.[9] Also, in most European countries, waiting lists for kidney transplantation are in a similar or worse condition than a decade ago,[6] making the severe shortage of cadaveric organ donors the major obstacle in preventing the full development of a transplant program and imposing a severe limit to the number of patients who benefit from this form of therapy worldwide. The challenge of expanding the donor pool has forced the scientific community to explore new avenues for organ replacement.

Stem Cells

Stem cells are defined as clonogenic cells that are capable of both self-renewal and multilineage differentiation.[10] The fertilized zygote has the highest developmental potential (totipotent stem cells), because it can generate all three embryonic germ layers and all extra-embryonic tissues, including the placenta. The same property is present in embryonic stem (ES) cells from morula (4–5 days after fecundation). Stem cells are pluripotent if they can form progenitors of all three embryonic germ layers, but not the extra-embryonic tissues. Currently, human pluripotent cells include embryonic carcinoma cells, derived from teratomas, embryonic germ cells, derived from primordial germ cells that populate the embryonic gonad, and ES cells.[11] ES cells are derived from the inner cell mass of the blastocyst stage embryos within the first 5–7 days after an egg is fertilized by the spermatozoon. ES cells can readily be cultured in an undifferentiated state for extended periods of time before a stimulus for differentiation is provided. Lower quantities of ES cells are present in fetal tissues (30–60 days of life). Many human ES cell lines have been derived worldwide, but only 78 cell lines met the eligibility criteria for federally funded research. A human ES cell registry is maintained by the National Institutes of Health, which collects the characteristics of some of these cell lines. To produce ES cell lines whose genetic material is identical to that of its source, nuclear cloning may be used. Two types of nuclear cloning, reproductive cloning and therapeutic cloning, have been described.[12] Reproductive cloning is used to generate an embryo that has the genetic material of the nucleus donor. This embryo can then be implanted into the uterus of a female to produce an infant that is a clone of the donor. Therapeutic cloning is used to generate early-stage embryos whose genetic material is identical to that of its intended recipient, allowing derivation of ES cell lines in vitro with a potential to become almost any type of cell in the adult body. Although presently exhibiting problems typical of cloning in general, including premature aging and high rate of mortality, this approach clearly might be useful in tissue and organ replacement applications.[12] Some applications might include the treatment of neurodegenerative diseases, diabetes, and end-stage kidney diseases. The use of transplantable tissues and organs derived from therapeutic cloning may lead to the avoidance of immune responses that are typically associated with transplantation of nonautologous tissues.

Finally, somatic stem cells have been identified in several organs of both aborted fetuses (>60 days of life) and adults. They have been shown to differentiate into a limited number of cell types. For example, neural stem cells produce neurons and glial cells, and bone marrow stem cells produce all types of blood cells.[13,14] However, some somatic stem cells are able to cross lineage boundaries under certain conditions. Perhaps the best example of adult stem cell plasticity is bone marrow stem cells. Bone marrow is the source of mesenchymal stem cells, which form cells of nonhematopoietic system, including cardiac myocytes, hepatocytes, endothelial cells, and epithelial cells of the gastrointestinal tract during tissue repair,[13,14] and hematopoietic stem cells, which are the ancestors of erythrocytes, granulocytes, monocytes, lymphocytes, and platelets. The use of human ES cells versus adult stem cells is under rigorous ethical debate, with the current political status strongly favoring adult stem cell processes.[11] The plasticity of adult stem cells to transdifferentiate from one lineage pathway to another is also under careful scientific scrutiny.[15,16]

Adult Stem and Progenitor Cells for Renal Repair

Repair of Endothelium

The kidney harbors several different types of endothelial cells, in particular the endothelium of the macrovasculature, the peritubular capillary endothelium, and the glomerular endothelium. Besides participation in the filtration, reabsorption, and nutrition of the renal tissue, endothelial cells have a key role in recovery from several renal diseases. The evident question therefore is whether endothelial progenitor cells (EPCs) can also participate in regeneration and maintenance of these renal endothelial cell types. Evidence for the existence of EPCs has mostly been derived from cardiovascular research on ischemia and angiogenesis.[17] Circulating progenitor cells for endothelial cells were first shown by Asahara et al.[18] In their experiments, CD34+ leukocytes were isolated from human adult peripheral blood. These cells were subsequently cultured and differentiated into an endothelial cell-like phenotype. That these EPCs are different from circulating mature endothelial cells was elegantly shown by Lin et al.[19] In bone marrow transplant patients, circulating endothelial cells from both donor (bone marrow-derived) and host origin were cultured from peripheral blood. Interestingly, the bone marrow-derived cells were markedly more proliferative than the host type cells and quickly outgrew circulating mature endothelial cells. EPCs can stimulate vascular repair processes in different ways. Several authors have shown that EPCs are involved in new vessel formation by incorporating in the vessel wall.[18] Furthermore, EPCs stimulate vessel formation by secreting pro-angiogenetic factors such as vascular endothelial growth factor and basic fibroblast growth factor, which subsequently enhance proliferation and migration of resident cells.[20]

A number of studies have addressed maintenance and regeneration of the specialized renal glomerular capillaries. Pabst and Sterzel[21] have reported that, in normal rats, the rate of total glomerular cell renewal is about 1% per day with the endothelial fraction being the most predominant cell type. However, in response to injury, the rate of vascular regeneration could well be increased. An established model to study glomerular injury and repair in rats is experimental anti-Thy1.1 glomerulonephritis. Injection of a complement-fixing antibody to the mesangial cell antigen Thy1.1 causes acute mesangiolysis and matrix dissolution, leading to ballooning of glomerular capillaries, formation of aneurysms, and loss of endothelial cells. In the subsequent repair phase, increased proliferation and migration of endothelial and mesangial cells are observed, resulting in partial restoration of glomerular structure and function. Using this model, it was shown that glomerular capillary repair is associated with a marked increase in endothelial cell proliferation.[22] Several studies have provided evidence that circulating EPCs may contribute to glomerular capillary repair. Recent experiments with rat hematopoietic chimeras demonstrated low levels of bone marrow-derived cells staining for the rat endothelial cell antigen RECA-1.[23] The number of these cells gradually increased over time suggesting that EPCs contribute to normal physiologic glomerular endothelial cell turnover. After anti-Thy1.1-induced glomerular injury, a fourfold increase in bone marrow-derived endothelial cells in the glomeruli was observed.[23] These data indicate that glomerular repair cannot only be attributed to migration and proliferation of resident endothelial cells but also involves bone marrow-derived cells.

Participation of circulating EPCs in renal regeneration has also been demonstrated in human adults. Williams and Alvarez[24] were the first to report the presence of host type endothelial cells in kidney allografts. Lagaaij et al.[25] reported that in human renal transplants the extent of replacement of donor endothelial cells lining the peritubular capillaries by cells originating from the recipient was related to the severity of vascular injury. They suggested that this endothelial replacement could be explained by the involvement of host-derived EPCs. Rookmaaker et al.[26] demonstrated male, donor-derived endothelial cells in the renal macrovasculature of a female patient who developed thrombotic microangiopathy after gender-mismatched bone marrow transplantation. Taken together, these observations confirm a novel role for bone marrow-derived endothelial cells in maintenance and repair of renal endothelium.

Repair of Mesangium

Glomerular mesangial cells provide structural capillary support to the glomerulus and display a pericyte- or smooth muscle cell-like phenotype. They have a central role in the pathogenesis of a number of human and experimental glomerular inflammatory diseases. In particular, mesangial hyperplasia is a prominent histopathologic feature associated with impaired glomerular function. Although transient hyperplasia is thought to reflect a physiologic response required for successful glomerular reconstitution and renal tissue repair, tight regulation of mesangial proliferation, function, and apoptosis is needed for recovery without fibrosis.

Initially, mesangial maintenance and repair after injury was thought to depend solely on proliferation of viable resident intraglomerular mesangial cells. These mature mesangial cells dedifferentiate before they proliferate, as is described by el Nahas.[27] Similar to the glomerular endothelial cells, in normal rats, mesangial cell turnover amounts to less then 1% per day.[21] Hugo et al.[28] demonstrated that during recovery of anti-Thy1.1 glomerulonephritis, proliferating immature mesangial cells migrated from the juxtaglomerular apparatus and hilar region into the glomerulus.

Reminiscent to mesangial cell recruitment during embryonic glomerulogenesis, the involvement of extraglomerular mesangial progenitor cells in glomerular repair was reported by several investigators.[29] Imasawa et al.[30] demonstrated the involvement of bone marrow-derived cells in normal mesangial cell turnover. Lethally irradiated mice transplanted with T cell-depleted bone marrow from syngeneic donors, transgenic for green fluorescent protein, manifested a time-dependent increase in green fluorescent protein-positive cells in their glomeruli. When isolated and cultured, these cells stained positive for the mesangial cell marker desmin and the cells contracted in response to angiotensin II, confirming that bone marrow-derived cells have the potential to differentiate into glomerular mesangial cells. Similar experiments with mice transplanted with purified clonally expanded hematopoietic progenitor cells were conducted by Masuya et al.[31] to confirm the hematopoietic origin of bone marrow-derived mesangial cells.

In similar experiments, using a rat allogenic bone marrow transplant model and antibodies to the mesangial cell-specific antigen Thy1 (ox7), Rookmaaker et al.[23] confirmed this time-dependent increase of bone marrow-derived mesangial cells in the glomerulus. Both Ito et al.[32] and Rookmaaker et al.[23] observed a major increase of bone marrow-derived mesangial cells during recovery from anti-Thy1.1-induced mesangiolysis in bone marrow transplantation models in rats.

Cornacchia et al.[33] demonstrated that glomerulosclerosis can be transmitted by bone marrow transplantation in mice. Transplantation of bone marrow cells from sclerosis-prone mice into normal recipients with the same genetic background, invoked glomerulosclerosis in the recipients. These data not only point to the contribution of bone marrow-derived cells to glomerular maintenance and repair but also show that dysfunctional or diseased mesangial progenitor cells can have a negative influence on the kidney.

Tubular Regeneration

The renal tubule is known for its high capacity for regeneration. Acute tubular necrosis, as a result of ischemia or toxic substances, can be followed by active migration and proliferation to restore normal tissue architecture and function.[34] Different sources of these proliferating progenitor cells have been reported. Humes et al.[3] isolated resident proliferative epithelial cells from the tubuli of mature rabbit kidneys and demonstrated that these cells displayed a high capacity for self-renewal and differentiated into complete three-dimensional tubular structures in vitro. Similar experiments were later performed with human epithelial cells.[4]

Bone marrow-derived extrarenal tubular progenitor cells were reported by Poulsom et al.[35] In female mouse recipients of male bone marrow grafts, colocalization of Y chromosomes and tubular epithelial cell markers was observed, suggesting participation of bone marrow-derived cells in normal tubular cell turnover. The potential importance of the role of bone marrow-derived cells in tubular repair was demonstrated by Kale et al.[36] When LacZ gene-positive bone marrow stem cells (Sca^+Lin^- hematopoietic stem cells) were transplanted into wild-type mice, renal ischemia was associated with the occurrence of LacZ-positive (bone marrow-derived) tubular cells. It was estimated that the majority of the tubular cells after tubular repair were bone marrow derived. Moreover, bone marrow ablation diminished functional recovery after tubular ischemia, whereas infusion of a progenitor cell reversed this effect, suggesting an important functional role for the hematopoietic stem cell in tubular repair. Furthermore, injection of mesenchymal stem cells of male bone marrow origin after renal injury induced in mice by the anticancer agent cisplatin remarkably protected cisplatin-treated syngeneic female mice from renal function impairment and severe tubular injury. Y chromosome-containing cells localized in the context of the tubular epithelial lining and displayed binding sites for Lens culinaris lectin, indicating that mesenchymal stem cells engraft the damaged kidney and differentiate into tubular epithelial cells, thereby restoring renal structure and function. Mesenchymal stem cells markedly accelerated tubular proliferation in response to cisplatin-induced damage, as revealed by higher numbers of Ki-67-positive cells within the tubuli with respect to cisplatin-treated mice that were given saline.[37] Also, in humans, there are some indications for bone marrow-derived tubular repair.[38] When male kidney transplant patients who received a female kidney and who recovered from acute tubular necrosis were studied, a Y chromosome could be demonstrated in few (less than 1%) of the tubular cells. Although the functional importance of this phenomenon in the human situation is still dubious, these experiments do provide a proof-of-principle observation on bone marrow-derived tubular repair.

To explore the presence of renal progenitor cells that are actively engaged in tubular regeneration after injury, the existence of label-retaining cells (LRCs; slow-cycling cells) in normal rat kidneys by in vivo bromodeoxyuridine labeling was examined. LRCs were scattered among renal epithelial tubular cells of normal rat kidneys. During the recovery after renal ischemia, LRCs underwent cell division and most of them became positive for proliferating cell nuclear antigen. At an early phase of tubular regeneration, descendants of LRCs expressed a mesenchymal marker, vimentin, and eventually became positive for an epithelial marker, E-cadherin, after multiple cell divisions. These findings suggested that LRCs function as a source for regenerating and replacing injured cells. Collectively, it was concluded that LRCs are renal progenitor-like tubular cells that provide regenerating cells, which actively proliferate and eventually differentiate into epithelial cells during tubular regeneration. Thus, intrinsic adult renal stem cells might also contribute to tubular repair. It may be possible to regenerate renal tubules in vivo through their activation or direct delivery to sites of disease.[39]

Fibroblasts

Renal fibrosis is a common denominator of most chronic renal diseases that progress to end-stage renal failure and is associated with major alterations in the tubular interstitial compartment. Increased numbers of fibroblasts producing excessive amounts of extracellular matrix molecules characterize interstitial pathology. Whether interstitial fibrosis is a cause or a consequence of renal pathology remains unclear. Recently, it was hypothesized that expansion of the cellular content of the interstitium could be an attempt to restore an embryonic environment supporting the repair of injured tubules.[40] Understanding the origin of interstitial fibroblasts may well contribute to our understanding of the role of these cells in renal pathology.

One hypothesis for the origin of interstitial fibroblasts proposes an epithelial–mesenchymal transition in the local formation of fibroblasts from organ epithelium. These transitions are particularly apparent during fibrogenesis: Fibrotic tissue repair after injury. Strutz et al.[41] first demonstrated de novo expression of a murine fibroblast-specific marker (FSP-1) in selected tubular epithelial cells during late stages of renal fibrogenesis. Ng et al.[42] showed that progressive renal failure is associated with the transdifferentiation of tubular cells into myofibroblasts. A second hypothesis for the origin of adult fibroblasts argues that marrow stromal cells are fibroblast progenitors that shuttle from the bone marrow through the circulation to populate peripheral organs. Accordingly, when circulating blood cells were labeled, they could be traced to sites of active wound healing and displaying a fibroblastic morphology. Bucala et al.[43] described a distinct population of human leukocytes that was able to differentiate into fibroblasts. In an animal wound healing model, the ability of fibroblast progenitor cells to home at sites of tissue injury and participate in scar formation was demonstrated. In a human study, Grimm et al.[44] assessed the relative participation of extrarenal derived–actin positive cells in the kidney. In renal transplanted patients, kidney biopsies were taken approximately 2 months after transplantation. The level of host-derived–actin positive cells in the kidney varied between 77% and 30%, indicating the existence of a circulating mesenchymal progenitor cell.

Finally, Iwano et al.[45] assessed the relative contribution of fibroblasts from both origins to the interstitial fibroblast content in normal and fibrotic murine kidneys. In the normal kidney, bone marrow-derived cells were responsible for 12% of total renal fibroblasts, whereas the remaining 88% were resident fibroblasts. In renal fibrosis, as a consequence of unilateral ureteral obstruction, these numbers were 15% and 49%, respectively. The remaining 36% was derived from epithelial–mesenchymal transdifferentiation. Furthermore, they showed that these transdifferentiated cells were actively involved in the fibrosis, producing abnormal amounts and types of collagen.

Pluripotent and Committed ES Cells for Renal Repair

Can a kidney be grown from pluripotent ES cells? Theoretically, human ES cells, which are derived from blastocysts, can form derivatives of all three germ layers and give rise to all cell types of the body.[11] Nevertheless, their in vivo use is limited; transplantation of human ES cells directly into adoptive hosts results in teratoma growth,[46] and they have to be initially programmed and differentiated in vitro into a specific cell lineage before transplantation,[47–49] a process that does not confer purity of a single cell type.[50] It remains to be determined whether human ES cells can be used as a starting material for creating complex functional three-dimensional organs in addition to their potential in generating individual cells.

Organ-specific stem/precursor cells (brain, lung, skin, kidney, etc.), which are thought to be able to directly generate many or the entire differentiated cell types in an organ, similar to hematopoietic stem cells which reconstitute the blood, may be ideal for tissue replacement (Figure 15.1). Although most adult organs, including the kidney, are mainly composed of terminally differentiated cells and the existence of an intrinsic stem cell population that supports regeneration is of debate, it might be useful to track down multipotent organ stem/

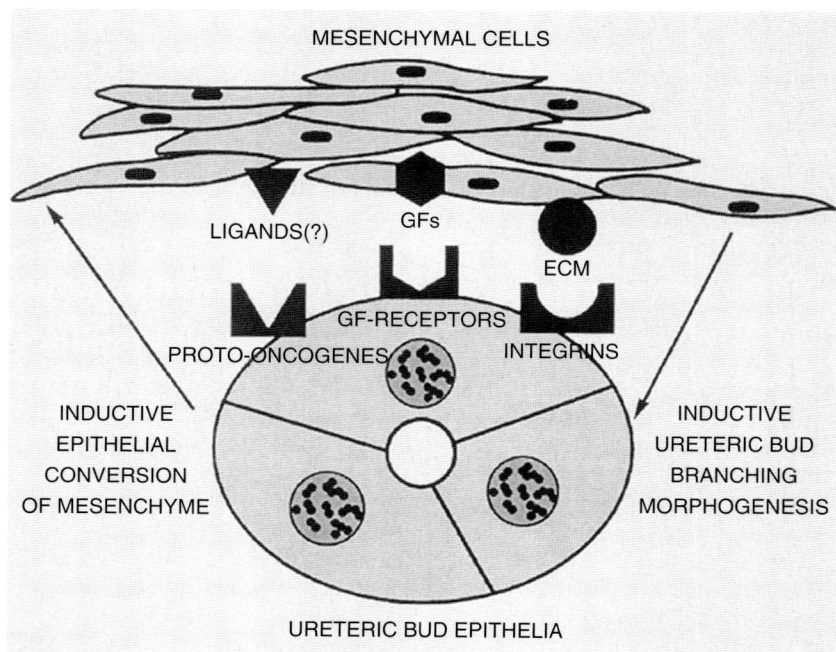

Figure 15.1. A simplified scheme of an embryonic renal progenitor unit consisting of metanephric mesenchymal stem cells and ureteric buds, which cross-talk via growth factors (GFs) and their receptors, molecules of the extracellular matrix (ECM) and specific integrins, proto-oncogenes and specific ligands and give rise to the differentiated cell types of the adult kidney (see text).

progenitor cells during embryonic life in areas where organogenesis is taking place. Such fetal organ committed progenitor cells are largely restricted to reconstitution of a specific organ, but they are pluripotent in their capacity to develop into a variety of different mature cell types in the growing organ.

Mammalian Kidney Development

In early embryonic life, there is a distinct stage that represents the direct developmental origin of the mature kidney[51,52] (Figure 15.1). This stage begins at 5 weeks of human gestation when a branch of the Wolffian duct, the ureteric bud, invades the metanephrogenic mesenchyme. Mutually inductive events cause the ureteric bud to branch serially (a process termed branching morphogenesis) to form the collecting ducts, renal pelvis, ureter, and bladder trigone, whereas the renal mesenchyme undergoes mesenchymal-to-epithelial conversion to form glomeruli, proximal and distal tubules, and loops of Henlé. Only at 9 weeks of human gestation will primitive glomeruli appear. In the developing human kidney, mesenchymal cells are induced into the nephrogenic pathway to form nephrons until 34 weeks of gestation.

The existence of renal ES cells in the metanephric mesenchyme is supported by several types of evidence. Previously, the presence of a single metanephric mesenchymal cell that can generate all the epithelial elements of the nephron, excluding the collecting tubule, was established using a lineage marker.[53] This indicated the presence of renal epithelial stem cells. Moreover, recent in vitro[54] and in vivo[55-57] data suggest that cells residing in the metanephric mesenchyme have, under various experimental conditions, the potential to differentiate, in addition to renal epithelia, into other professional cell types that participate in kidney organogenesis (myofibroblasts, smooth muscle, endothelium), as well as nonrenal derivatives including cartilage, bone, and blood.

Thus, the metanephric mesenchyme contains multipotent progenitors or embryonic renal stem cells with the ability to generate, in concert with the ureteric bud, many cell types in the mature kidney. Although the ultimate goal is the identification of a single nephrogenic stem cell that can build the entire organ, these precursor tissues offer excellent starting material to regenerate renal structures.

Over the past few years, we have studied the transplantability of human embryonic renal precursors in murine hosts.[56,58-60] Because of the difficulties in obtaining sufficient numbers of human embryos, as well as the ethical problems involved with the use of human embryonic tissue, we and others have used alternative embryonic donor tissue obtained from rodents[61-65] and pigs.[56,66]

Defining a Gestational Window for Optimal Growth and Differentiation of Embryonic Kidney Progenitors Free of Teratoma Risk

If embryonic kidney precursors were to be used for transplantation, extensive differentiation into nephrons along with the organization of a collecting system required for drainage of urine must take place in vivo. That is, most of the metanephric mesenchymal cells should convert into nephron epithelia and also form glomeruli after grafting, whereas ureteric buds should undergo branching morphogenesis. Theoretically, this could be more difficult to achieve for undifferentiated precursors derived from early embryos, which contain primarily metanephric blastema and a few ureteric buds, compared with later-gestation kidneys, which have already differentiated to a certain extent. Additional considerations should take into account properties that are inherent to undifferentiated and predifferentiated progenitor cells, such as the ability to differentiate to several lineages[67] and to undergo malignant transformation in the form of embryonic tumors after transplantation.[68]

Evidence for the tremendous capacity of kidney precursors to grow and differentiate after transplantation comes from studies with murine[61-65] and human tissues.[56,58-60] We initially transplanted human fetal kidney fragments derived from mid-gestation pregnancies (14–22 weeks) into immunodeficient mice and showed that they exhibit rapid growth and development.[58,59] Taking into account that branching and nephrogenesis continue to occur until 34 weeks of gestation, in the outer rim of the human kidney, the nephrogenic cortex, these grafts continued to mature in vivo. We then compared the differentiative capacity of kidney precursors obtained at different timepoints of gestation.[56] Whereas whole-organ grafting can be applied for the early kidney precursors, the development of areas of graft necrosis prevents the use of this methodology for later-gestation kidneys, and they have to be implanted in fragments, as previously described.[58] For organogenesis, the early undifferentiated kidney precursors (7–8 weeks' human gestation) were advantageous over later-gestation kidneys, significantly growing more in size and differentiating into a larger number of mature glomeruli and tubules[56] [Figure 15.2 (see color section)]. These findings are in accordance with several investigators,[61–65] which transplanted embryonic day 15 (E14–E15) mouse and rat kidney precursors and showed the latter to form mature glomeruli and tubules, as well as organized cortex and medulla.

To increase the donor pool, we have also analyzed the differentiative capacity of pig kidney precursors, obtained at different timepoints of gestation, in immunodeficient mice.[56] Similar to the human transplants, we could show that grafting of early pig kidney precursors, obtained from E27–E28 embryos, achieves organogenesis and leads to better growth and differentiation compared with later-gestation pig kidneys.

Because a pig gestation affords availability of very young embryos, we could perform grafting of very early pig kidney precursors (E21–E25) in immunodeficient mice. Here, grafts did not differentiate exclusively along the nephric lineage and other differentiated derivatives such as cartilage, bone, blood vessels, and myofibroblasts, could be found. As stated before, this finding complements recent in vitro[54] and in vivo[55] data to suggest that cells residing in the metanephric mesenchyme are pluripotent and can transdifferentiate into nonrenal derivatives especially of mesodermal origin.

Thus, we could define a window of opportunity for transplantation in which successful organogenesis is achieved when applying human or porcine stage-specific kidney precursors.

To gain insight into the molecular signals that stimulate the human kidney precursors to grow and develop after transplantation, we determined to what extent their transcriptional program resembles that involved in the induction of the normal human kidney or the transformation into an embryonic kidney malignancy (Wilms' tumor).[60] Grafts originating from a 10-week human gestation kidney were harvested at specific timepoints and cDNA was hybridized onto nylon arrays representing 1200 genes. Gene expression profiles were compared with those obtained for developing human gestation kidneys and Wilms' tumor. Strikingly, many of the details of the molecular program required to generate and build a human nephron after implantation into the mouse recipient were similar, in a global sense, to normal kidney induction. First, most of the "nephrogenesis" genes, classified under cell cycle regulators, transcription and growth factors, signaling, transport, adhesion, and extracellular matrix molecules, which were induced in the normal process, were also observed in the developing grafts. Aberrant gene expression in the developing transplants included a small group of molecules which function in oxidative stress and indicate possible early ischemia after the grafting procedure. Second, comparison of temporal expression profiles demonstrated that the time course for development of normal human kidneys is similar to that found in the development of transplanted kidney precursors. Our approach could also identify specific genes, including growth factors, the expression levels of which were lower in the transplants compared with the normal kidneys at specific timepoints. Development of strategies aimed at increasing the levels of such genes might further enhance the differentiative capacity of the developing grafts.

Host Versus Donor Vascularization of Embryonic Kidney Progenitors in Host Animals

Transplanted kidney precursors rely on the development of a vascular network in situ for their engraftment and growth. To improve the ability of the grafts to sustain angiogenesis in a foreign microenvironment, it is of great importance to determine the extent of vascularization and whether it is derived from host or donor endothelial cells. Moreover, hyperacute rejection is thought to be mediated via the interaction of preformed antibodies circulating in susceptible hosts with antigens present on the endothelium of a xenotransplanted donor organ.[69] In addition, donor endothelial cells act as antigen-presenting cells to mediate cellular rejection[70] and therefore represent an immunological barrier for xeno- and allotransplantation.

Classical studies with murine metanephric tissue grown in organ culture or on the avian chorioallantoic membrane have suggested that kidney endothelia arise from angiogenic ingrowth of extrinsic vessels.[71] However, when Hyink et al.[72] grafted E11–E12 kidneys from normal mice into anterior eye chambers of host transgenic mice expressing β-galactosidase in every cell, they found β-galactosidase activity in the peripheral vessels, but not in glomerular endothelial cells. Furthermore, Robert et al.[73] grafted E12 kidneys immunolabeled for the vascular endothelial growth factor receptor, flk-1, into kidney cortices of the adult and newborn β-galactosidase transgenic mice. In this model, cells expressing flk-1 but lacking galactosidase activity are indicative of donor vasculogenic angioblasts. Thus, when implanted into adult recipients, the grafts exhibited only few glomeruli containing host-derived endothelium, whereas a majority of glomeruli grafted into newborns contained host-derived cells. These results suggested that rather than ingrowth of vessels into the developing kidney, endothelial precursors residing in the metanephrogenic mesenchyme give rise, at least in part, to glomerular capillaries and microcirculation of the developed kidney.[52,72] In contrast, Rogers and Hammerman[65] using a non-cross-reactive anti-mouse PECAM-1 antibody to stain for host-type endothelial cells, showed that upon xenoimplantation of E15 rat kidney precursors into recipient mice, host-derived cells could be detected in external vessels as well as in some glomeruli.

We undertook the same approach to analyze for mouse-derived endothelial cells expressing PECAM-1 in developing transplants of human and pig kidney precursors.[56] Similar to Rogers et al.,[65] we found positive PECAM-1 immunoreactivity in external vessels as well as developing glomeruli and small capillaries of grafts of early human (7–8 weeks) and porcine (E27–E28) kidney precursors, whereas grafts of later-gestation kidneys had significantly reduced host-derived vessel counts composed mainly of external vessels. Our results suggested differential staining which was dependent on the gestational age of the donor at the time of grafting. Because later-gestation kidneys have already developed a vascular network including vascularized glomeruli (donor-derived), whereas the early kidney precursors are less vascularized, before transplantation, recipient mice have a larger contribution to vasculogenesis of the latter including the formation of the microcirculation, after grafting [Figure 15.3 (see color section)].

It seems prudent to conclude that transplanted early human and pig kidney precursors develop as chimeric organs in which blood vessels are of both donor and host origin, whereas external vessels required for graft maintenance are mostly host-derived. The exact relationship between donor and host-derived endothelial cells in the formation of the microcirculation is currently unknown.

Functionality of Embryonic Kidney Progenitors After Transplantation

In vivo differentiation of human kidney precursors into functional mature nephrons after transplantation is critical if such were to be applicable as donor tissue in clinical practice.

Studies in mice, using fluorescein isothiocyanate-labeled dextran as a marker of filtration into the proximal tubules, demonstrated glomerular filtration in donor nephrons of murine metanephric tissue implanted into the renal cortex of neonatal mice.[61] Similarly, intravenous injections of antilaminin immunoglobulin G into rats transplanted with fetal rat kidney tissue, resulted in labeling of glomerular basement membranes in the subcapsular grafted kidneys, confirming perfusion of the grafts.[62] Because previous transplantation studies of renal precursors obtained from murine embryos[61] were not able to demonstrate that donor nephrons become incorporated into the collecting system of hosts, Rogers et al.[63] transplanted E15 rat kidney precursors in the omentum of rat hosts (intraabdominal grafting), so as to render possible surgical anastomosis between the ureter (a ureteric bud derivative) which develops as part of the transplant and the host's ureter (ureteroureterostomy). After anastomosis, developing grafts were shown to produce urine and clear inulin infused into the host's circulation. Furthermore, inulin clearance, which was shown to be increased by constant infusion of insulin-like growth factor-1 (IGF-1) into hosts, began 4 weeks' postimplantation of E15 rat kidney precursors.[74] If the time course for development of normal rodent kidneys is applicable to the development of such grafts, the enhancement of inulin clearance resulting from IGF-1 administration occurred after nephrogenesis was complete (3 weeks after birth).

We analyzed tubular function in developing human kidney grafts established in immunodeficient mice, with 99technetium-DMSA renography, the uptake of which occurs through the peritubular side.[60] We could demonstrate positive uptake of the radioisotope only in tubules that matured in developed grafts. To further determine kidney functionality, we measured levels of urea nitrogen and creatinine in cyst fluid collected from cysts arising from transplants of the early human and pig kidney precursors.[56] Large cysts were mostly found in transplants established in the abdomen and therefore were not limited by the renal subcapsular space. Fluid was derived by insertion of a microcatheter into the developing renal grafts. Average levels of urea nitrogen and creatinine were higher in cyst fluid compared with those found in the sera of transplanted mice, indicating that the human and pig transplants had produced urine. Levels of urea nitrogen and creatinine in the cyst fluid were significantly lower compared with native bladder urine. The dilute urine in the cyst fluid is compatible with a reduced capacity of the fetal kidney to concentrate urine. Thus, similar to previous reports,[61–64] we were not able to demonstrate a connection between donor human and pig nephrons to the collecting system of hosts. However, our transplants did integrate into the host's microenvironment and use its blood vessels, and urine was produced separately from the native kidneys. Further experimentation needs to be developed to produce adequate urinary anastomosis and diversion of blood supply to the kidney grafts sufficient to correct biochemical aberrations in a uremic individual. Increasing the number of transplants and/or administering specific human growth factors might support functional replacement.

In Vitro Propagation of Embryonic Kidney Progenitors

Recent advances in the understanding of the molecular biology of rodent renal development have enabled separate culture of the components of the developing rat kidney, namely, the ureteric bud and the metanephric mesenchyme. Functionally recombining subcultures of each of these embryonic precursor tissues might lead to the formation of "neokidneys." In this context, Steer et al.[75] took advantage of recently identified factors that direct ureteric bud branching morphogenesis[76,77] and metanephric mesenchyme induction[78,79] and showed that the isolated rat ureteric bud and mesenchyme can be recombined in vitro and the resultant structure is morphologically and architecturally indistinguishable from a "normal" embryonic rat kidney precursor. In addition, the whole rat kidney rudiment in organ culture or the cultured isolated rat ureteric bud can be partitioned into smaller fragments and these subfractions can be propagated through several generations. These generations do not appear different from their progenitors. The subsequent generations of isolated rat ureteric bud can be recombined with fresh rat mesenchyme. Within the recombined rat neokidney, the ureteric buds branch into the mesenchyme and appear to induce the mesenchyme to epithelialize and form nephrons in a normal manner. The nascent tubular nephrons in the recombination experiments form contiguous connections with limbs of the branched UB, thereby leading to an intact aqueduct between tubule and collecting system.

Considering the limited availability of human fetal tissue, this method for subculturing and propagating whole rat metanephric rudiments in vitro might be applicable to humans and provide a large number of human kidney precursors derived from a single donor. Clearly, porcine early kidney precursors could afford an unlimited source for renal transplantation. Furthermore, the development of a large population of pig renal primordia derived from a single progenitor could potentially be manipulated in vitro before recombination, for instance, in ways that would enhance acceptance of the xenotransplants in immunocompetent hosts.

Generation of Histocompatible Kidney Progenitors Using Nuclear Transfer

Nuclear transfer denotes the introduction of a nucleus from an adult donor cell into an enucleated oocyte to generate a cloned embryo.[12] When transferred to the uterus of a female recipient, this embryo has the potential to grow into an infant that is a clone of the adult donor cell – a process termed "reproductive cloning." However, when explanted in culture, this embryo can give rise to ES cells that have the potential to become any or almost any type of cell present in the adult body ("therapeutic cloning"). ES cells derived from nuclear transfer are genetically identical to the donor's cells, thus eliminating the risk of immune rejection and the requirement for immunosuppression.[12] Consequently, the ability to turn cloned primordial stem cells into more complex functional structures such as kidneys would potentially overcome both immune rejection and organ shortage.

Lanza et al.[80] investigated the use of nuclear transfer to generate functional renal structures. Renal cells obtained from an early-stage cloned bovine fetus (embryonic day 56, cloned from adult bovine fibroblasts) were used to generate functional immune-compatible renal tissues. The cloned renal cells were expanded in vitro, seeded onto collagen-coated cylindrical polycarbonate membranes to form renal devices, and implanted back into the nuclear donor animal without immune destruction. The embryonic precursor cells organized themselves into glomeruli- and tubule-like structures with the ability to excrete toxic metabolic waste products through a urine-like fluid, establishing once more their high capacity to regenerate functional renal structures. Because the cloned cells were derived from early-stage fetuses, this approach is not an example of therapeutic cloning and would not be undertaken in humans. Furthermore, studies showing that cloned animals have common abnormalities, regardless of the type of donor cell or the species used, and that these abnormalities correlate with both subtle and gross errors in the nuclear DNA leading to aberrant gene expression, might limit this strategy for therapeutic applications.[12,81]

Conclusions

Regenerative medicine is focused on the development of cells, tissues, and organs for the purpose of restoring function through transplantation (Table 15.1).[2] The use of stem cells as starting material offers new and powerful strategies for future kidney tissue development and engineering. Currently, adult and ES cells are investigated to replace individual cells in a diseased organ,[10] i.e., insulin-producing pancreatic cells for type 1 diabetes mellitus or dopamine-producing brain cells for Parkinson's disease, but are not close to support creation of whole organs or even significant parts of such organs. The kidney is no exception; stem cell therapy of both renal or extrarenal origin to replace renal proximal tubular cells or glomerular mesangial and endothelial cells might delay the events leading to the deterioration of the organ and consequently decrease patients' demands for organ transplantation. Once chronic renal failure ensues, "neokidneys" will be needed to combat organ shortage. Vascularized organ xenotransplants, which are now genetically engineered not to elicit hyperacute rejection, represent one potential option.[82,83]

Organogenesis is an additional alternative. Organogenesis of complex tissues, such as the kidney, requires a coordinated sequential transformation process, with individual stages involving time-dependent expression of cell–cell, cell–matrix, and cell–signal interactions in three dimensions. Precursor tissues are composed of functionally diverse stem/progenitor cell types that are organized in spatially complex arrangements. When obtained at gestational-specific timepoints, the theme of temporal-spatial patterning of progenitor cell interactions is programmed in precursor tissues leading to their optimal growth and development. The findings summarized here raise hope that translation of organogenesis for purposes of organ replacement is within reach. Nevertheless, for renal replacement therapy ("neokidney"), further experimentation needs to be developed to enhance the function of the early human and porcine kidney grafts once matured. Producing a prolonged adequate urinary anastomosis of the growing kidney and deriving of blood supply sufficient to correct biochemical aberrations in a uremic individual is an important goal. Increasing the number of transplants and/or administering specific human growth factors might support functional replacement. Considering the limited availability of human fetal tissue, a method for subculturing and propagating whole metanephric rudiments in vitro recently developed in rats,[75] might provide a large number of human kidney progenitors derived from a single donor. Alternatively, pig early kidney precursors could afford an unlimited source for renal transplantation, provided that risk for porcine endogenous retrovirus could be eliminated.[84] Large-animal models are needed to test the relevance of these strategies for transplantation in humans.

Table 1. Published strategies for renal cell replacement using biologic material

Starting material	Method	Biologic mechanism	Targeted cell possible	Indication	Reference
Mouse adult HSCs	Intravenous transplantation	Transdifferentiation? Cell fusion? Epithelial stem cell?	Proximal tubular cells	Acute tubular necrosis	36
Mouse adult BMDCs	Intravenous transplantation	Bone marrow hemangioblast?	Glomerular endothelial cells	Acute/subacute glomerular injury	23, 26
Mouse adult MSCs	Intravenous transplantation	Plasticity?	Glomerular mesangial cells	Acute/subacute glomerular injury	32, 33
	Intrarenal		Renal tubular cells	Acute tubular necrosis	37
Embryonic kidney precursors (rat, pig, human)	Subcapsular/abdominal grafting	Mesenchymal-epithelial conversion Branching morphogenesis Angiogenesis	Neokidneys	ESRD	56, 58–64
Rat embryonic kidney precursors (UB-MM[SVM1])	In vitro propagation	Mesenchymal-epithelial conversion Branching morphogenesis	Neokidneys	ESRD	75
Bovine embryonic renal cells	Nuclear transfer Artificial membrane seeding Subcutaneous transplantation	Cell organization	Neokidneys	ESRD	80
Pig proximal tubular cells	Renal assist device Hemofiltration Extracorporeal circuit		Bioartificial kidneys	Acute renal failure Shock, sepsis	3, 4

HSCs, hematopoietic stem cells; MSCs, mesenchymal stem cells; BMDCs, bone marrow-derived cells.

References

1. Kasiske BL, Snyder J, Matas A, Collins A. The impact of transplantation on survival with kidney failure. Clin Transpl 2000:135–143.
2. Fodor WL. Tissue engineering and cell based therapies, from the bench to the clinic: the potential to replace, repair and regenerate. Reprod Biol Endocrinol 2003;1(1):102.
3. Humes HD, Buffington DA, MacKay SM, Funke AJ, Weitzel WF. Replacement of renal function in uremic animals with a tissue-engineered kidney. Nat Biotechnol 1999;17(5):451–455.
4. Humes HD, Fissell WH, Weitzel WF. The bioartificial kidney in the treatment of acute renal failure. Kidney Int Suppl 2002;80:121–125.
5. Perico N, Ruggenenti P, Scalamogna M, Remuzzi G. Tackling the shortage of donor kidneys: how to use the best that we have. Am J Nephrol 2003;23(4):245–259.
6. Matesanz R. International figures on organ donation and transplantation – 2000. Newslett Transplant 2001;6:1–41.
7. Cecka JM. The UNOS renal transplant registry. In: Cecka JM, Terasaki PI, eds. Clinical Transplants 2001. Los Angeles: UCLA Immunogenetics Center; 2002:1–18.
8. Renal Data System: USRDS 1998 Annual Data Report. Bethesda, MD: National Institute of Diabetes and Digestive Kidney Diseases; NIH Publ 98-3176, 1998:39.
9. UNOS Critical Data: Waiting List. http://www.unos.org. 2002. Last update Dec 2001.
10. Daley GQ, Goodell MA, Snyder EY. Realistic prospects for stem cell therapeutics. Hematology (Am Soc Hematol Educ Program) 2003:398–418.
11. Jones JM, Thomson JA. Human embryonic stem cell technology. Semin Reprod Med 2000;18(2):219–223.
12. Hochedlinger K, Jaenisch R. Nuclear transplantation, embryonic stem cells, and the potential for cell therapy. N Engl J Med 2003;349(3):275–286.
13. Kondo M, Wagers AJ, Manz MG, et al. Biology of hematopoietic stem cells and progenitors: implications for clinical application. Annu Rev Immunol 2003;21:759–806.
14. Fibbe W. Mesenchymal stem cells. A potential source for skeletal repair. Ann Rheum Dis 2002;61(suppl 2):ii29–31.
15. Wagers AJ, Sherwood RI, Christensen JL, Weissman IL. Little evidence for developmental plasticity of adult hematopoietic stem cells. Science 2002;297(5590):2256–2259.
16. Terada N, Hamazaki T, Oka M, et al. Bone marrow cells adopt the phenotype of other cells by spontaneous cell fusion. Nature 2002;416:542–545.
17. Carmeliet P. Mechanisms of angiogenesis and arteriogenesis. Nat Med 2000;6:389395.
18. Asahara T, Murohara T, Sullivan A, et al. Isolation of putative progenitor endothelial cells for angiogenesis. Science 1997;275:964–967.
19. Lin Y, Weisdorf D, Solovey A, Hebbel RP. Origins of circulating endothelial cells and endothelial outgrowth from blood. J Clin Invest 2000;105:71–77.
20. Kamihata H, Matsubara H, Nishiue T, et al. Implantation of bone marrow mononuclear cells into ischemic myocardium enhances collateral perfusion and regional function via side supply of angioblasts, angiogenic ligands, and cytokines. Circulation 2001;104:1046–1052.
21. Pabst R, Sterzel RB. Cell renewal of glomerular cell types in normal rats. An autoradiographic analysis. Kidney Int 1983;24:626–631.
22. Iruela-Arispe L, Gordon K, Hugo C, et al. Participation of glomerular endothelial cells in the capillary repair of glomerulonephritis. Am J Pathol 1995;147:1715–1727.
23. Rookmaaker MB, Smits AM, Tolboom H, et al. Bone marrow-derived cells contribute to glomerular endothelial repair in experimental glomerulonephritis. Am J Pathol 2003;163:553–562.
24. Williams GM, Alvarez CA. Host repopulation of the endothelium in allografts of kidneys and aorta. Surg Forum 1969;20:293–294.
25. Lagaaij EL, Cramer-Knijnenburg GF, van Kemenade FJ, et al. Endothelial cell chimerism after renal transplantation and vascular rejection. Lancet 2001;357:33–37.
26. Rookmaaker MB, Tolboom H, Goldschmeding R, et al. Bone-marrow-derived cells contribute to endothelial repair after thrombotic microangiopathy. Blood 2002;99:1095.
27. el Nahas AM. Plasticity of kidney cells: role in kidney remodeling and scarring. Kidney Int 2003;64:1553–1563.
28. Hugo C, Shankland SJ, Bowen-Pope DF, et al. Extraglomerular origin of the mesangial cell after injury. A new role of the juxtaglomerular apparatus. J Clin Invest 1997;100:786–794.
29. Takahashi T, Huynh-Do U, Daniel TO. Renal microvascular assembly and repair: power and promise of molecular definition. Kidney Int 1998;53:826–835.
30. Imasawa T, Utsunomiya Y, Kawamura T, et al. The potential of bone marrow-derived cells to differentiate to glomerular mesangial cells. J Am Soc Nephrol 2001;12:1401–1409.
31. Masuya M, Drake CJ, Fleming PA, et al. Hematopoietic origin of glomerular mesangial cells. Blood 2003;101:2215–2218.
32. Ito T, Suzuki A, Imai E, et al. Bone marrow is a reservoir of repopulating mesangial cells during glomerular remodeling. J Am Soc Nephrol 2001;12:2625–2635.
33. Cornacchia F, Fornoni A, Plati AR, et al. Glomerulosclerosis is transmitted by bone marrow-derived mesangial cell progenitors. J Clin Invest 2001;108:1649–1656.
34. Toback FG. Regeneration after acute tubular necrosis. Kidney Int 1992;41:226–246.
35. Poulsom R, Forbes SJ, Hodivala-Dilke K, et al. Bone marrow contributes to renal parenchymal turnover and regeneration. J Pathol 2001;195:229–235.
36. Kale S, Karihaloo A, Clark PR, et al. Bone marrow stem cells contribute to repair of the ischemically injured renal tubule. J Clin Invest 2003;112:42–49.
37. Morigi M, Imberti B, Zoja C, et al. Mesenchymal stem cells are renotropic, helping to repair the kidney and improve function in acute renal failure. J Am Soc Nephrol 2004;15(7):1794–1304.
38. Gupta S, Verfaillie C, Chmielewski D, et al. A role for extrarenal cells in the regeneration following acute renal failure. Kidney Int 2002;62:1285–1290.
39. Maeshima A, Yamashita S, Nojima Y. Identification of renal progenitor-like tubular cells that participate in the regeneration processes of the kidney. J Am Soc Nephrol 2003;14(12):3138–3146.
40. Herzlinger D. Renal interstitial fibrosis: remembrance of things past? J Clin Invest 2002;110:305–306.

41. Strutz F, Okada H, Lo CW, et al. Identification and characterization of a fibroblast marker: FSP1. J Cell Biol 1995;130:393–405.
42. Ng YY, Huang TP, Yang WC, et al. Tubular epithelial-myofibroblast transdifferentiation in progressive tubulointerstitial fibrosis in 5/6 nephrectomized rats. Kidney Int 1998;54:864–876.
43. Bucala R, Spiegel LA, Chesney J, et al. Circulating fibrocytes define a new leukocyte subpopulation that mediates tissue repair. Mol Med 1994;1:71–81.
44. Grimm PC, Nickerson P, Jeffery J, et al. Neointimal and tubulointerstitial infiltration by recipient mesenchymal cells in chronic renal-allograft rejection. N Engl J Med 2001;345:93–97.
45. Iwano M, Plieth D, Danoff TM, et al. Evidence that fibroblasts derive from epithelium during tissue fibrosis. J Clin Invest 2002;110:341–350.
46. Amit M, Carpenter MK, Inokuma MS, et al. Clonally derived human embryonic stem cell lines maintain pluripotency and proliferative potential for prolonged periods of culture. Dev Biol 2000;227:271–278.
47. Zhang SC, Wernig M, Duncan ID, Brustle O, Thomson JA. In vitro differentiation of transplantable neural precursors from human embryonic stem cells. Nat Biotechnol 2001;19(12):1129–1133.
48. Sottile V, Thomson A, McWhir J. In vitro osteogenic differentiation of human ES cells. Cloning Stem Cells 2003;5(2):149–155.
49. Rambhatla L, Chiu CP, Kundu P, Peng Y, Carpenter MK. Generation of hepatocyte-like cells from human embryonic stem cells. Cell Transplant 2003;12(1):1–11.
50. Vogel G. Stem cells: new excitement, persistent questions. Science 2000;290:1672.
51. Woolf AS. Embryology of the kidney. In: Barratt TM, Avner A, Harmon W, eds. Pediatric Nephrology. 4th ed. Baltimore: Williams & Wilkins; 1999:1–19.
52. Al-Awqati Q, Oliver JA. Stem cells in the kidney. Kidney Int 2002;61:387–395.
53. Herzlinger D, Koseki C, Mikawa T, et al. Metanephric mesenchyme contains multipotent stem cells whose fate is restricted after induction. Development 1992;114:565–572.
54. Oliver JA, Barasch J, Yang J, et al. Metanephric mesenchyme contains embryonic renal stem cells. Am J Physiol Renal Physiol 2002;283:F799–809.
55. Almeida-Porada G, El Shabrawy D, Porada C, et al. Differentiative potential of human metanephric mesenchymal cells. Exp Hematol 2002;30:1454–1462.
56. Dekel B, Burakova T, Arditti FD, et al. Human and porcine early kidney precursors as a new source for transplantation. Nat Med 2003;9:53–60.
57. Dekel B, Hochman E, Sanchez MJ, et al. Kidney, blood and endothelium: developmental expression of stem cell leukemia during nephrogenesis. Kidney Int 2004;65(4):1162–1169.
58. Dekel B, Burakova T, Ben-Hur H, et al. Engraftment of human kidney tissue in rat radiation chimera. II. Human fetal kidneys display reduced immunogenicity to adoptively transferred human peripheral blood mononuclear cells and exhibit rapid growth and development. Transplantation 1997;64:1550–1558.
59. Dekel B, Marcus H, Herzel BH, Bocher WO, Passwell JH, Reisner Y. In vivo modulation of the allogeneic immune response by human fetal kidneys: the role of cytokines, chemokines, and cytolytic effector molecules. Transplantation 2000;69:1470–1478.
60. Dekel B, Amariglio N, Kaminski N, et al. Engraftment and differentiation of human metanephroi into functional mature nephrons after transplantation into mice is accompanied by a profile of gene expression similar to normal human kidney development. J Am Soc Nephrol 2002;13(4):977–990.
61. Woolf AS, Palmer SJ, Snow ML, Fine LG. Creation of a functioning chimeric mammalian kidney. Kidney Int 1990;38:991–997.
62. Abrahamson DR, St. John PL, Pillion DL, Tucker DC. Glomerular development in intraocular and intra renal grafts of fetal kidneys. Lab Invest 1991;64:629–639.
63. Rogers SA, Lowell JA, Hammerman NA, Hammerman MR. Transplantation of developing metanephroi into adult rats. Kidney Int 1998;54:27–37.
64. Rogers SA, Liapis H, Hammerman MR. Transplantation of metanephroi across the major histocompatibility complex in rats. Am J Physiol Regul Integr Comp Physiol 2001;280:R132–136.
65. Rogers SA, Hammerman MR. Transplantation of rat metanephroi into mice. Am J Physiol Regul Integr Comp Physiol 2001;280:R1865–1869.
66. Rogers SA, Talcott M, Hammerman MR. Transplantation of pig metanephroi. ASAIO J 2003;49(1):48–52.
67. Galli R, Gritti A, Bonfanti L, Vescovi AL. Neural stem cells: an overview. Circ Res 2003;92(6):598–608.
68. Erdo F, Buhrle C, Blunk J, et al. Host-dependent tumorigenesis of embryonic stem cell transplantation in experimental stroke. J Cereb Blood Flow Metab 2003;23(7):780–785.
69. Cascalho M, Platt JL. The immunological barrier to xenotransplantation. Immunity 2001;14(4):437–446.
70. Kreisel D, Krupnick AS, Gelman AE, Engels FH, Popma SH, Krasinskas AM. Non-hematopoietic allograft cells directly activate CD8+ T cells and trigger acute rejection: an alternative mechanism of allorecognition. Nat Med 2002;8:233–239.
71. Sariola H, Ekblom P, Lehtonen E, Saxen L. Differentiation and vascularization of the metanephric kidney grafted on the chorioallantoic membrane. Dev Biol 1983;96:427–435.
72. Hyink DP, Tucker DC, St. John PL, et al. Endogenous origin of glomerular endothelial and mesangial cells in grafts of embryonic kidneys. Am J Physiol 1996;270: F886–F889.
73. Robert B, St. John PL, Hyink DP, Abrahamson DR. Evidence that embryonic kidney cells expressing flk-1 are intrinsic, vasculogenic angioblasts. Am J Physiol 1996;271:F744–F753.
74. Rogers SA, Powell-Braxton L, Hammerman MR. Insulin-like growth factor I regulates renal development in rodents. Dev Genet 1999;24:293–298.
75. Steer DL, Bush KT, Meyer TN, Schwesinger C, Nigam SK. A strategy for in vitro propagation of rat nephrons. Kidney Int 2002;62(6):1958–1965.
76. Sakurai H, Bush KT, Nigam SK. Identification of pleiotrophin as a mesenchymal factor involved in ureteric bud branching morphogenesis. Development 2001;128:3283–3293.
77. Qiao J, Bush KT, Steer DL, et al. Multiple fibroblast growth factors support growth of the ureteric bud but have different effects on branching morphogenesis. Mech Dev 2001;109:123–135.
78. Plisov SY, Yoshino K, Dove LF, et al. TGF beta 2, LIF and FGF2 cooperate to induce nephrogenesis. Development 2001;128:1045–1057.

79. Barasch J, Yang J, Ware CB, et al. Mesenchymal to epithelial conversion in rat metanephros is induced by LIF. Cell 1999;99:377–386.
80. Lanza RP, Chung HY, Yoo JJ, et al. Generation of histocompatible tissues using nuclear transplantation. Nat Biotechnol 2002;20:689–696.
81. Booth PJ, Viuff D, Tan S, et al. Numerical chromosome errors in day 7 somatic nuclear transfer bovine blastocysts. Biol Reprod 2003;68(3):922–928.
82. Cooper DK, Gollackner B, Sachs DH. Will the pig solve the transplantation backlog? Annu Rev Med 2002;53:133–147.
83. Cascalho M, Ogle BM, Platt JL. Xenotransplantation and the future of renal replacement. J Am Soc Nephrol 2004;15(5):1106–1112.
84. Blusch JH, Patience C, Martin U. Pig endogenous retroviruses and xenotransplantation. Xenotransplantation 2002;9(4):242–251.

16

Tissue Engineering – The Bladder

Anthony Atala

Patients with a variety of bladder pathologies may be treated with transplanted tissues and organs. However, there is a shortage of donor tissues and organs, which is worsening yearly because of the aging population. Scientists in the field of regenerative medicine and tissue engineering are applying the principles of cell transplantation, material science, and bioengineering to construct biological substitutes that will restore and maintain normal function in diseased and injured urologic tissues. This chapter reviews recent advances that have occurred in the science of tissue engineering and describes how these applications may offer novel therapies for patients with bladder disease or injury.

The bladder is exposed to a variety of possible injuries and anomalies from the time the fetus develops. Aside from congenital abnormalities, individuals may also have other disorders such as cancer, trauma, infection, inflammation, iatrogenic injuries, or other conditions that may lead to bladder tissue damage or loss, requiring eventual reconstruction. Bladder reconstruction may be performed with gastrointestinal tissues. However, a shortage of donor tissue may limit these types of reconstructions and there is a degree of morbidity associated with the harvest procedure. In addition, these approaches rarely replace the entire function of the original organ. The tissues used for reconstruction may lead to complications because of their inherently different functional parameters. In most cases, the replacement of lost or deficient tissues with functionally equivalent tissues would improve the outcome for these patients. This goal may be attainable with the use of tissue engineering techniques.

Tissue engineering, a component of regenerative medicine, follows the principles of cell transplantation, materials science, and engineering toward the development of biological substitutes that would restore and maintain normal function. Tissue engineering may involve matrices alone, wherein the body's natural ability to regenerate is used to orient or direct new tissue growth, or the use of matrices with cells. When cells are used for tissue engineering, donor tissue is dissociated into individual cells which are either implanted directly into the host, or expanded in culture, attached to a support matrix, and reimplanted after expansion. The implanted tissue can be heterologous, allogeneic, or autologous. Ideally, this approach might allow lost tissue function to be restored or replaced in toto and with limited complications.[1] The use of autologous cells would avoid rejection, wherein a biopsy of tissue is obtained from the host, the cells are dissociated and expanded in vitro, reattached to a matrix, and implanted into the same host.[1-20]

Cell Growth

One of the initial limitations of applying cell-based tissue engineering techniques to the bladder had been the previously encountered inherent difficulty of growing genitourinary-associated cells in large quantities. In the past, it was believed that urothelial cells had a natural senescence that was hard to overcome. Normal urothelial cells could be grown in the laboratory setting, but with limited expansion. Several protocols were developed over the last two decades that improved urothelial growth and expansion.[9,21–23] A system of urothelial cell harvest was developed that does not use any enzymes or serum and has a large expansion potential. Using these methods of cell culture, it is possible to expand a urothelial strain from a single specimen that initially covers a surface area of 1 cm^2 to one covering a surface area of 4202 m^2 (the equivalent area of one football field) within 8 weeks.[10] These studies indicated that it should be possible to collect autologous urothelial cells from human patients, expand them in culture, and return them to the human donor in sufficient quantities for reconstructive purposes. Bladder cells can be equally harvested, cultured, and expanded in a similar manner. Normal human bladder epithelial and muscle cells can be efficiently harvested from surgical material, extensively expanded in culture, and their differentiation characteristics, growth requirements, and other biological properties studied.[9,15,22–31]

Biomaterials

Biomaterials provide a cell-adhesion substrate and can be used to achieve cell delivery with high loading and efficiency to specific sites in the body. The configuration of the biomaterials can guide the structure of an engineered tissue. The biomaterials provide mechanical support against in vivo forces, thus maintaining a predefined structure during the process of tissue development. The biomaterials can be loaded with bioactive signals, such as cell-adhesion peptides and growth factors, which can regulate cellular function. The design and selection of the biomaterial is critical in the development of engineered tissues. The biomaterial must be capable of controlling the structure and function of the engineered tissue in a predesigned manner by interacting with transplanted cells and/or the host cells. Generally, the ideal biomaterial should be biocompatible, promote cellular interaction and tissue development, and possess proper mechanical and physical properties.

The selected biomaterial should be biodegradable and bioresorbable to support the reconstruction of a completely normal tissue without inflammation. The degradation products should not provoke inflammation or toxicity and must be removed from the body via metabolic pathways. The degradation rate and the concentration of degradation products in the tissues surrounding the implant must be at a nearly physiological level.[32] The mechanical support of the biomaterials should be maintained until the engineered tissue has sufficient mechanical integrity to support itself.[3] This can be potentially achieved by an appropriate choice of mechanical and degradative properties of the biomaterials.[33]

Generally, three classes of biomaterials have been used for engineering bladder tissues: Naturally derived materials (e.g., collagen and alginate), acellular tissue matrices (e.g., bladder submucosa and small intestinal submucosa), and synthetic polymers [e.g., polyglycolic acid (PGA), polylactic acid (PLA), and poly(lactic-co-glycolic acid) (PLGA)]. These classes of biomaterials have been tested in respect to their biocompatibility with primary human urothelial and bladder muscle cells.[34,35] Naturally derived materials and acellular tissue matrices have the potential advantage of biological recognition. Synthetic polymers can be produced reproducibly on a large scale with controlled properties of their strength, degradation rate, and microstructure.

Collagen is the most abundant and ubiquitous structural protein in the body, and may be readily purified from both animal and human tissues with an enzyme treatment and salt/acid extraction.[36] Collagen implants degrade through a sequential attack by collagenases. The in vivo resorption rate can be regulated by controlling the density of the implant and the extent of intermolecular crosslinking. The lower the density, the greater the interstitial space and generally the larger the pores for cell infiltration, leading to a higher rate of implant degradation. Collagen contains cell-adhesion domain sequences (e.g., RGD) that exhibit specific cellular interactions. This may assist to retain the phenotype and activity of many types of cells.

Polyesters of naturally occurring α-hydroxy acids, including PGA, PLA, and PLGA, are widely used in tissue engineering. These polymers have gained Food and Drug Administration approval for human use in a variety of applications, including sutures.[37] The ester bonds in these polymers are hydrolytically labile, and these polymers degrade by nonenzymatic hydrolysis. The degradation products of PGA, PLA, and PLGA are nontoxic natural metabolites and are eventually eliminated from the body in the form of carbon dioxide and water.[37] The degradation rate of these polymers can be tailored from several weeks to several years by altering crystallinity, initial molecular weight, and the copolymer ratio of lactic to glycolic acid. Because these polymers are thermoplastics, they can be easily formed into a three-dimensional scaffold with the desired microstructure, gross shape, and dimension by various techniques, including molding, extrusion,[38] solvent casting,[39] phase separation techniques, and gas foaming techniques.[40] Other biodegradable synthetic polymers, including poly(anhydrides) and poly(ortho-esters), can also be used to fabricate scaffolds for genitourinary tissue engineering with controlled properties.[41]

Regeneration of Bladder

Currently, gastrointestinal segments are often used as tissues for bladder replacement or repair. However, gastrointestinal tissues are designed to absorb specific solutes, whereas bladder tissue is designed for the excretion of solutes. Because of the problems encountered with the use of gastrointestinal segments, numerous investigators have attempted alternative materials and tissues for bladder replacement or repair.

Over the last few decades, several bladder wall substitutes have been attempted with both synthetic and organic materials. The first application of a free tissue graft for bladder replacement was reported by Neuhof[42] in 1917, when fascia was used to augment bladders in dogs. Since that first report, multiple other free graft materials have been used experimentally and clinically, including bladder allografts, small intestinal submucosa, pericardium, dura, and placenta.[14,43–51] In multiple studies using different materials as an acellular graft for cystoplasty, the urothelial layer was able to regenerate normally, but the muscle layer, although present, was not fully developed.[14,49,52,53] When using cell-free collagen matrices, scarring and graft contracture may occur over time.[54–59] Synthetic materials, which have been tried previously in experimental and clinical settings, include polyvinyl sponge, tetrafluoroethylene (Teflon), vicryl matrices, and silicone.[60-63] Most of the above attempts have usually failed because of mechanical, structural, functional, or biocompatibility problems. Usually, nondegrading synthetic materials used for bladder reconstruction succumb to mechanical failure and urinary stone formation whereas degradable materials lead to fibroblast deposition, scarring, graft contracture, and a reduced reservoir volume over time.

Engineering tissue using selective cell transplantation may provide a means to create functional new bladder segments.[1] The success of using cell transplantation strategies for bladder reconstruction depends on the ability to use donor tissue efficiently and to provide the right conditions for long-term survival, differentiation, and growth. Urothelial and muscle cells can be expanded in vitro, seeded onto the polymer scaffold, and allowed to attach and form sheets of cells. The cell-polymer scaffold can then be implanted in vivo. A series of in vivo urologic-associated cell-polymer experiments were performed. Histologic analysis of human urothelial, bladder muscle, and composite urothelial and bladder muscle-polymer scaffolds, implanted in athymic mice and retrieved at different time points, indicated that viable cells were evident in all three experimental groups.[8] Implanted cells oriented themselves spatially along the polymer surfaces. The cell populations appeared to expand from one layer to several layers of thickness with progressive cell organization with extended implantation times. Cell-polymer composite implants of urothelial and muscle cells, retrieved at extended times (50 days), showed extensive formation of multilayered sheet-like structures and well-defined muscle layers. Polymers seeded with cells and manipulated into a tubular configuration showed layers of muscle cells lining the multilayered epithelial sheets. Cellular debris appeared reproducibly in the luminal spaces, suggesting that epithelial cells lining the lumina are sloughed into the luminal space. Cell polymers implanted with human bladder muscle cells alone showed almost complete replacement of the polymer with sheets of smooth muscle at 50 days. This experiment demonstrated, for the first time, that composite tissue engineered structures could be created de novo. Before this study, only single cell type tissue engineered structures had been created.

Formation of Bladder Tissue Ex Situ

To determine the effects of implanting engineered tissues in continuity with the urinary tract, an animal model of bladder augmentation was used.[14] Partial cystectomies, which involved removing approximately 50% of the native bladders, were performed in 10 beagles. In five, the retrieved bladder tissue was microdissected and the mucosal and muscular layers were separated. The bladder urothelial and muscle cells were cultured using the techniques described above. Both urothelial and smooth muscle cells were harvested and expanded separately. A collagen-based matrix, derived from allogeneic bladder submucosa, was used for cell delivery. This material was chosen for these experiments because of its native elasticity. Within 6 weeks, the expanded urothelial cells were collected as a pellet. The cells were seeded on the luminal surface of the allogenic bladder submucosa and incubated in serum-free keratinocyte growth medium for 5 days. Muscle cells were seeded on the opposite side of the bladder submucosa and subsequently placed in Dulbecco's modified Eagle medium supplemented with 10% fetal calf serum for an additional 5 days. The seeding density on the allogenic bladder submucosa was approximately 1×10^7 cells/cm^2.

Preoperative fluoroscopic cystography and urodynamic studies were performed in all animals. Augmentation cystoplasty was performed with the matrix with cells in one group, and with the matrix without cells in the second group. The augmented bladders were covered with omentum, the membrane that encloses the bowel, in order to facilitate angiogenesis to the implant. Cystostomy catheters were used for urinary diversion for 10–14 days. Urodynamic studies and fluoroscopic cystography were performed at 1, 2, and 3 months postoperatively. Augmented bladders were retrieved 2 (n = 6) and 3 (n = 4) months after surgery and examined grossly, histologically, and immunocytochemically.

Bladders augmented with the matrix seeded with cells showed a 99% increase in capacity compared with bladders augmented with the cell-free matrix, which showed only a 30% increase in capacity. Functionally, all animals showed normal bladder compliance as evidenced by urodynamic studies; however, the remaining native bladder tissue may have accounted for these results. Histologically, the retrieved engineered bladders contained a cellular organization consisting of a urothelial lined lumen surrounded by submucosal tissue and smooth muscle. However, the muscular layer was markedly more prominent in the cell reconstituted scaffold.[14]

Most of the free grafts (without cells) used for bladder replacement in the past have been able to show adequate histology in terms of a well-developed urothelial layer; however, they have been associated with an abnormal muscular layer which may be developed to a variable extent.[2,3] It has been well established for decades that the bladder is able to regenerate generously over free grafts. Urothelium is associated with a high reparative capacity.[64] Bladder muscle tissue is less likely to regenerate in a normal manner. Both urothelial and muscle ingrowth are believed to be initiated from the edges of the normal bladder toward the region of the free graft.[65,66] Usually, however, contracture or resorption of the graft has been evident. The inflammatory response toward the matrix may contribute to the resorption of the free graft.

It was hypothesized that building the three-dimensional structure constructs in vitro, before implantation, would facilitate the eventual terminal differentiation of the cells after implantation in vivo, and would minimize the inflammatory response toward the matrix, thus avoiding graft contracture and shrinkage. This study demonstrated that there was a major difference evident between matrices used with autologous cells (tissue engineered) and matrices used without cells.[14] Matrices implanted with cells for bladder augmentation retained most of their implanted diameter, as opposed to matrices implanted without cells for bladder augmentation, wherein graft contraction and shrinkage occurred. The histomorphology demonstrated a marked paucity of muscle cells and a more aggressive inflammatory reaction in the matrices implanted without cells. Of interest is that the urothelial cell layers appeared normal, even though the underlying matrix was significantly inflamed. It was further hypothesized that having an adequate urothelial layer from the outset would limit the amount of urine contact with the matrix, and would therefore decrease the inflammatory response, and that the muscle cells were also necessary for bioengineering, because native muscle cells are less likely to regenerate over the free grafts. Further studies confirmed this hypothesis.[19] Thus, it seems that the presence of both urothelial and muscle cells on the matrices used for bladder replacement are important for successful tissue bioengineering.

Bladder Replacement Using Tissue Engineering

The results of initial studies showed that the creation of artificial bladders may be achieved in vivo; however, it could not be determined whether the functional parameters noted were attributable to the engineered segment or the intact native bladder tissue. To better address the functional parameters of tissue engineered bladders, an animal model was designed that required a subtotal cystectomy with subsequent replacement with a tissue engineered organ.[19]

A total of 14 beagle dogs underwent a trigone-sparing cystectomy. The animals were randomly assigned to one of three groups. Group A (n = 2) underwent closure of the trigone without a reconstructive procedure. Group B (n = 6) underwent reconstruction with a cell-free bladder shaped biodegradable polymer. Group C (n = 6) underwent reconstruction using a bladder shaped biodegradable polymer that delivered autologous urothelial cells and smooth muscle cells. The cell populations had been separately expanded from a previously harvested autologous bladder biopsy. Preoperative and postoperative urodynamic and radiographic studies were performed serially. Animals were sacrificed at 1, 2, 3, 4, 6, and 11 months postoperatively. Gross, histologic, and immunocytochemical analyses were performed.[19]

The cystectomy-only controls and polymer-only grafts maintained average capacities of 22% and 46% of preoperative values, respectively. An average bladder capacity of 95% of the original precystectomy volume was achieved in the tissue engineered bladder replacements. These findings were confirmed radiographically. The subtotal cystectomy reservoirs, which were not reconstructed, and polymer-only reconstructed bladders showed a marked decrease in bladder compliance (10% and 42%). The compliance of the tissue engineered bladders showed almost no difference from preoperative values that were measured when the native bladder was present (106%). Histologically, the polymer-only bladders presented a pattern of normal urothelial cells with a thickened fibrotic submucosa and a thin layer of muscle fibers. The retrieved tissue engineered bladders showed a normal cellular organization, consisting of a trilayer of urothelium, submucosa, and muscle [Figure 16.1 (see color section)]. Immunocytochemical analyses for desmin, alpha actin, cytokeratin 7, pancytokeratins AE1/AE3 and uroplakin III confirmed the muscle and urothelial phenotype. S-100 staining indicated the presence of neural structures. The results from this study showed that it is possible to tissue engineer bladders, which are anatomically and functionally normal.[19] Clinical trials for the application of this technology are currently being arranged.

Stem Cells for Regenerative Medicine

Most current strategies for engineering bladder tissues involve harvesting of autologous cells from the host diseased or injured organ. However, in situations wherein extensive end-stage organ failure is present, a tissue biopsy may not yield enough normal cells for expansion. Under these circumstances, the availability of pluripotent stem cells may be beneficial. Pluripotent embryonic stem cells are known to form teratomas in vivo, which are composed of a variety of differentiated cells. However, these cells are immunocompetent, and would require immunosuppression if used clinically.

The possibility of deriving stem cells from postnatal mesenchymal tissue from the same host, and inducing their differentiation in vitro and in vivo, was investigated. Stem cells were isolated from human foreskin-derived fibroblasts. Stem cell-derived chondrocytes were obtained through a chondrogenic lineage process. The cells were grown, expanded, seeded onto biodegradable scaffolds, and implanted in vivo, where they formed mature cartilage structures. This was the first demonstration that stem cells can be derived from postnatal connective tissue and can be used for engineering tissues in vivo ex situ.[67]

Conclusion

Regenerative medicine efforts are currently being undertaken for every type of tissue and organ, including the bladder, within the urinary system. Most of the effort expended to engineer bladder tissue has occurred within the last decade. Personnel who have mastered the techniques of cell harvest, culture, and expansion as well as polymer design are essential for the successful application of this technology. Various applications of engineered bladder tissues are at different stages of development, with some already being used clinically, a few in preclinical trials, and some in the discovery stage. Recent progress suggests that engineered bladder tissues may have an expanded clinical applicability in the future.

References

1. Atala A. Tissue engineering in the genitourinary system. In: Atala A, Mooney D, eds. Tissue Engineering. Boston: Birkhauser Press; 1997:149–150.
2. Atala A. Commentary on the replacement of urologic associated mucosa. J Urol 1995;156:338–339.
3. Atala A. Autologous cell transplantation for urologic reconstruction. J Urol 1998;159:2–3.
4. Atala A, Cima LG, Kim W, et al. Injectable alginate seeded with chondrocytes as a potential treatment for vesicoureteral reflux. J Urol 1993;150:745–747.
5. Atala A, Kim W, Paige KT, Vacanti CA, Retik AB. Endoscopic treatment of vesicoureteral reflux with chondrocyte-alginate suspension. J Urol 1994;152:641–643.
6. Kershen RT, Atala A. Advances in injectable therapies for the treatment of incontinence and vesicoureteral reflux. Urol Clin 1999;26:81–94.
7. Atala A, Peters CA, Retik AB, Mandell J. Endoscopic treatment of vesicoureteral reflux with a self-detachable balloon system. J Urol 1992;148:724–728.
8. Atala A, Freeman MR, Vacanti JP, Shepard J, Retik AB. Implantation in vivo and retrieval of artificial structures consisting of rabbit and human urothelium and human bladder muscle. J Urol 1993;150:608–612.
9. Cilento BG, Freeman MR, Schneck FX, Retik AB, Atala A. Phenotypic and cytogenetic characterization of human bladder urothelia expanded in vitro. J Urol 1994;152:655–670.
10. Yoo JJ, Atala A. A novel gene delivery system using urothelial tissue engineered neo-organs. J Urol 1997;158:1066–1070.
11. Machluf M, Atala A. Emerging concepts for tissue and organ transplantation. Graft 1998;1:31–37.
12. Yoo JJ, Lee I, Atala A. Cartilage rods as a potential material for penile reconstruction. J Urol 1998;160:1164–1168.
13. Fauza DO, Fishman S, Mehegan K, Atala A. Videofetoscopically assisted fetal tissue engineering: skin replacement. J Pediatr Surg 1998;33:357–361.
14. Yoo JJ, Meng J, Oberpenning F, Atala A. Bladder augmentation using allogenic bladder submucosa seeded with cells. Urology 1998;51:221–225.
15. Fauza DO, Fishman S, Mehegan K, Atala A. Videofetoscopically assisted fetal tissue engineering: bladder augmentation. J Pediatr Surg 1998;33:7–12.
16. Amiel GE, Atala A. Current and future modalities for functional renal replacement. Urol Clin 1999;2:235–246.
17. Yoo JJ, Park H, Lee I, Atala A. Autologous engineered cartilage rods for penile reconstruction. J Urol 1999;162:1119–1121.
18. Park HJ, Kershen R, Yoo J, Atala A. Reconstitution of human corporal smooth muscle and endothelial cells in vivo. J Urol 1999;162:1106–1109.
19. Oberpenning FO, Meng J, Yoo J, Atala A. De novo reconstitution of a functional urinary bladder by tissue engineering. Nat Biotechnol 1999;17:149–155.
20. Atala A. Future perspectives in reconstructive surgery using tissue engineering. Urol Clin 1999;26:157–165.
21. Scriven SD, Booth C, Thomas DF, Trejdosiewicz LK, Southgate J. Reconstitution of human urothelium from monolayer cultures. J Urol 1997;158:1147–1152.
22. Liebert M, Hubbel A, Chung M, et al. Expression of mal is associated with urothelial differentiation in vitro: identification by differential display reverse-transcriptase polymerase chain reaction. Differentiation 1997;61:177–185.
23. Puthenveettil JA, Burger MS, Reznikoff CA. Replicative senescence in human uroepithelial cells. Adv Exp Med Biol 1999;462:83–91.
24. Liebert M, Wedemeyer G, Abruzzo LV, et al. Stimulated urothelial cells produce cytokines and express an activated cell surface antigenic phenotype. Semin Urol 1991;9:124–130.
25. Tobin MS, Freeman MR, Atala A. Maturational response of normal human urothelial cells in culture is dependent on extracellular matrix and serum additives. Surg Forum 1994;45:786–789.
26. Freeman MR, Yoo JJ, Raab G, et al. Heparin-binding EGF-like growth factor is an autocrine factor for human urothelial cells and is synthesized by epithelial and smooth muscle cells in the human bladder. J Clin Invest 1997;99:1028–1036.
27. Nguyen HT, Park JM, Peters CA, et al. Cell-specific activation of the HB-EGF and ErbB1 genes by stretch in primary human bladder cells. In Vitro Cell Dev Biol 1999;35:371–375.
28. Harriss DR. Smooth muscle cell culture: a new approach to the study of human detrusor physiology and pathophysiology. Br J Urol 1995;75:18–26.
29. Solomon LZ, Jennings AM, Sharpe P, Cooper AJ, Malone PS. Effects of short-chain fatty acids on primary urothelial cells in culture: implications for intravesical use in enterocystoplasties. J Lab Clin Med 1998;132:279–283.
30. Lobban ED, Smith BA, Hall GD, et al. Uroplakin gene expression by normal and neoplastic human urothelium. Am J Pathol 1998;153:1957–1967.
31. Rackley RR, Bandyopadhyay SK, Fazeli-Matin S, Shin MS, Appell R. Immunoregulatory potential of urothelium: characterization of NF-kappaB signal transduction. J Urol 1999;162:1812–1816.
32. Bergsma JE, Rozema FR, Bos RRM, et al. Biocompatibility and degradation mechanism of pre-degraded and non-degraded poly(lactide) implants: an animal study. Mater Med 1995;6:715–724.
33. Kim BS, Mooney DJ. Development of biocompatible synthetic extracellular matrices for tissue engineering. Trends Biotechnol 1998;16:224–230.
34. Pariente JL, Kim BS, Atala A. In vitro biocompatibility assessment of naturally-derived and synthetic bioma-

34. terials using normal human urothelial cells. J Biomed Mater Res 2001;55:33–39.
35. Pariente JL, Kim BS, Atala A. In vitro biocompatibility evaluation of naturally derived and synthetic biomaterials using normal human bladder smooth muscle. J Urol 2002;167:1867–1871.
36. Li ST. Biologic biomaterials: tissue-derived biomaterials (collagen). In: Brozino JD, ed. The Biomedical Engineering Handbook. Boca Raton, FL: CRS Press; 1995:627–647.
37. Gilding DK. Biodegradable polymers. In: Williams DF, ed. Biocompatibility of Clinical Implant Materials. Boca Raton, FL: CRC Press; 1981:209–232.
38. Freed LE, Vunjak-Novakovic G, Biron RJ, et al. Biodegradable polymer scaffolds for tissue engineering. Biotechnology 1994;12:689–693.
39. Mikos AG, Thorsen AJ, Czerwonka LA, et al. Preparation and characterization of poly(L-lactic acid) foams. Polymer 1994;35:1068–1077.
40. Harris LD, Kim BS, Mooney DJ. Open pore biodegradable matrices formed with gas foaming. J Biomed Mater Res 1998;42:396–402.
41. Peppas NA, Langer R. New challenges in biomaterials. Science 1994;263:1715–1720.
42. Neuhof H. Fascial transplantation into visceral defects: an experimental and clinical study. Surg Gynecol Obstet 1917;25:383–387.
43. Piechota HJ, Dahms SE, Nunes LS, Dahiya R, Lue TF, Tanagho EA. In vitro functional properties of the rat bladder regenerated by the bladder acellular matrix graft. J Urol 1998;159:1717–1724.
44. Tsuji I, Ishida H, Fujieda J. Experimental cystoplasty using preserved bladder graft. J Urol 1961;85:42–44.
45. Kambic H, Kay R, Chen JF, Matsushita M, Harasaki H, Zilber S. Biodegradable pericardial implants for bladder augmentation: a 2.5-year study in dogs. J Urol 1992;148:539–543.
46. Kelami A, Ludtke-Handjery A, Korb G, Roll J, Schnell J, Danigel KH. Alloplastic replacement of the urinary bladder wall with lyophilized human dura. Eur Surg Res 1970;2:195–202.
47. Fishman IJ, Flores FN, Scott B, Spjut HJ, Morrow B. Use of fresh placental membranes for bladder reconstruction. J Urol 1987;138:1291–1294.
48. Probst M, Dahiya R, Carrier S, Tanagho EA. Reproduction of functional smooth muscle tissue and partial bladder replacement. Br J Urol 1997;79:505–515.
49. Sutherland RS, Baskin LS, Hayward SW, Cunha GR. Regeneration of bladder urothelium, smooth muscle, blood vessels, and nerves into an acellular tissue matrix. J Urol 1996;156:571–577.
50. Kropp BP, Sawyer BD, Shannon HE, et al. Characterization of using small intestine submucosa regenerated canine detrusor: assessment of reinnervation, in vitro compliance and contractility. J Urol 1996;156:599–607.
51. Vaught JD, Kroop BP, Sawyer BD, et al. Detrusor regeneration in the rat using porcine small intestine submucosal grafts: functional innervation and receptor expression. J Urol 1996;155:374–378.
52. Probst M, Dahiya R, Carrier S, Tanagho EA. Reproduction of functional smooth muscle tissue and partial bladder replacement. Br J Urol 1997;79:505–515.
53. Kropp BP, Rippy MK, Badylak SF, et al. Small intestinal submucosa: urodynamic and histopathologic evaluation in long term canine bladder augmentations. J Urol 1996;155:2098–2104.
54. Lai JY, Yoo JJ, Wulf T, Atala A. Bladder augmentation using small intestinal submucosa seeded with cells [abstract]. J Urol 2002;167:257.
55. Brown AL, Farhat W, Merguerian PA, Wilson GJ, Khoury AE, Woodhouse KA. 22 week assessment of bladder acellular matrix as a bladder augmentation material in a porcine model. Biomaterials 2002;23:2179–2190.
56. Reddy PP, Barrieras DJ, Wilson G, et al. Regeneration of functional bladder substitutes using large segment acellular matrix allografts in a porcine model. J Urol 2000;164:936–941.
57. Merguerian PA, Reddy PP, Barrieras DJ, et al. Acellular bladder matrix allografts in the regeneration of functional bladders: evaluation of large-segment (> 24 cm) substitution in a porcine model. BJU Int 2000;85:894–898.
58. Portis AJ, Elbahnasy AM, Shalhav AL, et al. Laparoscopic augmentation cystoplasty with different biodegradable grafts in an animal model. J Urol 2000, 164:1405–1411.
59. Portis AJ, Elbahnasy AM, Shalhav AL, et al. Laparoscopic midsagittal hemicystectomy and replacement of bladder wall with small intestinal submucosa and reimplantation of ureter into graft. J Endourol 2000;14:203–211.
60. Gleeson MJ, Griffith DP. The use of alloplastic biomaterials in bladder substitution. J Urol 1992;148:1377–1382.
61. Bona AV, De Gresti A. Partial substitution of urinary bladder with Teflon prothesis. Minerva Urol 1966;18:43–47.
62. Monsour MJ, Mohammed R, Gorham SD, French DA, Scott R. An assessment of a collagen/vicryl composite membrane to repair defects of the urinary bladder in rabbits. Urol Res 1987;15:235–238.
63. Rohrmann D, Albrecht D, Hannappel J, Gerlach R, Schwarzkopp G, Lutzeyer W. Alloplastic replacement of the urinary bladder. J Urol 1996;156:2094–2097.
64. De Boer WI, Schuller AG, Vermay M, van der Kwast TH. Expression of growth factors and receptors during specific phases in regenerating urothelium after acute injury in vivo. Am J Pathol 1994;145:1199–1207.
65. Baker R, Kelly T, Tehan T, Putman C, Beaugard E. Subtotal cystectomy and total bladder regeneration in treatment of bladder cancer. J Am Med Assoc 1955;168:1178–1185.
66. Gorham SD, French DA, Shivas AA, Scott R. Some observations on the regeneration of smooth muscle in the repaired urinary bladder of the rabbit. Eur Urol 1989;16:440–443.
67. Bartsch G, Yoo JJ, DeCoppi P, et al. Propagation, expansion, and multilineage differentiation of human somatic stem cells from dermal progenitors. Stem Cells Dev 2005;14:337–348.

Section 5

Eye

Section 5
Eye

Michael Belkin

Most of the information by which we live is received by the sense of vision through the eyes, optic nerves, and the visual processing parts of the brain. A complete loss of the ability to see is one of the most horrendous of human afflictions. Even partial sightedness lowers the ability of the affected individual considerably, preventing him from participating in and enjoying many of the activities that sighted individuals take for granted.

The great strides made in the field of ophthalmology in recent decades in combating loss of sight by curing or enabling the arrest or deceleration of the deterioration process of many eye diseases did not lead to a complete elimination of blindness and visual impairment, even in the parts of the world endowed with ample medical facilities. The main reason for this inability to cure the most common blinding eye conditions stems from the fact that these diseases are mostly afflictions of the retina and optic nerve. These tissues are, anatomically, histologically, and embryologically parts of the central nervous system and thus not considered by classical medicine to be amenable to regeneration after diseases or injuries.

There are three common blinding diseases in the developed world. The most important one is age-related macular degeneration (AMD), which is the leading cause of blindness and visual impairment. The disease is caused by a series of metabolic and histologic changes in the retina and underlying tissues that culminate in progressive retinal atrophy, and, in its most severe form, neovascularization. Because the lesion is often at or near the fovea, it gradually destroys the ability to see. AMD affects about 0.5% of people older than 40 years and its prevalence increases gradually with age to be about 40% in the over-70 age group. It is responsible for about a third of all cases of blindness and visual impairment in the developed world.

In contrast to the two other major blinding diseases, there is no treatment available or truly effective means of preventing AMD or of halting its inexorable progression. The medical, radiational, and surgical attempts at ameliorating AMD are thus barely effective.

The next most common blinding disease is glaucoma, which is often associated with increased intraocular pressure. Glaucoma affects about 2%–4% of the population older than 40 years and consists of progressive degeneration of the optic nerve fibers and their cell bodies in the retinal ganglion cell layer. The functional result of this degenerative process is progressive narrowing of the visual field which, if unchecked, leads to blindness. The disease is treatable, when diagnosed, by reducing the intraocular pressure, medically, by laser radiation, or surgically. However, existing damage to the retina cannot be cured and a considerable proportion of the patients deteriorate despite optimal pressure-lowering treatment. The problems associated with glaucoma are amplified by the fact that the disease in its common forms has no symptoms and thus is often diagnosed after the optic nerve fibers sustain irrevocable damage.

The third common blinding disease is diabetic retinopathy, which consists of microangiopathy leading to ischemia and larger vessel pathology and, in its more severe forms, macular edema, neovascularization, and scarring of the retina. The deterioration of the retina can be somewhat delayed by proper diabetic control and laser therapy. However, many people succumb to its relentless downhill course and diabetic retinopathy accounts for about 15% of blindness in the developed world.

There are other, mostly inherited, retinal degenerations, such as retinitis pigmentosa, which pursue a similar worsening course and are currently completely not amenable to treatment. The number of people affected by all those diseases, as is the case with all other major blinding diseases associated with the aging process, is expected to increase concomitantly with the aging of the population.

The predilection of the retina to succumb to blinding disease is attributed to its being part of the central nervous system and thus incapable of spontaneous regeneration. The new vistas opened by regenerative medicine enable us to hope that, in the not-too-distant future, the scourge of blindness resulting from retinal diseases can be at least partially checked. This is discussed in three chapters in this section. Barkana and Belkin describe the progress made in neuroprotection in ophthalmology whereby it is hoped that retinal and optic nerve degenerations resulting from diseases and injuries can be minimized and the regeneration processes augmented. A chapter by Schwartz and Kipnis describes the advanced research efforts to induce regeneration in the optic nerve, spinal cord, and other central nervous system tissues. Some of the fruits of this research are now in advanced clinical studies in the treatment of spinal cord injuries. The results of this and other preclinical research may in the future solve part of the retinal and optic nerve problems discussed above.

The chapter by Stern, Temple, and De delineate the hottest field in medical research today – that of stem cells – as it applies to ophthalmology. The cutting-edge investigations described in that chapter may soon lead to at least a partial cure of many hitherto untreatable maladies of the eye and brain.

Although most of the blinding eye diseases are those of the retina and optic nerve, diseases of the anterior part of the eye engender a not inconsiderable proportion of blindness. The particular problem in this part of the eye is that, for vision to be effective, the cornea has to be transparent. Hence, the scarring processes taking place after injuries or diseases, which may be beneficial in other parts of the body, tend to produce corneal opacities, which may lead to decline and loss of vision.

The article by Barequet describes the current state-of-art in therapy using stem cells from the corneal periphery and amniotic membranes that is now a routine clinical practice to overcome some of the scarring processes. This is a prime example of how stem cell therapy is in routine, effective clinical practice.

It is hoped that some of the other methods described in the ophthalmology chapter of this book will also yield clinically meaningful results and save many patients from impaired vision and blindness.

17

Neuroprotection in Ophthalmology: A Review

Yaniv Barkana and Michael Belkin

Regardless of the cause and nature of neuronal injury, the lesion spreads not only to other parts of the affected cells but also beyond the directly injured neurons to affect neighboring neurons that escaped or were only partially affected by the primary insult. The primary insult, whether mechanical, ischemic, degenerative, or radiational, leads to changes in the extracellular environment, which in turn engender degeneration of adjacent neurons that escaped the primary injury.[1-4] The purpose of neuroprotective therapy is to minimize this process of secondary degeneration – to reduce the ensuing morphologic and functional damage as well as maximize the recovery of a neural system after acute or chronic insult. This feat can be brought about by lessening the noxiousness of the extracellular milieu caused by substances secreted from the primarily injured axons, by preventing the adverse effect of those substances on healthy adjacent neurons, by assisting the latter to resist these effects, by minimizing the spread of damage in the injured neurons and encouraging them to regenerate.

The term neuroprotection should only be used to designate interference with processes that occur after the primary neural insult. That is, neuroprotection interferes with processes associated with secondary degeneration, not with the direct effects of the primary insult. For instance, in the case of glaucoma, neuroprotection should not be used to describe the use of ocular hypotensive drugs. Rather, in this context, neuroprotection means the use of modalities that, by ameliorating secondary degeneration processes in the optic nerve and retinal ganglion cell (RGC) layer, will arrest or diminish the progress of glaucomatous neuropathy.

Many compounds are involved in the process of secondary neuronal degeneration. Those neurotoxic substances include, among others, excitatory amino acids (e.g., glutamate), free radicals, nitric oxide, lipid peroxidation products (e.g., polyunsaturated fatty acid), eicosanoids, cations, monoamines (e.g., 5-hydroxytryptamine), and opioids. Thus, modalities that can inhibit the synthesis, release, spread, or interaction of these compounds with neighboring neurons have been investigated as potential neuroprotective drugs. Hundreds of agents have been tested in animals, but only a few have reached phase III clinical trials and only two have achieved Food and Drug Administration (FDA) approval for clinical use: Riluzole for amyotrophic lateral sclerosis[5] and memantine for moderate to severe Alzheimer's disease.[6]

Although many agents have been associated with secondary degeneration, they cause neuronal death by only a few common final pathways. The most prevalent and best-known one is apoptosis. Apoptotic death of RGCs was shown, for example, in animal models of pressure-induced glaucoma and after optic nerve axotomy.[7,8] When in excessive concentration, the most common retinal neurotransmitter, glutamate, induces apoptosis in retinal cells as a mediator of an ischemic insult through hyperactivation of the N-methyl-D-aspartate (NMDA) receptor,[9] and NMDA has shown a similar effect directly.[10] Recent studies have provided evidence of apoptosis associated with RGC death in human eyes with glaucoma[11] and ischemic optic neuropathy.[12]

In theory, many ophthalmic diseases can be treated to an extent hitherto impossible if efficacious clinical neuroprotection becomes available. Diseases of the retina that could be a target for neuroprotective therapy include age-related and other forms of degeneration, diabetic retinopathy, arterial and venous occlusions, retinal trauma including that caused by surgery, retinal ischemia, retinal edema, and damage induced by photocoagulation or accidental laser injuries. Optic nerve diseases that could potentially be treated include glaucomatous neuropathy, ischemic optic neuropathy, optic nerve trauma and surgery, optic neuritis, and damage from increased intracranial pressure. The neural lesions of these diseases are currently untreatable and as a consequence they account for a major proportion of the cases of blindness and visual disability in the world. Three diseases, age-related macular degeneration, glaucoma, and diabetic retinopathy cause the vast majority of yet untreatable blindness and visual impairment in the industrial world.[13,14] In the less developed parts of the globe, although cataract is the main cause of visual function decrement, the retinal diseases listed above account for a very considerable proportion of visual disability. The worldwide toll on vision by those diseases is expected to increase with the aging of the population and the increase in prevalence of diabetes.

This review will briefly summarize the relevance and potential applications of neuroprotection in ophthalmology, the preclinical research performed on animal models of eye diseases, and the beginning of research in clinical ophthalmology. An attempt will be made to explain the fact that, despite the enormous promise, extensive laboratory and clinical research, and the expenditure of enormous financial resources associated with neuroprotection as a therapeutic modality, there is almost a complete lack of clinical success of neuroprotective therapies in neurologic and ophthalmic diseases. Finally, a new, immune-based approach to the subject, which holds promise of solving some of the problems that plague the clinical development of neuroprotection, will be described.

Animal Models for Testing Neuroprotection

Retinal Ischemia

Acute ischemia and reperfusion is the most commonly used model of retinal neuronal injury because it is technically relatively easy (Table 17.1). It is performed by increasing the intraocular pressure (IOP) above systolic blood pressure for a limited, predefined duration, usually 30 to 60 minutes. During the weeks after the insult, neurons, mainly in the inner retina, die, a process which is morphologically quantifiable by histologic assays or functionally by electroretinography (ERG).[15,16]

Ischemia can be also modeled by inducing vascular occlusion, such as ligating ophthalmic or carotid vessels, or producing vascular thrombosis.[17–20] These procedures lead to a prolonged but less precisely controllable retinal ischemia.

Exposure to Endogenous Excitotoxins

Exposing the retina to a measurable high concentration of a noxious substance is facilitated by the ease of in vitro retinal exposure or injections into the vitreous body. The endogenous excitotoxin most widely investigated is the neurotransmitter glutamic acid which, when present in excessive concentrations, is a major cause of cytotoxicity leading to secondary degeneration after brain injury and in brain disorders.[21–23] The direct detrimental effect of glutamate on RGCs and other cell types is observed by exposing the retina to high glutamate concentrations in vitro[24,25] or in animal models where glutamate is injected intravitreally.[26] Because the neuro-

Table 17.1. Models of neurotoxicity

Model	References
Retinal ischemia	9, 15–20, 27, 54
Retinal exposure to glutamate	24–26, 30
Retinal exposure to NMDA	1, 27–29, 63, 70
Retinal laser injury	38, 42, 43
Acute partial crush lesion of the optic nerve	52, 53
Primate glaucoma model	44–47
Rat glaucoma model	7, 48–50

toxic effect of glutamate is mediated primarily through its NMDA receptors, similar models involve injection of NMDA.[27–29] Whereas most of those models attempt to mimic acute pathological conditions, "chronic" exposure to relatively low-dose intravitreal glutamate for 3 months was described.[30] In this connection, it is interesting to note that an increase in intraocular glutamate has been reported in the eyes of humans and monkeys with glaucoma[31] and in the crush-injured optic nerve of the rat.[32]

Retinal Laser Injury

Laser photocoagulation of the retina is used extensively in the treatment of many vision-impairing retinal disorders, such as diabetic retinopathy and age-related macular degeneration.[33–35] Clinical experience has shown that this treatment is associated with some loss of vision, especially when treatment is applied to subfoveal or juxtafoveal lesions. Spreading of the destructive effect to adjacent retinal tissue not directly destroyed by the laser beam has been demonstrated.[36–38]

The latest method of laser treatment of retinal diseases, photodynamic therapy, although purportedly limiting the damage to blood vessels, is associated with a considerable number of visual side effects, probably resulting from neuronal damage.[39–41]

Neuroprotective therapy that preserves the neurosensory retina from the injurious effect would protect the patient's sight and allow the irradiation to be applied closer to the fovea, thereby enhancing the beneficial effects of laser treatment. Thus, models of laser-induced injury of the rat retina are useful animal models of acute retinal damage, which are accurately quantifiable both with respect to lesion diameter and to the number of cells injured and rescued.[42,43] Furthermore, they mimic precisely the prevalent clinical problem on which they are based.

Animal Models of Glaucoma

There are many glaucoma models in which the optic neuropathy is induced by increasing IOP, although none of them emulate precisely the pathogenesis and chronic development of primary open-angle glaucoma. The most commonly used glaucoma model in primates is laser photocoagulation of the trabecular meshwork, resulting in its blockage, failure of aqueous humor outflow, and consequently an increase in IOP and neuropathy.[44–47] This model was used in numerous studies of pressure-induced changes in the optic nerve, such as histologic changes in RGC populations, as well as changes in pattern-evoked retinal potentials, blood flow in the optic nerve head, and in the extracellular matrix. This model is also in common use for pharmacologic studies.

Rat models offer clear advantages of availability, cost, and ease of handling without the need for general anesthesia of primates. An increase in IOP in rats' eyes can be induced by various techniques of blood flow obstruction in the episcleral veins[7,48,49] or laser photocoagulation of the trabecular meshwork.[50] The rat glaucoma model has become even more useful since the development of the TonoPen tonometer with its small applanation tip, which greatly facilitates the measurement of IOP in this animal.

Optic Nerve Injury

One of the models of the primary, initial glaucomatous neuropathy lesion[51] consists of a reproducible, well-calibrated, and partial crush injury of the optic nerve of the adult rat.[52] Because the initial mechanical neuronal loss is controlled, the secondary loss can easily be quantified. The measurement is performed by retrograde labeling of RGCs after applying a dye distal to the site of the lesion and counting the labeled ganglion cell bodies in the corresponding retina. Another method to quantify the neuronal loss is to measure the change in action potential in response to electrical stimulation of the excised nerve or the visual evoked potential response to light. These amplitudes are proportional to the numbers of excitable fibers left in the optic nerve.

Levkovitch-Verbin et al.[53] described a monkey model in which the upper third of the optic nerve was partially transected. Because there is vertical topographic separation of RGCs in the primate retina and their corresponding axons in the optic nerve, the observed loss of RGCs in the inferior retina was attributed to secondary degeneration.

Compounds Investigated in Neuroprotection Research

NMDA Receptor Antagonists

MK-801 is one of the first neuroprotective compounds to be developed. It is a potent noncompetitive NMDA receptor blocker, shown to be effective in protecting retinal cells in various animal models (Table 17.2).

Solberg et al.,[43] using a rat model of argon laser irradiation-induced retinal lesion, found significant beneficial effects of MK-801 on the diameter of the retinal lesions and the percentage of surviving photoreceptor cells in the outer nuclear layer of the retina. The treated rats also showed a pronounced, dose-dependent inhibition of proliferation of the retinal pigment epithelium (RPE), fibrosis, and neovascularization. Similarly, MK-801 significantly inhibits the death of RGCs in models of ischemia in the rat and cat.[9,19,27,54] MK-801 is also effective in treating partial crush injury of the rat optic nerve where it triples the survival rate of neurons.[55] MK-801 also prevents cellular loss[29] and apoptosis[10] after intravitreal injection of NMDA in rats. The compound, although quite effective as a neuroprotectant, cannot be used in humans because it was found to have psychotropic side effects in clinical trials.[56]

NMDA receptors are very common on RGC bodies, suggesting that they might be the site for MK-801 and other NMDA antagonist-induced protection of optic neurons from secondary degeneration.

There are other NMDA receptor antagonists that were tested for retinal neuroprotective activity. Dextromethorphan was found to protect the rabbit retina from ischemia[57] and laser-induced injury.[58] Flupirtine protected rabbit retina from ischemia,[59] and rat RGCs from both ischemia and NMDA-induced toxicity.[60]

Riluzole antagonizes glutamate excitotoxicity by inhibiting its release rather than binding to the glutamate receptor. In a rat model of retinal ischemia/reperfusion, riluzole attenuated damage, measured by indices of retinal cellular necrosis and apoptosis and by reduction of ERG a and b waves.[61] This drug was the first FDA-approved neuroprotective drug. It is used for the treatment of amyotrophic lateral sclerosis but is not very effective, prolonging life of the patients by an average of 2 months.[5]

The most currently clinically relevant neuroprotective drug to ophthalmology is memantine, which is in an advanced phase III clinical trial for glaucoma. It is a noncompetitive and low- to moderate-affinity NMDA antagonist, but seems to lack the central nervous system (CNS) side effects associated with other NMDA antagonists.[62] Memantine is the only neuroprotective compound approved by the FDA for clinical use in Alzheimer's disease, as its clinical benefit is clearly similar to those observed with acetylcholinesterase inhibitors.[63]

In ophthalmology, memantine was shown to protect rat and rabbit retinal cells after ischemia/reperfusion injury.[64] It also protected ganglion cells in a model of chronic (3-month) elevation in vitreal glutamate.[30] Of more clinical relevance is the investigation showing that it was safe and effective in reducing damage in a monkey model of glaucoma as evinced by histologic measurements of RGC survival as well as tomographic measurements of nerve head topography without affecting IOP.[65] Its short-term effectiveness was demonstrated in the same model by conventional and multifocal recordings of the electroretinogram (ERG).

Table 17.2. Neuroprotective agents

Agent	References
MK-801	9, 10, 19, 27, 29, 43, 54–56
Dextromethorphan	57, 58
Flupirtine	59, 60
Memantine	6, 30, 49, 62, 64–66, 78, 101
Riluzole	61
Corticosteroids	42, 74–81
Brimonidine	82–85
Betaxolol	15, 16, 86, 87
Flunarizine	54, 89, 90
Brain-derived neurotrophic factor	104–107, 110
Pigment epithelium-derived factor	50
Aminoguanidine	98
Minocycline	99–103
Autoimmune T cells	15, 21, 39, 41, 106, 111, 112, 117–120, 128
Copaxone	121, 123–126

There was no effect on the visually evoked cortical potential.[66] Memantine was effective in clinical trials of a variety of dementias, mainly Alzheimer's disease, without causing the toxic side effects of MK-801 and earlier NMDA antagonists.[6,67] It is also somewhat effective in Parkinson's disease.[68]

However, it is not effective in the treatment of other neural diseases such as in ameliorating the symptoms of patients with phantom pains after upper limb amputation.[69]

Prednisolone

Prednisolone is a potent corticosteroid that exerts a variety of physiological and cellular reactions, such as inhibition of arachidonic acid metabolism, stabilization of lysosomal membranes, modification of edema formation, and antioxidant activity. High-dose methylprednisolone therapy is effective in the treatment of CNS injury in different animal models[70–72] and in controlled clinical trials for spinal cord trauma for which high doses are the standard treatment in the acute stage.[73]

Treatment with corticosteroids has been investigated in animal models of laser injury to the eye, with mixed results. Lam et al.[42] reported a beneficial effect of treatment with methylprednisolone administered as an intravenous bolus of 30 mg/kg and a maintenance dose of 5.4 mg/kg per hour in laser injuries of nonhuman primate retina. Morphologically, the treated retina showed rapid reestablishment of retinal and choroidal vasculature, proliferation, and organization of the RPE and reformation of the outer limiting membrane, less macrophage activity, and reduced photoreceptor damage at the periphery of the lesion.[42,74] After a single retinal argon laser lesion, Naveh and Weissman[75] found that vitreal accumulation of protein and prostaglandin E_2 was reduced in rabbits treated daily with intramuscular dexamethasone (0.5 mg/kg weight). Wilson et al.[76] showed that breakdown of the blood–retinal barrier after panretinal photocoagulation was reduced by intravitreal injection of triamcinolone. Ishibashi et al.[77] reported that continuous intravitreal infusion of steroids inhibits subretinal neovascularization after laser induction of retinal lesions in monkeys.

However, there are compelling doubts regarding the efficacy of corticosteroids as neuroprotective drugs for minimizing visual loss in laser-induced retinal injuries. Rosner et al.[78] reported that systemic corticosteroids had only a short-term effect on argon-laser-induced lesions in the retinas of pigmented rats. Corticosteroids were shown to promote sparing of neurons after mechanical injury but to interfere with regeneration of neural tissue, for which inflammation was necessary.[79] Marshall[80] reported that steroids slowed the regeneration of the outer blood–retinal barrier by RPE cells and suggested that steroids not be used to treat retinal laser burns until more data become available. Schuschereba et al.[81] reported a deleterious effect of mega doses of intravenous steroids on the prognosis of argon-laser-induced retinal injuries in rabbits. On the whole, it seems that corticosteroids are not an effective neuroprotectant in ophthalmic diseases.

Adrenergic Agonists and Antagonists

The α_2-adrenergic agonist brimonidine, a commercially available topical ocular hypotensive glaucoma drug, has been associated with a neuroprotective effect on RGCs. Yoles et al.[82] found that a single injection of brimonidine (and other α_2-adrenergic agonists) resulted in a significantly smaller loss of RGCs and lesser reduction in action potential amplitude after partial crush injury of the rat optic nerve. Timolol, a β-receptor blocker that similarly lowers IOP, had no such protective effect in that model.[82] Donello et al.[83] showed in a rat model of acute retinal ischemia that pretreatment with brimonidine has a marked protective role on RGC loss, as evaluated by histology, cell labeling, and ERG. Furthermore, brimonidine treatment prevented an increase in the vitreous body of glutamate and aspartate, indicating interference with the excitotoxic mechanism of secondary degeneration. However, it seems likely that it exerts its neuroprotective effect by another mechanism, not demonstrated for other ophthalmic neuroprotective compounds. Gao et al.[84] showed that brimonidine promotes the production of the growth factor brain-derived neurotrophic factor (BDNF) in RGCs, a finding that may account for its significant neuroprotective efficacy.

The neuroprotective capabilities of this drug have been further demonstrated by improving, in an IOP independent manner, the contrast sensitivity of glaucoma patients.[85] The most compelling evidence for the effects of topical brimonidine in reducing the rate of ganglion cell loss in severe glaucoma was reported by Gandolfi et al. in the 2004 meeting of the Association for Research in Vision and Ophthalmology. He studied 52 high-risk eyes on two antihypertensive drugs in a masked manner. All eyes exhibited progressive visual field loss during the 18 months preceding the trial. The subjects were randomly assigned to treatment with topical brimonidine or to undergo laser trabeculoplasty without changing the hypertensive treatment. Eighteen further months later, the brimonidine-treated eyes showed significantly less visual field loss than the laser-treated eyes although the extent of IOP reduction was lower in the former eyes.

Adrenergic antagonists have also shown neuroprotective capability in animal experiments. Osborne et al.[86] reported that betaxolol, a β_1-adrenergic receptor blocker, protects rat RGCs from ischemia/reperfusion insult when injected intraperitoneally or intravitreally and that topical use of betaxolol significantly reduces the death of RGCs after ischemia/reperfusion in rabbit eyes and after intravitreal injection of NMDA into the rat eye.[87] The neuroprotective effect of betaxolol was attributed to the drug's action as a calcium channel blocker, reducing excessive influx of calcium into stressed cells, and was thought to be unrelated to its β_1 receptor-mediated reduction of IOP.

Betaxolol has also been shown by others to have a neuroprotective effect when applied topically before or after an ischemic insult.[15,16]

Calcium Channel Blockers

Calcium ions, when entering a cell through either voltage-sensitive or receptor-operated channels have a cardinal role in the pathophysiology of apoptosis leading to tissue destruction after CNS insult of all types. The increase in intracellular calcium exerts a neurotoxic effect through the activation of Ca^{2+}-dependent catabolic enzymes, leading to lethal alteration of the cell's metabolism.[88]

It was therefore thought that blocking calcium ions egress into cells would prevent their death, providing neuroprotection. Indeed, flunarizine, a potent antagonist of the neuronal voltage-dependent calcium channel, when administered daily to rats after unilateral axotomy of the optic nerve, was found to somewhat enhance RGC survival which was measured 14 days after the injury.[89] Both flunarizine and another calcium blocking drug, lomerizine, have a protective effect after induction of retinal ischemia in rats by temporary increase of the IOP.[54,90]

The beneficial effect of treatment with Ca^{2+} channel blockers was shown in one moderate-term clinical trial of patients with normal-tension glaucoma.[91] The relevance of the results of this trial is still moot. Even if further clinical evidence will accumulate for calcium channel blockers having beneficial effects on glaucoma, it is still uncertain whether the observed effects are neuroprotective in nature or operate via a different mechanism such as vasodilation.

Nitric Oxide Synthase Inhibitors

Nitric oxide has multiple physiological roles in the normal metabolism of various tissues, including neural ones. As is the case with excitotoxic amino acids, its presence in high concentrations is noxious to cells. Consequently, many research projects were devoted to understanding the cellular origins and synthetic mechanisms of the compound and its function as a neurotoxin in animal models of human neural degenerative diseases, including glaucoma.[92–95] Shareef et al.[96] demonstrated that, in the rat model of gradual chronic IOP elevation, isoforms of the enzyme nitric oxide synthase are induced in optic nerve astrocytes, such as nitric oxide synthase 2. The induction of this enzyme is in turn predicated on activation of epidermal growth factor receptor-induced nitric oxide synthase-2 in the astrocytes.[97]

These authors subsequently showed that aminoguanidine, a relatively specific inhibitor of this isoform, reduces the loss of RGCs in this model.[98]

Minocycline

This second-generation tetracycline antibiotic is an inhibitor of caspase-3, an essential enzyme in the apoptosis pathway, and thus is anti-apoptotic in neural and non-neural cells. Quite a few promising preliminary studies showed this drug to be effective as a neuroprotectant in neurodegenerative diseases animal models. The ophthalmic models included light-induced retinal degeneration,[99] retinal cell culture,[100] and retinal degeneration.[101]

However, some negative results using minocycline were obtained in animal testing as well as serious side effects,[102] casting doubt on the future of minocycline as a neuroprotectant drug.[103]

Neurotrophic Factors

BDNF, a member of the nerve growth factor family of proteins, is highly effective in reducing the rate of RGC death after optic nerve axotomy in rats[104–106] and optic nerve crush in cats.[107] These findings may be particularly pertinent to the therapy of glaucoma, where death of RGCs may be partly attributed to a decrease in axonal transport of trophic factors.[107–109]

Experiments with other growth factors also indicate that the growth factors are potent agents for providing neuroprotection and inducing regeneration in neural tissues after insults. Intravitreal injection of adenovirus vectors containing pigment epithelium-derived growth factor 4 days before inducing retinal ischemia was found to preserve inner retinal thickness and cell density in the ganglion cell layer, and to decrease cell apoptosis.[50]

The problem associated with the clinical use of BDNF and any other protein with neuroprotective and regeneration enhancement property in neurologic and ophthalmic diseases is the inability of large molecules to penetrate the blood–brain barrier or the blood–retina barrier in sufficient quantities to exert significant clinical impact. Those compounds, therefore, have to be delivered intravitreally or intrathecally. Indeed, in the clinical trials in using BDNF, e.g., for amyotrophic lateral sclerosis, the compound is injected intrathecally.[110]

Apoptosis Prevention

Another possible approach to neuroprotection is interference with the final common pathway of apoptosis, or programmed cell death, shown to occur in RGCs under a variety of conditions, both naturally occurring and experimental.[7–12] As the genetic and molecular mechanisms of apoptosis are gradually elucidated, new targets for neuroprotection appear. Current research efforts are aimed at up-regulating anti-apoptotic proteins such as BCLX, and inhibiting the promoters of apoptosis such as BAX and the executors of apoptosis, the caspase proteases.

Immune-Based Neuroprotection

A very promising, experimentally advanced technique for providing neuroprotection to injured neural tissues utilizes the body's immune system to supply the necessary neuroprotective compounds, at the proper regimen, to the site of the primary insult. This potential therapy is based on the novel insights gained and promulgated by Schwartz[111] on the nature of autoimmunity. Autoimmunity in general, and in the CNS in particular, has long been considered to be harmful and this was considered the reason for the CNS "immune free" status. Schwartz has shown that the adaptive immune response displayed by regulatory T cells directed against self-antigens ("autoimmune" T cells) is essential for body homeostasis in the eye and other parts of the CNS.[112] The autoimmune system is activated after CNS trauma[113] and can be therapeutically manipulated to provide more effective neuroprotection than it affords without such medical maneuvers.[114–116]

This immune mechanism was demonstrated to be effective in preventing secondary degeneration and promoting significant recovery from axonal injuries more than other neuroprotective modalities.[111] It was first demonstrated in rodents who underwent optic nerve crush injury and were injected systemically with T cells that recognize CNS self-antigens such as myelin basic protein. The resulting protection of RGCs was demonstrated by morphologic and electrophysiological means.[117–119] The neuroprotection afforded by the T cells was shown not only by passive T cell transfer, but also by active vaccination with the relevant antigens.[120] Of even greater immediate clinical relevance is the pronounced neuroprotection achieved using Copaxone, a drug that prevents the development of experimental autoimmune encephalomyelitis in rodents and is clinically used to ameliorate multiple sclerosis in humans[121] as a vaccine that preferentially directed T cells unto the lesion site.[122]

Protection of RGCs by vaccination with Copaxone was also observed in rats into whose vitreous a toxic dose of glutamate was injected. From the clinical point of view, an even more directly pertinent finding was that in a rat model of glaucoma the RGCs were saved from destruction by Copaxone vaccination, even if the IOP was not reduced,[123] giving a prospect of developing vaccination against glaucoma,[124,125] a treatment for other optic nerve diseases and injuries,[126] and other retinal diseases.

The possible mechanism whereby the system functions when activated at the lesion site, is by local secretion of neurotrophic factors and other agents which lessen the secondary degeneration and promote healing and regeneration. This secretion is effected either directly or through interaction with microglia.[127] The advantage of the neuroprotective immunity is in its ability to circumvent the blood–brain barrier and provide large molecules such as growth factors in the lesion site.[128] Neuroprotective vaccination has another major advantage over other neuroprotective modalities, each of which addresses one secondary degeneration agent of the multiple compounds involved in the process of secondary degeneration. In contradistinction to those, the T cells at the lesion site presumably secrete the right mix of factors according to their proper timing, dosage, and duration.[129]

Neuroprotective Therapy – A Thumbnail History and State of Art

A therapeutic idea that would have been called today neuroprotection was put forward by Dr. Bernard Becker in the early 1970s who suggested using the antiepileptic drug phenytoin for glaucoma control (personal communication by Paul Palmberg, 2004). The concept underlying neuroprotection, secondary degeneration, was described by Astrup in 1979 who described an area which he later termed the ischemic penumbra around the primary infarct in stroke.[130] In the same year, barbiturates were tried to ameliorate the functional effects of stroke, with the same idea in mind.[131] The first ophthalmic experiments were performed by Tso who tried the use of ascorbate to treat a model of a photic injury of the retina.[132] The term neuroprotection was first used in 1987 to describe the effect of MK-801 on brain ischemia, and the first reasoned suggestion for the use of the technique to moderate glaucomatous neuropathy was made by Schwartz in 1996.[133]

During all this period, to the present day, there has been a continuous effort to translate the vast scientific knowledge collected over recent decades on the subject of neuroprotection into clinical therapeutic reality. As a part of the research aimed at developing neuroprotective drugs for neural diseases, hundreds of compounds have been subjected to preclinical testing, scores have reached clinical trials, and many have made it to phase III testing. Yet, only two drugs of this class have been approved by the FDA, namely, riluzole for amyotrophic lateral sclerosis, and memantine for moderate to severe Alzheimer's disease. Both drugs, especially the former, are of marginal clinical value and have not manifested the great hopes associated with neuroprotection.

This meager clinical return for enormous decades-long research efforts is attributable to many factors. The main one is probably the fact that the secondary degeneration of neurons is mediated by many noxious agents. Thus, mitigating the harmful effects of one of them is insufficient to produce meaningful clinical effects. Furthermore, all of the agents that induce secondary degeneration are compounds intimately involved with the normal functioning of the nervous system. Their degeneration-inducing effects are attributable to their presence at abnormally high concentrations in the injury site. The primary example of this problem is glutamate, which is a major neurotransmitter in the retina and elsewhere. It becomes toxic as a result of its release at abnormally high concentrations from the primarily injured neurons into the extracellular environment. Blocking the effects of glutamate and the other secondary degeneration agents too intensively is liable to produce severe side effects, as was the case with MK-801. Furthermore, to achieve clinically relevant neuroprotection, the activities of some of the agents of secondary degeneration would have to be blocked to the right extent and with the appropriate timing. Finding the proper combination of drugs, and ensuring that they all act according to the proper sequence, concentration, and timing is impossible by present-day medical practice. Other reasons for the almost uniform failure of neuroprotective therapy as a medical modality are associated with the differences between preclinical testing and medical practice. The animal models used are mostly acute and do not represent the human disease accurately. The animals tested do not adequately represent the patient population, the former being of uniform strain, age, sex, and extent of lesion. For acute diseases, there is the problem of the "window of opportunity," the time interval after the onset of the disease during which the process of secondary degeneration can be arrested or decelerated. The animals are always treated within this window, whereas most patients do not seek treatment nor are diagnosed within this time period. The clinical trial population differs considerably from the animal population in being young and healthy in phase I, too few in phase II, and old, heterogeneous and with comorbidities in phase III.

Despite all the difficulties and disappointing track record, the search for new means of providing neuroprotection to neural diseases and injuries is continuing, because the concept holds a promise to reduce morbidity and mortality from some of humanity's most devastating diseases. It seems, however, that new approaches to the problem are required and interfering with a single secondary degeneration agent will not be useful as a clinical modality. Methods of providing generalized, timely amelioration of the secondary degeneration and of promoting regeneration, as described above, will possibly provide effective neuroprotection in the not too distant future.

References

1. Faden AI. Pharmacotherapy in spinal cord injury: a critical review of recent developments. Clin Neuropharmacol 1987;10:193–204.
2. Faden AI, Salzman S. Pharmacological strategies in CNS trauma. Trends Pharmacol Sci 1992;13:29–35.
3. Lynch DR, Dawson TM. Secondary mechanisms in neuronal trauma. Curr Opin Neurol 1994;7:510–516.
4. McIntosh TK. Novel pharmacologic therapies in the treatment of experimental traumatic brain injury: a review. J Neurotrauma 1993;10:215–261.
5. Miller RG, Mitchell JD, Lyon M, Moore DH. Riluzole for amyotrophic lateral sclerosis (ALS)/motor neuron disease (MND). Amyotroph Lateral Scler Other Motor Neuron Disord 2003;4:191–206.
6. Tariot PN, Farlow MR, Grossberg GT, et al. Memantine treatment in patients with moderate to severe Alzheimer disease already receiving donepezil: a randomized controlled trial. JAMA 2004;291(3):317–324.
7. Garcia Valenzuela E, Shareef S, Walsh J, Sharma SC. Programmed cell death of retinal ganglion cells in experimental glaucoma. Exp Eye Res 1995;61:33–44.
8. Quigley HA, Nickells RW, Kerrigan LA, et al. Retinal ganglion cell death in experimental glaucoma and after axotomy occurs by apoptosis. Invest Ophthalmol Vis Sci 1995;36:774–786.
9. Joo CK, Choi JS, Ko H, et al. Necrosis and apoptosis after retinal ischemia: involvement of NMDA-mediated excitotoxicity and p53. Invest Ophthalmol Vis Sci 1999;40:713–720.
10. Lam TT, Abler AS, Kwong JM, Tso MO. N-methyl-D-aspartate (NMDA)-induced apoptosis in rat retina. Invest Ophthalmol Vis Sci 1999;40:2391–2397.
11. Kerrigan LA, Zack DJ, Quigley HA, et al. TUNEL-positive ganglion cells in human primary open-angle glaucoma. Arch. Ophthalmol. 1997;115:1031–1035.
12. Levin LA, Louhab A. Apoptosis of retinal ganglion cells in anterior ischemic optic neuropathy. Arch Ophthalmol 1996;114:488–491.
13. Bamashmus MA, Matlhaga B, Dutton GN. Causes of blindness and visual impairment in the West of Scotland. Eye 2004;18(3):257–261.
14. Farber MD. National Registry for the Blind in Israel: estimation of prevalence and incidence rates and causes of blindness. Ophthalmic Epidemiol 2003;10(4):267–277.
15. Sakamoto K, Yonoki Y, Kuwagata M, Saito M, Nakahara T, Ishii K. Histological protection against ischemia-reperfusion injury by early ischemic preconditioning in rat retina. Brain Res 2004;1015:154–160.
16. Cheon EW, Kim HY, Cho YY, et al. Betaxolol, a beta1-adrenoceptor antagonist, protects a transient ischemic injury of the retina. Exp Eye Res 2002;75:591–601.
17. Barnett NL, Osborne NN. Redistribution of GABA immunoreactivity following central retinal artery occlusion. Brain Res 1995;677:337–340.
18. Barnett NL, Osborne NN. Prolonged bilateral carotid artery occlusion induces electrophysiological and immunohistochemical changes to the rat retina without causing histological damage. Exp Eye Res 1995;61:83–90.
19. Mosinger JL, Price MT, Bai HY, et al. Blockade of both NMDA and non-NMDA receptors is required for optimal protection against ischemic neuronal degeneration in the in vivo adult mammalian retina. Exp Neurol 1991;113:10–17.
20. Osborne NN, Casson RJ, Wood JP, et al. Retinal ischemia: mechanisms of damage and potential therapeutic strategies. Prog Retin Eye Res 2004;23:91–147.
21. Choi D, Rothman SM. The role of glutamate neurotoxicity in hypoxic-ischemic neuronal death. Annu Rev Neurosci 1990;13:171–182.
22. Choi DW. Glutamate neurotoxicity and diseases of the nervous system. Neuron 1988;1:623–634.
23. Meldrum B, Garthwaite J. Excitatory amino acid neurotoxicity and neurodegenerative disease. Trends Pharmacol Sci 1990;11:379–387.
24. Hahn JS, Aizenman E, Lipton SA. Central mammalian neurons normally resistant to glutamate toxicity are made sensitive by elevated extracellular Ca^{2+}: toxicity is blocked by the N-methyl-D-aspartate antagonist MK-801. Proc Natl Acad Sci USA 1988;85:6556–6560.

25. Levy DI, Lipton SA. Comparison of delayed administration of competitive and uncompetitive antagonists in preventing NMDA receptor-mediated neuronal death. Neurology 1990;40:852–855.
26. Sisk DR, Kuwabara T. Histologic changes in the inner retina of albino rats following intravitreal injection of monosodium L-glutamate. Graefes Arch Clin Exp Ophthalmol 1985;223:250–258.
27. Adachi K, Kashii S, Masai H, et al. Mechanism of the pathogenesis of glutamate neurotoxicity in retinal ischemia. Graefes Arch Clin Exp Ophthalmol 1998;236: 766–774.
28. Sabel BA, Sautter J, Stoehr T, Siliprandi R. A behavioral model of excitotoxicity: retinal degeneration, loss of vision, and subsequent recovery after intraocular NMDA administration in adult rats. Exp Brain Res 1995;106:93–105.
29. Siliprandi R, Canella R, Carmignoto G, et al. N-methyl-D-aspartate-induced neurotoxicity in the adult rat retina. Vis Neurosci 1992;8:567–573.
30. Vorwerk CK, Lipton SA, Zurakowski D, et al. Chronic low-dose glutamate is toxic to retinal ganglion cells. Toxicity blocked by memantine. Invest Ophthalmol Vis Sci 1996;37:1618–1624.
31. Dreyer EB, Zurakowski D, Schumer RA, et al. Elevated glutamate levels in the vitreous body of humans and monkeys with glaucoma. Arch Ophthalmol 1996;114: 299–305.
32. Yoles E, Schwartz M. Elevation of intraocular glutamate levels in rats with partial lesion of the optic nerve. Arch Ophthalmol 1998;116:906–910.
33. Photocoagulation treatment of proliferative diabetic retinopathy: the second report of diabetic retinopathy study findings. Ophthalmology 1978;85:82–106.
34. The Macular Photocoagulation Study Group. Laser photocoagulation of subfoveal neovascular lesions in age-related macular degeneration. Results of a randomized clinical trial. Arch Ophthalmol 1991;109: 1220–1231.
35. The Macular Photocoagulation Study Group. Krypton laser photocoagulation for neovascular lesions of age-related macular degeneration. Results of a randomized clinical trial. Arch Ophthalmol 1990;108:816–824.
36. Brancato R, Pece A, Avanza P, Radrizzani E. Photocoagulation scar expansion after laser therapy for choroidal neovascularization in degenerative myopia. Retina 1990;10:239–243.
37. Dastgheib K, Bressler SB, Green WR. Clinicopathologic correlation of laser lesion expansion after treatment of choroidal neovascularization. Retina 1993;13:345–352.
38. Kyoko M, Noriko U, Tomohiro Otani, Shoji K. Progressive enlargement of scattered photocoagulation scars in diabetic retinopathy. Retina 2004;24: 507–511.
39. Lai TYY, Chan WM, Lam DSC. Transient reduction in retinal function revealed by multifocal electroretinogram after photodynamic therapy. Am J Ophthalmol 2004;137:826–833.
40. Treatment of Age-related Macular Degeneration with Photodynamic Therapy (TAP) Study Group and Verteporfin in Photodynamic Therapy (VIP) Study Group. Acute severe visual acuity decrease after photodynamic therapy with verteporfin: case reports from randomized clinical trials – TAP and VIP report no. 3. Am J Ophthalmol 2004;137:683–696.
41. Verteporfin in Photodynamic Therapy Study Group. Verteporfin therapy of subfoveal choroidal neovascularization in age-related macular degeneration: two-year results of a randomized clinical trial including lesions with occult with no classic choroidal neovascularization – verteporfin in photodynamic therapy report 2. Am J Ophthalmol 2001;131:541–560.
42. Lam TT, Fu J, Takahashi K, Tso MOM. Methylprednisolone therapy in laser injury of the retina Graefes Arch Clin Exp Ophthalmol 1993;231: 729–736.
43. Solberg Y, Rosner M, Turetz J, Belkin M. MK-801 has neuroprotective and antiproliferative effects in retinal laser injury. Invest Ophthalmol Vis Sci 1997;38: 1380–1389.
44. Gaasterland D, Kupfer C. Experimental glaucoma in the rhesus monkey. Invest Ophthalmol Vis Sci 1974;13:455–457.
45. Pederson JE, Gaasterland DE. Laser-induced primate glaucoma. I. Progression of cupping. Arch Ophthalmol 1984;102:1689–1692.
46. Quigley HA, Hohman RM. Laser energy levels for trabecular meshwork damage in the primate eye. Invest Ophthalmol Vis Sci 1983;24:1305–1307.
47. Radius RL, Pederson JE. Laser-induced primate glaucoma. II. Histopathology. Arch Ophthalmol 1984;102: 1693–1698.
48. Morrison JC, Moore CG, Deppmeier LM, et al. A rat model of chronic pressure-induced optic nerve damage. Exp Eye Res 1997;64:85–96.
49. Shareef SR, Garcia-Valenzuela E, Salierno A. Chronic ocular hypertension following episcleral venous occlusion in rats. Exp Eye Res 1995;61:379–382.
50. Takita H, Yoneya S, Gehlbach PL, et al. Retinal neuroprotection against ischemic injury mediated by intraocular gene transfer of pigment epithelium-derived factor. Invest Ophthalmol Vis Sci 2003;44: 4497–4504.
51. Yoles E, Schwartz M. Potential neuroprotective therapy for glaucomatous optic neuropathy. Surv Ophthalmol 1998;42(4):367–372.
52. Duvdevani R, Rosner M, Belkin M, et al. Graded crush of the rat optic nerve as a brain injury model: combining electrophysiological and behavioral outcome. Restor Neurol Neurosci 1990;2:31–38.
53. Levkovitch-Verbin H, Quigley HA, Kerrigan-Baumrind LA, et al. Optic nerve transection in monkeys may result in secondary degeneration of retinal ganglion cells. Invest Ophthalmol Vis Sci 2001;42: 975–982.
54. Toriu N, Akaike A, Yasuyoshi H. Lomerizine, a Ca2+ channel blocker, reduces glutamate-induced neurotoxicity and ischemia/reperfusion damage in rat retina. Exp Eye Res 2000;70:475–484.
55. Yoles E, Muller S, Schwartz M. NMDA-receptor antagonist protects neurons from secondary degeneration after partial optic nerve crush. J Neurotrauma 1997;14:665–675.
56. Muir KW, Lees KR. Clinical experience with excitatory amino acid antagonist drugs. Stroke 1995;26:503–513.
57. Yoon YH, Marmor MF. Dextromethorphan protects retina against ischemic injury in vivo. Arch Ophthalmol 1989;107:409–411.
58. Calzada JI, Jones BE, Netland PA, Johnson DA. Glutamate-induced excitotoxicity in retina: neuroprotection with receptor antagonist, dextromethorphan,

58. but not with calcium channel blockers. Neurochem Res 2002;27:79–88.
59. Osborne NN, Schwarz M, Pergande G. Protection of rabbit retina from ischemic injury by flupirtine. Invest Ophthalmol Vis Sci 1996;37:274–280.
60. Nash MS, Wood JP, Melena J, Osborne NN. Flupirtine ameliorates ischaemic-like death of rat retinal ganglion cells by preventing calcium influx. Brain Res 2000;856:236–239.
61. Ettaiche M, Fillacier K, Widmann C, et al. Riluzole improves functional recovery after ischemia in the rat retina. Invest Ophthalmol Vis Sci 1999;40:729–736.
62. Nat Rev Drug Discov 2004;3:S38–S40.
63. Livingston G, Katona C. The place of memantine in the treatment of Alzheimer's disease: a number needed to treat analysis. Int J Geriatr Psychiatry 2004;19:919–925.
64. Osborne NN. Memantine reduces alterations to the mammalian retina, in situ, induced by ischemia. Vis Neurosci 1999;16:45–52.
65. Hare WA, WoldeMussie E, Weinreb RN, et al. Efficacy and safety of memantine treatment for reduction of changes associated with experimental glaucoma in monkey. II. Structural measures. Invest Ophthalmol Vis Sci 2004;45:2640–2651.
66. Hare WA, WoldeMussie E, Lai RK, et al. Efficacy and safety of memantine treatment for reduction of changes associated with experimental glaucoma in monkey. I. Functional measures. Invest Ophthalmol Vis Sci 2004;45:2625–2639.
67. Jain KK. Evaluation of memantine for neuroprotection in dementia. Expert Opin Investig Drugs 2000;9:1397–1406.
68. Merello M, Nouzeilles MI, Cammarota A, Leiguarda R. Effect of memantine (NMDA antagonist) on Parkinson's disease: a double-blind crossover randomized study. Clin Neuropharmacol 1999;22:273–276.
69. Wiech K, Kiefer RT, Topfner S, et al. A placebo-controlled randomized crossover trial of the N-methyl-D-aspartic acid receptor antagonist, memantine in patients with chronic phantom limb pain. Anesth Analg 2004;98:408–413.
70. Green BA, Kahn T, Klose KJ. A comparative study of steroid therapy in acute experimental spinal cord injury. Surg Neurol 1980;13:91–97.
71. Hall ED. High-dose glucocorticoid treatment improves neurological recovery in head-injured mice. J Neurosurg 1985;62:882–887.
72. Means ED, Anderson DK, Waters TR, Kalaf L. Effect of methylprednisolone in compression trauma to the feline spinal cord. J Neurosurg 1981;55(2):200–208.
73. Bracken MB, Shepard MJ, Collins WF, et al. A randomized, controlled trial of methylprednisolone or naloxone in the treatment of acute spinal-cord injury. Results of the Second National Acute Spinal Cord Injury Study. N Engl J Med 1990;322:1405–1411.
74. Takahashi K, Lam TT, Fu J, Tso MOM. The effect of high-dose methylprednisolone on laser-induced retinal injury in primates: an electron microscopic study. Graefes Arch Clin Exp Ophthalmol 1997;235:723–732.
75. Naveh N, Weissman C. Corticosteroid treatment of laser retinal damage affects prostaglandin E2 response. Invest Ophthalmol Vis Sci 1990;31:9–13.
76. Wilson CA, Berkowitz BA, Sato Y, et al. Treatment with intravitreal steroid reduces blood-retinal breakdown due to retinal photocoagulation. Arch Ophthalmol 1992;110:1155–1159.
77. Ishibashi T, Miki K, Sorgente N, et al. Effects of intravitreal administration of steroids on experimental subretinal neovascularization in the subhuman primate. Arch Ophthalmol 1985;103:708–711.
78. Rosner M, Solberg Y, Turetz J, Belkin M. Neuroprotective therapy for argon-laser induced retinal injury. Exp Eye Res 1997;65:485–495.
79. Hirschberg DL, Yoles E, Belkin M, Schwartz M. Inflammation after axonal injury has conflicting consequences for recovery of function: rescue of spared axons is impaired but regeneration is supported. J Neuroimmunol 1994;50:9–11.
80. Marshall J. Structural aspects of laser induced damage and their functional implications. Health Phys 1989;56:617–624.
81. Schuschereba ST, Cross ME, Pizarro JAM, et al. High dose methylprednisolone treatment of laser-induced retinal injury exacerbates acute inflammation and long-term scarring [abstract]. Int Symp Biomed Optics 1999:40.
82. Yoles E, Wheeler LA, Schwartz M. Alpha2-adrenoreceptor agonists are neuroprotective in a rat model of optic nerve degeneration. Invest Ophthalmol Vis Sci 1999;40:65–73.
83. Donello JE, Padillo EU, Webster ML, et al. Alpha(2)-adrenoceptor agonists inhibit vitreal glutamate and aspartate accumulation and preserve retinal function after transient ischemia. J Pharmacol Exp Ther 2001;296:216–223.
84. Gao H, Qiao X, Cantor LB, WuDunn D. Up-regulation of brain-derived neurotrophic factor expression by brimonidine in rat retinal ganglion cells. Arch Ophthalmol 2002;120(6):797–803.
85. Evans DW, Hosking SL, Gherghel D, Bartlett JD. Contrast sensitivity improves after brimonidine therapy in primary open angle glaucoma: a case for neuroprotection. Br J Ophthalmol 2003;87:1463–1465.
86. Osborne NN, Cazevieille C, Carvalho AL, et al. In vivo and in vitro experiments show that betaxolol is a retinal neuroprotective agent. Brain Res 1997;751:113–123.
87. Osborne NN, DeSantis L, Bae JH, et al. Topically applied betaxolol attenuates NMDA-induced toxicity to ganglion cells and the effects of ischaemia to the retina. Exp Eye Res 1999;69:331–342.
88. Choi DW. Calcium-mediated neurotoxicity: relationship to specific channel types and role in ischemic damage. Trends Neurosci 1988;11:465–469.
89. Eschweiler GW, Bähr M. Flunarizine enhances rat retinal ganglion cell survival after axotomy. J Neurol Sci 1993;116:34–40.
90. Takahashi K, Lam TT, Edward DP, et al. Protective effects of flunarizine on ischemic injury in the rat retina. Arch Ophthalmol 1992;110:862–870.
91. Netland PA, Chaturvedi N, Dreyer EB. Calcium channel blockers in the management of low-tension and open-angle glaucoma. Am J Ophthalmol 1993;115:608–613.
92. Dawson VL, Dawson TM, Bartley DA, et al. Mechanisms of nitric oxide-mediated neurotoxicity in primary brain cultures. J Neurosci 1993;13:2651–2661.
93. Malinski T, Bailey F, Zhang ZG, Chopp M. Nitric oxide measured by a porphyrinic microsensor in rat brain after transient middle cerebral artery occlusion. J Cereb Blood Flow Metab 1993;13:355–358.

94. Neufeld AH. Nitric oxide: a potential mediator of retinal ganglion cell damage in glaucoma. Surv Ophthalmol 1999;43(suppl 1):S129–135.
95. Neufeld AH, Hernandez MR, Gonzalez M. Nitric oxide synthase in the human glaucomatous optic nerve head. Arch Ophthalmol 1997;115:497–503.
96. Shareef S, Sawada A, Neufeld AH. Isoforms of nitric oxide synthase in the optic nerves of rat eyes with chronic moderately elevated intraocular pressure. Invest Ophthalmol Vis Sci 1999;40:2884–2891.
97. Liu B, Neufeld AH. Activation of epidermal growth factor receptor signals induction of nitric oxide synthase-2 in human optic nerve head astrocytes in glaucomatous optic neuropathy. Neurobiol Dis 2003;13:109–123.
98. Neufeld AH, Sawada A, Becker B. Inhibition of nitric-oxide synthase 2 by aminoguanidine provides neuroprotection of retinal ganglion cells in a rat model of chronic glaucoma. Proc Natl Acad Sci USA 1999;96:9944–9948.
99. Zhang C, Lei B, Lam TT, Yang F, Sinha D, Tso MO. Neuroprotection of photoreceptors by minocycline in light-induced retinal degeneration. Invest Ophthalmol Vis Sci 2004;45:2753–2759.
100. Baptiste DC, Hartwick AT, Jollimore CA, Baldridge WH, Seigel GM, Kelly ME. An investigation of the neuroprotective effects of tetracycline derivatives in experimental models of retinal cell death. Mol Pharmacol 2004;66:1113–1122.
101. Hughes EH, Schlichtenbrede FC, Murphy CC, et al. Minocycline delays photoreceptor death in the rds mouse through a microglia-independent mechanism. Exp Eye Res 2004;78:1077–1084.
102. Tsuji M, Wilson MA, Lange MS, Johnston MV. Minocycline worsens hypoxic-ischemic brain injury in a neonatal mouse model. Exp Neurol 2004;189:58–65.
103. Diguet E, Gross CE, Tison F, Bezard E. Rise and fall of minocycline in neuroprotection: need to promote publication of negative results. Exp Neurol 2004;189:1–4.
104. Mansour-Robaey S, Clarke DB, Wang YC, et al. Effects of ocular injury and administration of brain-derived neurotrophic factor on survival and regrowth of axotomized retinal ganglion cells. Proc Natl Acad Sci USA 1994;91:1632–1636.
105. Peinado-Ramon P, Salvador M, Villegas-Perez MP, et al. Effects of axotomy and intraocular administration of NT-4, NT-3, and brain-derived neurotrophic factor on the survival of adult rat retinal ganglion cells. A quantitative in vivo study. Invest Ophthalmol Vis Sci 1996;37:489–500.
106. Sawai H, Clarke DB, Kittlerova P, et al. Brain derived growth factor and neurotrophin 4/5 stimulate growth of axonal branches from regenerating retinal ganglion cells. J Neurosci 1996;16:3887–3894.
107. Chen H, Weber AJ. BDNF enhances retinal ganglion cell survival in cats with optic nerve damage. Invest Ophthalmol Vis Sci 2001;42:966–974.
108. Quigley HA, McKinnon SJ, Zack DJ, et al. Retrograde axonal transport of BDNF in retinal ganglion cells is blocked by acute IOP elevation in rats. Invest Ophthalmol Vis Sci 2000;41:3460–3466.
109. Isenmann S, Kretz A, Cellerino A. Molecular determinants of retinal ganglion cell development, survival, and regeneration. Prog Retin Eye Res 2003;22:483–543.
110. Kalra S, Genge A, Arnold DL. A prospective, randomized, placebo-controlled evaluation of corticoneuronal response to intrathecal BDNF therapy in ALS using magnetic resonance spectroscopy: feasibility and results. Amyotroph Lateral Scler Other Motor Neuron Disord 2003;4:22–26.
111. Schwartz M. Neurodegeneration and neuroprotection in glaucoma: development of a therapeutic neuroprotective vaccine. The Friedenwald lecture. Invest Ophthalmol Vis Sci 2003;44:1407–1411.
112. Bakalash S, Kipnis J, Yoles E, Schwartz M. Resistance of retinal ganglion cells to an increase in intraocular pressure is immune-dependent. Invest Ophthalmol Vis Sci 2002;43:2648–2653.
113. Yoles E, Hauben E, Palgi O. Protective autoimmunity is a physiological response to CNS trauma. J Neurosci 2001;21:3740–3748.
114. Schwartz M, Kipnis J. Self and non-self discrimination is needed for the existence rather than deletion of autoimmunity: the role of regulatory T cells in protective autoimmunity. Cell Mol Life Sci 2004;61:2285–2289.
115. Nevo U, Golding I, Neumann AU, Schwartz M, Akselrod S. Autoimmunity as an immune defense against degenerative processes: a primary mathematical model illustrating the bright side of autoimmunity. J Theor Biol 2004;21;227:583–592.
116. Kipnis J, Avidan H, Markovich Y, et al. Low-dose gamma-irradiation promotes survival of injured neurons in the central nervous system via homeostasis-driven proliferation of T cells. Eur J Neurosci 2004;19:1191–1198.
117. Hirschberg DL, Moalem G, He J, et al. Accumulation of passively transferred primed T cells independently of their antigen specificity following central nervous system trauma. J Neuroimmunol 1998;89:88–96.
118. Moalem G, Leibowitz-Amit R, Yoles E. Autoimmune T cells protect neurons from secondary degeneration after central nervous system axotomy. Nat Med 1999;5:49–55.
119. Moalem G, Yoles E, Leibowitz-Amit R, et al. Autoimmune T cells retard the loss of function in injured rat optic nerves. J Neuroimmunol 2000;106:189–197.
120. Fisher J, Levkovitch-Verbin H, Schori H, et al. Vaccination for neuroprotection in the mouse optic nerve: implications for optic neuropathies. J Neurosci 2001;21:136–142.
121. Schori H, Kipnis J, Eti Yoles E, et al. Vaccination for protection of retinal ganglion cells against death from glutamate cytotoxicity and ocular hypertension: implications for glaucoma. Proc Natl Acad Sci USA 2001;98:3398–3403.
122. Schwartz M, Kipnis J. A common vaccine for fighting neurodegenerative disorders: recharging immunity for homeostasis. Trends Pharmacol Sci 2004;25:407–412.
123. Schori H, Kipnis J, Eti Yoles E, et al. Vaccination for protection of retinal ganglion cells against death from glutamate cytotoxicity and ocular hypertension: implications for glaucoma. Proc Natl Acad Sci USA 2001;98:3398–3403.
124. Schwartz M. Vaccination for glaucoma: dream or reality? Brain Res Bull 2004;15(62):481–484.
125. Bakalash S, Kessler A, Mizrahi T, Nussenblatt R, Schwartz M. Antigenic specificity of immunoprotec-

tive therapeutic vaccination for glaucoma. Invest Ophthalmol Vis Sci 2003;44:3374–3381.
126. Scwartz M. Optic nerve crush: protection and regeneration. Brain Res Bull 2004;15(62):467–471.
127. Shaked I, Porat Z, Gersner R, Kipnis J, Schwartz M. Early activation of microglia as antigen-presenting cells correlate with T cell-mediated protection and repair of the injured central nervous system. J Neuroimmunol 2004;146:84–93.
128. Moalem G, Gdalyahu A, Shani Y, et al. Production of neurotrophins by activated T cells: implications for neuroprotective autoimmunity. J Autoimmun 2000;15:331–345.
129. Schwartz M, Shaked I, Fisher J, Mizrahi T, Schori H. Protective autoimmunity against the enemy within: fighting glutamate toxicity. Trends Neurosci 2003;26: 297–302.
130. Symon L, Astrup J. Phenomena associated with focal ischaemia in the central nervous system. Acta Neurochir Suppl (Wien) 1979;28(1):215–217.
131. Agnoli A, Palesse N, Ruggieri S, Leonardis G, Benzi G. Barbiturate treatment of acute stroke. Adv Neurol 1979;25:269–274.
132. Li ZY, Tso MO, Wang HM, Organisciak DT. Amelioration of photic injury in rat retina by ascorbic acid: a histopathologic study. Invest Ophthalmol Vis Sci 1985;26:1589–1598.
133. Schwartz M, Belkin M, Yoles E, Solomon A. Potential treatment modalities for glaucomatous neuropathy: neuroprotection and neuroregeneration. J Glaucoma 1996;5:427–432.

18

Autoimmunity for Central Nervous System Maintenance, Regeneration, and Renewal: Development of a T Cell-Based Vaccination Against Neurodegeneration

Michal Schwartz and Jonathan Kipnis

The adult central nervous system (CNS), despite its need for plasticity, has a poor capacity for cell renewal, regeneration, and repair. It also poorly tolerates immune activity, the body's machinery for defense and repair. This latter feature, coupled with the limited immune responsiveness characteristic of immune-privileged sites such as the healthy CNS, seemed to substantiate the traditional view that any immune response in the CNS would do more harm than good, and therefore the less immune intervention the better. Accumulating evidence indicates, however, that well-controlled immune activity promotes neuroprotection, neuroregeneration, and – as recently discovered – renewal of neural cells under acute or chronic degenerative conditions. Innate immunity, represented by well-controlled activated macrophages, can facilitate regeneration in the severed spinal cord. Adaptive immunity, represented by T cells specific to self-antigens that reside in sites of CNS damage, facilitates neuronal survival and renewal by suitably activating the resident microglia. Adaptive immunity, moreover, can be safely boosted by means of T cell-mediated therapeutic vaccination. This review summarizes the findings, the concept, and the challenges in connection with boosting of the immune activity as a way to promote and control plasticity in the healthy CNS, and repair in the case of CNS injury or disease.

The limited immune activity in the CNS is manifested by low expression of class I and II major histocompatibility complex proteins (MHC-I and MHC-II). A unique immunologic feature of the brain, possibly evoked as partial compensation for the limited immune activity, is the abundant presence of resident innate immune cells (microglia), which account for approximately 12% of the total brain-cell population. Under neurodegenerative conditions, activated microglia are often seen in damaged sites. These activated microglia have therefore traditionally been perceived as inflammation-related, and hence as part of the pathology. Data obtained in our laboratory and elsewhere over the last few years suggest, however, that macrophages are needed for CNS repair after axotomy, that T cells specific to certain self-antigens are essential for controlling brain-resident microglia, and that microglia are key players in these processes, provided that they are well controlled and properly activated by the adaptive immune system.

Implantation of Activated Macrophages Promotes CNS Regrowth

The peripheral nervous system (PNS), in contrast to the CNS, can regenerate after injury. Therefore, comparison of the inflammatory responses of the CNS and the PNS to injury has proved helpful in identifying factors that are important for recovery of neural tissue. Relative to the PNS, the macrophage response to injury in the CNS is sluggish. Moreover, although microglia are activated after injury, their activity is significantly lower than that of peripheral-blood macrophages and is transient. The question then arises: Can this limitation in macrophage and microglial activity explain, at least in part, the failure of the CNS to regenerate and repair itself?

Findings in our laboratory led to the suggestion that in the injured CNS, as in other injured tissues, activated macrophages are needed at an early postinjury stage for tissue healing.[1,2] In addition, healing of the CNS might be adversely affected by the late arrival of macrophages at the site of injury, their limited spread within the injured tissue, and their restricted activity. This hypothesis was substantiated in a spinal cord model by incubation of peripheral blood macrophages with PNS tissue, followed by application of the macrophages to the site of injury. Some functional recovery was demonstrated in studies of adult rat spinal cord, in which local application of PNS-activated macrophages to the completely transected spinal cord was found to lead to the partial recovery of otherwise paraplegic rats. Recovery was manifested by acquisition of locomotor activity, which was tested in an open field by measurement of the generation of motor-elicited potential responses in the hindlimb muscles and verified by morphologic alterations that met specific criteria.[3] Subsequent studies conducted with skin-activated macrophages showed that the timing, site, and dose of the macrophages critically affected the outcome.[4] Moreover, the macrophages demonstrated features reminiscent of antigen-presenting cells, not of classically activated cytotoxic/phagocytic cells.[4]

The above data supported three conclusions. First, the CNS is not intrinsically refractory to the processes of healing and regrowth. Second, the ability of well-regulated activated macrophages to promote CNS healing and regrowth is, in principle, not unlike that promoted by the innate immune response in other organs. Third, the failure of the CNS to regrow can be attributed, at least in part, to a relative inability of the damaged CNS to recruit and activate a local immune response whose activity, type, level, and timing are geared to protection and repair.

Adaptive Autoimmunity and CNS Repair

Macrophages do not bear receptors for antigens and they lack immune memory, thus representing the nonadaptive, innate arm of the immune response. T cells, in contrast, respond to specific antigens and "remember" past experience, and so represent part of the adaptive arm of the immune response. When activated, T cells can kill their target cells or produce signal molecules that activate or suppress the growth, movement, or differentiation of other cells. Thus, T cells have an important role in protecting the individual against foreign invaders, as well as in maintaining body function. The blood–brain barrier of the CNS is normally impermeable to resting T cells, but is permeable to activated T cells. Activated T cells, however, do not accumulate in the healthy CNS unless they recognize and are able to react to their specific antigen there.[5]

Comparative studies of the T cell response at sites of optic and sciatic nerve injury, using T cell immunocytochemistry, revealed a significantly greater accumulation of endogenous T cells in the injured PNS than in the injured CNS. Moreover, the CNS shows a marked propensity for elimination of T cells via apoptosis, whereas this mechanism is less effective in the PNS and is almost absent in other tissues such as muscle and skin.[6] These findings suggested that the T cell response in the traumatized CNS is both restricted and tightly regulated.

To determine whether an increase in accumulated T cells is beneficial or harmful to the injured CNS, our group used a model of a partial lesion of the rat optic nerve, which allows assessment of nerve maintenance after traumatic axonal injury. Axonal injury was followed by a transient accumulation of endogenous T cells at the site of the lesion. Passive administration of activated syngeneic T cells specific to a CNS self-antigen such as myelin basic protein (MBP), or to a non-self-antigen such as ovalbumin, resulted in an increased local accumulation of T cells.[7,8] Although both T cell lines accumulated at the site of the lesion, there was a clear difference in their effects on the maintenance of the damaged tissue, as manifested by their ability to affect the progression of degeneration. Two weeks after injury, the rats injected with T_{MBP} cells showed significantly less degeneration than rats injected with phosphate-buffered saline or with T cells specific to the foreign antigen ovalbumin. This neuroprotective property of the T_{MBP} cells was demonstrated using criteria derived from morphometric and electrophysiological studies.[8] Thus, both the numbers of retinal ganglion cells and the degree of optic nerve conduction (measured by its compound action potential) were significantly higher in the rats injected with T_{MBP} cells than in the other groups of rats. The neuroprotective effect was discernible despite the fact that the transferred T_{MBP} cells induced the transient monophasic paralytic disease experimental autoimmune encephalomyelitis (EAE). Symptoms of EAE appeared 2 days after cell injection, peaked on day 6, and terminated around day 10. It should be emphasized that the adoptive transfer of EAE to Lewis rats by T_{MBP} cells does not involve structural demyelination.[9]

Interestingly, protection of neurons from posttraumatic degeneration was not related to the intrinsic pathogenicity of the T_{MBP} cells. The EAE induced by T cells specific to a cryptic epitope of MBP, p51–70, was significantly milder, if seen at all, than that induced by the T_{MBP} cells. Nevertheless, this weakly pathogenic anti-p51–70 T cell line was as effective in reducing secondary degeneration as the highly pathogenic T_{MBP} cell line.[8] Thus, induction of clinical autoimmune disease was not a prerequisite for the T_{MBP} cell-mediated protection against secondary degeneration. Subsequent studies have proven that a similar benefit of autoimmunity is seen after spinal cord injury with meaningful and significant effect on functional and morphologic recovery.[10–13]

These results prompted our group to address the following question: After an insult, is protective autoimmunity a physiological response that is amenable to boosting? If so, what controls autoimmunity so that it is expressed or suppressed according to need? What is the antigenic specificity of the response? What mechanism underlies protection? What is the role, if any, of these autoimmune T cells in neuronal plasticity in health? These and other questions were addressed by our group and others over the last few years. The results are summarized below.

Protective Autoimmunity – A Physiological Response

The adaptive immune response has generally been considered as an immune activity evoked to enable the organism to cope with stressful conditions caused by pathogens. One suggestion was that an adaptive immune response would be evoked unless the pathogen was recognized as self.[14] Opinions differ as to the mechanisms by which self becomes invisible to the immune system (for example, by clonal deletion, anergy, or tolerance).[15-23] Some authors proposed that autoimmunity, once established, might be at best harmless.[24-27] Until recently, however, none had described a situation in which the body calls for help from an anti-self response.

The finding that passive transfer of autoimmune T cells promotes recovery of damaged myelinated axons prompted our group to investigate whether the observed response is physiological or a reflection of experimental manipulation. Several lines of research led to the conclusion that the T cell response to self-antigens is a physiological defense mechanism to insults, at least in the CNS. First, in most strains, recovery after a CNS insult, in the absence of intervention, is worse if the animals are immune deficient, for example in mice with severe combined immune deficiency (SCID mice, which lack both T and B cells) or deprived of T cells only (nude mice). We further found that the specificity of the T cells needed for spontaneous recovery is toward self-antigens residing in the site of stress; in rats that were tolerized to self-antigens as newborns, the spontaneous recovery from CNS insults as adults was worse than in normal mice.[10,28,29] Thus, specificity of the response is determined not by the type of threat but by its location, implying that insults of different types (mechanical, ischemic, biochemical), if they occur at the same site, will recruit help from T cells of the same specificity.[30] Whether the effect of the autoimmune T cell response will be beneficial or harmful seems to depend, moreover, on the timing of its onset and shutoff.[31] A response that is delayed or excessive might not only lead to a lack of benefit but even result in an autoimmune disease.[11]

The Mechanism Underlying Protective Autoimmunity

There are different subpopulations of CD4+ T cells, each responsible for a certain type of immune response. T-helper (Th)1 cells, for example, reinforce innate immunity and activate CD8+ T cells, whereas Th2 cells recruit and activate B cells. Studies have shown that controlled levels of the autoimmune CD4+ T cells (effector T cells) locally boost and control resident microglia and infiltrating blood-borne monocytes. This effect helps the microglia/macropages to acquire an activity that allows them to fight off degenerative conditions requiring removal of dead cells and cell debris, as well as to buffer toxic compounds without producing inflammation-associated compounds, such as tumor necrosis factor-α, nitric oxide, or cyclooxygenase-2.[32-35] Thus, according to these findings, the role of CD4+ T cells directed against self-antigens is to activate in a well-controlled way the innate response, enabling it to recognize the threat to the tissue not as a pathogen that it must destroy, but as a toxic substance that it must neutralize or buffer. In addition, the autoimmune T cells, upon encountering their specific antigens presented by antigen-presenting cells at the lesion site, can produce protective compounds such as growth factors and neurotrophins.[36-38] All of these tasks can be accomplished by a well-controlled response of Th cells. More recent studies have shown that both Th1 and Th2 cells, directed to self-antigens via different mechanisms, benefit the damaged nerve. Thus, whereas Th1 cells activate microglia to buffer glutamate via interferon-γ secretion, Th2 cells produce insulinlike growth factor-I via microglia activated by interleukin-4 (Butovsky et al., unpublished observations) abstract neuroscience.

Naturally Occurring CD4+CD25+ Regulatory T Cells: A Compromise Between the Need for Autoimmunity and the Risk

After the discovery that autoimmunity is the body's defense mechanism against its own self-compounds, and that in principle T cells are spontaneously recruited in individuals with a genetic tendency toward autoimmune disease development, it became apparent that a constitutively operating mechanism maintains a balance between the need for autoimmunity on the one hand and its attendant risks on the other.[39] This regulatory mechanism was shown to be displayed by a subpopulation of T cells, previously identified as naturally occurring CD4+CD25+ regulatory T cells (Treg cells).[40] One of the molecular signals responsible for the activity of these cells was found to be the stress-related compound dopamine.[41] Interaction between dopamine and Treg cells via the dopamine type 1 receptor family down-regulates Treg-cell activity.[41] Elimination or down-regulation of Treg cells can be viewed as a means of boosting a physiological protective autoimmune response.[41,42] According to these findings, it is clear that the CD4+CD25+ cells, traditionally viewed as suppressors of autoimmune T cells that escaped neonatal deletion, are the very cells that keep the autoimmune T cells under tight control and are themselves amenable to control upon need.

Immune-Based Manipulations Leading to Boosting of Antigen-specific T Cells at the Site of Injury

Any immune manipulation that activates the immune system to induce a well-controlled increase in the likelihood that relevant T cells will home to an injury site can be expected to be beneficial. Our group examined three ways to obtain the desired effect: by active vaccination with self or self-like antigens, by induction of lymphopenia, and by depletion or functional inactivation of naturally occurring regulatory CD4+CD25+ T cells.

The search for a way to boost autoimmunity without incurring the risk of autoimmune disease led us to seek "safe" antigens. Safe antigens can be weak agonists of encephalitogenic peptides, cryptic epitopes, or peptides that can cross-react weakly with safe synthetic antigens such as copolymer-1 (Cop-1). T cells specific to self-antigens can be made available either by the use of compounds that transiently weaken the mechanism that normally keeps autoimmunity suppressed, such as dopamine or its relevant agonists,[42] or by active vaccination with relevant self-antigens. The autoimmune T cell population needed to fight off neurotoxic self-agents can, in principle, be boosted by immunization with a nonpathogenic agonist of the relevant self-antigens.[44,45] In seeking such an agonist for vaccination, we used Cop-1, a synthetic copolymer that was originally designed to mimic the T cell-receptor-binding site of a dominant epitope of MBP, and was serendipitously found, in experiments with rodents, to prevent the development of EAE.[46–48] Cop-1 is now an approved drug for the treatment of multiple sclerosis.[49] When vaccinated according to a different regimen, it was beneficial also in various types of acute or chronic CNS injury by preserving both the morphology and the function of threatened neurons.[44,45,50–53]

Induction of lymphopenia significantly increases immunoreactivity toward cancer-specific proteins and efficiently suppresses cancer.[54] A sudden decrease in the pool of peripheral T lymphocytes stimulates their homeostasis-driven proliferation in order to restore the pool. In response to the stimulus of lymphopenia, naive peripheral T cells proliferate and acquire a phenotype reminiscent of memory T cells.[55] The induced proliferation predisposes the individual to development of an autoimmune response because, under lymphopenic conditions, T cells can proliferate upon interaction with MHC-II molecules alone, with no need for a costimulatory signal.[56–58] If at the time of lymphopenia induction the body undergoes stress that leads to the exposure of certain self-antigens (e.g., antigens related to tissue injury or cancer), an autoimmune response to those antigens will occur, resulting in a high overall incidence of proliferation of the relevant T lymphocytes.[59] We found that in rodents having acute or chronic neurodegenerative conditions, induction of lymphopenia significantly benefits postinjury neuronal survival.[53] Lymphopenia and the subsequent homeostatic proliferation can be induced in a number of ways, the most clinically relevant being low-dose irradiation of the lymphoid organs. Because of the lymphopenia, T cells proliferate and become activated. They patrol the body, and their patrol route includes the CNS. On reaching the lesion site, and after being activated by the resident cells that present self-antigens in the MHC-II groove, these lymphopenia-derived T cells perform their effector functions, similarly to T cells obtained by immunization with self- or altered self-proteins.[41]

Because the aim is to achieve activation of T cells that cross-react with self-antigens at the site of injury, this can also be done by weakening the naturally occurring Treg cells. In an experimental context, nude mice (devoid of mature T cells) repopulated with a T cell population that did not contain Treg cells[60] showed better recovery from a CNS insult than wild-type mice of the same strain. For clinical use, however, what is needed is a reagent that will weaken Treg cells. Dopamine was found both to weaken the activity and to reduce the trafficking of Treg cells.[41] It is possible that dopamine represents a family of physiological compounds capable of controlling Treg-cell activity and therefore allowing speedy recruitment of the relevant autoimmune T cells. Development of synthetic compounds that can reproduce the dopamine effect is another apparently feasible approach in which a common immune-based therapy could be used to fight off neurodegenerative diseases, irrespective of etiology. Although such compounds might weaken Treg cells nonselectively (i.e., regardless of their antigenic specificity), the subsequently evoked autoimmunity will be restricted to CD4+ cells that encounter their relevant antigens, and will consequently be associated with the site under stress.

Recent data suggest that the very same cells that support survival also support cell renewal (Butovsky et al., unpublished data, Ziv et al. unpublished observations). This opens up new avenues of treatment by immune-based manipulation, not only to remedy the loss of neural tissue resulting from injury or disease but also to counteract age or disease-related loss of brain plasticity.

References

1. Miller C, Tsatas O, David S. Dibutyryl cAMP, interleukin-1 beta, and macrophage conditioned medium enhance the ability of astrocytes to promote neurite growth. J Neurosci Res 1994 38:56–63.
2. Stoll G, Trapp BD, Griffin JW. Macrophage function during Wallerian degeneration of rat optic nerve: clearance of degenerating myelin and Ia expression. J Neurosci 1989;9:2327–2335.
3. Rapalino O, Lazarov-Spiegler O, Agranov E, et al. Implantation of stimulated homologous macrophages results in partial recovery of paraplegic rats. Nat Med 1998;4:814–821.
4. Bomstein Y, Marder JB, Vitner K, et al. Features of skin-coincubated macrophages that promote recovery from spinal cord injury. J Neuroimmunol 2003;142:10–16.

5. Hickey WF, Hsu BL, Kimura H. T-lymphocyte entry into the central nervous system. J Neurosci Res 1991;28:254–260.
6. Gold R, Hartung HP, Lassmann H. T-cell apoptosis in autoimmune diseases: termination of inflammation in the nervous system and other sites with specialized immune-defense mechanisms. Trends Neurosci 1997;20:399–404.
7. Hirschberg DL, Moalem G, He J, Mor F, Cohen IR, Schwartz M. Accumulation of passively transferred primed T cells independently of their antigen specificity following central nervous system trauma. J Neuroimmunol 1998;89:88–96.
8. Moalem G, Leibowitz-Amit R, Yoles E, Mor F, Cohen IR, Schwartz M. Autoimmune T cells protect neurons from secondary degeneration after central nervous system axotomy. Nat Med 1999;5:49–55.
9. Meeson AP, Piddlesden S, Morgan BP, Reynolds R. The distribution of inflammatory demyelinated lesions in the central nervous system of rats with antibody-augmented demyelinating experimental allergic encephalomyelitis. Exp Neurol 1994;129:299–310.
10. Hauben E, Butovsky O, Nevo U, et al. Passive or active immunization with myelin basic protein promotes recovery from spinal cord contusion. J Neurosci 2000;20:6421–6430.
11. Hauben E, Agranov E, Gothilf A, et al. Posttraumatic therapeutic vaccination with modified myelin self-antigen prevents complete paralysis while avoiding autoimmune disease. J Clin Invest 2001;108:591–599.
12. Hauben E, Ibarra A, Mizrahi T, Barouch R, Agranov E, Schwartz M. Vaccination with a Nogo-A-derived peptide after incomplete spinal-cord injury promotes recovery via a T-cell-mediated neuroprotective response: comparison with other myelin antigens. Proc Natl Acad Sci USA 2001;98:15173–15178.
13. Hauben E, Gothilf A, Cohen A, et al. Vaccination with dendritic cells pulsed with peptides of myelin basic protein promotes functional recovery from spinal cord injury. J Neurosci 2003;23:8808–8819.
14. Fabbri M, Smart C, Pardi R. T lymphocytes. Int J Biochem Cell Biol 2003;35:1004–1008.
15. Benson JM, Whitacre CC. The role of clonal deletion and anergy in oral tolerance. Res Immunol 1997;148:533–541.
16. Goodnow CC. Balancing immunity, autoimmunity, and self-tolerance. Ann NY Acad Sci 1997;815:55–66.
17. Koh DR. Oral tolerance: mechanisms and therapy of autoimmune diseases. Ann Acad Med Singapore 1998;27:47–53.
18. Wood KJ. New concepts in tolerance. Clin Transplant 1996;10:93–99.
19. Weigle WO. Immunologic tolerance: development and disruption. Hosp Pract (Off Ed) 1995;30:81–84, 89–92.
20. Lafferty KJ, Gill RG. The maintenance of self-tolerance. Immunol Cell Biol 1993;71(pt 3):209–214.
21. Lo D. T-cell tolerance. Curr Opin Immunol 1992;4: 711–715.
22. Siegel RM, Katsumata M, Komori S, et al. Mechanisms of autoimmunity in the context of T-cell tolerance: insights from natural and transgenic animal model systems. Immunol Rev 1990;118:165–192.
23. Urbain J, Urbain-Vansanten G, De Wit D. Self non self discrimination within the immune system: a view from the bridge. Nephrologie 1989;10:99–101.
24. Cohen IR. The cognitive paradigm and the immunological homunculus. Immunol Today 1992;13:490–494.
25. Cohen IR. The cognitive principle challenges clonal selection. Immunol Today 1992;13:441–444.
26. Gallucci S, Matzinger P. Danger signals: SOS to the immune system. Curr Opin Immunol 2001;13:114–119.
27. Matzinger P. An innate sense of danger. Semin Immunol 1998;10:399–415.
28. Kipnis J, Yoles E, Schori H, Hauben E, Shaked I, Schwartz M. Neuronal survival after CNS insult is determined by a genetically encoded autoimmune response. J Neurosci 2001;21:4564–4571.
29. Yoles E, Hauben E, Palgi O, et al. Protective autoimmunity is a physiological response to CNS trauma. J Neurosci 2001;21:3740–3748.
30. Mizrahi T, Hauben E, Schwartz M. The tissue-specific self-pathogen is the protective self-antigen: the case of uveitis. J Immunol 2002;169:5971–5977.
31. Shaked I, Porat Z, Gersner R, Kipnis J, Schwartz M. Early activation of microglia as antigen-presenting cells correlates with T cell-mediated protection and repair of the injured central nervous system. J Neuroimmunol 2004;146:84–93.
32. Basu A, Krady JK, Enterline JR, Levison SW. Transforming growth factor beta1 prevents IL-1beta-induced microglial activation, whereas TNFalpha- and IL-6-stimulated activation are not antagonized. Glia 2002;40:109–120.
33. Janabi N. Selective inhibition of cyclooxygenase-2 expression by 15-deoxy-Delta(12,14)(12,14)-prostaglandin J(2) in activated human astrocytes, but not in human brain macrophages. J Immunol 2002;168:4747–4755.
34. Levi G, Minghetti L, Aloisi F. Regulation of prostanoid synthesis in microglial cells and effects of prostaglandin E2 on microglial functions. Biochimie 1998;80:899–904.
35. Schwartz M, Shaked I, Fisher J, Mizrahi T, Schori H. Protective autoimmunity against the enemy within: fighting glutamate toxicity. Trends Neurosci 2003;26:297–302.
36. Gielen A, Khademi M, Muhallab S, Olsson T, Piehl F. Increased brain-derived neurotrophic factor expression in white blood cells of relapsing-remitting multiple sclerosis patients. Scand J Immunol 2003;57: 493–497.
37. Hammarberg H, Lidman O, Lundberg C, et al. Neuroprotection by encephalomyelitis: rescue of mechanically injured neurons and neurotrophin production by CNS-infiltrating T and natural killer cells. J Neurosci 2000;20:5283–5291.
38. Moalem G, Gdalyahu A, Shani Y, et al. Production of neurotrophins by activated T cells: implications for neuroprotective autoimmunity. J Autoimmun 2000;15:331–345.
39. Shevach EM. Regulatory T cells in autoimmunity. Annu Rev Immunol 2000;18:423–449.
40. Thornton AM, Shevach EM. CD4+CD25+ immunoregulatory T cells suppress polyclonal T cell activation in vitro by inhibiting interleukin 2 production. J Exp Med 1998;188:287–296.
41. Kipnis J, Cardon M, Avidan H, et al. Dopamine, through the extracellular signal-regulated kinase pathway, downregulates CD4+CD25+ regulatory T-cell activity: implications for neurodegeneration. J Neurosci 2004;24:6133–6143.

42. Kipnis J, Avidan H, Caspi RR, Schwartz M. Dual effect of CD4+CD25+ regulatory T cells in neurodegeneration: pro- and anti-inflammatory cytokines determine microglial activity. Proc Natl Acad Sci USA 2004;101(suppl 2):14663–14669.
43. Schwartz M. Protective autoimmunity as a T-cell response to central nervous system trauma: prospects for therapeutic vaccines. Prog Neurobiol 2001;65:489–496.
44. Kipnis J, Yoles E, Porat Z, et al. T cell immunity to copolymer 1 confers neuroprotection on the damaged optic nerve: possible therapy for optic neuropathies. Proc Natl Acad Sci USA 2000;97:7446–7451.
45. Schori H, Kipnis J, Yoles E, et al. Vaccination for protection of retinal ganglion cells against death from glutamate cytotoxicity and ocular hypertension: implications for glaucoma. Proc Natl Acad Sci USA 2001;98:3398–3403.
46. Arnon R, Teitelbaum D, Sela M. Suppression of experimental allergic encephalomyelitis by COP1: relevance to multiple sclerosis. Isr J Med Sci 1989;25:686–689.
47. Sela M. Specific vaccines against autoimmune diseases. C R Acad Sci III 1999;322:933–938.
48. Teitelbaum D, Arnon R, Sela M. Copolymer 1: from basic research to clinical application. Cell Mol Life Sci 1997;53:24–28.
49. Sela M. Structural components responsible for peptide antigenicity. Appl Biochem Biotechnol 2000;83:63–70; discussion 145–153.
50. Angelov DN, Waibel S, Guntinas-Lichius O, et al. Therapeutic vaccine for acute and chronic motor neuron diseases: implications for ALS. Proc Natl Acad Sci USA 2003;100:4790–4795.
51. Benner EJ, Mosley RL, Destache CJ, et al. Therapeutic immunization protects dopaminergic neurons in a mouse model of Parkinson's disease. Proc Natl Acad Sci USA 2004;101:9435–9440.
52. Kipnis J, Nevo U, Panikashvili D, et al. Therapeutic vaccination for closed head injury. J Neurotrauma 2003;20:559–569.
53. Kipnis J, Avidan H, Markovich Y, et al. Low-dose gamma-irradiation promotes survival of injured neurons in the central nervous system via homeostasis-driven proliferation of T cells. Eur J Neurosci 2004;19:1191–1198.
54. Dummer W, Niethammer AG, Baccala R, et al. T cell homeostatic proliferation elicits effective antitumor autoimmunity. J Clin Invest 2002;110:185–192.
55. Ma J, Urba WJ, Si L, Wang Y, Fox BA, Hu HM. Antitumor T cell response and protective immunity in mice that received sublethal irradiation and immune reconstitution. Eur J Immunol 2003;33:2123–2132.
56. Elflein K, Rodriguez-Palmero M, Kerkau T, Hunig T. Rapid recovery from T lymphopenia by CD28 superagonist therapy. Blood 2003;102:1764–1770.
57. Gudmundsdottir H, Turka LA. A closer look at homeostatic proliferation of CD4+ T cells: costimulatory requirements and role in memory formation. J Immunol 2001;167:3699–3707.
58. Sara E, Kotsakis A, Souklakos J, et al. Post-chemotherapy lymphopoiesis in patients with solid tumors is characterized by CD4+ cell proliferation. Anticancer Res 1999;19:471–476.
59. Gelinas S, Martinoli MG. Neuroprotective effect of estradiol and phytoestrogens on MPP+-induced cytotoxicity in neuronal PC12 cells. J Neurosci Res 2002;70:90–96.
60. Bakalash S, Kipnis J, Yoles E, Schwartz M. Resistance of retinal ganglion cells to an increase in intraocular pressure is immune-dependent. Invest Ophthalmol Vis Sci 2002;43:2648–2653.

19

Retinal Repair by Stem Cell Transplantation

Jeffrey H. Stern, Sally Temple, and Soma De

The retina is an accessible and highly structured central nervous system (CNS) tissue with the well-defined function of processing early visual signals. Two distinct layers with closely related neural origins make up the retina: the sensory retinal layer, which is also referred to simply as "retina," or "neural retina," and the retinal pigment epithelial (RPE) layer that is separated from the sensory retina by a potential space. The sensory retina mediates visual excitation whereas the RPE processes visual pigment and participates in visual adaptation as well as providing diurnal metabolic support to the photoreceptor cells. In the sensory retina, three cellular layers directly transmit visual signals: an outermost layer of photoreceptor cells that transduce light into a neural signal and a middle layer of bipolar cells that convey the visual signal to an inner layer of ganglion cells with axons that output via the optic nerve. Two additional sensory retinal layers, the horizontal cell and amacrine cell layers, process rather than directly transmit visual signals. Specialized glial cells termed Muller cells span the retinal layers.[1] The sensory retina is composed of neurons and glial cells whereas the RPE is composed of an epithelial monolayer apposing the photoreceptor cells present in the outermost sensory retina [Figure 19.1 (see color section)].

Several techniques enable imaging of living human retina through a dilated pupil, and surgical manipulation of the retina is undertaken with relative ease compared with most other areas of the human CNS. Because the retina has a well-defined function that allows objective and subjective testing, and can be easily manipulated and observed, pioneering transplantation studies have been performed in the eye that are arguably at the forefront of progress in CNS transplantation. The retina is therefore an important host tissue in which to study the role of stem cells in regenerative medicine, an emerging cell technology. Not unexpectedly, given that retina has pioneered transplantation, discussions concerning ethical considerations of CNS transplantation, which are part of the active debate surrounding stem cells, have already been initiated in the eye literature.[2-4] Weighing up the benefits and pitfalls of adding exogenous cells into such a delicate and crucial part of the CNS is a complex and emotive issue. On one hand, patients are highly motivated to submit to these experimental treatments. On the other, the fact that cell implantation could cause unwanted outcomes, for example, caused by cell overproliferation, formation of aberrant neural connections, or by creating a detrimental immune response, urges caution. Animal models continue to provide much valuable information regarding technique optimization and about how particular donor cell types behave after implantation. Nevertheless, some studies have to be done in humans, given that there are known species differences in donor and host tissue behavior. This is especially true for the development of cell transplant therapies for diseases that are not easily modeled in animals, such as macular degeneration. We have to acknowledge that the establishment of any successful transplant surgery protocol necessarily involves, at early stages, experimental surgery on human subjects. The technologies for generating and genetically manipulating suitable retinal donor cells, for surgical transplantation and for tracking outcome, are becoming increasingly well developed, and recent studies indicate that we can be cautiously optimistic about the eventual establishment of transplantation therapies for retinal repair.

Retinal regeneration occurs in lower vertebrates after injury or transplantation of embryonic tissue, and this repair recreates functional retina even in adulthood. The activation of progenitor cells is thought to mediate regeneration, and the nature of the involved cell type, stem or progenitor, is actively studied.[5] In this chapter, "progenitor cell" is used as a blanket term to describe any type of proliferating precursor cell that generates differentiated progeny, and "stem cell" is used to describe a subtype of progenitor cell that is capable of self-renewal (perpetuating itself) as well as generating differentiated progeny. This is a rather basic and broadly encompassing definition of stem cells, but serves while more rigorous molecular definitions are being developed, understanding that important distinctions that define the general stem cell and stem cell subpopulations may emerge from future studies.[6]

In contrast to lower vertebrates, injury in mammals does not regenerate functional retinal tissue. In fact, activation of mammalian retinal progenitor cells does not generally restore, but rather destroys retinal function. Some remodeling of existing retinal circuits may occur[7-9] but overall cellular plasticity results in functional damage. For example, in retinal detachment, neural and fibrous proliferation known as proliferative vitreoretinopathy consumes the remaining retina,[10] in proliferative diabetic retinopathy (PDR), fibrovascular proliferation can destroy the remaining functional retina,[11] and in exudative macular degeneration (wet AMD), fibrovascular and undefined proliferative responses lead to loss of the overlying neural retina.[12] Several proliferating cell types have been implicated in these retinopathies and, in each case, the proliferation has a destructive effect on the structural and functional integrity of the retina. The destructive response of progenitor cell activation in human retina contrasts sharply with lower vertebrates where activation of retinal progenitors leads to functional repair. Our hope is that conditions exist that permit reparative mechanisms to dominate in humans.

Understanding the conditions that regulate the proliferative response of progenitor cells may lead to therapy based on controlling the pathological proliferation that underlies disorders such as proliferative vitreoretinopathy, PDR, and wet AMD. Vascular endothelial growth factor (VEGF) inhibition with anti-VEGF antibody or aptamer has proven clinically useful in slowing neovascular ingrowth in wet AMD[13] and may have application for treating vascular proliferation in PDR.[14] The extraordinary clinical gains emerging from anti-VEGF therapy of vascular retinal progenitor cell populations has increased research interest in the nonvascular retinal progenitors that are also involved in proliferative retinopathy and in the interactions between the neural and vascular retinal progenitor cells.

In contrast to the proliferative retinopathies, the degenerative retinopathies are mediated by the loss of a retinal layer rather than by abnormal proliferation. In turn, activation rather than inhibition of the involved retinal progenitor cells is sought as potential therapy for the degenerative disorders. In this chapter, we focus on two major degenerative retinopathies, retinitis pigmentosa (RP), which involves the loss of the single outer retinal layer of photoreceptor cells, and nonexudative or dry AMD, which has a primary defect in the loss of the underlying RPE. RP and dry AMD are major blinding conditions arising from a defect in a homogeneous cell population that is located in a well-defined retinal layer and, thereby, raise the possibility that progenitor cell transplantation can repopulate, or improve survival in, the dystrophic layer to preserve or restore visual function. Glaucoma is another major blinding condition primarily involving the degeneration of a single homogeneous retinal layer, the ganglion cell layer, and there is also a strong interest in utilizing stem cell transplantation to replace or preserve the affected retinal ganglion cell layer.[15]

Transplantation of retinal progenitor cells holds hope for discovering therapeutic conditions for retinal degeneration via two basic strategies: Implanting cells for cell replacement therapy and implantation of cells as factories for cell-mediated delivery of growth factors. Great progress has been made to prevent or recover retinal degeneration in animal models, even long-term cures in some models. The current stage of progress in humans is that retinal transplantation is feasible and relatively safe, and the efficacy of preserving or restoring vision is being assessed. These early transplantation studies help define the obstacles that need to be overcome if this new therapeutic strategy is to become an effective treatment for human retinal disease and hold great hope for advancing our ability to treat otherwise inexorable retinal conditions.

Progenitor Cell Sources for Retina and RPE Repair

Degenerative retinal diseases such as RP and dry AMD are generally irreparable and clinical emphasis is placed on prevention, delay, and symptom management. Basic research in developmental neuroscience in vertebrates has helped define progenitor cell populations that could conceivably be used to repair lost neural cells in the eye. Early transplantations used arguably the most logical donor cell source, which is embryonic retinal tissue. More recent research has uncovered a subpopulation of highly prolific cells residing in several areas of the CNS, including retina: Stem cells. Moreover, stem cells reside in a number of non-neural tissues, raising the possibility that stem cells derived from an easily accessible tissue source, such as bone marrow or skin could transdifferentiate into neural cells. Early studies were enthusiastic, but problems in reproducibility and the discovery that some so-called transdifferentiation events were actually caused by fusion of stem cells with existing cells[16] have dampened enthusiasm for using non-neural cells as neural cell sources at this juncture. However, these stem cells may be useful in helping to repair other tissues in the eye such as vasculature, which can itself slow retinal degeneration.[17] For retinal cell replacement therapy, researchers are looking to stem cells derived from the nervous system or embryonic stem (ES) cells as more realistic sources of neural cells. It is important to recognize that even if a stem cell is derived from the nervous system, this is no guarantee that it can generate retina or RPE cells. As progenitor cell research advances, we have come to appreciate that there are many different types of stem cells, even within the nervous system, which vary in their efficiency of making retinal and RPE progeny.

ES Cells

The major neural-derived cells in the eye (retina and RPE) are normally generated in embryonic and early postnatal life, and given that these tissues have little regenerative power in adulthood, the most obvious stem cell source for retinal cells is the embryo. ES cells are derived from the preimplantation embryo at the blastocyst stage.[18] This early hollow ball of approximately 100 cells contains a smaller cluster of cells inside called the inner cell mass (ICM). ICM cells are pluripotent, being able to contribute progeny to all tissues of the embryo and they can efficiently generate all types of neural tissue, including retina and RPE. Although the ICM is a transient structure, and the stem cells within it normally succumb rapidly to developmental diversification and restriction, they can be maintained in their pluripotent state by artificially promoting self-renewal in the culture dish, enabling massive, long-term expansion. The resulting ES cell lines are being actively explored as a source of neural cells, especially with the advent of human ES lines, which are increasing in number and availability.[19]

Research progress in the ES field is providing essential information about how these highly plastic cells can be maintained in a pluripotent state. Importantly, the factors required to expand mouse ES cells and human ES cells are different. Mouse ES cell self-renewal in vitro is stimulated by a combination of leukemia inhibitory factor, via STAT-3 signaling, and bone morphogenetic protein (BMP),[20] or by the canonical Wnt signaling pathway.[21] In contrast, human ES cell self-renewal does not require leukemia inhibitory factor or STAT-3 signaling,[21-23] and BMP stimulates them to generate endoderm.[24,25] The fact that mouse and human differ widely in other aspects of gene expression[26] underlines the necessity of studying human ES lines. Progress is being made in establishing human feeder lines and culture conditions to create xeno-free conditions to optimize transplantation success.[27]

Mouse and human ES cells can be stimulated to generate neural progeny by factors such as retinoic acid, increased beta-catenin signaling, and feeder cells.[28,29] Usually, these differentiation protocols are applied while the ES cells are grown in nonattached culture as so-called embryoid bodies, to enhance their differentiation. Mouse ES cells can be induced to generate retinal cell subtypes.[30] Surprisingly, they can generate eye-like structures in vitro containing lens, neural retina, and pigmented retinal cells.[31] This occurs in a Pax-6-dependent manner (a gene essential for eye development in a variety of species[32]), suggesting that the differentiation of eye tissues from ES cells recapitulates normal developmental processes. It should thus be possible to draw upon the knowledge of these evolutionarily conserved developmental pathways to direct eye cell formation from ES cells from various species. Indeed, induced expression of the early retinal Rx/rax transcription factor in mouse ES cells promotes their differentiation into retinal cell types in vitro and after transplantation in vivo, producing cells with marker profiles and electrophysiological characteristics of ganglion cells.[33] Although much of the groundbreaking studies on ES cells have been done in murine models, the field is moving toward use of human ES cells. Primate ES cells cocultured with feeder cells spontaneously generate RPE progeny,[34] and we can anticipate a similar result from human ES cells in the near future, providing a potentially invaluable source of human eye neural cells.

Although ES cells robustly produce retinal and RPE progeny, they have drawbacks: They tend to generate tumors after transplantation in vivo, interestingly more virulent in homologous than xenografted hosts, and can produce inappropriate types of progeny, e.g., non-neural cells after placement in the CNS.[35,36] Genetic mechanisms for selecting neural lineages, for example by using sox gene promoters,[37] can help eliminate undesirable lineages, and this strategy could be used in the future to select for retinal or RPE lineages.

Embryonic Neural Stem Cells

An alternative source of neural cells is embryonic neural stem (ENS) cells [Figure 19.2 (see color section)]. These have the advantage over ES cells of being restricted to generating neural progeny, and they do not show evidence of tumor formation after transplantation in vivo.[38] In addition, there is evidence that these cells lack immunogenicity, having poor expression of MHC class I or class II, and therefore have inherent immune privilege,[39] a characteristic that is also found in neural stem cells derived from the adult CNS.[40] ENS cells were originally described in embryonic murine forebrain[41,42] and have since been found in a wide number of embryonic CNS regions including midbrain,[43] spinal cord,[44] and retina.[45] The cells can be grown in vitro as adherent cultures or as nonadherent neurospheres, which consist of floating balls of stem cells and their progeny. ENS cells have been obtained from human forebrain, maintained in culture for long periods, and survive freezing, providing a bankable tissue source.[38,46-48]

Although ENS cells are derived from the embryo, they are still regionally specified, i.e., they are primed to produce different cell types depending on their origination site in vivo.[49-52] Furthermore, ENS cells alter their behavior as development proceeds[52,53]: For example, at early stages, forebrain ENS cells proliferate in response to fibroblast growth factor (FGF)2 but not epidermal growth factor (EGF), whereas at later stages they acquire EGF responsiveness, and at early stages they are primed to generate neurons and at later stages, glia. Whereas ENS cells can produce both projection neurons and interneurons, their counterparts in the adult seem restricted to producing interneurons. Moreover, neural stem cell activity declines with aging and can be altered by environmental factors such as exercise.[54-59] Consequently, ENS are not equivalent: They vary in their biological properties and most importantly, they vary in "potency," which is defined as the types of progeny they can give rise to. Although self-renewal is the most accepted defining feature of stem cells, the term itself is somewhat misleading because it implies that stem cells remain unchanged throughout their lifespan. But it is now clear that stem cells, although perpetuating extensively, do not in fact renew themselves exactly at each cell division, but become specified for particular tasks. The question becomes to what extent ENS cells exhibit plasticity, and can be pushed to generate appropriate neural cells for a particular application, e.g., retinal or RPE transplantation. Of course, progenitor cells derived from embryonic eye obviate the need for regional transdifferentiation.

Embryonic Retinal Progenitor Cells

The vertebrate retina, derived from the neural tube as an evagination from the diencephalon in embryonic development, is initially produced by progenitor cells similar to those that generate the neurons and glia of other areas of the CNS.[60] The growing optic vesicle initially contains bipotential progenitors that can give rise to both neuroretina and RPE cell types. External cues such as FGFs secreted from surface ectoderm promote neuroretinal cell fate, and transforming growth factor β secreted from ocular mesenchyme directs RPE formation.[61,62] Multipotent progenitor cells that generate neuroretina are present during embryogenesis and early postnatal stages, and undergo temporal waves of competence to generate different types of retinal cells.[63,64] The neuroretina comprises six major classes of neurons and one class of glia that are generated in an order that seems generally conserved across all species: Ganglion cells and horizontal cells differentiate first, followed by, in overlapping phases, cone photoreceptors, amacrine cells, rod photoreceptors, bipolar cells, and finally Müller cells. Genes encoding Otx, Pax, Six, Rx, and Emx and Lhx families of transcription factors,[65,66] as well as environmental factors that regulate the expression of these transcription factors, such as BMP[67] and sonic hedgehog (Shh) signaling,[68] impart specific characteristics to progenitor cells in the developing eye.

Retinal cell types are born on a precise time schedule, and the progenitor populations within the eye change over time to reflect this. Most of the progenitor cells in the retina seem restricted to generating one or a few cell types.[64] In broad terms, there is a population of progenitor cells that can generate retinal cell types produced in the early embryonic period, and another population that generates late-embryonic and postnatal retinal cell types. Interestingly, both early and late progenitors can coexist in the early retina, indicating that they can be specified as separate populations in the embryonic period.[69,70] Whereas environmental factors may push an early progenitor to select between a variety of early fates and a late progenitor to select between a variety of late fates, it is difficult to environmentally shift a cell from the early to late category or vice versa.[64] Nevertheless, it has been reported that late progenitors can be stimulated to generate early-born retinal ganglion cells in vitro,[71] which indicates a degree of plasticity persists beyond the normal period of cell generation in vivo.

Among the majority of restricted progenitor cells present in the developing retina, a subpopulation of progenitors have stem-like properties, being able to generate spheres when grown in culture, but only if plated at high density. However, the spheres have limited ability to passage, indicating they are not lifelong stem cells, unlike the stem cells derived from the adult ciliary epithelium, which we will describe later. These embryonic retinal stem-like cells are able to generate progeny that bear a variety of retinal markers in vitro, and after transplantation in vivo.[72] However, long-term expansion as neurospheres with EGF or FGF2 can alter their properties, leading to a loss of regional specificity.[73] Human embryonic retinal progenitors that retained multilineage potential up to at least eight passages have been described in cultures containing serum and FGF2.[74] Whereas embryonic retinal cells can make neurons, later retinal progenitors become primed to produce glial cells.[75] The observation that late-born retinal progenitors tend to lose the ability to make early-born cell types and become primed to make glia is seen in ENS cells as described earlier, so this might be a general feature of some embryonic progenitor cells.

Most of the human retinal transplantations to date have used human embryonic retinal sheets or semi-dissociated embryonic retina. From the foregoing description, it is clear that this donor tissue contains a mixture of progenitor cell types, most being restricted progenitors and a minor population of more multipotent stem-like cells. Thus, it is likely that the transplant behavior is dominated by the restricted progenitors that are most prevalent in the mixture, and it will be beneficial to study the behavior of purified retinal stem cell populations in human transplant paradigms.

Adult Neural Stem Cells

In the adult CNS, neurogenesis continues in specific regions of the nervous system [Figure 19.2 (see color section)]. In mammals, new neuron production has been reported in hippocampus and the forebrain striatal lateral ventricle subventricular zone (SVZ)[76] and there have been controversial reports of neurogenesis in cerebral cortex.[77,78] The neurogenic cells derived from adult hippocampus and SVZ have properties that identify them as adult neural stem (ANS) cells. Surprisingly, in murine species, SVZ stem cells express GFAP, placing them in the astrocyte lineage.[79–81] These cells also express the surface marker LeX/SSEA-1, a marker of ES cells, and other markers often found in neural stem cells, such as the RNA-binding protein Musashi, allowing them to be prospectively isolated.[82,83] Neural stem cells lack many markers of differentiated neural cells, enabling their enrichment as a LIN-negative population.[84]

Humans possess a ribbon of astrocytes in the SVZ, and neurosphere-generating cells that make both neurons and glia in vitro can be derived from that region, but endogenous neuron production has not been detected from these cells in vivo.[85] In contrast, new neurons are produced throughout life in human hippocampus.[86] Adult hippocampal progenitor cells show remarkable proliferative ability, and have been maintained as primary lines for many passages.[87] ANS cells normally generate solely interneurons in vivo, and we do not know how effectively they can produce projection neurons or other neuron classes that are normally born in the embryonic period. However, exogenous supplies of brain-derived neurotrophic factor and noggin can stimulate striatal projection neuron formation in vivo.[88]

Although endogenous neurogenic sites in the adult CNS are very limited, stem cells can be extracted from normally non-neurogenic regions such as spinal cord and cultured as sphere-forming cells that retain the ability to make neurons.[44] However, to be a useful source of new neural eye cells, just as we described for ENS, these ANS cells must regionally and temporally transdifferentiate to produce retinal and RPE cells normally laid down early in the developing eye. Hence, it was particularly exciting to discover that the adult eye retains a source of stem-like cells that would at least avoid regional respecification.

Adult Ciliary and Iris Epithelium-Derived Stem Cells

Fish and amphibians continually grow eye neural tissue from the peripheral region of the retina, the ciliary margin zone.[89,90] Adult mammals seem to have a vestigial source of stem cells located in the ciliary epithelium, which is an anterior structure that in humans is separated from the retina by the ora serrata (Figure 19.3).[91–93] These cells, present at very low frequency in the ciliary epithelium, are normally quiescent, but when extracted and placed in vitro they are stimulated to divide by FGF2, or even with no additional growth factors, and generate multi-cell spheres.[91,92] Spheres form when the cells are plated as single cells in isolated wells, indicating that unlike embryonic retinal stem cells, cell–cell interactions are not as significant in maintaining CE cells. These cells, which share some features of other neural stem cells including Nestin and LeX/SSEA-1 expression,[94] produce progeny that express markers for all major retinal cell types but do not make oligodendrocytes.[75] Cells in this region are increased in number and persist longer in mice heterozygous for the *patched* receptor, indicating an important role for the growth factor *hedgehog* in their maintenance.[95] Microarray analysis of ciliary epithelial spheres grown in proliferating and differentiating conditions led to identification of a number of putative stem cell maintenance genes.[96] Among these is the receptor for stem cell factor, c-kit, which functions along with activated Notch receptor.[96] Interestingly, although in post-hatch chicks these ciliary epithelial cells only make amacrine and bipolar neurons, they can be induced to generate retinal ganglion cells by addition of insulin and FGF, showing that environmental factors can increase the repertoire of neuron types generated.[97] It will be very important to test the ability of ciliary epithelial stem cells to make retinal cells in transplantation paradigms.

Adult iris pigment epithelium also contains cells with stem-like properties that can generate spheres in vitro and progeny expressing retinal markers,[98] although their ability to self-renew has not been tested in the long-term. They have a similar profile of production of neurotrophic factors as RPE cells, and are being considered as a source for autologous stem cell transplant.[99]

Maintaining Self-Renewal and Neurogenesis of Neural Stem Cells

Typically, the number of highly prolific progenitor cells that can be extracted is too low for

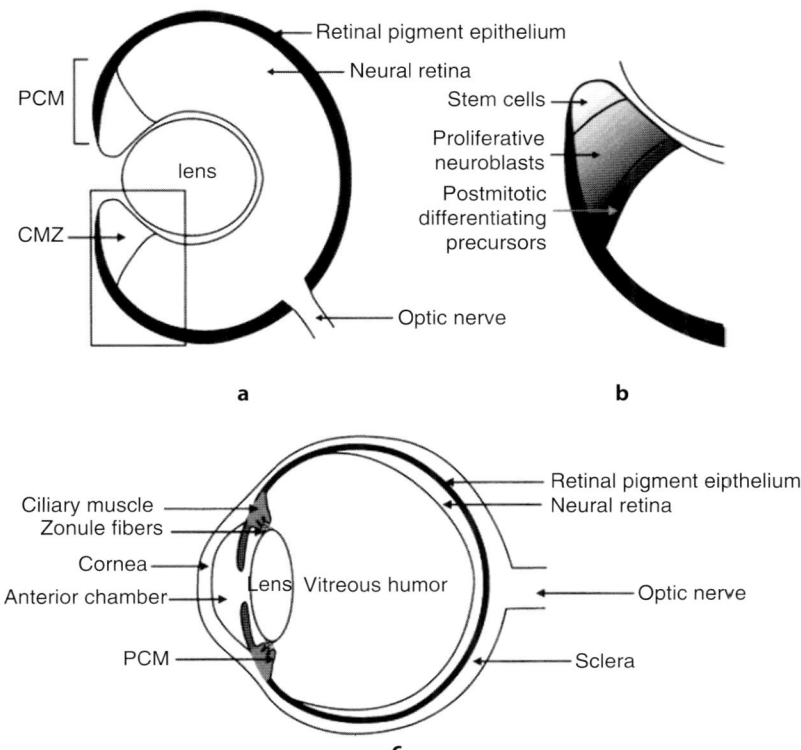

Figure 19.3. Schematic diagram of a section of the amphibia Xenopus retina. The ciliary marginal zone (CMZ) is located at the periphery of the retina, surrounded by a pigmented ciliary margin (PCM). The boxed area in a is magnified in b. The retinal stem-cell containing region is located at the peripheral edge of the CMZ. More centrally, progenitors mature progressively and new neurons are added at the most central region of the CMZ. c, Schematic diagram of a section of an adult mouse retina. The PCM, overlying the ciliary muscle, contains stem cells. (Reproduced from Perron and Harris,[90] 2000, BioEssays, with permission.)

immediate transplantation, and the cells have to be expanded in tissue culture. The traditional method of expanding neural stem cells is to grow them as neurospheres in FGF2 and/or EGF. However, neurosphere-expanded neural stem cells have proven disappointing as a source of neurons after transplantation, because most generate astrocytes in vivo, whereas neuron production is poor.[52] This may be because the culture conditions generally used to expand these cells do not prevent the normal changes in developmental profile of stem cells alluded to earlier: ENS grown under these conditions become progressively gliogenic and restricted in neurogenic potential. As yet unidentified environmental factors could delay the loss of neurogenicity, allowing more effective in vitro expansion of ENS or ANS cells.

In vivo, stem cells reside in specialized niches that regulate their proliferation and differentiation.[100,101] In the adult murine SVZ, for example, localized noggin from the nearby ependymal cells antagonizes glia-inducing BMP signals, and helps to maintain neuron generation in that region. However, exogenously applied noggin is not able to induce neuron generation from stem cells injected into sites that do not normally support endogenous neurogenesis in the adult; other environmental factors must be key. ANS cells in hippocampus[102] and SVZ[82] lie close to blood vessels, and coculture of ENS or ANS cells, either in adherent or neurosphere conditions, with endothelial cells can delay their normal loss of neurogenic potential[103] and thus expand their self-renewal. This and other techniques for maintaining neural stem cells self-renewing and neurogenic, if applicable to humans, will be a valuable mechanism for providing large numbers of stem cells for retinal and RPE repair.

Progenitor Cell Organization: Retinal Rosettes, Aggregates, and Layers

Besides establishing a suitable source of donor cells, another major hurdle is to ensure that progenitor cells transplanted into the eye migrate to the right locale and function appropriately. For therapies in which the intended function of implanted cells is growth factor production, a location close to dystrophic tissue might be chosen. However, where implanted progenitor cells are intended to substitute for missing retinal or RPE cells, the donor cells are required to generate missing neural cell types in appropriate numbers, to disperse them in the correct layers, and then have them functionally integrate.

Neural retina has been widely used as a model for constructing brain layers, and hence numerous efforts have been directed to reconstruct normal retinal layered structures in culture. Pioneered by Moscona, the reaggregation approach was applied to retinal cells, based on capacities of dissociated cells for cell–cell recognition, aggregation, sorting-out, proliferation, and establishment of specific cell–cell contacts. Histotypic areas resembling the original retinal tissue and having all major retinal cell types were detected in the reaggregates.[104–108] These rosettes arise through activation of progenitor cells in the embryonic source tissue, which proliferate and generate retinal cell types that assemble into layers through migration and integration. This process resembles normal retinal development in several aspects, but the layers are inverted: Photoreceptor outer segments are aligned toward the center of the rosette and synaptic connections are made to the surface cells [Figure 19.4 (see color section)].[109–112] Interestingly, when retinal cells as well as RPE cells from embryonic chick eye margin were dissociated and reaggregated, a complete reorganization of fully laminated spheres expressing all three retinal cell layers in the correct polarity was observed, with ganglion cells located inside the sphere, whereas photoreceptors faced the culture medium. Neither isolated RPE cells from the central retina alone or in combination with retinal stem cells nor isolated stem cells from the eye periphery alone gave rise to this kind of sphere. Such a laminar reorganization of retinal spheres can also be induced by conditioned media from RPE cells, Müller glia,[113] and from another type of radial glial cell similar to Müller cells: Cerebellar Bergmann glia.[114,115] This finding demonstrates that particular cell–cell interactions have critical roles in organizing retinal progenitors to make three-dimensional layers.

Occurrence of Rosettes In Vivo

Retinal rosettes can be observed in vivo under various pathological and experimental conditions. Rosettes are a classical histopathological finding in retinoblastoma and other retinal malignancies. Developmental disorders such as retinal dysplasia, as well as injury to normal tissue such as occurs in retinal detachment, lead to rosette formation via unknown mechanisms. So far, no genetic mutation has been linked to rosette formation, although in the absence of Numb function, a gene critical for asymmetric cell division, the cerebral cortex, another layered region, develops rosette-like structures.[116] This suggests a role for organized cell divisions in generating rosette layers. In support of this, if embryonic cell proliferation is blocked early in the development, huge rosettes are formed throughout the retina as though rosette formation is a default pathway of retinal histogenesis.[117,118]

In an attempt to understand the origin and characteristics of tumor rosettes formed in different human retinal malignancies, the tumor rosettes from retinoblastoma cells were compared with those of dysplastic rosettes seen in retinal dysplasia.[119] Whereas tumor rosettes from retinoblastoma include glial, neuronal, RPE, and photoreceptor cell markers, dysplastic rosettes diffusely express neuron-specific enolase and retinal S-antigen, but no retinal markers. Moreover, rosettes in retinal tissue, e.g., in retinoblastoma, are distinct from rosettes in other tissues, representing true Flexner-Wintersteiner rosettes.[120] In these rosettes, the cells are better differentiated and the presence of circles of primitive photoreceptors indicates an outer nuclear layer origin. They are not common in other brain regions, whereas in brain and other tumors, Homer-Wright rosettes are frequent.[121] Photoreceptor rosettes, with a row of predominantly blue cones or rods arranged radially around a central lumen have also been described in several cases of RP.[122–124] It is an important challenge to elucidate mechanisms of retinal rosette formation as the maldevelopment of rosette formation emerges as a major obstacle to successful integration of embryonic retinal transplants. Interestingly, purified retinal stem cells do not form rosettes but rather form neurospheres of relatively homogeneous composition when grown in vitro that lack recognizable retinal layers.[45,72,91,92,94,125] As described later in this chapter, the use of stem cells rather than more differentiated source tissue for transplantation into retina avoids rosette formation and thereby promotes transplant integration.

Signaling Molecules for Rosette Formation/Laminar Organization

Retinal rosettes could be instrumental for regenerative medicine including stem cell-based tissue engineering by revealing constraints/determinants of layered tissue formation. It has been speculated for a long time that extracellular molecules prevent rosette formation and permit the generation of layered structures during normal retinal development.[109,113,114,126–129] The molecular nature of the laminar-inducing activity has so far remained elusive.[130] It has been shown recently that rosette formation is inhibited when pellets of dissociated retinal progenitor cells are cocultured with explants of the anterior rim of the retina.[131] Instead, the rosette-forming cells were rearranged into a neuroepithelial structure characteristic of the undifferentiated retinal layer. The rosette-inhibiting activity was shown to be mediated by Wnt-2b, a secreted signaling molecule expressed in the anterior rim of the embryonic retina, and could be neutralized by a soluble form of the Frizzled extracellular domain, which works as a Wnt antagonist. In addition, the epithelial structure induced by Wnt-2b subsequently generated the correct retinal layers in rotation cultures. The idea that there is a requirement for an epithelial structure for retinal laminar formation is supported by the fact that blocking epithelial adhesion junctions led to retinal rosette formation.[132–135]

It is intriguing that the Wnt-2b rosette-inhibiting activity of the anterior rim is a short-range effect because the central neural retina may be too distant to receive these signals. RPE cells, shown to inhibit rosette formation, thus may have an important role in maintaining the epithelial organization in this central region of the neural retina. It will be important to characterize the signaling molecule from RPE to understand how retinal layer formation is regulated by signals from the surrounding tissues. The growth factor sonic hedgehog expressed in retinal ganglion cells, for example, was shown to be required for the maintenance of Müller cell organization, which is necessary for the laminated organization of the retina.[136]

The basic helix-loop-helix (bHLH) transcription factor Hes1, a downstream target of the Notch receptor, has an important role in maintenance of retinal precursors and morphogenesis of the retina. Hes1 expression initially occurs in precursors and later transiently in developing Müller glial cells to disappear by approximately postnatal day 10 in mouse.[137] Hes1 inhibits neuronal differentiation and in Hes1-null retina, precursors prematurely differentiate into neurons and form abnormal rosette-like structures at the expense of normal laminar architecture. Further gain-of-function and loss-of-function studies showed that mis-expression of Hes1 generates precursor-like or Müller glial-like cells, whereas in the absence of Hes1, precursors prematurely differentiate into ganglion cells. Because of the premature ganglion cell genesis, precursors are lost and the outer limiting membrane is broken in some regions. This may allow prematurely differentiated ganglion cells to erupt into the subretinal space as abnormal rosette structures in the Hes1-null retina.[138]

It is becoming evident that the mechanisms of rosette genesis have an important role in retinal progenitor transplantation. Rosette formation occurs under most transplantation procedures. Much progress has been made to refine transplantation techniques so that integration rather than rosette formation occurs. The refinements to transplant technique have not yet included the molecular mechanisms discovered by studying in vitro rosette formation. We speculate that the in vitro techniques for manipulating rosette structure may find application in promoting integration of transplanted retinal tissue into the host retina.

Studies of Transplantation of Progenitor Cells into Retina

Retinal transplantation as therapy for retinal degeneration has generated increasing interest over the past 20 years. Fetal retinal explants were found to survive after transplantation in early studies that used mice, rats, rabbits, and monkeys[139-145] and later humans.[143,146-149] These studies demonstrated that transplantation of retinal cells is technically feasible and relatively safe. Graft success, in terms of donor cell survival, proliferation, and integration, was enhanced when using donor tissue younger than embryonic day 15,[150-152] suggesting that progenitor cells, enriched in embryonic tissue, have an important role in retinal transplantation. We begin this section with a brief review of the pioneering embryonic retinal graft experiments. For other reviews of retinal transplantation, see references 93, 153–160.

In general, transplantation of embryonic retinal tissue results in long-term survival of the graft. Significant immune rejection does occur but only when the blood–retina barrier has been badly compromised such as in neovascular AMD. The immunologic issues in retinal transplantation are not addressed in this chapter but have been well reviewed recently.[160]

Retinal cells survive after transplantation, with proliferation and appropriate differentiation of the transplanted tissue observed under selected conditions. In many experiments, the functional success of the graft has been limited, however, by a lack of integration of donor tissue into the host retinal structure. Partial integration does occur but complete integration is inhibited by several mechanisms. Rather than fully integrating into host tissue, the transplanted cells often form rosettes.[161-164] Although rosettes can synapse with host retinal circuitry, the synapses are limited in extent and have not been demonstrated to recreate pathways that carry visual signals.[165-167] In addition to impeding synapse formation, rosette formation limits other cell–cell interactions between the donor and host tissue. For example, the outer limiting membrane of the rosette acts as a barrier[105,106,115,168] to block photoreceptors from contacting the RPE, which is necessary for their normal function. The rosette structure and limiting membrane may also affect cell adhesion and soluble factor gradients thought to influence the normal migration and integration of cells in retinal development.

Strategies have been adopted to promote the integration of transplanted embryonic retinal tissue into the existing host structure. Disruption of the host retina results in greater integration of source tissue, and transplantation of embryonic retina into sites of surgical injury results in significant repair and preservation of the injured host retina.[125,141,169] Disrupting the normal laminar retinal architecture may promote integration by exposing the edges of host lamina to the graft. In addition to this mechanical mechanism for improved integration, injury of the host retina has been found to stimulate growth factor production that may promote survival, proliferation, or integration of transplanted cells via alteration of the host biochemical niche.[170,171] These results suggest that components of the regenerative response seen after retinal injury in lower vertebrates are conserved in mammals and raises the possibility that injury creates a niche that guides transplanted progenitor cell migration to result in appropriate integration.

Another strategy to limit rosette formation and promote integration of transplanted embryonic retina is to transplant intact sheets of embryonic retina as source tissue[165,172]; recently reviewed by Aramant and Seiler.[159] Initially, fetal retina was sliced into thin slivers that were then injected into the subretinal space. Some slivers oriented correctly and showed photoreceptor cells integrating with the adjacent host RPE.[173-175] Techniques have been developed to obtain large sheets of embryonic donor retinal layers, with or without the RPE for subretinal transplantation.[159,172,176] Scrolls of sectioned embryonic retina can be injected through a small retinotomy for larger animals.[158,177] The excimer laser has been used to ablate selected retinal layers in human embryonic wholemounts, and sheets of embryonic retina with layers selected by this technique have been transplanted to humans.[149] Transplanted embryonic retinal sheets have been shown to incorporate well into the host retina, surviving and even forming synapses under the appropriate conditions. Rosette formation is minimized when the inner nuclear layer and supportive Müller cells are included in the donor retinal sheets.[152]

The use of dissociated embryonic retinal cell sources without encountering rosette formation after transplantation has also been reported to occur under certain conditions. When retinal progenitors were dissociated from ongoing cultures and transplanted at low density into the subretinal space of the rat, the transplanted cells survived, differentiated, and became incorporated in the host retina with little rosette formation.[178] In another case, rosette formation was avoided by enriching the donor cells for progenitor cells using culture conditions that did not promote survival of differentiated neurons.[72] The progenitor-rich source tissue did integrate and did not form rosettes. Thus, cultured, relatively immature retinal progenitor and stem cells are less prone to form rosettes and integrate well into host retina.

Transplantation of Embryonic Retina into Degenerating Retina

RP is particularly well suited for cell replacement therapy because the photoreceptor layer's main synaptic connection is via short afferent axons to the adjacent bipolar cell layer, so that long-distance connectivity, which in itself is a major hurdle in CNS repair, is not necessary to achieve functional integration. There are indications that such short synaptic connections can reestablish under appropriate conditions.[179] Studies of neural progenitor cells injected into the outer retina have, indeed, shown promise for restoring visual function in animal models of RP, and progenitor cell transplant experiments have been initiated in RP and AMD patients.

One series of transplantation experiments utilized animal models of RP such as the rd mouse. This model has a primary photoreceptor layer defect with the remaining inner retina well preserved.[180] Newborn mouse retinal microaggregates were transplanted under the rd retina to replace the degenerated photoreceptors.[181,182] The dissociated donor retina survived indefinitely and integrated into the host retina. Differentiation of photoreceptor cells occurred and synapses between the host and donor cells were thought to underlie a mild behavioral visual improvement.[183] Definite improvement in the electrophysiological response of ganglion cells to light after transplantation into young mice was found but integration of the transplanted retina was believed to be incomplete and rescue of the host retinal photoreceptor cells was raised as a possible mechanism for the observed visual improvement.[184] Another report indicated that the synapses between host and donor were too few to mediate vision and suggested that the grafted retinal microaggregates improved vision by rescue of the host photoreceptor cells via a trophic effect.[185] As with normal mice, rosette formation occurred and may have limited integration of the transplanted cells into the host. The problem of rosette formation was overcome by transplanting flat sheets of embryonic retina. Indeed, the flat tissue did not form rosettes and, remarkably, resulted in improved retinal function after transplantation into the rd mouse model of RP.[186] These authors, however, found that visual recovery was greater when the host retina was disorganized than when the sheet differentiated into organized retinotypic layers and were unable to determine whether the visual recovery measured was the result of integration of the graft into the retinal circuit or of a trophic effect of the engrafted embryonic retinal sheets. Visual recovery by transplanted embryonic or early postnatal retina has also been reported using the light-damaged rat retina as a model system.[151,187,188] The functional success in animal models for RP kindled great hope that this progress could be translated to treat the devastating human condition.

A rapid transfer of retinal transplantation technology to study the potential for treating human retinal degenerations was undertaken. Suspensions of dissociated human embryonic retina were transplanted into the subretinal space of RP and AMD patients by de Juan and del Cerro in 1995. Transplantation of human embryonic retinal tissue into the subretinal space of RP patients was found to be a feasible and safe procedure in this pioneering study. Seven patients in Baltimore and 12 in Prassad, India were transplanted with suspensions of fetal human retina.[153] A lasting and significant improvement in visual acuity occurred after a 4- to 6-month delay in several patients.

In 2000, one AMD patient from the Baltimore study expired and histologic examination of the transplanted eye was undertaken. This patient had both microaggregate and retinal sheet transplantated from a 16-week fetus. The microaggregate transplant showed rosette-like structure formation although complete differentiation of photoreceptor cells was not observed. The fetal sheet that was transplanted elsewhere in the retina showed good survival and integration with little rosette formation or immune rejection. The transplanted fetal retinal sheet did develop differentiated retinal neurons and layers but photoreceptor differentiation was incomplete.[189] The lack of photoreceptor differentiation may have resulted from the lack of underlying RPE in this elderly AMD patient who had previously undergone submacular hematoma evacuation.

Kaplan et al.[149,190] transplanted sensory retinal sheets that were enriched for photoreceptor cells into the subretinal space of RP patients but found that visual acuity did not, on average, improve. This human transplantation study also indicated that retinal transplantation was feasible and safe but did not demonstrate an average visual benefit.

It should be noted that in each of the early human studies, the RP patients who volunteered for transplantation all had end-stage RP in which 95% or more of the photoreceptors were lost so that there was little expectation for visual recovery from rescue of surviving host photoreceptor cells. The human studies did achieve the design endpoints demonstrating feasibility and safety.

A recent study of human embryonic retinal transplantation in an RP patient reported both objective and subjective improvement in vision. The volunteer patient was transplanted with full-thickness sheets of embryonic retina containing both sensory retina and RPE. A significant subjective recovery of visual acuity was described. Scanning laser microperimetry and focal electrophysiology were used for objective measurement of vision after transplantation with the contralateral eye serving as control. Objective recovery of vision was measured using the scanning laser only from the subretinal graft eye.[191] Clearly, it is important to reproduce and refine this measurement of vision seen after transplantation; for example, the reported variability of visual change between transplanted patients may be a significant factor.[192]

In the single report of objective visual improvement,[191] visualization of the laser microperimetry target was localized outside the edge of the graft and little visual improvement was observed in the sensory retina directly overlying the graft. This raises the possibility that the mechanism for visual improvement was the result of release of trophic factors from the surgical graft site rather than from neural integration of the graft into the retinal circuitry. Synapses do form between transplanted embryonic retina and host retina in animals.[172,179,185,193,194] Ribbon synapses characteristic of photoreceptor cells were observed but these have not been demonstrated to transmit visual information. If synaptic connectivity of the grafted sheet to the host retina neural network were the mechanism for visual field improvement, one would expect vision to occur over rather than near the graft. Because this was not the case, a neurotrophic mechanism is more likely than direct synaptic transmission to be the mechanism underlying the reported objective visual improvement.

In summary, the pioneering studies of human embryonic retinal transplantation establish a benchmark for the safety and feasibility of subretinal cell transplantation in RP patients, and identify problems that can be addressed. Rosette formation has emerged to be a common problem in both animals and humans preventing donor integration into host retina. Rosette formation is minimized and integration promoted by using immature progenitor cells or embryonic retinal sheets. Another problem identified by the early human studies relates to difficulty in obtaining and handling fresh preparations of source tissue. Proper timing of the harvest and transplant is challenging when adequate screening for potential pathogens in the host is necessary. The tissue acquisition problems can be effectively addressed by banking retinal stem cells in self-perpetuating cultures that are screened before transplantation, and the use of stem cells or another type of early embryonic retinal precursor would likely improve the degree of donor cell integration that occurs after transplantation.

Transplantation of Embryonic Retinal Cells to Replace RPE

Another series of retinal transplant experiments utilize animal models where the primary defect is in the RPE rather than in the photoreceptor layer. The RPE transplant studies are aimed at macular degeneration and less common forms of RP that involve a primary RPE defect. The main animal model is the RCS rat that has a primary RPE defect with consequent loss of the photoreceptor layer. RPE transplantation is conceptually simpler than sensory transplantation because the RPE monolayer supports photoreceptor functions by close apposition, and a neural network or synaptic connectivity is not present.

Transplantation of embryonic RPE sheets or fresh suspensions of embryonic RPE cells into the subretinal space of RCS rats prevents photoreceptor loss.[195-198] Unlike embryonic sensory retina, transplanted RPE does not readily form rosettes. Similar to embryonic sensory retinal transplants, immunologic rejection of RPE is variable and depends on the status of the blood–retina barrier. In the RCS rat, the primary RPE defect causes photoreceptor cell loss to occur during the first few months of life. If the wild-type RPE is transplanted into the subretinal space before complete photoreceptor cell death occurs, then the remaining photoreceptor cells are rescued. Morphologic changes that occur in the photoreceptor cell outer segments are reversed and the rescued cells have apparently normal metabolic and visual function indefinitely. The success of RPE transplantation at preserving the RCS retina that is otherwise destined to degenerate is remarkable, clearly demonstrating effective neural cell rescue by transplantation in this animal model.

Extension of the RPE transplantation experiments to macular degeneration patients is at an early stage of development. The feasibility and safety of RPE transplantation has been demonstrated in 17 patients with advanced macular degeneration.[199] Significant immune rejection was inferred from the development of macular edema only in patients with the wet form of AMD. In dry AMD, where the immune privilege conferred by the retina–blood barrier is less disrupted, transplanted RPE survived without signs of rejection. All patients studied had advanced forms of AMD with severe tissue loss in multiple retinal layers so that visual recovery was expected to be minimal. Indeed, no visual improvement was found during long-term follow-up of the original 17 study patients. Related studies transplanting fetal RPE to dry AMD patients also showed no overall visual improvement.[148] These studies show that RPE transplantation is feasible and safe in AMD patients.

To improve screening and availability of donor RPE, animal RPE transplantation experiments have utilized cells that can be passaged in vitro such as RPE cell lines.[200] Problems of tumor formation and immune rejection are, however, associated with the transplantation of cell lines. This concern may be addressed using genetically normal stem cells that are already committed to an RPE fate for transplantation. As discussed, only the most primitive types of ES cells form tumors after neural transplantation, and more specified stem cells tend to be less tumor-genic.

Recent work has demonstrated that primate[34] and human ES stem cells are readily driven to differentiate into RPE cells. These ES RPE lines have been developed for transplantation to retinal and nonretinal neural tissue. As with sensory retina, and neural stem cell transplantation in general, it may be more desirable to utilize stems cell more committed to producing the intended cell type to promote integration and avoid issues of non-neural differentiation and tumor formation. The RPE stem cell, however, has not yet been characterized and the types of progenitor cells that were present in the RPE source tissue that was used in completed RPE transplantation studies is also unknown. There is ongoing interest in identifying the appropriate RPE cell for future transplantation studies of primary diseases of the RPE and stem cells should be prominent in these research efforts.

Transplantation of Stem Cells into Retina

The advance of retinal transplantation techniques has allowed early testing of various stem cell populations in the eye. There is much interest in using the most basic stem cell type: ES cells, which as described above can unequivocally generate retina and RPE progeny. Important questions remain as to whether they can do this without inappropriate differentiation and hyperproliferation after transplantation in vivo. More committed stem cells such as brain-derived stem cells or retinal stem cells may be more likely to produce appropriate progeny with appropriate integration and proliferation in response to the host environmental needs.

An important point to bear in mind when analyzing transplant data is the recent discovery that stem cells can fuse with existing cells in vitro and in vivo.[201,202] The resulting chimeric cells can have the morphology of the preexisting cell, and some features, e.g., genetic markers, of the donor cells. Although fusion is a very rare event, it can be a possible explanation for some results of transplantation. More recent publications often assess whether fusion could account for some observations, for example, by examining cell ploidy.

ES-derived neural progeny will functionally integrate after transplantation into the immature, developing nervous system, and differentiate to express appropriate neurotransmitters and active synapses.[203] Appropriate integration and differentiation is also found when ES cells are transplanted into various regions of the damaged adult CNS but not when transplanted to normal adult CNS.[204] The same general requirement for either a developing or damaged environment has been found for neural stem cells to integrate into retina.[125,205–208] However, one study using ES cells demonstrated their ability to integrate even into normal retina. When mouse ES cells that were undifferentiated (and therefore able to generate all cell types in the body) were transplanted into the vitreous of normal adult mice, they were seen as undifferentiated cells at 5 days. By 30 days, surprisingly, some cells had integrated into the inner retinal layers and acquired complex morphologies.[209] Some had ganglion cell-like characteristics and even developed processes that synapsed with recipient processes in the inner plexiform layer. Only cells at the inner surface differentiated into neurons, and the authors speculated that close proximity to the retinal vasculature might have a key role in directing the fate of the ES cells. In deeper retinal layers, the transplanted ES cells did not integrate but rather formed teratoma-like tumors containing many inappropriate cell types. Thus, some primitive ES cells did integrate even in normal hosts, but the ES cells that did not integrate hyperproliferated to cause destructive tumors.

Transplantation of ES cells pretreated with retinoic acid to encourage neural differentiation has also been investigated. Retinoic acid-exposed ES cells have been transplanted into the eyes of mutant rd1 mice, an RP model with rapid retinal degeneration.[210] This mouse has a mutation in the gene encoding the β-subunit of rod photoreceptor cyclic GMP phosphodiesterase, resulting in the loss of rods from the retina shortly after birth whereas the remaining inner retina remains. After injection into the vitreous of 5-week-old rd1 mice, the cells were not integrated by 4 days, but by 6 weeks most had become neuronal-like and had created a network on the retinal surface. Some cells had penetrated and were present in retinal ganglion or inner plexiform layers, but few were in the inner nuclear layer. The differentiated cells expressed markers of neurons and glia but not oligodendrocytes. Markers for specific retinal cell types were not assessed. Although penetration to outer layers was not detected, the authors reported preliminary data in which these cells were injected into the mnd mouse in which photoreceptor loss is delayed, and were able to penetrate outer regions making cells with bipolar and horizontal morphologies, but not photoreceptors. These data indicate that particular types of retinal damage create factors that can stimulate migration to particular layers. Obviously, more targeted transplantation could help direct cell integration. For example, when transplanted directly into the subretinal space of the immature, 20-day-old RCS rat, mouse ES cells pretreated for neural differentiation in vitro significantly retarded photoreceptor loss, resulting in up to eight photoreceptor rows compared with complete photoreceptor loss in control 2 months after transplantation.[211]

Transplantation of stem cells from sources with developmental fates that are closer to the retina such as neural stem cells (from embryos or adults) has not been found to result in tumor formation. In addition, neural stem cells do not form rosettes when grown in culture or after transplantation. ENS cells are frequently forebrain-derived, and there is the question as to whether these can make retinal neurons and glia. One study showed that injection of rat embryonic forebrain-derived ENS cells into the subretinal space enhances retinal differentiation, indicating a degree of plasticity[212] and another using neonatal brain-derived NS cells resulted in neuronal and astrocytic differentiation in damaged RCS rat, rds mouse, and, surprisingly, even normal mouse retina.[213] Neonatal murine brain progenitor cells cultured as neurospheres were transplanted into retinas of the Brazilian opossum, which is born in an immature state and is therefore a useful model for retinal development studies.[206] Implanted cells only integrated into young retinas, and the degree of incorporation was impressive: Cells acquired retinal morphologies, and even expressed some retinal markers, including calretinin and recoverin. These studies again point to critical environmental cues being present developmentally that are needed for stem cell integration.

When adult hippocampal stem cells are transplanted into rat eyes, proliferation occurs without rosette formation. Hippocampal-derived ANS cells differentiate into retinal cell types but the retinal cell characteristics are relatively immature and seen only after transplantation into neonatal or damaged host eyes.[205] They can integrate and give cells of retinal-like morphologies only after transplantation into a host with mechanical injury,[85] ischemic retinal injury,[214] or in a genetic dystrophic retina.[215] Hippocampal ANS cells injected into the vitreous of adult RCS rats with degenerating RPE and photoreceptor layers resulted in integration into appropriate retinal layers. Furthermore, integrated graft cells developed processes that arborized in appropriate retinal plexiform layers suggesting synapse formation.[215] However, these cells did not fully acquire characteristic retinal markers, such as HPC-1, and rhodopsin, indicating their plasticity is limited. Human neural stem cells pretreated with transforming growth factor and then injected into rat vitreous were also found to migrate and differentiate into opsin-positive retinal cells.[216] Thus, the use of neural stem cells with fates closer to the retina than that of ES cells overcomes the problem of tumor formation and results in a limited degree of respecification of cells to produce ones more closely resembling retinal cell types.

Stem cells derived from the sensory retina form more completely differentiated retinal cell types. Cultures enriched for embryonic retinal stem cells with EGF were transplanted into the subretinal space of normal postnatal rats. The donor cells differentiated to produce the photoreceptor marker opsin but these embryonic retinal stem cells did not integrate well into the normal host retina.[72] When the host retina was injured or diseased, however, the embryonic retinal stem cells did integrate well.[71,93] Integration into the inner retina was greater than into the outer retina, and the grafted cells acquired markers appropriate to their retinal lamina [Figure 19.5 (see color section)]. Stem or stem-like progenitors from the limbal epithelium, the ciliary epithelium, and the retina itself were studied. Similar results were obtained for each ocular stem cell, although the non-neural limbal stem cells integrated with a significant delay compared with the neural ciliary or retinal stem cells.[125] The differentiated photoreceptor cell marker opsin stained stem cells that migrated to the outermost photoreceptor cell layer whereas amacrine or bipolar cell markers stained stem cells that migrated to those retinal layers. That injury induces a microenvironment directing the transplanted retinal stem cells to incorporate and differentiate appropriately within the injured tissue is reminiscent of injury in lower vertebrates in which injury causes endogenous retinal stem cell activation that mediates functional repair of the damaged retina.

Cell Transplantation for Growth Factor Delivery

When embryonic retina was transplanted into the subretinal space of RP patients, visual fields were maximal at the edge of the graft. The possibility was raised that the localized, relative visual field improvement occurred because the surgical graft induced a reparative response in neighboring tissue rather than by functional integration of the graft into the host retinal circuit.[191] That is, the surgical implantation itself stimulated a regenerative response, or the transplanted tissue released a trophic stimulus resulting in recovery of nearby native retina. Visual recovery after embryonic retinal transplantation in animal models also extended beyond the transplanted region.[217] A trophic effect is also thought to cause improvement in retinal function surrounding but not overlying photosensitive chips implanted in the subretinal space of RP patients.[218] Indeed, disturbance in the growth factor microenvironment has an important role in mediating animal models of retinal degeneration.[219,220] Basic FGF (bFGF) rescues photoreceptors in a rat RP model[221] but causes pathological retinal neovascularization. Ciliary neurotrophic factor (CNTF) delays morphologic loss of photoreceptors in animal models[222] but may decrease retinal function by an unknown mechanism.[223,224] Rod photoreceptor cells release a diffusible factor that slows the degeneration of neighboring cone photoreceptors in an animal model of RP[225] and transplanted rod photoreceptor cells slows cone loss in the rd mouse presumably by release of a rod-dependent cone survival factor[226] that has been recently isolated.[227] The findings of neural rescue in retina surrounding a surgical transplantation site or after injection of growth factors raise the exciting possibility that the transplantation of cells engineered to produce these factors may become a valuable tool for long-term delivery of factors to degenerating retina.

Rat RPE cells have been genetically altered to produce selected growth factors. Transplantation of these lines into the subretinal space leads to immune rejection for lines producing CNTF or bFGF but RPE cells producing brain-derived neurotrophic factor are not rejected and continue to produce factor at significant levels in the subretinal space.[228] These experiments were conducted using primary or early passage cultures of RPE cells that proliferated and therefore likely contained RPE progenitor or stem cells.

A neural cell line modified to produce CNTF within an encapsulated delivery device has been surgically implanted into the vitreous cavity of rabbits,[229] and human trials with the surgically implanted device are in early stages. Transplantation of transformed cell lines is a promising mechanism for factor delivery but may be limited in terms of safety and immune reactivity. In the future, stem cells may replace cell lines to deliver factors to degenerating retina to minimize tumor formation and immune rejection that have been observed after the transplantation of transformed cell lines.

Conclusions

Retinal degeneration is an ideal subject for stem cell transplantation studies. Success in reversing retinal degeneration in animal models of RP and AMD contribute to the great hope that advances in stem cell biology combined with the lessons already obtained from clinical retinal transplantation studies will lead to a breakthrough that makes retinal transplantation effective at treating human retinal degeneration. Retinal progenitor cell transplantation has been accomplished in humans and found to be feasible with manageable safety and immune issues. The stage has been set for future progress in this exciting field, but it is likely that problems will arise to slow our progress. Although some will point to such impediments as reason to deter the effort toward developing this technology, others will continue to surmount these problems and find increased enthusiasm in each success.

To summarize the current state of progress in stem cell transplantation for retinal degeneration: If we consider appropriate proliferation, differentiation, and integration as the three variables that need to be solved together for a graft to be successful, then conditions have been discovered that solve any two of the variables, but a simultaneous solution for all three remains elusive. Efforts to accomplish each in harmony are increasing. Aspects of the growth factor microenvironment and cell–cell interactions that orchestrate and coordinate proliferation, integration, and differentiation in normal development, and retinal regeneration in lower animals, have been discovered. Similar factors have been found to regulate stem cells transplanted into injured tissue and, importantly, aspects of the mechanisms that inhibit repair and regeneration in higher vertebrates are emerging. Each step toward enabling stem cells to behave appropriately after transplantation into degenerate retina is significant. The hope that progress in this field will generate therapy does already provide comfort to many patients experiencing retinal degeneration.

References

1. Dowling JE. Organization of vertebrate retinas. Invest Ophthalmol 1970;9(9):655–680.
2. Berson EL, Jakobiec FA. Neural retinal cell transplantation: ideal versus reality. Ophthalmology 1999; 106(3):445–446.
3. Gouras P. Neural retinal cell transplantation. Ophthalmology 1999;106(10):1855; author reply 1857.
4. Wong F. Neural retinal cell transplantation. Ophthalmology 1999;106(10):1855–1857; author reply 1857.
5. Otteson DC, Hitchcock PF. Stem cells in the teleost retina: persistent neurogenesis and injury-induced regeneration. Vision Res 2003;43(8):927–936.
6. Cai J, Weiss ML, Rao MS. In search of "stemness." Exp Hematol 2004;32(7):585–598.
7. Li ZY, Possin DE, Milam AH. Histopathology of bone spicule pigmentation in retinitis pigmentosa. Ophthalmology 1995;102(5):805–816.
8. Lewis GP, Linberg KA, Fisher SK. Neurite outgrowth from bipolar and horizontal cells after experimental retinal detachment. Invest Ophthalmol Vis Sci 1998;39(2):424–434.
9. Marc RE, Jones BW. Retinal remodeling in inherited photoreceptor degenerations. Mol Neurobiol 2003; 28(2):139–147.
10. Chandler DB, Quansah FA, Hida T, Machemer R. A refined experimental model for proliferative vitreoretinopathy. Graefes Arch Clin Exp Ophthalmol 1986;224(1):86–91.
11. Wiedemann P. Growth factors in retinal diseases: proliferative vitreoretinopathy, proliferative diabetic retinopathy, and retinal degeneration. Surv Ophthalmol 1992;36(5):373–384.
12. Gass JDM. Drusen and discuform macular detachment and degeneration. Tr Am Soc 1972;LXX: 409–436.
13. Eyetech. Anti-vascular endothelial growth factor therapy for subfoveal choroidal neovascularization secondary to age-related macular degeneration: phase II study results. Ophthalmology 2003;110(5): 979–986.
14. Duh EJ, Yang HS, Haller JA, et al. Vitreous levels of pigment epithelium-derived factor and vascular endothelial growth factor: implications for ocular angiogenesis. Am J Ophthalmol 2004;137(4):668–674.
15. Levin LA, Ritch R, Richards JE, Borras T. Stem cell therapy for ocular disorders. Arch Ophthalmol 2004;122(4):621–627.

16. Wagers AJ, Weissman IL. Plasticity of adult stem cells. Cell 2004;116(5):639–648.
17. Otani A, Dorrell MI, Kinder K, et al. Rescue of retinal degeneration by intravitreally injected adult bone marrow-derived lineage-negative hematopoietic stem cells. J Clin Invest 2004;114(6):765–774.
18. Pera MF, Reubinoff B, Trounson A. Human embryonic stem cells. J Cell Sci 2000;113(pt 1):5–10.
19. Cowan CA, Klimanskaya I, McMahon J, et al. Derivation of embryonic stem-cell lines from human blastocysts. N Engl J Med 2004;350(13):1353–1356.
20. Ying QL, Nichols J, Chambers I, Smith A. BMP induction of Id proteins suppresses differentiation and sustains embryonic stem cell self-renewal in collaboration with STAT3. Cell 2003;115(3):281–292.
21. Sato N, Meijer L, Skaltsounis L, Greengard P, Brivanlou AH. Maintenance of pluripotency in human and mouse embryonic stem cells through activation of Wnt signaling by a pharmacological GSK-3-specific inhibitor. Nat Med 2004;10(1):55–63.
22. Sumi T, Fujimoto Y, Nakatsuji N, Suemori H. STAT3 is dispensable for maintenance of self-renewal in non-human primate embryonic stem cells. Stem Cells 2004;22(5):861–872.
23. Daheron L, Opitz SL, Zaehres H, et al. LIF/STAT3 signaling fails to maintain self-renewal of human embryonic stem cells. Stem Cells 2004;22(5):770–778.
24. Schuldiner M, Yanuka O, Itskovitz-Eldor J, Melton DA, Benvenisty N. Effects of eight growth factors on the differentiation of cells derived from human embryonic stem cells. Proc Natl Acad Sci USA 2000;97(21):11307–11312.
25. Pera MF, Andrade J, Houssami S, et al. Regulation of human embryonic stem cell differentiation by BMP-2 and its antagonist noggin. J Cell Sci 2004;117(pt 7):1269–1280.
26. Ginis I, Luo Y, Miura T, et al. Differences between human and mouse embryonic stem cells. Dev Biol 2004;269(2):360–380.
27. Lee JB, Lee JE, Park JH, et al. Establishment and maintenance of human embryonic stem cell lines on human feeder cells derived from uterine endometrium under serum-free condition. Biol Reprod 2005;72(1):42–49.
28. Nakayama T, Momoki-Soga T, Yamaguchi K, Inoue N. Efficient production of neural stem cells and neurons from embryonic stem cells. Neuroreport 2004;15(3):487–491.
29. Otero JJ, Fu W, Kan L, Cuadra AE, Kessler JA. Beta-catenin signaling is required for neural differentiation of embryonic stem cells. Development 2004;131(15):3545–3557.
30. Zhao X, Liu J, Ahmad I. Differentiation of embryonic stem cells into retinal neurons. Biochem Biophys Res Commun 2002;297(2):177–184.
31. Hirano M, Yamamoto A, Yoshimura N, et al. Generation of structures formed by lens and retinal cells differentiating from embryonic stem cells. Dev Dyn 2003;228(4):664–671.
32. Gehring WJ, Ikeo K. Pax 6: mastering eye morphogenesis and eye evolution. Trends Genet 1999;15(9):371–377.
33. Tabata Y, Ouchi Y, Kamiya H, Manabe T, Arai K, Watanabe S. Specification of the retinal fate of mouse embryonic stem cells by ectopic expression of Rx/rax, a homeobox gene. Mol Cell Biol 2004;24(10):4513–4521.
34. Haruta M, Sasai Y, Kawasaki H, et al. In vitro and in vivo characterization of pigment epithelial cells differentiated from primate embryonic stem cells. Invest Ophthalmol Vis Sci 2004;45(3):1020–1025.
35. Tzukerman M, Rosenberg T, Ravel Y, Reiter I, Coleman R, Skorecki K. An experimental platform for studying growth and invasiveness of tumor cells within teratomas derived from human embryonic stem cells. Proc Natl Acad Sci USA 2003;100(23):13507–13512.
36. Erdo F, Buhrle C, Blunk J, et al. Host-dependent tumorigenesis of embryonic stem cell transplantation in experimental stroke. J Cereb Blood Flow Metab 2003;23(7):780–785.
37. Li M, Pevny L, Lovell-Badge R, Smith A. Generation of purified neural precursors from embryonic stem cells by lineage selection. Curr Biol 1998;8(17):971–974.
38. Kelly S, Bliss TM, Shah AK, et al. Transplanted human fetal neural stem cells survive, migrate, and differentiate in ischemic rat cerebral cortex. Proc Natl Acad Sci USA 2004;101(32):11839–11844.
39. Hori J, Ng TF, Shatos M, Klassen H, Streilein JW, Young MJ. Neural progenitor cells lack immunogenicity and resist destruction as allografts. Stem Cells 2003;21(4):405–416.
40. Klassen H, Imfeld KL, Ray J, Young MJ, Gage FH, Berman MA. The immunological properties of adult hippocampal progenitor cells. Vision Res 2003;43(8):947–956.
41. Temple S. Division and differentiation of isolated CNS blast cells in microculture. Nature 1989;340(6233):471–473.
42. Reynolds BA, Tetzlaff W, Weiss S. A multipotent EGF-responsive striatal embryonic progenitor cell produces neurons and astrocytes. J Neurosci 1992;12(11):4565–4574.
43. Studer L, Tabar V, McKay RD. Transplantation of expanded mesencephalic precursors leads to recovery in parkinsonian rats. Nat Neurosci 1998;1(4):290–295.
44. Shihabuddin LS, Horner PJ, Ray J, Gage FH. Adult spinal cord stem cells generate neurons after transplantation in the adult dentate gyrus. J Neurosci 2000;20(23):8727–8735.
45. Ahmad I, Dooley CM, Thoreson WB, Rogers JA, Afiat S. In vitro analysis of a mammalian retinal progenitor that gives rise to neurons and glia. Brain Res 1999;831(1–2):1–10.
46. Svendsen CN, Caldwell MA, Shen J, et al. Long-term survival of human central nervous system progenitor cells transplanted into a rat model of Parkinson's disease. Exp Neurol 1997;148(1):135–146.
47. Tamaki S, Eckert K, He D, et al. Engraftment of sorted/expanded human central nervous system stem cells from fetal brain. J Neurosci Res 2002;69(6):976–986.
48. Vescovi AL, Galli R, Gritti A. Clonal analyses and cryopreservation of neural stem cell cultures. Methods Mol Biol 2002;198:115–123.
49. Hitoshi S, Tropepe V, Ekker M, van der Kooy D. Neural stem cell lineages are regionally specified, but not committed, within distinct compartments of the developing brain. Development 2002;129(1):233–244.
50. Smith R, Bagga V, Fricker-Gates RA. Embryonic neural progenitor cells: the effects of species, region, and culture conditions on long-term proliferation and

50. neuronal differentiation. J Hematother Stem Cell Res 2003;12(6):713–725.
51. Horiguchi S, Takahashi J, Kishi Y, et al. Neural precursor cells derived from human embryonic brain retain regional specificity. J Neurosci Res 2004;75(6):817–824.
52. Temple S. The development of neural stem cells. Nature 2001;414(6859):112–117.
53. Kruger GM, Mosher JT, Bixby S, Joseph N, Iwashita T, Morrison SJ. Neural crest stem cells persist in the adult gut but undergo changes in self-renewal, neuronal subtype potential, and factor responsiveness. Neuron 2002;35(4):657–669.
54. Limke TL, Rao MS. Neural stem cells in aging and disease. J Cell Mol Med 2002;6(4):475–496.
55. Maslov AY, Barone TA, Plunkett RJ, Pruitt SC. Neural stem cell detection, characterization, and age-related changes in the subventricular zone of mice. J Neurosci 2004;24(7):1726–1733.
56. Heine VM, Maslam S, Joels M, Lucassen PJ. Prominent decline of newborn cell proliferation, differentiation, and apoptosis in the aging dentate gyrus, in absence of an age-related hypothalamus-pituitary-adrenal axis activation. Neurobiol Aging 2004;25(3):361–375.
57. Kim YP, Kim H, Shin MS, et al. Age-dependence of the effect of treadmill exercise on cell proliferation in the dentate gyrus of rats. Neurosci Lett 2004;355(1–2):152–154.
58. Kempermann G, Gast D, Gage FH. Neuroplasticity in old age: sustained fivefold induction of hippocampal neurogenesis by long-term environmental enrichment. Ann Neurol 2002;52(2):135–143.
59. Zitnik G, Martin GM. Age-related decline in neurogenesis: old cells or old environment? J Neurosci Res 2002;70(3):258–263.
60. Chow RL, Lang R.A. Early eye development in vertebrates. Annu Rev Cell Dev Biol 2001;17:255–296.
61. Pittack C, Grunwald GB, Reh TA. Fibroblast growth factors are necessary for neural retina but not pigmented epithelium differentiation in chick embryos. Development 1997;124(4):805–816.
62. Fuhrmann S, Levine EM, Reh TA. Extraocular mesenchyme patterns the optic vesicle during early eye development in the embryonic chick. Development 2000;127(21):4599–4609.
63. Reh TA, Levine EM. Multipotential stem cells and progenitors in the vertebrate retina. J Neurobiol 1998;36(2):206–220.
64. Livesey FJ, Cepko CL. Vertebrate neural cell-fate determination: lessons from the retina. Nat Rev Neurosci 2001;2(2):109–118.
65. Ashery-Padan R, Gruss P. Pax6 lights-up the way for eye development. Curr Opin Cell Biol 2001;13(6):706–714.
66. Chuang JC, Raymond PA. Embryonic origin of the eyes in teleost fish. Bioessays 2002;24(6):519–529.
67. Adler R, Belecky-Adams TL. The role of bone morphogenetic proteins in the differentiation of the ventral optic cup. Development 2002;129(13):3161–3171.
68. Perron M, Boy S, Amato MA, et al. A novel function for Hedgehog signalling in retinal pigment epithelium differentiation. Development 2003;130(8):1565–1577.
69. Cayouette M, Barres BA, Raff M. Importance of intrinsic mechanisms in cell fate decisions in the developing rat retina. Neuron 2003;40(5):897–904.
70. Turner DL, Snyder EY, Cepko CL. Lineage-independent determination of cell type in the embryonic mouse retina. Neuron 1990;4(6):833–845.
71. James J, Das AV, Bhattacharya S, Chacko DM, Zhao X, Ahmad I. In vitro generation of early-born neurons from late retinal progenitors. J Neurosci 2003;23(23):8193–8203.
72. Chacko DM, Rogers JA, Turner JE, Ahmad I. Survival and differentiation of cultured retinal progenitors transplanted in the subretinal space of the rat. Biochem Biophys Res Commun 2000;268(3):842–846.
73. Akagi T, Haruta M, Akita J, Nishida A, Honda Y, Takahashi M. Different characteristics of rat retinal progenitor cells from different culture periods. Neurosci Lett 2003;341(3):213–216.
74. Yang P, Seiler MJ, Aramant RB, Whittemore SR. In vitro isolation and expansion of human retinal progenitor cells. Exp Neurol 2002;177(1):326–331.
75. Engelhardt M, Wachs FP, Couillard-Despres S, Aigner L. The neurogenic competence of progenitors from the postnatal rat retina in vitro. Exp Eye Res 2004;78(5):1025–1036.
76. Cameron HA, McKay R. Stem cells and neurogenesis in the adult brain. Curr Opin Neurobiol 1998;8(5):677–680.
77. Gould E, Reeves AJ, Graziano MS, Gross CG. Neurogenesis in the neocortex of adult primates. Science 1999;286(5439):548–552.
78. Rakic P. Neurogenesis in adult primate neocortex: an evaluation of the evidence. Nat Rev Neurosci 2002;3(1):65–71.
79. Doetsch F, Caille I, Lim DA, Garcia-Verdugo JM, Alvarez-Buylla A. Subventricular zone astrocytes are neural stem cells in the adult mammalian brain. Cell 1999;97(6):703–716.
80. Gotz M. Glial cells generate neurons: master control within CNS regions – developmental perspectives on neural stem cells. Neuroscientist 2003;9(5):379–397.
81. Laywell ED, Steindler DA. Glial stem-like cells: implications for ontogeny, phylogeny, and CNS regeneration. Prog Brain Res 2002;138:435–450.
82. Capela A, Temple S. LeX/ssea-1 is expressed by adult mouse CNS stem cells, identifying them as nonependymal. Neuron 2002;35(5):865–875.
83. Keyoung HM, Roy NS, Benraiss A, et al. High-yield selection and extraction of two promoter-defined phenotypes of neural stem cells from the fetal human brain. Nat Biotechnol 2001;19(9):843–850.
84. Rietze RL, Valcanis H, Brooker GF, Thomas T, Voss AK, Bartlett PF. Purification of a pluripotent neural stem cell from the adult mouse brain. Nature 2001;412(6848):736–739.
85. Sanai N, Tramontin AD, Quinones-Hinojosa A, et al. Unique astrocyte ribbon in adult human brain contains neural stem cells but lacks chain migration. Nature 2004;427(6976):740–44.
86. Eriksson PS, Perfilieva E, Bjork-Eriksson T, et al. Neurogenesis in the adult human hippocampus. Nat Med 1998;4(11):1313–1317.
87. Gage FH, Kempermann G, Palmer TD, Peterson DA, Ray J. Multipotent progenitor cells in the adult dentate gyrus. J Neurobiol 1998;36(2):249–266.
88. Chmielnicki E, Benraiss A, Economides AN, Goldman SA. Adenovirally expressed noggin and brain-derived neurotrophic factor cooperate to induce new medium spiny neurons from resident progenitor cells in the

89. Reh TA, Fischer AJ. Stem cells in the vertebrate retina. Brain Behav Evol 2001;58(5):296–305.
90. Perron M, Harris WA. Retinal stem cells in vertebrates. Bioessays 2000;22(8):685–688.
91. Tropepe V, Coles BL, Chiasson BJ, et al. Retinal stem cells in the adult mammalian eye. Science 2000; 287(5460):2032–2036.
92. Ahmad I, Tang L, Pham H. Identification of neural progenitors in the adult mammalian eye. Biochem Biophys Res Commun 2000;270(2):517–521.
93. Klassen H, Sakaguchi DS, Young MJ. Stem cells and retinal repair. Prog Retin Eye Res 2004;23(2): 149–181.
94. Ahmad I, Das AV, James J, Bhattacharya S, Zhao X. Neural stem cells in the mammalian eye: types and regulation. Semin Cell Dev Biol 2004;15(1):53–62.
95. Moshiri A, Reh TA. Persistent progenitors at the retinal margin of ptc+/− mice. J Neurosci 2004;24(1): 229–237.
96. Das AV, James J, Zhao X, Rahnenfuhrer J, Ahmad I. Identification of c-Kit receptor as a regulator of adult neural stem cells in the mammalian eye: interactions with Notch signaling. Dev Biol 2004;273(1):87–105.
97. Fischer AJ, Reh TA. Exogenous growth factors stimulate the regeneration of ganglion cells in the chicken retina. Dev Biol 2002;251(2):367–379.
98. Haruta M, Kosaka M, Kanegae Y, et al. Induction of photoreceptor-specific phenotypes in adult mammalian iris tissue. Nat Neurosci 2001;4(12):1163–1164.
99. Arnhold S, Semkova I, Andressen C, et al. Iris pigment epithelial cells: a possible cell source for the future treatment of neurodegenerative diseases. Exp Neurol 2004;187(2):410–417.
100. Alvarez-Buylla A, Lim DA. For the long run: maintaining germinal niches in the adult brain. Neuron 2004;41(5):683–686.
101. Doetsch F. A niche for adult neural stem cells. Curr Opin Genet Dev 2003;13(5):543–50.
102. Palmer TD, Willhoite AR, Gage FH. Vascular niche for adult hippocampal neurogenesis. J Comp Neurol 2000;425(4):479–494.
103. Shen Q, Goderie SK, Jin L, Karanth N, et al. Endothelial cells stimulate self-renewal and expand neurogenesis of neural stem cells. Science 2004;304(5675):1338–1340.
104. Sheffield JB, Moscona AA. Electron microscopic analysis of aggregation of embryonic cells: the structure and differentiation of aggregates of neural retina cells. Dev Biol 1970;23(1):36–61.
105. Akagawa K, Hicks D, Barnstable CJ. Histiotypic organization and cell differentiation in rat retinal reaggregate cultures. Brain Res 1987;437(2):298–308.
106. Watanabe T, Raff MC. Rod photoreceptor development in vitro: intrinsic properties of proliferating neuroepithelial cells change as development proceeds in the rat retina. Neuron 1990;4(3):461–467.
107. Vardimon L, Fox LE, Cohen-Kupiec R, Degenstein L, Moscona AA. Expression of v-src in embryonic neural retina alters cell adhesion, inhibits histogenesis, and prevents induction of glutamine synthetase. Mol Cell Biol 1991;11(10):5275–5284.
108. Layer PG, Willbold E. Histogenesis of the avian retina in reaggregation culture: from dissociated cells to laminar neuronal networks. Int Rev Cytol 1993; 146:1–47.
109. Rothermel A, Willbold E, Degrip WJ, Layer PG. Pigmented epithelium induces complete retinal reconstitution from dispersed embryonic chick retinae in reaggregation culture. Proc Biol Sci 1997;264(1386):1293–1302.
110. Rothermel A, Layer P.G. Photoreceptor plasticity in reaggregates of embryonic chick retina: rods depend on proximal cones and on tissue organization. Eur J Neurosci 2001;13(5):949–958.
111. Wolburg H, Willbold E, Layer P.G. Muller glia endfeet, a basal lamina and the polarity of retinal layers form properly in vitro only in the presence of marginal pigmented epithelium. Cell Tissue Res 1991;264(3): 437–451.
112. Hering H, Kroger S. Synapse formation and agrin expression in stratospheroid cultures from embryonic chick retina. Dev Biol 1999;214(2):412–428.
113. Willbold E, Rothermel A, Huhn J, Reinicke M, Layer PG. Cerebellar glia cells induce a correct laminar organization in chicken retinal reaggregates. Cells Tissues Organs 2001;169(2):104–112.
114. Willbold E, Rothermel A, Tomlinson S, Layer PG. Muller glia cells reorganize reaggregating chicken retinal cells into correctly laminated in vitro retinae. Glia 2000;29(1):45–57.
115. Layer PG, Willbold E. Embryonic chicken retinal cells can regenerate all cell layers in vitro, but ciliary pigmented cells induce their correct polarity. Cell Tissue Res 1989;258(2):233–242.
116. Li HS, Wang D, Shen Q, et al. Inactivation of Numb and Numblike in embryonic dorsal forebrain impairs neurogenesis and disrupts cortical morphogenesis. Neuron 2003;40(6):1105–1118.
117. Shimada M, Wakaizumi S, Kasubuchi Y, Kusunoki T, Nakamura T. Cytosine arabinoside and rosette formation in mouse retina. Nature 1973;246(5429):151–152.
118. Liu L, Halfter W, Layer PG. Inhibition of cell proliferation by cytosine-arabinoside and its interference with spatial and temporal differentiation patterns in the chick retina. Cell Tissue Res 1986;244(3):501–513.
119. Ohira A, Yamamoto M, Honda O, Ohnishi Y, Inomata H, Honda Y. Glial-, neuronal- and photoreceptor-specific cell markers in rosettes of retinoblastoma and retinal dysplasia. Curr Eye Res 1994;13(11): 799–804.
120. al-Ubaidi MR, Font RL, Quiambao AB, et al. Bilateral retinal and brain tumors in transgenic mice expressing simian virus 40 large T antigen under control of the human interphotoreceptor retinoid-binding protein promoter. J Cell Biol 1992;119(6):1681–1687.
121. Schmidt D, Herrmann C, Jurgens H, Harms D. Malignant peripheral neuroectodermal tumor and its necessary distinction from Ewing's sarcoma. A report from the Kiel Pediatric Tumor Registry. Cancer 1991;68(10):2251–2259.
122. Apple DJ, Rabb MF. Retinoblastoma, leukokoria, and phakomatoses. In: Apple DJ, Rabb MF, eds. Ocular Pathology: Clinical Applications and Self-assessment. New York: Elsevier Science; 1998:484–488.
123. Tulvatana W, Adamian M, Berson EL, Dryja TP. Photoreceptor rosettes in autosomal dominant retinitis pigmentosa with reduced penetrance. Arch Ophthalmol 1999;117(3):399–402.
124. Milam AH, Jacobson SG. Photoreceptor rosettes with blue cone opsin immunoreactivity in retinitis pigmentosa. Ophthalmology 1990;97(12):1620–1631.

125. Chacko DM, Das AV, Zhao X, James J, Bhattacharya S, Ahmad I. Transplantation of ocular stem cells: the role of injury in incorporation and differentiation of grafted cells in the retina. Vision Res 2003;43(8):937–946.
126. Fujisawa H. A complete reconstruction of the neural retina of chick embryo grafted onto the chorio-allantoic membrane. Dev Growth Differ 1971;13(1):25–36.
127. Vollmer G, Layer PG, Gierer A. Reaggregation of embryonic chick retina cells: pigment epithelial cells induce a high order of stratification. Neurosci Lett 1984;48(2):191–196.
128. Vollmer G, Layer PG. An in vitro model of proliferation and differentiation of the chick retina: coaggregates of retinal and pigment epithelial cells. J Neurosci 1986;6(7):1885–1896.
129. Layer PG, Alber R, Mansky P, Vollmer G, Willbold E. Regeneration of a chimeric retina from single cells in vitro: cell-lineage-dependent formation of radial cell columns by segregated chick and quail cells. Cell Tissue Res 1990;259(2):187–198.
130. Layer PG, Robitzki A, Rothermel A, Willbold E. Of layers and spheres: the reaggregate approach in tissue engineering. Trends Neurosci 2002;25(3):131–134.
131. Nakagawa S, Takada S, Takada R, Takeichi M. Identification of the laminar-inducing factor: Wnt-signal from the anterior rim induces correct laminar formation of the neural retina in vitro. Dev Biol 2003;260(2):414–425.
132. Erdmann B, Kirsch FP, Rathjen FG, More MI. N-cadherin is essential for retinal lamination in the zebrafish. Dev Dyn 2003;226(3):570–577.
133. Matsunaga M, Hatta K, Takeichi M. Role of N-cadherin cell adhesion molecules in the histogenesis of neural retina. Neuron 1988;1(4):289–295.
134. Horne-Badovinac S, Lin D, Waldron S, et al. Positional cloning of heart and soul reveals multiple roles for PKC lambda in zebrafish organogenesis. Curr Biol 2001;11(19):1492–1502.
135. Wei X, Malicki J. nagie oko, encoding a MAGUK-family protein, is essential for cellular patterning of the retina. Nat Genet 2002;31(2):150–157.
136. Wang YP, Dakubo G, Howley P, et al. Development of normal retinal organization depends on Sonic hedgehog signaling from ganglion cells. Nat Neurosci 2002;5(9):831–832.
137. Tomita K, Ishibashi M, Nakahara K, et al. Mammalian hairy and Enhancer of split homolog 1 regulates differentiation of retinal neurons and is essential for eye morphogenesis. Neuron 1996;16(4):723–734.
138. Takatsuka K, Hatakeyama J, Bessho Y, Kageyama R. Roles of the bHLH gene Hes1 in retinal morphogenesis. Brain Res 2004;1004(1–2):148–155.
139. Royo PE, Quay WB. Retinal transplantation from fetal to maternal mammalian eye. Growth 1959;23:313–336.
140. del Cerro M, Gash DM, Rao GN, Notter MF, Wiegand SJ, Gupta M. Intraocular retinal transplants. Invest Ophthalmol Vis Sci 1985;26(8):1182–1185.
141. Turner JE, Blair JR. Newborn rat retinal cells transplanted into a retinal lesion site in adult host eyes. Brain Res 1986;391(1):91–104.
142. Gouras P, Flood MT, Kjeldbye H. Transplantation of cultured human retinal cells to monkey retina. An Acad Bras Cienc 1984;56(4):431–443.
143. Gouras P, Algvere P. Retinal cell transplantation in the macula: new techniques. Vision Res 1996;36(24):4121–4125.
144. Wasselius J, Ghosh F. Adult rabbit retinal transplants. Invest Ophthalmol Vis Sci 2001;42(11):2632–2638.
145. Seiler M, Aramant RB, Ehinger B, Adolph AR. Transplantation of embryonic retina to adult retina in rabbits. Exp Eye Res 1990;51(2):225–228.
146. Radtke ND, Seiler MJ, Aramant RB, Petry HM, Pidwell DJ. Transplantation of intact sheets of fetal neural retina with its retinal pigment epithelium in retinitis pigmentosa patients. Am J Ophthalmol 2002;133(4):544–550.
147. Algvere PV, Berglin L, Gouras P, Sheng Y. Transplantation of fetal retinal pigment epithelium in age-related macular degeneration with subfoveal neovascularization. Graefes Arch Clin Exp Ophthalmol 1994;232(12):707–716.
148. Weisz JM, Humayun MS, De Juan E Jr, et al. Allogenic fetal retinal pigment epithelial cell transplant in a patient with geographic atrophy. Retina 1999;19(6):540–545.
149. Kaplan HJ, Tezel TH, Berger AS, Wolf ML, Del Priore LV. Human photoreceptor transplantation in retinitis pigmentosa. A safety study. Arch Ophthalmol 1997;115(9):1168–1172.
150. Aramant R, Seiler M, Turner JE. Donor age influences on the success of retinal grafts to adult rat retina. Invest Ophthalmol Vis Sci 1988;29(3):498–503.
151. del Cerro M, Ison JR, Bowen GP, Lazar E, del Cerro C. Intraretinal grafting restores visual function in light-blinded rats. Neuroreport 1991;2(9):529–532.
152. Silverman MS, Hughes SE, Valentino TL, Liu Y. Photoreceptor transplantation: anatomic, electrophysiologic, and behavioral evidence for the functional reconstruction of retinas lacking photoreceptors. Exp Neurol 1992;115(1):87–94.
153. del Cerro M, Lazar ES, Diloreto D Jr. The first decade of continuous progress in retinal transplantation. Microsc Res Tech 1997;36(2):130–141.
154. Adolph AR, Zucker CL, Ehinger B, Bergstrom A. Function and structure in retinal transplants. J Neural Transplant Plast 1994;5(3):147–161.
155. Sharma RK, Ehinger B. Retinal cell transplants: how close to clinical application? Acta Ophthalmol Scand 1997;75(4):355–363.
156. Litchfield TM, Whiteley SJ, Lund RD. Transplantation of retinal pigment epithelial, photoreceptor and other cells as treatment for retinal degeneration. Exp Eye Res 1997;64(5):655–666.
157. Kaplan HJ, Tezel TH, Berger AS, Del Priore LV. Retinal transplantation. Chem Immunol 1999;73:207–219.
158. Ghosh F, Ehinger B. Full-thickness retinal transplants: a review. Ophthalmologica 2000;214(1):54–69.
159. Aramant RB, Seiler MJ. Retinal transplantation: advantages of intact fetal sheets. Prog Retin Eye Res 2002;21(1):57–73.
160. Lund RD, Ono SJ, Keegan DJ, Lawrence JM. Retinal transplantation: progress and problems in clinical application. J Leukoc Biol 2003;74(2):151–160.
161. del Cerro M, Notter MF, Seigel G, Lazar E, Chader G, del Cerro C. Intraretinal xenografts of differentiated human retinoblastoma cells integrate with the host retina. Brain Res 1992;583(1–2):12–22.
162. Szel A, Juliusson B, Bergstrom A, Wilke K, Ehinger B, van Veen T. Reversed ratio of color-specific cones in rabbit retinal cell transplants. Brain Res Dev Brain Res 1994;81(1):1–9.

163. Grasbon T, Grasbon-Frodl EM, Juliusson B, et al. CuZn superoxide dismutase transgenic retinal transplants. Graefes Arch Clin Exp Ophthalmol 1999;237(4):336–341.
164. Larsson J, Juliusson B, Ehinger B. Survival and MHC-expression of embryonic retinal transplants in the choroid. Acta Ophthalmol Scand 1998;76(4):417–421.
165. Sharma RK, Bergstrom A, Ehinger B. Influence of technique and transplantation site on rosette formation in rabbit retinal transplants. Acta Ophthalmol Scand 1997;75(1):3–10.
166. Seiler MJ, Aramant RB, Bergstrom A. Co-transplantation of embryonic retina and retinal pigment epithelial cells to rabbit retina. Curr Eye Res 1995;14(3):199–207.
167. Khodair MA, Zarbin MA, Townes-Anderson E. Synaptic plasticity in mammalian photoreceptors prepared as sheets for retinal transplantation. Invest Ophthalmol Vis Sci 2003;44(11):4976–4988.
168. Sheffield JB. Studies on aggregation of embryonic cells: initial cell adhesions and the formation of intercellular junctions. J Morphol 1970;132(3):245–263.
169. Turner JE, Seiler M, Aramant R, Blair JR. Embryonic retinal grafts transplanted into the lesioned adult rat retina. Prog Brain Res 1988;78:131–139.
170. Vinores SA, Youssri AI, Luna JD, et al. Upregulation of vascular endothelial growth factor in ischemic and non-ischemic human and experimental retinal disease. Histol Histopathol 1997;12(1):99–109.
171. Cao W, Wen R, Li F, Lavail MM, Steinberg RH. Mechanical injury increases bFGF and CNTF mRNA expression in the mouse retina. Exp Eye Res 1997;65(2):241–248.
172. Silverman MS, Hughes SE. Photoreceptor transplantation in inherited and environmentally induced retinal degeneration: anatomy, immunohistochemistry and function. Prog Clin Biol Res 1989;314:687–704.
173. Gouras P, Du J, Kjeldbye H, Yamamoto S, Zack DJ. Long-term photoreceptor transplants in dystrophic and normal mouse retina. Invest Ophthalmol Vis Sci 1994;35(8):3145–3153.
174. Ivert L, Gouras P, Naeser P, Narfstrom K. Photoreceptor allografts in a feline model of retinal degeneration. Graefes Arch Clin Exp Ophthalmol 1998;236(11):844–852.
175. Gouras P, Cao H, Sheng Y, Tanabe T, Efremova Y, Kjeldbye H. Patch culturing and transfer of human fetal retinal epithelium. Graefes Arch Clin Exp Ophthalmol 1994;232(10):599–607.
176. Aramant RB, Seiler MJ. Progress in retinal sheet transplantation. Prog Retin Eye Res 2004;23(5):475–494.
177. Ghosh F, Arner K, Ehinger B. Transplant of full-thickness embryonic rabbit retina using pars plana vitrectomy. Retina 1998;18(2):136–142.
178. Juliusson B, Bergstrom A, van Veen T, Ehinger B. Cellular organization in retinal transplants using cell suspensions or fragments of embryonic retinal tissue. Cell Transplant 1993;2(5):411–418.
179. Gouras P, Du J, Gelanze M, et al. Survival and synapse formation of transplanted rat rods. J Neural Transplant Plast 1991;2(2):91–100.
180. Drager UC, Hubel DH. Studies of visual function and its decay in mice with hereditary retinal degeneration. J Comp Neurol 1978;180(1):85–114.
181. Jiang LQ, del Cerro M. Reciprocal retinal transplantation: a tool for the study of an inherited retinal degeneration. Exp Neurol 1992;115(3):325–334.
182. Gouras P, Du J, Kjeldbye H, Yamamoto S, Zack DJ. Reconstruction of degenerate rd mouse retina by transplantation of transgenic photoreceptors. Invest Ophthalmol Vis Sci 1992;33(9):2579–2586.
183. Kwan AS, Wang S, Lund RD. Photoreceptor layer reconstruction in a rodent model of retinal degeneration. Exp Neurol 1999;159(1):21–33.
184. Radner W, Sadda SR, Humayun MS, et al. Light-driven retinal ganglion cell responses in blind rd mice after neural retinal transplantation. Invest Ophthalmol Vis Sci 2001;42(5):1057–1065.
185. Gouras P, Tanabe T. Survival and integration of neural retinal transplants in rd mice. Graefes Arch Clin Exp Ophthalmol 2003;241(5):403–409.
186. Arai S, Thomas BB, Seiler MJ, et al. Restoration of visual responses following transplantation of intact retinal sheets in rd mice. Exp Eye Res 2004;79(3):331–341.
187. del Cerro M, Notter MF, Grover DA, et al. Retinal transplants for cell replacement in phototoxic retinal degeneration. Prog Clin Biol Res 1989;314:673–686.
188. Seiler MJ, Aramant RB. Intact sheets of fetal retina transplanted to restore damaged rat retinas. Invest Ophthalmol Vis Sci 1998;39(11):2121–2131.
189. del Cerro M, Humayun MS, Sadda SR, et al. Histologic correlation of human neural retinal transplantation. Invest Ophthalmol Vis Sci 2000;41(10):3142–3148.
190. Berger AS, Tezel TH, Del Priore LV, Kaplan HJ. Photoreceptor transplantation in retinitis pigmentosa: short-term follow-up. Ophthalmology 2003;110(2):383–391.
191. Radtke ND, Aramant RB, Seiler MJ, Petry HM, Pidwell D. Vision change after sheet transplant of fetal retina with retinal pigment epithelium to a patient with retinitis pigmentosa. Arch Ophthalmol 2004;122(8):1159–1165.
192. Yanai D, Lakhanpal RR, Weiland JD, et al. The value of preoperative tests in the selection of blind patients for a permanent microelectronic implant. Trans Am Ophthalmol Soc 2003;101:223–228; discussion 228–230.
193. del Cerro M, Notter MF, del Cerro C, Wiegand SJ, Grover DA, Lazar E. Intraretinal transplantation for rod-cell replacement in light-damaged retinas. J Neural Transplant 1989;1(1):1–10.
194. Zucker CL, Ehinger B, Seiler M, Aramant RB, Adolph AR. Ultrastructural circuitry in retinal cell transplants to rat retina. J Neural Transplant Plast 1994;5(1):17–29.
195. Li LX, Turner JE. Transplantation of retinal pigment epithelial cells to immature and adult rat hosts: short- and long-term survival characteristics. Exp Eye Res 1988;47(5):771–785.
196. Lopez R, Gouras P, Kjeldbye H, et al. Transplanted retinal pigment epithelium modifies the retinal degeneration in the RCS rat. Invest Ophthalmol Vis Sci 1989;30(3):586–588.
197. Sheedlo HJ, Li L, Turner JE. Photoreceptor cell rescue at early and late RPE-cell transplantation periods during retinal disease in RCS dystrophic rats. J Neural Transplant Plast 1991;2(1):55–63.
198. Lavail MM, Li L, Turner JE, Yasumura D. Retinal pigment epithelial cell transplantation in RCS rats: normal metabolism in rescued photoreceptors. Exp Eye Res 1992;55(4):555–562.

199. Algvere PV, Berglin L, Gouras P, Sheng Y, Kopp ED. Transplantation of RPE in age-related macular degeneration: observations in disciform lesions and dry RPE atrophy. Graefes Arch Clin Exp Ophthalmol 1997;235(3):149–158.
200. Kanuga N, Winton HL, Beauchene L, et al. Characterization of genetically modified human retinal pigment epithelial cells developed for in vitro and transplantation studies. Invest Ophthalmol Vis Sci 2002;43(2):546–555.
201. Ying QL, Nichols J, Evans EP, Smith AG. Changing potency by spontaneous fusion. Nature 2002;416(6880): 545–548.
202. Alvarez-Dolado M, Pardal R, Garcia-Verdugo JM, et al. Fusion of bone-marrow-derived cells with Purkinje neurons, cardiomyocytes and hepatocytes. Nature 2003;425(6961):968–973.
203. Wernig M, Benninger F, Schmandt T, et al. Functional integration of embryonic stem cell-derived neurons in vivo. J Neurosci 2004;24(22):5258–5268.
204. Harkany T, Andang M, Kingma HJ, et al. Region-specific generation of functional neurons from naive embryonic stem cells in adult brain. J Neurochem 2004;88(5):1229–1239.
205. Takahashi M, Palmer TD, Takahashi J, Gage FH. Widespread integration and survival of adult-derived neural progenitor cells in the developing optic retina. Mol Cell Neurosci 1998;12(6):340–348.
206. Van Hoffelen SJ, Young MJ, Shatos MA, Sakaguchi DS. Incorporation of murine brain progenitor cells into the developing mammalian retina. Invest Ophthalmol Vis Sci 2003;44(1):426–434.
207. Lu B, Kwan T, Kurimoto Y, Shatos M, Lund RD, Young MJ. Transplantation of EGF-responsive neurospheres from GFP transgenic mice into the eyes of rd mice. Brain Res 2002;943(2):292–300.
208. Nishida A, Takahashi M, Tanihara H, et al. Incorporation and differentiation of hippocampus-derived neural stem cells transplanted in injured adult rat retina. Invest Ophthalmol Vis Sci 2000;41(13): 4268–4274.
209. Hara A, Niwa M, Kunisada T, et al. Embryonic stem cells are capable of generating a neuronal network in the adult mouse retina. Brain Res 2004;999(2):216–221.
210. Meyer JS, Katz ML, Maruniak JA, Kirk MD. Neural differentiation of mouse embryonic stem cells in vitro and after transplantation into eyes of mutant mice with rapid retinal degeneration. Brain Res 2004;1014(1–2):131–144.
211. Schraermeyer U, Thumann G, Luther T, et al. Subretinally transplanted embryonic stem cells rescue photoreceptor cells from degeneration in the RCS rats. Cell Transplant 2001;10(8):673–680.
212. Enzmann V, Howard RM, Yamauchi Y, Whittemore SR, Kaplan HJ. Enhanced induction of RPE lineage markers in pluripotent neural stem cells engrafted into the adult rat subretinal space. Invest Ophthalmol Vis Sci 2003;44(12):5417–5422.
213. Mizumoto H, Mizumoto K, Shatos MA, Klassen H, Young MJ. Retinal transplantation of neural progenitor cells derived from the brain of GFP transgenic mice. Vision Res 2003;43(16):1699–1708.
214. Kurimoto Y, Shibuki H, Kaneko Y, et al. Transplantation of adult rat hippocampus-derived neural stem cells into retina injured by transient ischemia. Neurosci Lett 2001;306(1–2):57–60.
215. Young MJ, Ray J, Whiteley SJ, Klassen H, Gage FH. Neuronal differentiation and morphological integration of hippocampal progenitor cells transplanted to the retina of immature and mature dystrophic rats. Mol Cell Neurosci 2000;16(3):197–205.
216. Dong X, Pulido JS, Qu T, Sugaya K. Differentiation of human neural stem cells into retinal cells. Neuroreport 2003;14(1):143–146.
217. Sahel JA, Mohand-Said S, Leveillard T, Hicks D, Picaud S, Dreyfus H. Rod-cone interdependence: implications for therapy of photoreceptor cell diseases. Prog Brain Res 2001;131:649–661.
218. Chow AY, Packo KH, Pollack JS, Schuchard RA. Subretinal artificial silicone retinal microchip for the treatment of retinitis pigmentosa in 10 patient: long term followup. ASRS Abstracts 2003:68.
219. Chong NH, Alexander RA, Waters L, Barnett KC, Bird AC, Luthert PJ. Repeated injections of a ciliary neurotrophic factor analogue leading to long-term photoreceptor survival in hereditary retinal degeneration. Invest Ophthalmol Vis Sci 1999;40(6):1298–1305.
220. Wahlin KJ, Adler R, Zack DJ, Campochiaro PA. Neurotrophic signaling in normal and degenerating rodent retinas. Exp Eye Res 2001;73(5):693–701.
221. Faktorovich EG, Steinberg RH, Yasumura D, Matthes MT, LaVail MM. Photoreceptor degeneration in inherited retinal dystrophy delayed by basic fibroblast growth factor. Nature 1990;347(6288):83–86.
222. LaVail MM, Unoki K, Yasumura D, Matthes MT, Yancopoulos GD, Steinberg RH. Multiple growth factors, cytokines, and neurotrophins rescue photoreceptors from the damaging effects of constant light. Proc Natl Acad Sci U S A 1992;89(23): 11249–11253.
223. Liang FQ, Aleman TS, Dejneka NS, et al. Long-term protection of retinal structure but not function using RAAV.CNTF in animal models of retinitis pigmentosa. Mol Ther 2001;4(5):461–472.
224. Bok D, Yasumura D, Matthes MT, et al. Effects of adeno-associated virus-vectored ciliary neurotrophic factor on retinal structure and function in mice with a P216L rds/peripherin mutation. Exp Eye Res 2002;74(6):719–735.
225. Mohand-Said S, Deudon-Combe A, Hicks D, et al. Normal retina releases a diffusible factor stimulating cone survival in the retinal degeneration mouse. Proc Natl Acad Sci USA 1998;95(14):8357–8362.
226. Mohand-Said S, Hicks D, Dreyfus H, Sahel JA. Selective transplantation of rods delays cone loss in a retinitis pigmentosa model. Arch Ophthalmol 2000;118(6):807–811.
227. Leveillard T, Mohand-Said S, Lorentz O, et al. Identification and characterization of rod-derived cone viability factor. Nat Genet 2004;36(7):755–759.
228. Saigo Y, Abe T, Hojo M, Tomita H, Sugano E, Tamai M. Transplantation of transduced retinal pigment epithelium in rats. Invest Ophthalmol Vis Sci 2004;45(6):1996–2004.
229. Tao W, Wen R, Goddard MB, et al. Encapsulated cell-based delivery of CNTF reduces photoreceptor degeneration in animal models of retinitis pigmentosa. Invest Ophthalmol Vis Sci 2002;43(10):3292–3298.

20

Induction of Ocular Surface Regeneration

Irina S. Barequet

The ocular surface consists of the cornea, the conjunctiva, and the intervening transition area (the limbus) (Figure 20.1). The avascular cornea is continuous with the sclera, forming together the outer envelop of the eyeball [Figure 20.1 and 20.2 (see color section)]. The transparent cornea is the gateway for the entrance of images into the eye, and accounts for more than two thirds of the total refractive power of the eye. The cornea consists of five layers: The epithelium, Bowman's layer, the stroma, Descemet's membrane, and the endothelium. The corneal transparency is essentially maintained by its avascularity, an intact epithelium, and a normal morphology and function of its other layers. These components of the ocular surface are essential for vision, the integrity of the eye, and for preventing ocular infections.

Injury to the ocular surface may be caused by physical or chemical agents, infectious, oculocutaneous disorders, drugs, or systemic disorders. A variety of physical agents may induce tissue damage: Thermal burns, microwaves, lasers, ionizing radiation. Chemical agents are a common cause for severe ocular surface injury: Acids tend to precipitate tissue proteins and cause coagulation and necrosis, thus creating a barrier against deeper penetration, and damaging mainly the external eye; in alkali burns, the hydroxyl ions saponify lipids in the corneal epithelium, denature proteins, and cause tissue melting and may penetrate into the deeper layers. Various microorganisms may be associated with damage to the ocular surface, such as herpes zoster virus that may cause a chronic conjunctivitis with submucosal scarring, hypoesthesia, and lid impairment caused by cicatrization. Chlamydia trachomatis (serotypes A, B, Ba, and C) is a major cause for blindness in developing countries because of the infection of conjunctival cells that initiates an inflammatory response with fibrosis of the subconjunctival tissue, and cicatrizing process of the external eye. A wide range of dermatologic conditions are associated with ocular surface injury. They include mainly ocular cicatricial pemphigoid and Stevens-Johnson syndrome. In ocular cicatricial pemphigoid, a condition with an autoimmune origin, chronic conjunctival inflammation is progressive with exacerbations; the disease is usually bilateral and can lead to severe scarring of the conjunctiva and adherence between bulbar and palpebral conjunctiva (symblepharon) with limitation of ocular motility and to vascularization of the cornea, which may progress to blindness. The ocular manifestations of Stevens-Johnson syndrome are a pseudomembranous conjunctivitis in the acute stage, and in the later phase, conjunctival cicatrization with involvement of the limbus and the cornea are predominant. Moreover, genetic diseases such as aniridia also result in disruption of the normal ocular surface.

Ocular surface reconstruction (OSR) has recently become a common methodology in the regenerative treatment of severe ocular surface disease. The challenge in this field was motivated by the necessity to find a cure for patients as mentioned above, affected by severe and difficult

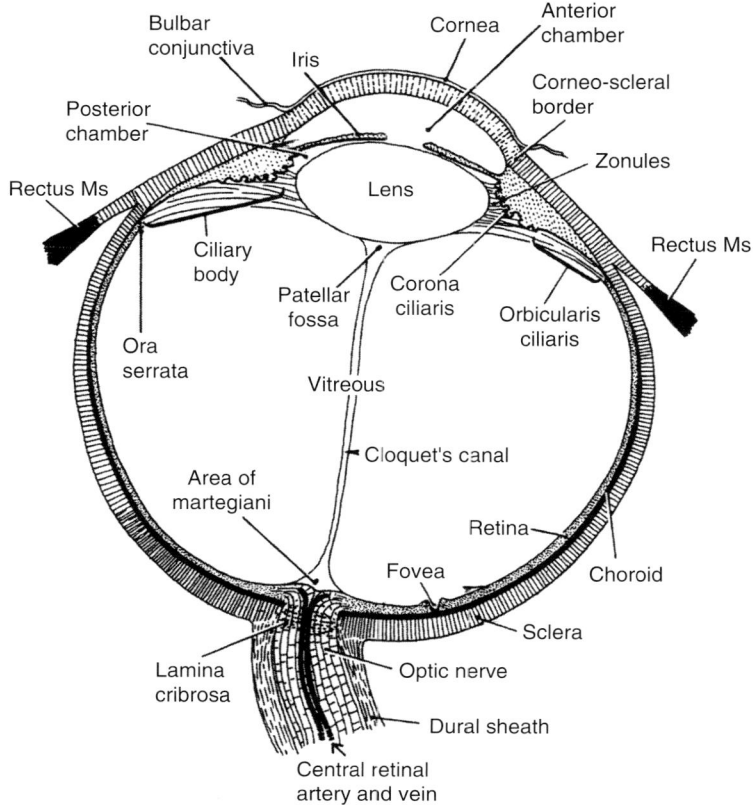

Figure 20.1. Limbal autografts, early postoperative and the donor eye. [From Basti S, Rao SK. Current status of limbal conjunctival autograft. Curr Opin Ophthalmol 2000;11:224-232.]

to treat diseases that damage the integrity of the ocular surface.

The most important breakthrough in OSR came when the limbus was identified as the anatomic location of the corneal epithelial stem cells, which led to the development of various effective techniques of limbal stem cell transplantation. These developments further benefited from the realization that the tears are vital for ocular surface integrity in addition to their lubrication and optical functions, and the use of amniotic membrane (AM) as a basement membrane substitute and other physiologic functions.[1] This review will describe the various current methodologies for induction of ocular surface regeneration and its reconstruction and those in process of clinical development.

The Corneal Epithelium

The role of the corneal epithelium, which forms 10% of the total corneal thickness, is to absorb nutrients and oxygen while protecting the eye by acting as a barrier to fluid loss and pathogen entrance. The corneal epithelium is composed of basal cells, wing cells, and stratified nonkeratinizing squamous cells. The corneal epithelium is constantly renewing itself and regenerating. The cells in the most superficial layer of the epithelium are continuously desquamated from the surface and replaced by proliferating cells. The proliferation of the cells is probably limited to the basal layer of the epithelium.[2] The basal cells rest on a basement membrane and are connected through an adhesion complex (hemidesmosomes) to the underlying connective tissue stroma. Only cells that are in contact with the basement membrane have the ability for mitotic cell division, whereas cells that are displaced into the suprabasal layers become postmitotic and lose their capability for cell division.[3]

The kinetics of the maintenance of the corneal epithelial mass consists of a vertical movement caused by the proliferative pressure of the basal cell layer, and a horizontal movement from the periphery of the cornea toward its center. Also, transient amplifying cells that are found in the basal layers and are generated by stem cells (see below) have a role in corneal epithelial wound healing.[3]

The Limbus

The corneal limbus is the transition zone between the corneal and neighboring conjunctival epithelium. Davanger and Evensen[4] proposed that the corneal epithelium is renewed from a source of cells located at the limbus. They observed that pigment in the epithelium in heavily pigmented eyes migrated in lines from the limbus to the central cornea in healed eccentric corneal epithelial defects. Melanin pigmentation of the limbus provides the resident cells with protection from potential damage by ultraviolet light, a sensible strategy for an area thought to harbor stem cells although this does not occur in Caucasians. Cotsarelis et al.[5] reported the existence of slow-cycling limbal epithelial basal cells that retained tritiated thymidine label for long time periods.

Adult stem cells are defined as clonogenic, self-renewing progenitor cells that can generate one or more specialized types of cells. However, major obstacles in this field have been a lack of molecular markers to identify stem cells (most available markers identify proliferating cells rather than stem cells) and uncertainty regarding the precise location of the putative stem cells in vivo.

Although the stem cell itself is yet to be fully characterized, circumstantial evidence in favor of the limbal location of stem cells has been reported in the literature, and they were identified as the source of corneal epithelial cells.[6,7] These stem cells are responsible for repopulation of the corneal epithelial cells, and maintain high capacity of self-renewal throughout the adult's life. The stem cells are a small subpopulation of the total epithelial tissue and consist between 0.5% and 10% of the total cell population.

There is more evidence supporting the location of corneal epithelial stem cells at the limbus: In culture, limbal basal cells have the highest proliferative capacity[8–11] and surgical removal of the limbus results in delayed healing taking place by noncorneal epithelium.[12–15] It is widely believed that the maintenance of stem cells is controlled by their particular microenvironments (or "niches"), which are best thought of as clusters of environmental cues affecting the state and behavior of the cell.[16]

Limbal Stem Cell Deficiency

There are both primary and acquired causes of limbal stem cell deficiency in the cornea, which can be focal or diffuse, depending on the extent of limbal involvement with underlying disease processes.

Another approach to the classification of limbal deficiency is based on its pathogenic nature of the limbal involvement.[3] Category I is characterized by a clear pathogenic cause responsible for the destruction of the limbal stem cell population. This includes chemical or thermal injury, radiation injury, Stevens-Johnson syndrome (in which severe conjunctivitis and keratitis are common complications of stem cell deficiency), multiple surgeries in the limbal area, or cryotherapy applied at the limbus region. Rare causes are contact lens-induced keratopathy, lens-wearing injuries, or toxic effects from lens-cleaning solutions. Category II includes diverse causes with a dysfunction of stromal microenvironment of limbal stem cells, such as aniridia, chronic limbitis, neurotrophic keratopathy, and pterygium/pseudopterygium, or immunologic conditions, such as ocular cicatricial pemphigoid. In this category, a milder form of corneal diseases, in which limbal stem cell dysfunction is not the result of the total loss of limbal stem cells, but rather is associated with either a gradual loss of stem cell population or poor transient amplifying cell generation and amplification. Because it has not resulted from traumatic loss, the underlying pathogenesis might stem from deficient microenvironment support for limbal stem cells or transient amplifying cells, or a poor regulatory mechanism. In the case of aniridia (a heritable disease in which the eye develops with a vestigial iris only), in which the stem cells are dysfunctional, such poor regulation is probably associated with microenvironmental alteration caused by the anomalous development of the adjacent angle-iris structures. Poor nutritional supply of endocrine factors and of trophic cytokines might be the basis for the development of limbal stem cell deficiency in keratitis associated with multiple endocrine deficiency and neurotrophic keratopathy derived from a primary neuronal or ischemic component, respectively. The introduction of adverse undesirable cytokines secreted by chronic inflammation of various etiologies might inhibit or antagonize normal regulators and create a state of limbal stem cell dysfunction. These mechanisms might explain the poor support of stem cell function in clinical examples of chronic limbitis and pterygium or pseudopterygium.

In each of the limbal deficiency conditions mentioned above, patients may experience severe photophobia, pain, reduced visual acuity, and even blindness. The common pathology in these diverse diseases is depletion of the corneal stem cell population in the limbus. When limbal stem cell deficiency occurs, the neighboring conjunctival epithelium, which is normally prevented from encroaching on the corneal surface by the limbal cells, migrates over the corneal stroma. This process is known as conjunctivalization. This may seem to be a useful strategy to protect the stroma, except that the conjunctival epithelial cells do not share the same phenotypic properties as corneal epithelial cells. The conjunctival cells are not able to fully transdifferentiate into corneal epithelial cells and they express different proteins and keratins.[17–19] In addition, mucin-producing goblet cells of conjunctival origin are present in the epithelium covering the corneal stroma. The result is corneal opacity and therefore very poor vision, vascularization,[19] an unstable surface prone to epithelial breakdown, irregular corneal epithelium, and patient discomfort.

These eyes are poor candidates for the conventional treatment of corneal opacities – corneal transplantation. After a standard penetrating keratoplasty in such cases, the transplanted corneal button is invariably replaced by invading vascularized tissue, which is further complicated by immunologic rejection and secondary glaucoma. This occurs because of the fact that the limbal stem cells are not part of the graft, and the corneal button contains only transient amplifying cells. Also, the preexisting corneal vascularization and inflammation increases the risk of allograft rejection, and the loss of stem cell function leads to recurrent conjunctivalization.

Ocular Surface Reconstruction

Over the past few years, OSR has become a widespread method in the treatment of severe ocular surface disease. A number of therapeutic strategies have been adopted to treat limbal stem cell deficiency, using several techniques with the same aim of restoring stem cell function. Limbal stem cell transplantation aims to replace the absent or damaged cells that are incapable of differentiating into normal corneal epithelium, in order to regenerate corneal-like epithelium.[20] It is required to restore the ocular surface of patients with stem cell deficiency covering the whole cornea.[21] Penetrating keratoplasty and lamellar keratoplasty in these eyes have recently regained their status as a surgical tool to provide the essential clarity of the cornea, only in conjunction with limbal transplantation.

The major breakthroughs in OSR were: 1) the identification of the limbus as the anatomic location of corneal epithelial stem cells[22]; 2) the realization that tears are not only for lubrication but that many physiologic components of tears are vital for ocular surface integrity[23,24]; and 3) the use of AM as a basement membrane substitute,[25] as well as provider of other physiologic functions.

Moreover, restoration of the adnexal anatomical and functional integrity also has an important role in the long-term reconstruction of the ocular surface. Thus, lid morphology and the proper alignment of the lid margin are important to the tear meniscus.

Initially, the term OSR was used synonymously with limbal, or stem cell, transplantation. The cases presented in the literature varied greatly, ranging from mild forms of stem cell deficiency, such as aniridia, to severe cases in the form of Stevens-Johnson syndrome. Early attempts were made to restore changes in the ocular surface by limbal transplantation.[26] After years of follow-up, certain factors that had to be addressed came to the attention of anterior segment surgeons. There was a need to standardize terminology used to describe OSR techniques. Holland and Schwartz[27] proposed a classification of the surgical techniques in order to standardize the nomenclature. This classification is based not only on the carrier tissue of the limbal stem cells (conjunctiva or cornea) but also on the origin of the tissue (autograft or allograft). They thus separated limbal transplantation into the following four categories: Conjunctival limbal autograft, living-relative conjunctival limbal allograft, cadaveric conjunctival limbal allograft, and cadaveric keratolimbal allograft (Table 20.1).

Amniotic Membrane Transplantation

The amniotic membrane (AM) constitutes the inner wall of the fetal membranes, and consists of a single layer of epithelium with an underlying stroma rich in extracellular matrix and collagens. Although first used in the 1940s, this method was abandoned, and then reintroduced for ophthalmic use in 1995 by Kim and Tseng.[25] In a rabbit model, 40% of corneas with total limbal deficiency could be reconstructed by replacing the conjunctivalized surface with a preserved human AM. Since then, AM has proven to be an integral part of OSR. AM can easily be obtained from seronegative mothers undergoing routine Cesarean delivery. The AM is usually used after cryopreservation, but fresh AM seems to work as well.[28]

The AMT can be used for several indications, either as a graft to replace the damaged ocular surface stromal matrix or as a patch (dressing) to prevent unwanted inflammatory insults from gaining access to the damaged ocular surface, or a combination of both. Reports indicated that potential action mechanisms might include reduction of inflammation, vascularization and scarring, and facilitation of epithelialization.

Compositionally, the basement membrane of the AM resembles that of the conjunctiva. The basement side of the membrane can act as a substrate for supporting the growth of epithelial progenitor cells by prolonging their lifespan and maintaining their clonogenicity. This may support the idea of using AM transplantation (AMT) to expand the remaining limbal stem cells and corneal transient amplifying cells during the treatment of partial limbal deficiency[29] and to facilitate epithelialization for persistent corneal epithelial defects with stromal ulceration.[30-32] In tissue cultures, AM supports epithelial cell grown from explant cultures[33-35] or other cultures,[36,37] and maintains their normal epithelial morphology and differentiation.[34,35] The resultant epithelial cells–AM can be transplanted back to reconstruct the damaged corneal surface in humans[38] and in rabbits.[36] The AM can also be used to promote non-goblet cell differentiation of the conjunctival epithelium.[34]

The stromal side of the membrane contains a unique matrix component that suppresses transforming growth factor β signaling, and proliferation and myofibroblast differentiation of normal human corneal and limbal fibroblasts[37] and of normal conjunctival fibroblasts and pterygium body fibroblasts.[39] This may explain the scar reduction during conjunctival surface reconstruction,[40,41] recurrent scarring prevention after pterygium removal,[37-46] and corneal haze reduction after phototherapeutic keratectomy and photorefractive keratectomy.[47,48] Although such an action is more potent when fibroblasts are in contact with the stromal matrix, a lesser effect is also noted when fibroblasts are separated from the membrane by a distance,[37] suggesting that some diffusible factors might also be involved besides the insoluble matrix components in the membrane.

Table 20.1. Classification of surgical procedures for the management of severe ocular surface disease

Procedure	Abbrev	Donor	Transplanted tissue
Conjunctival transplantation			
Conjunctival autograft	CAU	Fellow eye	Conjunctiva
Living-related conjunctival allograft	lr-CAL	Living relative	Conjunctiva
Limbal transplantation			
Conjunctival limbal autograft	CLAU	Fellow eye	Limbus/conjunctiva
Cadaveric conjunctival limbal allograft	c-CLAL	Cadaveric whole globe	Limbus/conjunctiva
Living related conjunctival limbal allograft	lr-CAL	Living relative	Limbus/conjunctiva
Keratolimbal allograft	KLAL	Cadaverie stored tissue	Limbus/cornea
Ex-vivo expanded limbal autograft	EVELAU	Fellow eye	Ex-vivo expanded limbal cells
Living related ex-vivo expanded limbal allograft	lr-EVELAL	Living-relative	Ex-vivo expanded limbal cells
Amniotic membrane transplantation	AMT	Stored human amniotic membrane	Human amniotic membrane

Source: Holland EJ, Schwartz GS. The Paton lecture: ocular surface transplantation: 10 years' experience. Cornea 2004;23:425-431.

Several growth factors have been identified in the AM.[49] The stromal matrix of the membrane can also exclude inflammatory cells by stimulating them into rapid apoptosis[48] and contains various forms of protease inhibitors.[50] This can explain the reduction of stromal inflammation after AMT[29,30] and corneal neovascularization,[51] actions important for preparing the stroma for supporting limbal stem cells to be transplanted either at the same time or later.[29,44,52-55]

AMT can facilitate epithelialization, maintain normal conjunctival epithelium phenotype (with goblet cells when performed on conjunctiva[56]), and reduce inflammation, vascularization, and scarring. Based on these therapeutic effects, one can envision that AMT can be used for conjunctival surface reconstruction to restore normal stroma and provide a healthy basement membrane for renewed epithelial proliferation and differentiation. Several reports showed that AMT can be used to reconstruct the conjunctival surface as an alternative to conjunctival graft after removal of large conjunctival lesions such as pterygium,[42-46] conjunctival intraepithelial neoplasia and tumors,[40] scars and symblepharon,[43-45] and conjunctivochalasis.[57] These results indicate that the reconstructed area can be very large so long as the underlying bed is not ischemic and the bordered conjunctiva has a normal conjunctival epithelium and subconjunctival stroma.

AM acts as a basement membrane allowing the migration of epithelial cells over areas of bare sclera, and can avert impending perforation of the cornea. A report by Chen et al.[31] shows the efficacy of AMT as a substrate in the treatment of neurotrophic ulcers of the cornea. More than 70% of patients in this series healed by AMT, after a mean follow-up of 18.8 months. The significance of focusing on neurotrophic ulcers is the fact that these patients present one of the most difficult cases to manage. The success of AMT in neurotrophic ulcers leads one to speculate that humoral factors of AM origin may also be involved in the healing process.

Segments of AM can also be used as a filling in localized stromal deficiencies, even when accompanied by perforation.[32] Small segments of AM in this case are stuffed under an overlying layer of AM that acts as a basement membrane. This procedure can also be done with the use of surgical adhesion glue.[58,59] The possibility of patching a perforation with AM can save the eye in many ways. Institutions without the immediate availability of donor tissue can buy time before performing a therapeutic keratoplasty.[32]

The AM has been used as a graft in adjunction to limbal stem cell transplantation,[20,26,29] intended to restore the damaged limbal stromal environment, as a support to restoration of the limbal stem cell population. Reported clinical experience showed that this combined approach is effective in treating various extents of limbal deficiency according to the following parameters: The extent of limbal deficiency, presence or absence of the central corneal transient amplifying cells, and depth of central corneal involvement.[41] AMT is an important adjunct in limbal transplantation for both transplanted limbal stem cells to expand on the recipient eye and the residual stem cells to expand in the donor eye.

Partial limbal deficiency can be reconstructed by AMT without the use of limbal transplantation.[60] This result first observed in rabbit experiments at the time when no explanation was available,[25] indicates that partial limbal deficiency can be treated without long-term use of immunosuppression with oral cyclosporin.

AM can also be applied to treat corneal surface diseases as a graft. When used as a graft or a patch, AM can promote healing of persistent corneal ulcers from different causes including neurotrophic keratopathy caused by various underlying etiologies,[30,31,44] and band keratopathy.[61,62] This approach is superior to conjunctival flaps or tarsorrhaphy because it preserves a cosmetically more acceptable appearance.

AM can also be used as a patch in a temporary or prolonged manner. Experimentally, when used as a patch on a temporary basis, this membrane has been shown to reduce corneal haze after photorefractive keratectomy or phototherapeutic keratectomy,[46,62] an effect verified in human patients.[48,64] As a temporary patch, AM can reduce inflammation, facilitate epithelialization, and prevent scarring caused by acute chemical burns in a rabbit model[44] and in human patients.[65,66] AM as a patch was also used successfully in the acute stage of Stevens-Johnson syndrome[52] and to suppress refractory inflammation in various ocular surface disorders.[67]

The fact that the AM can help preserve and expand limbal epithelial stem cells indicates that it can also be used as a carrier to expand them in in vitro culture. This new approach is applicable to those patients with limited limbal reserve or who are concerned about having a large part of the healthy limbus removed from the fellow eye or from a living-related donor. In this case, a small limbal biopsy will be performed and the sample will be placed on the AM and appropriately cultured. Within 3 to 4 weeks, such an ex vivo expanded culture together with the AM can then be transplanted to restore the normal corneal surface on limbal deficient corneas. The feasibility of this new approach based on an autologous source has been demonstrated in a short-term rabbit study[38] and in long-term human patients.[36,68,69] This new approach paves the way to use AM as a tissue engineering substrate and may open up new therapeutics by incorporating gene therapies in the future.

There are certain limitations to AMT because this is a substrate transplantation and thus cannot be used to treat ocular surface disorders that are characterized with a total loss of limbal epithelial stem cells or conjunctival epithelial stem cells. Because AMT still relies on the host tissue to supply epithelial and mesenchymal cells, it cannot be used to reconstruct the ocular surface that has severe aqueous tear deficiency, diffuse keratinization,[55] absence of blinking in severe neurotrophic state, and stromal ischemia. If not overcome, these conditions present as contraindications for AMT.

Limbal Autografts

In cases of unilateral limbal stem cell deficiency, a limbal conjunctival autograft (CLAU) can be harvested from the healthy eye. The transplantation limbal tissue from the fellow eye, using adjacent conjunctiva as the carrier tissue, was first reported by Kenyon and Tseng[20] in 1989. CLAU has become the popular choice in the treatment of unilateral limbal deficiency. Reports continue to support CLAU as the treatment of choice for unilateral disease such as chemical and thermal burns[70,71] [Figures 20.3 (see color section)].

The principles of the standard procedure is to transplant two segments of conjunctival limbal tissue at the 12 and 6 o'clock positions, mainly because these areas are protected by the lids, and are often the sights of conjunctival invasion. The procedure is performed under general or bilateral retrobulbar and/or topical anesthesia. In the injured eye, a 360° conjunctival peritomy 2 mm posterior to the limbus is performed. Bare scleral dissection to the limbus is performed, and the ring of tissue is removed. This is followed by removal of abnormal corneal epithelium and vascular tissue (pannus). The donor limbal epithelium is harvested from the noninjured fellow eye. Two grafts, each with about a 4–clock hour circumferential length, are taken. The two incisions, conjunctival and corneal, are then joined by a radial incision at each end. The graft extends 0.5 mm onto clear cornea and 2 mm onto the bulbar conjunctiva. It therefore includes limbal stem cells. The donor site is left open and heals rapidly. The donor tissue is transplanted to the injured eye. It is sutured to the cornea. The donor tissue size of two 4–clock hour circumference provides a sufficient number of stem cells to the injured eye and avoids limbal deficiency in the donor eye. Postoperative care consists of topical antibiotics, steroids, cycloplegics, and nonpreserved artificial tears [Figure 20.3 (see color section)]. The presence of limbal tissue may act as a physical barrier against invading tissue. Dua et al.[38] recommended that any invading conjunctiva after CLAU be removed, so that corneal epithelium of donor origin may migrate to reepithelialize the entire cornea.

The use of CLAU for recurrent pterygia[72] is also effective in preventing recurrence. However, whether stem cells are in fact required in this case is still debatable. Healthy limbal tissue in pterygia patients is usually sufficient in providing transient amplifying cells to cover for resected pterygium tissue.

Although CLAU cannot be used in bilateral disease, conjunctival limbal allograft tissue from living relatives (lr-CLAL) is an alternative method, especially when the same human leukocyte antigen haplotypes are available (i.e., siblings).[73] Although there are no incidents of limbal dysfunction after procurement of donor tissue from a healthy eye, caution is required in cases with unilateral chemical burns, because claims that only one eye was inflicted may not be entirely true. Removal of limbal tissue from a partially stem cell-deficient eye may cause irreversible damage.

The most significant advantage of CLAU is the abolishment of any risks of immunologic rejection. However, persistent inflammation of the ocular surface cause by the original disease or surgical trauma can also cause loss of donor limbal tissue, and care must be taken to control the original disease and inflammation in these patients.

Limbal Allografts

In cases of bilateral disease, a living relative may provide healthy stem cells (lr-CLAL).[73,74] However, reports of studies in the rabbit eye have shown that the removal of two thirds of the limbal zone can result in delayed epithelial healing, vascularization, and conjunctival epithelial ingrowth.[76] Because of this potential complication and because a healthy contralateral conjunctiva is not always available, allograft limbal transplantation with cadaver eyes may be considered.[77] In such cases, either a conjunctival limbal allograft (c-CLAL) or a keratolimbal allograft (KLAL) is performed.[78]

Conjunctival limbal allograft[79] is technically similar to conjunctival limbal autograft, except for the need for a living donor[80] or a cadaver.[81]

Keratoepithelioplasty was first described by Thoft.[82] In this technique, four lenticules of peripheral corneal epithelium with superficial corneal stroma are harvested from a fresh donor eye. Originally, limbal tissue was not harvested with the lenticules. Only later was the technique modified to include limbal tissue.[83,84] The lenticules are secured to the corneoscleral limbus on the recipient eye 90° apart. Limbal transplant from cadaveric donors (KLAL) is the treatment of choice in bilateral disease, and can restore a cornea epithelial phenotype in approximately 50% to 70% of cases.[85] In KLAL, cadaveric limbal tissue is transplanted by using the peripheral cornea as carrier tissue, and therefore the procedure has two specific advantages over other limbal stem cell techniques: Stored donor tissue is readily available, and because three separate 180° segments of limbal tissue are used, KLAL affords the largest number of transplanted limbal stem cells compared with any other limbal stem cell transplantation technique. Although encouraging results have been reported,[86] dry eye and preoperative conjunctival keratinization were initially associated with poor results after keratolimbal allografts.[86]

With allografts, either from a living relative or from cadaver eyes, the possibility of rejection and/or infection must be considered. The combination of allograft limbal transplantation, AMT, treating severe conjunctival scarring and limbal stem cell deficiency in cases of cicatricial pemphigoid and Stevens-Johnson syndrome was reported.[87] However, longer follow-up in these patients showed that many of the severe patients with Stevens-Johnson syndrome and ocular cicatricial pemphigoid, are at risk of vessel invasion and conjunctivalization after months of a seemingly smooth course. Chronic deterioration of donor stem cells can be caused by a number of factors, many of which still need to be addressed. Discontinuation of immunosuppression may cause rejection of grafts (see below, immunotherapy). Lid deformities and dry eye may inflict chronic mechanical damage leading to persistent epithelial defects and stem cell depletion. Recurrence of original disease may cause nonspecific inflammation, triggering any number of events leading to graft failure. The limbus acting as a physical barrier may also be important, because a single-piece lamellar keratoplasty (LKP) and KLAL graft (large graft) had less success than a two-piece or a two-stage procedure (KLAL and LKP).[88,89] There is a controversy regarding the staging of the procedure. Ilary and Daya[90] reported no difference in KLAL survival whether it was performed simultaneously with a keratoplasty or as a later procedure. However, KLAL combined with keratoplasty seemed to have a shorter survival time than KLAL followed by keratoplasty. Holland and Schwartz[91] suggested waiting at least 3 months after an epithelial transplantation before considering a corneal graft to allow stabilization of the transplanted epithelial tissue. Conversely, Rao et al.[73] advocated a combined approach with the rationale of avoiding the need for a second procedure and preserving donor transient amplifying cells. Because successful epithelial transplantation often obviates the need for keratoplasty, Daya and Ilari[92] recommended waiting at least 1 year before performing a keratoplasty, and, in cases in which there is a normal endothelium, a deep lamellar keratoplasty is preferable in their opinion.

Holland et al.[93] reported the results of KLAL in aniridia (Figures 20.4 and 20.5); the outcome seemed improved if surgery was performed earlier in the disease process – specifically, before vision was impaired from irreversible stromal opacification. Because aniridic keratopathy involves only the corneal epithelium in the early stages, KLAL alone may be sufficient for visual rehabilitation when performed on younger aniridic patients. However, if an aniridic patient is merely observed through young adulthood, the epithelial keratopathy will typically lead to stromal scarring, and the patient will likely need PK in addition to KLAL to restore baseline visual acuity.

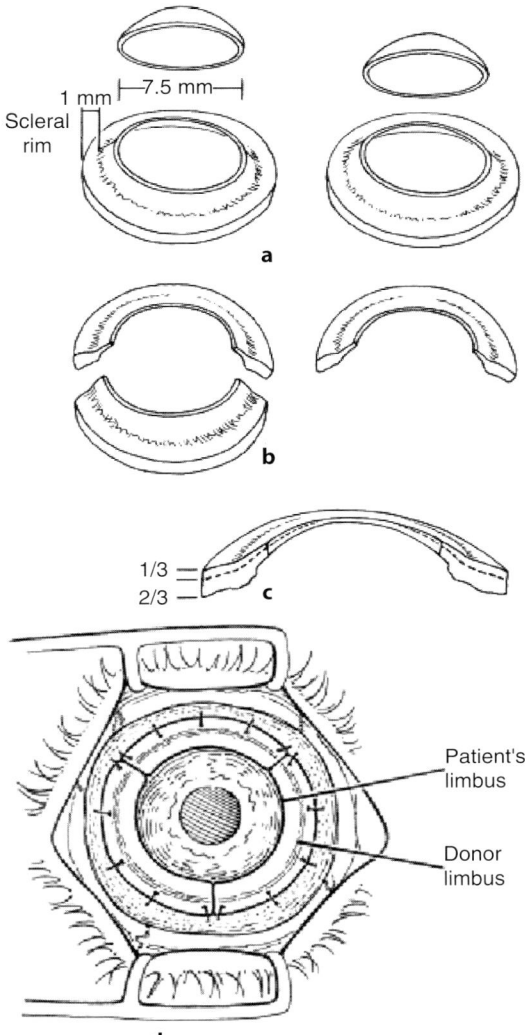

Figure 20.4. Diagram of key steps in preparation of tissue for keratolimbal allograft and **a** recipient eye with three keratolimbal crescents sutured in place. **b** The central corneal button is removed with a trephine. **c** The remaining limbal ring is divided into two 180° crescents. **d** The crescents are thinned by removing the posterior two-thirds of the corneoscleral tissue via sharp dissection. [Reprinted from Holland EJ, Djalilian AR, Schwartz GS. Management of aniridic keratopathy with keratolimbal allograft: a limbal stem cell transplantation technique. Ophthalmology 2003;110:126–127, Figures 2 and 3. With permission from the American Academy of Opthalmology.]

The identification of allograft rejection is of high priority because failure to diagnose rejection will compromise graft survival. Daya et al.[94] showed pathologic findings of clinically diagnosed KLAL rejection. Donor limbal segments removed during a second KLAL showed infiltration of T cells, and loss of corneal epithelium-like cells that express cornea-specific keratin. Clinical signs associated with these pathologic findings were intense sectoral injection, perilimbal conjunctival injection, limbal edema, and cellular infiltration of KLAL grafts. These signs are followed by persistent epithelial defects, vessel invasion, and keratinization. It is not known whether rejection in KLAL occurs via a similar mechanism as penetrating keratoplasty. The incidence of rejection does not need to involve both tissues at the same time, and has been observed to occur in only one of the grafts. In fact, immunologic rejection to the central graft seems to be higher when accompanied by KLAL.[95]

The usefulness of Cyclosporine A as an immunosuppressant agent has shown conflicting results. The rationale for the use of immunosuppressants is to increase graft survival rate by decreasing progressive destruction of limbal stem cells from acute or chronic allograft rejection. Acute allograft rejection rate as reported by others varies from none[82] to 30%,[96] and in this study it was 39.4%. There is no consensus regarding specific immunosuppressive regimens after KLAL. Systemic Cyclosporine A was used in more severe cases and in higher doses where there was recurrent inflammation. In the study published by Ilari and Daya,[90] no difference in KLAL survival was found between patients treated or not treated with long-term Cyclosporine A, primary failure excluded. However, there was a higher rate of acute allograft rejections in patients treated with oral Cyclosporine A as compared with the patients not receiving Cyclosporine A, and this probably reflected patient selection for using oral Cyclosporine A. In their study, although there were fewer episodes of acute rejection in the group not receiving Cyclosporine A, KLAL survival was shorter (13.5 months compared with 22 months). This possibly reflects a process of chronic low-grade rejection as suggested by Daya et al.[94] and Holland and Schwartz,[91] which may be prevented or delayed by the use of Cyclosporine A.

In addition, management of all other aspects of the patient's ocular health is essential to ensure the best opportunity for allograft survival (Table 20.2). The presence and severity of glaucoma need to be elucidated, because it is important that the management of intraocular pressure be stable before limbal allograft is performed. Holland and Schwartz[97] recommended aggressive and early

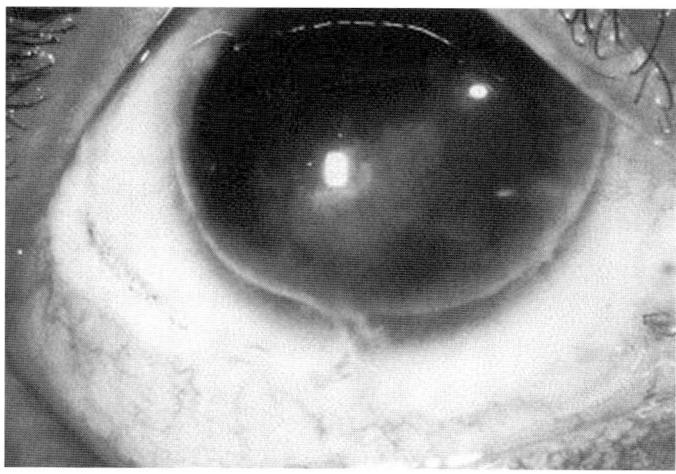

Figure 20.5. Slit lamp photograph of severe aniridic keratopathy, prior and 1 year after keratolimbal allograft. [Reprinted from Holland EJ, Djalilian AR, Schwartz GS. Management of aniridic keratopathy with keratolimbal allograft: a limbal stem cell transplantation technique. Ophthalmology 2003;110:126–127, Figures 1 and 4.]

placement of a tube shunt in patients receiving more than one topical glaucoma medication. The rationale for this aggressive approach is that an increase in intraocular pressure after limbal allograft is quite common. In addition, multiple topical medications and their preservatives can be toxic to the transplanted epithelial surface. Next, the status of the eyelids and lashes are evaluated. Surgical correction of existing exposure, lagophthalmos, and ectropion as well as aggressive management of trichiasis and distichiasis must be performed before limbal allograft. Failure of the ocular surface secondary to nonimmune inflammation can occur from exposure and trauma secondary to misdirected eyelashes. Aggressive management of preoperative inflammation is the next factor that must be considered and aggressively managed before limbal allograft. Limbal allografts that are transplanted into an inflamed ocular surface have a significantly poorer prognosis than those in which the inflammation has been minimized. Therefore, topical and systemic immunosuppression are initiated weeks to months before limbal allograft to achieve the greatest chance for success. Once the glaucoma is stabilized, the lid anatomy is restored, and the ocular inflammation is reasonably controlled, a limbal transplantation technique will be performed. The selection of which ocular surface procedure to be used is based on several factors. If the patient has unilateral disease, Holland and Schwartz recommended CLAU as the procedure of choice because this procedure does not run the risk of failure secondary to immune rejection. For patients with bilateral disease, the choice is between KLAL and lr-CLAL. For the majority of patients with limbal deficiency without extensive conjunctival disease, the authors advocated KLAL, because of the availability of cadaver donor tissue as well as the increased quantity of stem cells available for transplantation (18 clock hours of limbus). However, if the patient has extensive conjunctival disease, they recommended lr-CLAL procedure,

Table 20.2 Algorithm for an approach to treat patients with severe ocular surface disease

1. Management of glaucoma
    a. Tube shunt for patients on more than 1 topical medication
2. Correction of eyelid and eyelash abnormalities
    a. Exposure: lagophthalmos, ectropion
    b. Misdirected lashes: entropion, trichiasis, distichiasis
3. Suppression of inflammation
    a. Topical corticosteroids and cyclosporin A
    b. Systemic immunosuppression
        i. Oral corticosteroids
        ii. Tacrolimus or cyclosporin A
        iii. Mycophenolate or azathioprine
4. Ocular surface transplantation
    a. Conjunctival limbal autograft (CLAU) for unilateral disease
    b. Keratolimbal allograft (KLAL) for bilateral limbal deficiency with minimal to moderate conjunctival disease
    c. Living-related conjunctival limbal allograft (lr-CLAL) for bilateral limbal deficiency with moderate to severe conjunctival disease
    d. Combined conjunctival-keratolimbal allograft (C-KLAL) for bilateral limbal deficiency with severe conjunctival disease
5. Keratoplasty
    a. Lamellar (LK) for patients with stromal opacification with normal endothelium
    b. Penetrating (PK) for patients with stromal opacification with loss of endothelial function

Source: Holland EJ, Schwartz GS. The Paton lecture: ocular surface transplantation: 10 years' experience. Cornea 2004;23:425-431.

because it provides much needed healthy conjunctival cells in addition to limbal tissue. More recently, we have combined KLAL and lr-CLAL in patients with the most severe ocular surface disease to maximize the advantages inherent in each procedure. In those patients in whom a stable ocular surface has been obtained, consideration of a subsequent keratoplasty can be entertained. If the patient has significant stromal scarring with good endothelial function, a lamellar keratoplasty should be considered. In patients with stromal and endothelial disease, penetrating keratoplasty is often required for visual rehabilitation.

Stem Cell Therapy

As an alternative to limbal grafting, corneal stem cell therapy may be considered for some patients. The aims of stem cell therapy are to promote reepithelialization of the cornea, provide stable corneal epithelium, prevent regression of new vessels, and restore epithelial clarity. A pioneering approach published by Rheinwald and Green[98] that optimized the production of cultured cutaneous epithelium suitable for grafting burn patients has been successfully adopted for the culture of multilayered corneal epithelium.[99] Pellegrini et al.[100] have shown that this can be produced for grafting of corneal patients with unilateral limbal stem cell deficiency. The discovery that cultured limbal cells include stem cells, detectable as holoclones (clones that are derived from human epithelial stem cells and that have high proliferative potential), permitted the development of limbal cultures for the treatment of patients with a partial deficiency of limbal stem cells. Limbal epithelial cells were obtained from a small biopsy specimen from a healthy area of the patient's cornea; after culturing, these cells developed into corneal epithelium, which was successfully transplanted back into the patient. Further results have shown clinical improvement of the corneal surface after application of cultured autologous corneal epithelial cells.[68] Recent work has also shown the potential for using limbal tissue stored in eye banks as a source of cells for producing cultured corneal epithelial allografts.[101] Providing the cultured epithelium with a basement membrane is likely to improve graft "take" and may even promote survival of any cultured stem cells, allowing them to establish themselves in the host stem cell niche. Tseng et al.[102] have developed a technique in which epithelial cells from a limbal biopsy are explanted directly onto AM in culture. After 2 to 3 weeks, the composite graft is then ready for the patient. Significant improvements in corneal clarity and surface stability have been achieved using this technique. This technique of ex vivo expanded limbal transplantation provides a novel method for transplantation of either an autograft (EVELAU), using the patient's own limbal stem cells, or from a living-related donor (lr-EVELAU).

Tissue Engineering

The next stage in OSR is the identification of corneal epithelial stem cells and the transplantation of bioengineered tissue, including isolated stem cells. Because the potential markers for stem cell identification have been reported,[103,104] the next challenge will be to isolate these cells, and to maintain cell cultures with the potential to provide an unlimited stock of undifferentiated cells. Culture conditions can be modified to induce these cells to differentiate as required. Stem cells may be further engineered for low immunogenicity by the induction of genes, and perhaps express genes that will help these cells proliferate.

The AM has a thick basement membrane that is able to support the growth of corneal epithelial cells.[36] This will allow AM to be used as a carrier for transplanting cultured cells, and in fact, animal studies[35] and clinical reports[38,68,105] show that cultured epithelial transplants using AM substrate are effective in selected cases. However, the long-term results of this procedure are unknown, and yet we still await the demonstration of the stem cell itself. There is no guarantee that these transplantable sheets of epithelium contain stem cells, even though the cells may be of limbal origin. An entirely different strategy will be required for developing epithelial transplants to be used as a temporary graft, and those that are intended to seed stem cells.

A possible alternative is under development of natural and/or synthetic biopolymers that will support cellular components of the cornea. An *in vitro* model of such design is already a reality,[106] and further studies in polymer design and cell cultures may someday produce a transplantable artificial cornea.

Summary

Visual function requires an intact ocular surface. The integrity of this surface is maintained in humans by two highly specialized epithelia – the conjunctival epithelium and the limbal corneal epithelium. Although anatomically continuous with each other at the corneoscleral limbus, the two cell phenotypes represent quite distinct subpopulations. A population of keratinocyte stem cells in defined locations governs the renewal of these stratified epithelia. Stem cells for the cornea reside at the corneoscleral limbus. Corneal stem cells are segregated in the basal layer of the limbus, the transitional zone between the cornea (the transparent part of the ocular surface) and the bulbar conjunctiva (which covers the white part of the ocular surface). The microenvironment of the limbus is considered to be important in maintaining the stemness of stem cells. These stem cells generate transient amplifying cells that terminally differentiate after a discrete number of cell divisions. Limbal stem cells also act as a "barrier" to conjunctival epithelial cells and normally prevent them from migrating onto the corneal surface. Under certain conditions, however, the limbal stem cells may be partially or totally depleted, resulting in varying degrees of stem cell deficiency with resulting abnormalities in the corneal surface. Such deficiency of limbal stem cells leads to "conjunctivalization" of the cornea with vascularization, appearance of goblet cells, and an irregular and unstable epithelium. This results in ocular discomfort and reduced vision. Partial stem cell deficiency can be managed by removing the abnormal epithelium and allowing the denuded cornea, especially the visual axis, to resurface with cells derived from the remaining intact limbal epithelium. In total stem cell deficiency, several surgical techniques have been developed. Conjunctival transplantation procedures can be either autografts or allografts, depending on the source of donor tissue. A conjunctival autograft (CAU) uses tissue from the fellow or same eye. A conjunctival allograft can use donor tissue from a cadaver or living relative and be designated as a cadaveric conjunctival allograft (c-CAL) or living-related conjunctival allograft (lr-CAL). Limbal transplantation procedures can be subdivided based on the donor and the carrier tissue. A conjunctival limbal autograft (CLAU) uses tissue from the fellow eye, and conjunctiva is the carrier. A cadaveric conjunctival limbal allograft (c-CLAL) uses a cadaveric donor for conjunctiva and limbus. A living-related conjunctival limbal allograft (lr-CLAL) is a procedure in which a living relative donates conjunctiva and limbal tissue. A keratolimbal allograft (KLAL) utilizes a cadaveric donor, and peripheral cornea is used to transfer the limbal stem cells. With the latter option, systemic immunosuppression is required: The initial systemic immunosuppression protocol consisted of oral prednisone, cyclosporine A, and azathioprine. Later, the protocol was changed to oral prednisone, tacrolimus, and mycophenolate.

Ex vivo expanded limbal transplantation is the newest technique to provide a source of donor limbal tissue. With this technology, limbal tissue from a donor is expanded in culture before transplantation. In ex vivo expanded limbal autograft (EVELAU), the source of tissue is the patient's own limbal stem cells. In living-related ex vivo expanded limbal allograft (lr-EVELAL), the source of tissue is the limbus of a living relative.

Amniotic membrane (AM) has also been used in OSR. AM is harvested from human placenta and can be stored frozen for extended periods of time. AM provides basement membrane and can be used for conjunctival replacement or as an adjunct to limbal stem cell transplantation. This tissue provides substrate for epithelial growth without providing epithelial stem cells.

In conclusion, ocular surface transplantation has now progressed to the point of achieving a reasonable success rate even in the most severely diseased patients. Careful preoperative evaluation and postoperative management with a team approach to address not only corneal and ocular surface problems but also glaucoma and oculoplastic issues improves long-term success. Control of inflammation both pre- and postoperatively with systemic immunosuppression is imperative for the successful management of these patients. Although great strides have been achieved, significant challenges still exist. What are needed to further advance the success rate are safer systemic immunosuppression to minimize long-term effects to the patient, a better conjunctival replacement for those patients with severe conjunctival disease, and further evaluation and implementation of recipient-derived bone marrow pluripotent stem cells as a source of ocular surface tissue because rejection remains a major cause of failure.

References

1. Shimmura S, Tsubota K. Ocular surface reconstruction update. Curr Opin Ophthalmol 2002;13:213–219.
2. Nishida T. Cornea. In: Krachmer JH, Mannis MJ, Holland EJ, eds. Cornea Fundamentals of Cornea and External Disease. St. Louis: Mosby; 1997:7–10.
3. Sangwan VS. Limbal stem cells in health and disease. Biosci Rep 2001;21:385–404.
4. Davanger M, Evensen A. Role of the pericorneal structure in renewal of corneal epithelium. Nature 1971;229:560–561.
5. Cotsarelis SZ, Cheng G, Dong G, Sun TT, Lavker RM. Existence of slow-cycling limbal epithelial basal cells that can be preferentially stimulated to proliferate: implications on epithelial stem cells. Cell 1989;57:201–209.
6. Cotsarelis G, Dong G, Sun TT, Lavker RW. Differential response of limbal and corneal epithelia to phorbol myristate acetate [abstract]. Invest Ophthalmol Vis Sci 1987;28(suppl):1.
7. Lavker RW, Dong G, Cotsarelis G, Sun TT. Limbal basal epithelial cells display characteristics consistent with stem cells from various stratifying epithelia. Invest Ophthalmol Vis Sci 1938;29(suppl):191.
8. Schermer A, Galvin S, Sun TT. Differentiation-related expression of a major 64K corneal keratin in vivo and in culture suggests limbal location of corneal epithelial stem cells. J Cell Biol 1986;103:49–62.
9. Ebato B, Friend J, Thoft RA. Comparison of limbal and peripheral human corneal epithelium in tissue culture. Invest Ophthalmol Vis Sci 1988;29:1533–1537.
10. Lindberg K, Brown ME, Chaves HV, Kenyon KR, Rheinwald JG. In vitro propagation of human ocular surface epithelial cells for transplantation. Invest Ophthalmol Vis Sci 1993;34:2672–2679.
11. Pellegrini G, Golisano O, Paterna P, et al. Location and clonal analysis of stem cells and their differentiated progeny in the human ocular surface. J Cell Biol 1999;145:769–782.
12. Chen JJ, Tseng SC. Abnormal corneal epithelial wound healing in partial-thickness removal of limbal epithelium. Invest Ophthalmol Vis Sci 1991;32:2219–2233.
13. Huang AJ, Tseng SC. Corneal epithelial wound healing in the absence of limbal epithelium. Invest Ophthalmol Vis Sci 1991;32:96–105.
14. Puangsricharern V, Tseng SC. Cytologic evidence of corneal diseases with limbal stem cell deficiency. Ophthalmology 1995;102:1476–1485.
15. Kruse FE, Chen JJ, Tsai RJ, Tseng SC. Conjunctival transdifferentiation is due to the incomplete removal of limbal basal epithelium. Invest Ophthalmol Vis Sci 1990;31:1903–1913.
16. Pellegrini G. Changing the cell source in cell therapy. N Engl J Med 2004;35:1170–1172.
17. Chen WY, Mui MM, Kao WW, Liu CY, Tseng SC. Conjunctival epithelial cells do not transdifferentiate in organotypic cultures: expression of K12 keratin is restricted to corneal epithelium. Curr Eye Res 1994;13:765–778.
18. Dua HS. The conjunctiva in corneal epithelial wound healing. Br J Ophthalmol 1998;82:1407–1411.
19. Tseng SC, Hirst LW, Farazdaghi M, Green WR. Goblet cell density and vascularization during conjunctival transdifferentiation. Invest Ophthalmol Vis Sci 1984;25:1168–1176.
20. Kenyon KR, Tseng SC. Limbal autograft transplantation for ocular surface disorders. Ophthalmology 1989;96:709–722.
21. Dua HS. Stem cells of the ocular surface. Scientific principles and clinical applications. Br J Ophthalmol 1995;79:968–969.
22. Schermer A, Galvin S, Sunday TT. Differentiation-related expression of a major 64K corneal keratin in vivo and in culture suggests limbal location of corneal epithelial stem cells. J Cell Biol 1986;103:49–62
23. Tsubota K, Goto E, Fujita H, et al. Treatment of dry eye by autologous serum application in Sjogren's syndrome. Br J Ophthalmol 1999;83:390–395.
24. Tsubota K, Goto E, Shimmura S, et al. Treatment of persistent corneal epithelial defect by autologous serum application. Ophthalmology 1999;106:1984–1989.

25. Kim JC, Tseng SCG. Transplantation of preserved human amniotic membrane for surface reconstruction in severely damaged rabbit corneas. Cornea 1995;14:472–484.
26. Tsubota K, Satake Y, Kaido M, et al. Treatment of severe ocular-surface disorders with corneal epithelial stem-cell transplantation. N Engl J Med 1999;340:1697–1703.
27. Holland E, Schwartz G. Changing concepts in the management of severe ocular surface disease over twenty-five years. Cornea 2000;19:688–698.
28. Mejia LF, Acosta C, Santamaria JP. Use of non preserved human amniotic membrane for the reconstruction of the ocular surface. Cornea 2000;19:288–291.
29. Tseng SCG, Prabhasawat P, Barton K, Gray T, Meller D. Amniotic membrane transplantation with or without limbal allografts for corneal surface reconstruction in patients with limbal stem cell deficiency. Arch Ophthalmol 1998;116:431–441.
30. Lee SH, Tseng SCG. Amniotic membrane transplantation for persistent epithelial defects with ulceration. Am J Ophthalmol 1997;123:303–312.
31. Chen HJ, Pires RT, Tseng SC. Amniotic membrane transplantation for severe neurotrophic corneal ulcers. Br J Ophthalmol 2000;84:826–833.
32. Kruse FE, Rohrschneider K, Volcker HE. Multilayer amniotic membrane transplantation for reconstruction of deep corneal ulcers. Ophthalmology 1999;106:1504–1511.
33. Cho BJ, Djalilian AR, Obritsch WF, Matteson DM, Chan CC, Holland EJ. Conjunctival epithelial cells cultured on human amniotic membrane fail to transdifferentiate into corneal epithelial-type cells. Cornea 1999;18:216–224.
34. Meller D, Tseng SCG. Conjunctival epithelial cell differentiation on amniotic membrane. Invest Ophthalmol Vis Sci 1999;40:879–886.
35. Koizumi N, Inatomi T, Quantock AJ, Fullwood N J, Dota A, Kinoshita S. Amniotic membrane as a substrate for cultivating limbal corneal epithelial cells for autologous transplantation in rabbits. Cornea 2000;19:65–71.
36. Koizumi N, Fullwood NJ, Bairaktaris G, Inatomi T, Kinoshita S, Quantock AJ. Cultivation of corneal epithelial cells on intact and denuded human amniotic membrane. Invest Ophthalmol Vis Sci 2000;41:2506–2513.
37. Tseng SCG, Li DQ, Ma X. Suppression of transforming growth factor isoforms, TGF-β receptor II, and myofibroblast differentiation in cultured human corneal and limbal fibroblasts by amniotic membrane matrix. J Cell Physiol 1999;179:325–335.
38. Schwab IR. Cultured corneal epithelia for ocular surface disease. Trans Am Ophthalmol Soc 1999;97:891–986.
39. Lee SB, Li DQ, Tan DTH, Meller D, Tseng SCG. Suppression of TGF-β signaling in both normal conjunctival fibroblasts and pterygial body fibroblasts by amniotic membrane. Curr Eye Res 2000;20:325–334.
40. Tseng SCG, Prabhasawat P, Lee SH. Amniotic membrane transplantation for conjunctival surface reconstruction. Am J Ophthalmol 1997;124:765–774.
41. Azuara-Blanco A, Pillai CT, Dua, HS. Amniotic membrane transplantation for ocular surface reconstruction. Br J Ophthalmol 1999;8339:399–402.
42. Prabhasawat P, Barton K, Burkett G, Tseng SCG. Comparison of conjunctival autografts, amniotic membrane grafts and primary closure for pterygium excision. Ophthalmology 1997;104:974–985.
43. Shimazaki J, Shinozaki N, Tsubota K. Transplantation of amniotic membrane and limbal autograft for patients with recurrent pyterygium associated with symblepharon. Br J Ophthalmol 1998;82:235–240.
44. Kim JC, Lee D, Shyn KH. Clinical uses of human amniotic membrane for ocular surface diseases. In: Lass JH, ed. Advances in Corneal Research. New York: Plenum Press; 1997:117–134.
45. Solomon A, Pires RTF, Tseng SCG. Amniotic membrane transplantation after extensive removal of primary and recurrent pterygia. Ophthalmology 2001;108:449–460.
46. Ma DHK, See LC, Liau SB, Tsai RJF. Amniotic membrane graft for primary pterygium: comparison with conjunctival autograft and topical mitomycin C treatment. Br J Ophthalmol 2000;84:973–978.
47. Wang MX, Gray TB, Park WC, et al. Reduction in corneal haze and apoptosis is reduced by amniotic membrane matrix in excimer laser protoablation in rabbits. J Cataract Refract Surg 2001;27:310–319.
48. Park WC, Tseng SCG. Modulation of acute inflammation and keratocyte death by suturing, blood and amniotic membrane in PRK. Invest Ophthalmol Vis Sci 2000;41:2906–2914.
49. Koizumi N, Inatomi T, Sotozono C, Fullwood NJ, Quantock AJ, Kinoshita S. Growth factor mRNA and protein in preserved human amniotic membrane. Curr Eye Res 2000;20:173–177.
50. Kim JS, Kim JC, Na BK, Jeong JM, Song CY. Amniotic membrane patching promotes healing and inhibits proteinase activity on wound healing following acute corneal alkali burn. Exp Eye Res 2000;70:329–337.
51. Kim JC, Tseng SCG. The effects of inhibition of corneal neovascularization after human amniotic membrane transplantation in severely damaged rabbit corneas. Korean J Ophthalmol 9:32–46.
52. Tsubota K, Satake Y, Ohyama M, et al. Surgical reconstruction of the ocular surface in advanced ocular cicatricial pemphigoid and Stevens-Johnson syndrome. Am J Ophthalmol 1996;122:38–52.
53. Shimazaki J, Yang HY, Tsubota K. Amniotic membrane transplantation of ocular surface reconstruction in patients with chemical and thermal burns. Ophthalmology 1997;104:2068–2076.
54. Tsubota K, Satake Y, Kaido M, et al. Treatment of severe ocular surface disorders with corneal epithelial stem-cell transplantation. N Engl J Med 1999;340:1697–1703.
55. Tsubota K, Shimazaki J. Surgical treatment of children blinded by Stevens-Johnson syndrome. Am J Ophthalmol 1999;128:573–581.
56. Prabhasawat P, Tseng SCG. Impression cytology study of epithelial phenotype of ocular surface reconstructed by preserved human amniotic membrane. Arch Ophthalmol 1997;115:1360–1367.
57. Meller D, Maskin SL, Pires RTF, Tseng SCG. Amniotic membrane transplantation for symptomatic conjunctivochalasis refractory to medical treatments. Cornea 2000;19:796–803.
58. Su CY, Lin CP. Combined use of an amniotic membrane and tissue adhesive in treating corneal perforation: a case report. Ophthalmic Surg Lasers 2000;31:151–154.

59. Duchesne B, Tahi H, Galand A. Use of human fibrin glue and amniotic membrane transplant in corneal perforation. Cornea 2001;20:230–232.
60. Anderson DF, Ellies P, Pires RT, Tseng SC. Amniotic membrane transplantation for partial limbal stem cell deficiency. Br J Ophthalmol 2001;85:567–575.
61. Anderson DF, Prabhasawat P, Alfonso E, Tseng SC. Amniotic membrane transplantation after the primary surgical management of band keratopathy. Cornea 2001;20:354–361.
62. Kwon YS, Song YS, Kim JC. New treatment for band keratopathy: superficial lamellar keratectomy, EDTA chelation and amniotic membrane transplantation. J Korean Med Sci 2004;19:611–615.
63. Choi YS, Kim JY, Wee WR, Lee JH. Effect of the application of human amniotic membrane on rabbit corneal wound healing after excimer laser photorefractive keratectomy. Cornea 1998;17:389–395.
64. Lee HK, Kim JK, Kim EK, Kim GO, Lee IS. Phototherapeutic keratectomy with amniotic membrane for severe subepithelial fibrosis following excimer laser refractive surgery. J Cataract Refract Surg 2003l;29:1430–1435.
65. Kim JS, Kim JC, Na BK, Jeong JM, Song CY. Amniotic membrane patching promotes healing and inhibits protease activity on wound healing following acute corneal alkali burns. Exp Eye Res 1948;70:329–337.
66. Meller D, Pires RT, Mack RJ, et al. Amniotic membrane transplantation for acute chemical or thermal burns. Ophthalmology 2000;107:980–990.
67. Hanada K, Shimazaki J, Shimmura S, et al. Multilayered amniotic membrane transplantation for severe ulceration of the cornea and sclera. Ophthalmology 2001;131:324–331.
68. Tsai RJF, Li LM, Chen JK. Reconstruction of damaged corneas by transplantation of autologous limbal epithelial cells. N Engl J Med 2000;343:86–93.
69. Schwab IR, Reyes M, Isseroff RR. Successful transplantation of bioengineered tissue replacements in patients with ocular surface disease. Cornea 2000;19:421–426.
70. Dua HS, Azuara-Blanco A. Autologous limbal transplantation in patients with unilateral corneal stem cell deficiency. Br J Ophthalmol 2000;84:273–278.
71. Nuijts RM. Autologous limbal transplantation in unilateral chemical burns. Doc Ophthalmol 1999;98:257–266.
72. Gris O, Guell JL, del Campo Z. Limbal-conjunctival autograft transplantation for the treatment of recurrent pterygium. Ophthalmology 2000;107:270–273.
73. Rao SK, Rajagopal R, Sitalakshmi G, et al. Limbal allografting from related live donors for corneal surface reconstruction. Ophthalmology 1999;106:822–828.
74. Rao SK, Rajagopal R, Sitalakshmi G, Padmanabhan P. Limbal allografting from related live donors for corneal surface reconstruction. Ophthalmology 1999;106:822–828.
75. Daya SM, Ilari FA. Living related conjunctival limbal allograft for the treatment of stem cell deficiency. Ophthalmology 2001;108:126–133.
76. Chen JJ, Tseng SCG. Corneal epithelial wound healing in partial limbal deficiency. Invest Ophthalmol Vis Sci 1990;31:1301–1314.
77. Tan DTH, Ficker LA, Buckley RJ. Limbal transplantation. Ophthalmology 1996;103:29–36.
78. Turgeon PW, Nauheim RC, Roat MI, et al: Indications for keratoepithelioplasty. Arch Ophthalmol 1990;108:233–236.
79. Kwitko S, Marinho D, Barcaro S, et al. Allograft conjunctival transplantation for bilateral ocular surface disorders. Ophthalmology 1995;102:1020–1025.
80. Weise RA, Mannis MJ, Vastine DW, et al. Conjunctival transplantation. Autologous and homologous grafts. Arch Ophthalmol 1985;103:1736–1740.
81. Pfister RR. Corneal stem cell disease: concepts, categorization, and treatment by auto- and homotransplantation of limbal stem cells. CLAO J 1994;20:64–72.
82. Thoft RA. Keratoepithelioplasty. Am J Ophthalmol 1984;97:1–6.
83. Tsai RJF, Tseng SCG. Human allograft limbal transplantation for corneal surface reconstruction. Cornea 1994;13:389–400.
84. Tsubota K, Toda I, Saito H, et al. Reconstruction of the corneal epithelium by limbal allograft transplantation for severe ocular surface disorders. Ophthalmology 1995;102:1486–1496.
85. Tsubota K, Satake Y, Ohyama M, et al. Surgical reconstruction of the ocular surface in advanced ocular cicatricial pemphigoid and Stevens-Johnson syndrome. Am J Ophthalmol 1996;122:38–52.
86. Kinoshita S, Ohashi Y, Ohji M, Manabe R. Long-term results of keratoepithelioplasty in Mooren's ulcer. Ophthalmology 1991;98:438–445.
87. Holland EJ, Schwartz GS. The evolution of epithelial transplantation for severe ocular surface disease and a proposed classification system. Cornea 1996;15:549–556.
88. Tsubota K, Satake Y, Kaido M, et al. Stem cell transplantation of corneal epithelium for the treatment of severe ocular surface disorders. N Engl J Med 1999;340:1697–1703.
89. Shimmura S, Ando M, Shimazaki J, et al. Complications with one-piece lamellar keratolimbal grafts for simultaneous limbal and corneal pathologies. Cornea 2000;19:439–442.
90. Ilari L, Daya SM. Long-term outcomes of keratolimbal allograft for the treatment of severe ocular surface disorders. Ophthalmology 2002;109:1278–1284.
91. Holland EJ, Schwartz GS. Epithelial stem-cell transplantation for severe ocular-surface disease. N Engl J Med 1999;340:1752–1753.
92. Daya SM, Ilari L. Living related conjunctival limbal allograft (lrCLAL) for the treatment of stem cell deficiency. Ophthalmology 2001;108:126–133.
93. Holland EJ, Djalilian AR, Schwartz GS. Management of aniridic keratopathy with keratolimbal allograft: a limbal stem cell transplantation technique. Ophthalmology 2003;110:125–130.
94. Daya SM, Bell RW, Habib NE, et al. Clinical and pathologic findings in human keratolimbal allograft rejection. Cornea 2000;19:443–450.
95. Shimazaki J, Maruyama F, Shimmura S, et al. Immunologic rejection of the central graft after limbal allograft transplantation combined with penetrating keratoplasty. Cornea 2001;20:149–152.
96. Tseng SCG, Chen JJY, Huang AJW, et al. Classification of conjunctival surgeries for corneal disease based on stem cell concept. Ophthalmol Clin North Am 1990;3:595–610.
97. Holland EJ, Schwartz GS. The Paton lecture: ocular surface transplantation – 10 years' experience. Cornea 2004;23:425–431.

98. Rheinwald JG, Green H. Serial cultivation of strains of human epidermal keratinocytes: the formation of keratinizing colonies from single cells. Cell 1975;6:331–343.
99. Lindberg K, Brown ME, Chaves HV, Kenyon KR, Rheinwald JG. In vitro propagation of human ocular surface epithelial cells for transplantation. Invest Ophthalmol Vis Sci 1993;34:2672–2679.
100. Pellegrini G, Traverso CE, Franzi AT, Zingirian M, Cancedda R, De Luca M. Long-term restoration of damaged corneal surfaces with autologous cultivated human epithelium. Lancet 1997;349:990–993.
101. James SE, Rowe A, Ilari L, Daya S, Martin R. The potential for eye bank limbal rings to generate cultured corneal epithelial allografts. Cornea. 2001;20:488–494.
102. Tseng SC, Prabhasawat P, Barton K, Gray T, Meller D. Amniotic membrane transplantation with or without limbal allografts for corneal surface reconstruction in patients with limbal stem cell deficiency. Arch Ophthalmol 1998;116:431–441.
103. Sunday L, Sunday TT, Lavker RM. CLED: a calcium-linked protein associated with early epithelial differentiation. Exp Cell Res 2000;259:96–106.
104. Pellegrini G, Dellambra E, Golisano O, et al. p63 identifies keratinocyte stem cells. Proc Natl Acad Sci USA 2001;98:3156–3161.
105. Koizumi N, Inatomi T, Suzuki T, et al. Cultivated corneal epithelial stem cell transplantation in ocular surface disorders. Ophthalmology 2001;108:1569–1574.
106. Griffith M, Osborne R, Munger R, et al. Functional human corneal equivalents constructed from cell lines. Science 1999,286:2169–2172.

Section 6

Pancreas

Section 6

Pancreas

Shimon Efrat

The pancreas is composed of two main cell populations: The majority of the pancreas is made up of acinar cells, which produce and release digestive enzymes into the gastrointestinal tract. Approximately 1% of the pancreas consists of the islets of Langerhans, including four cell types that are in charge of endocrine regulation of carbohydrate homeostasis. Approximately 80% of the islet cells are insulin-producing β cells, whereas the remainder are divided among α, δ, and pancreatic polypeptide (PP) cells, which produce glucagon, somatostatin, and pancreatic polypeptide, respectively. The most common disorder associated with failure of pancreatic function is diabetes. Type 1 (insulin-dependent) diabetes afflicts approximately 0.5% of the world population. It is caused by an autoimmune destruction of pancreatic islet β cells, resulting in an absolute insulin deficiency. Treatment of type 1 diabetes has not changed much since the discovery of insulin more than 80 years ago. Insulin administration cannot mimic the tightly regulated physiological release of the hormone, resulting in episodes of hypoglycemia and hyperglycemia. The latter are responsible in the long run for microvascular complications, resulting in failure of key organs, morbidity, and mortality. Type 2 diabetes, which is 10-fold more common than type 1, and its incidence is increasing in epidemic proportions as the result of modern lifestyle, is caused by peripheral insulin resistance, coupled with an eventual failure to compensate for it by increased insulin production. Approximately 40% of patients with type 2 diabetes require exogenous insulin administration.

The efforts to preserve or restore normal β-cell function in type 1 diabetes have centered on three approaches: Prevention, regeneration, and transplantation. Prevention of islet damage is difficult, because overt hyperglycemia is manifested when more than 90% of the β cells are destroyed. There are a number of genetic and serologic markers, but at present they do not provide a high degree of confidence in diagnosis of people predisposed to develop the disease. Even if early detection were possible, intervention approaches for preventing the autoimmune islet damage are in an early stage of development in animal models and still far from clinical application.

The adult pancreas is made up primarily of postmitotic cells with a slow turnover rate under normal circumstances. However, as described in the chapter by Bonner-Weir et al., it maintains a considerable regeneration capacity. This is manifested in animal models of partial pancreatectomy, and in physiological conditions such as pregnancy and obesity, which involve a large increase in the islet mass. Although the cells responsible for this increase have not been clearly identified, a major goal of diabetes research is learning to utilize this capacity to stimulate islet regeneration in type 1 diabetes. It is quite likely that newly formed islets, whether by physiological or induced mechanisms, would be targeted by recurring autoimmunity. Therefore, this approach must be coupled with manipulation of the immune system to prevent destruction of regenerated islets.

Immunologic issues are a major barrier also for pancreas and islet transplantation. Pancreas transplantation is quite successful, but requires continuous immunosuppression. Islet transplantation has met with greater difficulties. Although it involves a simpler surgical procedure, its success rate is lower, because of the difficulty to maintain cell function during the isolation and implantation procedures. Another possibility is a greater susceptibility of isolated islets to both immune effector mechanisms and immunosuppressive drugs, compared with intact pancreas. Even with islets from two to three donors per recipient, this loss of cell viability and function results in eventual graft failure. In addition, this donor-to-recipient ratio underscores the organ donor shortage, which has severely limited both pancreas and islet transplantation. Although xenografts remain a viable alternative to human tissue, at present this option is hindered by concerns regarding presence of infectious agents, limited physiological compatibility, and vigorous immune rejection. Thus, the search is on for an abundant source of human insulin-producing cells for transplantation.

A normal adult human pancreas contains approximately 10^9 islet cells. The need to develop an unlimited supply of human surrogate β cells has led investigators to attempt islet expansion in tissue culture, as well as differentiation of other cells into insulin-producing cells. So far, islet expansion has proven to be quite challenging, because the cells do not grow well and tend to dedifferentiate. Thus, the focus at present is on differentiation of stem cells, which can be easily expanded in vitro. Manipulation of their culture conditions, as well as the introduction of transcription factor genes capable of reprogramming cell differentiation, hold the promise of inducing stable phenotypic changes in stem cells to convert them into β-like insulin-producing cells. The chapter by Browning et al. evaluates the potential of human embryonic stem cells to be induced to preferentially differentiate into surrogate β cells. Finally, the chapter by Efrat describes efforts to utilize stem/progenitor cells already committed to other tissues, such as liver and bone marrow, in an attempt to divert their development into β-like cells, which may allow the use of autologous cells. Although the expansion capacity of stem cells may solve the quantitative limits to islet transplantation, the goal of reconstructing a complete, stable β-cell phenotype in a non-β-cell is a tall order. In particular, regulated insulin secretion, which is orchestrated in β cells by continuous integration of multiple nutrient, hormonal, and neural signals, is likely to prove a difficult feature to recreate. However, this is a must, without which cell replacement therapy will not represent an improvement over insulin administration. In addition, it is important to assure that the differentiated cells maintain a stable phenotype and do not replicate out of control after transplantation. An open question is whether transplantation of β cells, and their placement in a nonpancreatic site, is sufficient, or whether intact islets or pancreas are needed for proper function. As in the case of pancreas and islet transplantation, transplantation of β-like cells derived from stem cells will face the challenge of prevention of graft rejection and recurring autoimmunity. Despite these difficulties, the intense research efforts promise rapid progress and exciting developments in the coming years.

21

Insulin-Producing Cells Generated from Nonpancreatic Tissues

Shimon Efrat

β-Cell replacement is considered the most promising approach for long-term treatment of type 1 diabetes. However, its application on a large scale is limited by the availability of tissue donors and by recurring autoimmunity. The difficulty of expanding mature β cells and their pancreatic precursors has focused attention on the potential of generating surrogate β cells from cells of other tissues. Stem/progenitor cells, which can be propagated and differentiated in tissue culture, offer the promise of an abundant source of cells for transplantation. Recent work has demonstrated that cells from a number of nonpancreatic tissues can be induced to produce, process, and store insulin, release it in response to physiological signals, and restore euglycemia in hyperglycemic rodents. The change in cell phenotype has been achieved by ectopic expression of dominant transcription factor genes, and by exposure of the cells to specific tissue culture conditions or to differentiation signals in vivo. In addition to cell propagation and differentiation, the cultivation of surrogate β cells in vitro offers an opportunity for enhancing their resistance to immune destruction, by genetic modifications or cell encapsulation.

Type 1 (insulin-dependent) diabetes is caused by destruction of the pancreatic islet insulin-producing β cells by autoimmunity. Insulin administration does not constitute a cure of the disease, because it usually fails to prevent diabetes complications. This is attributed to the difficulty of adjusting the precise insulin dosage in response to changing physiological conditions.

Efforts for developing an insulin pump connected in a closed loop to a glucose sensor have not succeeded yet in producing a working "artificial pancreas." Restoration of a long-term tight regulation of insulin delivery by replacement of the damaged β cells with intact β cells represents the most promising approach for a future cure of type 1 diabetes. Pancreas transplantation, although quite successful, represents a rather invasive intervention, which is restricted to patients with advanced complications, requires constant immunosuppression, and is severely limited by donor availability. Recent progress in human islet isolation and in immunosuppression protocols[1] resulted in restoration of euglycemia in patients who received islets from 2–3 pancreas donors. This progress underscores the urgent need for alternative sources of human β cells.

Forced expansion of mature β cells in tissue culture by expression of oncogenes has been successful in rodents[2]; however, in human β cells, it resulted in a significant irreversible dedifferentiation.[3] The remarkable progress in stem cell biology in recent years has raised new hopes for the generation of surrogate β cells from stem/progenitor cells, which can be expanded in tissue culture with relative ease. Cells with stem cell properties have been described in the pancreatic ducts,[4,5] and in both exocrine[6] and endocrine[7] pancreas (see chapter by Bonner-Weir et al.); however, their expansion capacity has been quite limited. A recent report has challenged the notion that mature β cells can emerge in the adult from pancreatic precursors which do not express insulin.[8]

The derivation of pluripotent human embryonic stem (ES) cells,[9] and the suggestion of a broad differentiation spectrum of stem/progenitor cells from a number of fetal and adult tissues,[10-13] have opened the way for generation of surrogate β cells from nonpancreatic tissues. ES cells are capable of spontaneous differentiation into virtually all cell types, including insulin-producing cells[14,15] (see chapter by Browning et al.). In addition, they can be induced to preferentially differentiate into insulin-containing cells by tissue culture conditions[16,17] and genetic manipulations.[18,19] However, these results have been challenged by findings that the insulin content is an artifact, resulting from uptake from the culture medium. In addition, the risk of uncontrolled proliferation of residual undifferentiated ES cells, as well as the ethical controversy surrounding the use of ES cells, has prompted the evaluation of the potential of tissue stem cells for cell replacement therapy.

Expansion and Transdifferentiation of Tissue Stem Cells

A number of fetal and adult tissues[20-23] have been shown to contain stem/progenitor cells, which are responsible for normal tissue repair and renewal, and fulfill the criteria of stem cells as defined by Weissman[24]: Self-renewal, multipotency, and tissue reconstitution. The growth capacity of these cells is considered to be limited, compared with that of ES cells, and to diminish with age. Although this property restricts their utility as an abundant source of cells for transplantation, it may represent a safety advantage. In addition to a lower risk of uncontrolled proliferation, tissue stem cells offer the possibility of using autologous cells, with the likely advantage of improved graft tolerance, compared with an allograft.

The replication limit of somatic cells has been attributed to telomere shortening in the absence of telomerase reverse transcriptase (TERT) activity.[25] Activation or overexpression of TERT has been shown to be effective in extending the replication capacity of a number of human cell types,[26-28] without compromising their ability to undergo contact inhibition in culture, changing their karyotype, or increasing their neoplastic potential in vivo.[29-31] Thus, introduction of the TERT gene into tissue stem cells may extend their replication capacity in tissue culture to resemble that of ES cells. However, because TERT activation is a hallmark of many tumors, the risks of neoplasia need to be carefully evaluated in each modified cell source.

The prospect of generation of β-like cells from other cell types depends not only on the ability to induce insulin biosynthesis in non-β cells, but also on the activation in such cells of multiple additional β-cell functions, such as the correct processing of proinsulin, storage of mature insulin, and regulated insulin secretion in response to physiological signals. Using a source of cells lacking these properties would not represent a significant advantage over insulin administration.

Achieving such a profound transdifferentiation relies on the ability of tissue stem cells to undergo nuclear reprogramming in response to natural or artificial signals. Until recently, tissue stem cells were thought to be committed and therefore restricted, compared with ES cells, with respect to the number of different cell types that they can generate. In recent years, this concept has been challenged by reports demonstrating that cells from adult organs can give rise to unrelated cell types, both in vivo and in culture, in response to appropriate stimuli.[10-13] At present, the transdifferentiation potential of tissue stem cells remains poorly defined and the subject of heated debate. It is unclear whether the different reports of transdifferentiation represent: 1) The direct change of a differentiated cell type A into a differentiated cell type B; 2) dedifferentiation of a differentiated cell type A into a common progenitor cell type, followed by differentiation into cell type B; 3) de novo differentiation of pluripotent cells which persist in adult tissues; or 4) fusion of such cells with already differentiated cells (Figure 21.1). Further work using cell lineage tracing approaches is needed to distinguish among these possibilities.

Regardless of their physiological differentiation spectrum, recent work has demonstrated that cells from both fetal and adult tissues can undergo forced nuclear reprogramming in vitro under the influence of dominant transcription factor genes introduced into the cells, or after cell exposure to growth conditions and factors in the tissue culture medium, which may activate such genes endogenously. In the case of mouse pancreatic islet cells, the cascade of tran-

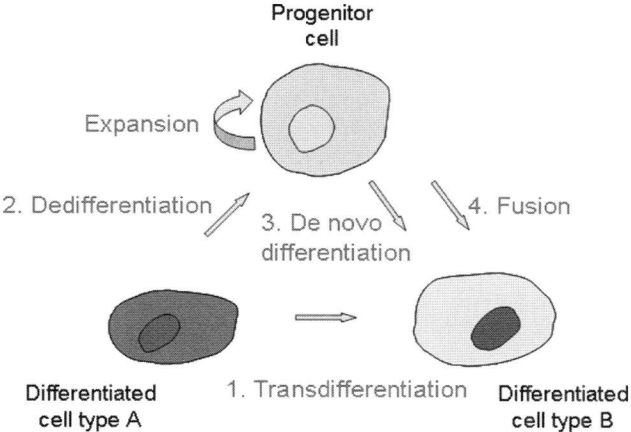

Figure 21.1. Possible pathways for generation of differentiated cells from cells derived from a different tissue. 1) True transdifferentiation of a differentiated cell type A into a differentiated cell type B; 2) dedifferentiation of a differentiated cell type A into a common progenitor cell type, followed by differentiation into cell type B; 3) de novo differentiation of pluripotent cells which persist in adult tissues; 4) fusion of pluripotent cells with already differentiated cells. [Reprinted from Efrat S. Curr Diab Rep 2004;4:298–303, with permission.]

scription factors that are responsible for endocrine pancreas development and gene expression in differentiated islets has been described in considerable detail (see references 32–34 for reviews). Some of these transcription factors may be capable of switching on the entire β-cell developmental program. They could be ectopically expressed in non-β cells using transient or stable gene transfer, or as demonstrated in the case of one factor, pancreatic duodenal homeobox 1 (Pdx1), by transduction with the protein itself.[35] Below, I will review the progress in the derivation of insulin-producing cells from three different tissues: Liver, intestine, and bone marrow (BM).

Insulin-Producing Cells Derived from Liver Cells

The developmental origin of the pancreas in the embryonic gut makes other tissues derived from the same origin, such as liver and intestine, good candidates for transdifferentiation into β-like cells. Mature hepatocytes are glucose sensitive and share similarities in gene expression with mature β cells, including the glucose transporter GLUT2 and the glucose phosphorylating enzyme glucokinase, which are involved in sensing extracellular glucose levels. In addition, hepatocytes are a primary target of insulin, which is delivered from the pancreas through the portal vein.

However, hepatocytes do not possess a regulated secretory pathway, the induction of which may represent a high hurdle for cell engineering.

Rodent liver cells have been shown to give rise to insulin-producing cells in vivo, and after genetic manipulations both in vivo and in vitro. Cells derived from mouse fetal liver differentiate in vivo into a number of hepatic, pancreatic, and intestinal cell types.[36] In addition, adult rat hepatic stem cells termed oval cells give rise to pancreatic endocrine cells in vitro.[37] Mouse[38] and Xenopus[39] liver cells were shown to activate β-cell gene expression in vivo following expression of Pdx1, a transcription factor that has key roles in pancreas development and gene expression in mature β cells. Similarly, expression of another β-cell transcription factor, NeuroD/Beta2, in mouse liver cells in vivo resulted in reversal of hyperglycemia.[40]

The isolation and propagation of human fetal liver cells[41] allowed us to evaluate the potential of these cells to be reprogrammed into insulin-producing cells by dominant transcription factors that direct the development of endocrine pancreas. These cells express markers of hepatocytes, bile duct cells, and oval cells, and are capable of differentiation into mature hepatocytes in vivo. Their replication capacity was extended by introduction of the TERT gene, without evidence for neoplastic cell transformation in either in vitro or in vivo assays.[42] We have recently shown that these cells can be induced by ectopic expression of Pdx1 to produce and store mature insulin in amounts up to a third of those produced by normal β cells, release it in response to physiological glucose levels (Figure 21.2), and replace β-cell function in streptozotocin (STZ)-treated nonobese diabetic severe combined immunodeficient (NOD-scid) mice (Figure 21.3).[43] The modified cells expressed multiple β-cell genes; however, they also activated genes expressed in other islet cells and exocrine pancreas, and continued to express some hepatic genes. Although multiple lines of evidence suggested that Pdx1 expression induced a regulated secretory pathway in the fetal liver cells, this remains to be directly demonstrated by ultrastructural and biochemical analyses. Manipulation of the culture conditions of the Pdx1-expressing human fetal liver cells was shown to further promote the differentiation of these cells toward the β-cell phenotype, as judged by gene expression and insulin content.[43]

Insulin-Producing Cells Derived from Intestine Epithelial Cells

Intestine epithelial cells, just like liver and pancreas cells, are derived from the primordial gut. In addition to sharing a common developmental origin with the pancreas, the endocrine cells in the intestine epithelium possess a regulated secretory pathway, which may allow them to store insulin and release it in response to physiological signals. Ectopic expression of Pdx1, in combination with treatment with betacellulin, a β-cell mitogenic and differentiation factor, or coexpression of another β-cell transcription factor, Isl1, in a rat enterocyte cell line, IEC-6, resulted in activation of insulin expression.[44] However, the subcellular compartment in which insulin was stored in these cells was not determined. In another study using the same cells and inductive elements, the presence of insulin

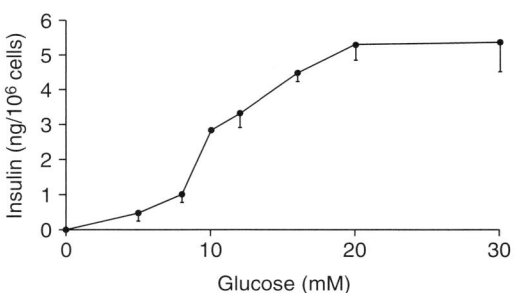

Figure 21.2. Glucose-induced insulin secretion from human fetal liver cells expressing Pdx1. Values are mean ± SEM (n = 9) of secretion during a 2-hour static incubation period. [Reprinted from Zalzman et al.,[43] with permission.]

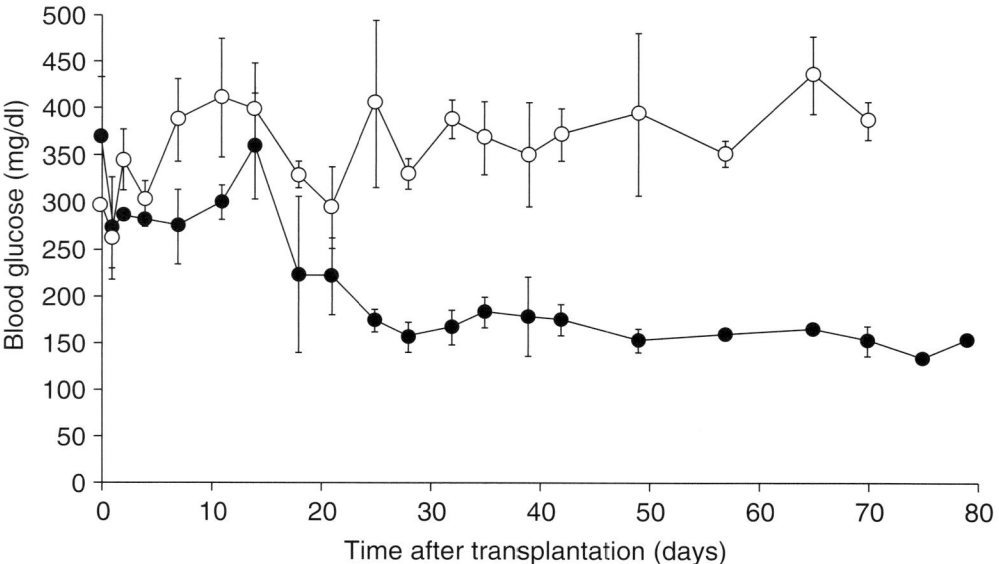

Figure 21.3. Insulin-producing cells derived from human fetal liver cells expressing Pdx1 replace β-cell function in NOD-scid mice made diabetic by STZ injection. Closed circles, transplanted mice (n = 3); open circles, untransplanted mice (n = 4). Values are mean ± SEM. The differences between the two groups were significant on days 25–70 posttransplantation ($P < 0.0001$). [Reprinted from Zalzman et al.,[43] with permission.]

secretory granules was shown by electron microscopy; however, insulin secretion was constitutive.[45] Finally, in a study utilizing primary mouse intestinal cells, insulin production was induced after treatment with glucagon-like peptide 1, which activated the expression of Ngn3, a transcription factor acting as a master regulator of endocrine pancreas development.[46] Transplantation of these cells into STZ-diabetic mice resulted in normalization of blood glucose levels 8 weeks later. This relatively long lag period suggests that additional cell differentiation and/or proliferation were required in vivo to achieve sufficient insulin production. These studies suggest that intestinal cells represent a potential cell source for development of surrogate insulin-producing cells. However, intestinal endocrine cells are quite rare, and the intestinal epithelium is not easily accessible for biopsy. Thus, realization of their potential will likely require in vivo gene targeting, or the use of allogeneic donor cells.

Insulin-Producing Cells Derived from BM

Adult BM has been shown in recent years to constitute a promising source of tissue stem cells. BM cells contain at least two types of stem cells with pluripotent capacities, hematopoietic stem cells, and stromal or mesenchymal stem cells. BM transplantation results in differentiation of the transplanted cells into a variety of ectodermal, mesodermal, and endodermal tissues, in both mice and humans.[47] Although a number of reports have challenged these results by demonstrating that they were likely caused by fusion of BM cells with differentiated cells, rather than a direct differentiation of BM cells, other rigorous studies support the wide differentiation potential of BM stem cells. It is possible that adult BM cells serve as a major source for continuous renewal of other tissue stem cells, including those in the pancreas. A recent report has suggested that insulin-positive cells, which appear in a number of tissues in STZ-treated mice, originate from BM.[48] It is possible that in patients with type 1 diabetes, the endogenous BM provides cells for continuous islet renewal; however, newly formed β cells are rapidly destroyed by autoimmunity. BM cells represent an attractive source for autologous stem cells, because they can be biopsied with relative ease.

Two studies have recently demonstrated that grafted mouse BM cells can differentiate into endocrine pancreas cells,[49] as well as induce regeneration of endogenous islets in STZ-diabetic mice.[50] Cell fusion was rigorously excluded in the first study.[49] In contrast, both Choi et al.[51] and Lechner et al.,[52] using mouse BM cells labeled with green fluorescent protein, concluded that these cells did not contribute to islet repopulation after STZ-induced damage to β cells. In addition to these in vivo models, Tang et al.[53] demonstrated that a clonal population of adult murine BM stem cells (probably mesenchymal) could be induced to differentiate in vitro into insulin-producing cells by culture in a high-glucose medium, followed by transfer to a low-glucose medium containing nicotinamide and exendin 4, two agents known to promote β-cell function. Although their insulin content was quite low, these cells were capable of correcting hyperglycemia in vivo.[53] Similar results were reported by Oh et al.,[54] using rat BM cultured under somewhat different conditions. Taken together, these studies support the potential of BM cells to differentiate into surrogate β cells. However, further work is clearly needed to determine to what extent BM-derived insulin-producing cells can mimic the function of mature β cells, as judged by the ability to store large amounts of insulin and release it in response to the array of physiological signals that regulate insulin secretion from normal β cells.

Protection of Engineered Insulin-Producing Cells from Immune Destruction

Transplanted surrogate β cells are likely to be exposed to recurring autoimmune responses, as well as to allograft rejection. Generation of insulin-producing cells from nonpancreatic tissues in tissue culture may offer a number of ways for avoiding the immune responses directed against β cells. The antigenic targets of these immune responses remain largely unknown. However, it is possible that cells induced to differentiate into insulin-producing cells will not express these antigens. Even if some of these antigens are expressed, and these cells are targeted by autoimmunity, it is possible that the cells will be more resistant to apoptosis induced by cytokines and free radicals, compared with normal β cells, which express relatively low levels of free-radical scavenging enzymes. Moreover, propagation of these cells in tissue culture provides an opportunity for increasing their resistance to immune responses, by introduction of antiapoptotic genes (reviewed in reference 55), or by cell encapsulation in semipermeable membrane devices.[56]

Future Prospects

The difficulty of expanding mature β cells or their pancreatic precursors has forced investigators to explore the potential of cells from other tissues, which can be more readily obtained and expanded, to develop into surrogate β cells. The ability to induce the key properties of β cells in cells from other tissues by several genetic and/or epigenetic manipulations has been confirmed by work in recent years. Cells from a number of tissues were capable of acquiring the ability to produce, process, and store large amounts of insulin, release it in response to physiological signals, and replace β-cell function in rodents. In most cases, the precise identity of the cells that acquired the β-cell phenotype remained unknown. One possibility is that these were differentiated cells that transdifferentiated directly into insulin-producing cells. In some cases, the modified cells were shown to maintain part of the properties associated with their original phenotype.[43] Alternatively, the transdifferentiation process may involve dedifferentiation of differentiated cells into a progenitor cell type, which is then induced to differentiate into insulin-producing cells. Another possibility is that the documented cases of transdifferentiation into insulin-producing cells reflect the presence of pluripotent stem cells in these tissues, which undergo de novo differentiation in response to appropriate signals, or that of tissue-restricted multipotent progenitor cells common to tissues that share a developmental origin with the pancreas. If the former is correct, cells capable of differentiation into β-like cells may not be restricted to tissues derived from the primordial gut, and may also be found in tissues from mesodermal or ectodermal origin. The ability of BM cells to differentiate into insulin-producing cells supports this possibility. Such pluripotent stem cells are likely to be more abundant in fetal tissues, compared with adult tissues. However, the use of fetal tissue raises ethical reservations, and may preclude the use of autologous cells.

The use of autologous versus allogeneic cells remains an open question. The relative efficiency of recurring autoimmunity against insulin-producing cells derived from autologous tissues, compared with that against allogeneic surrogate β cells, is unknown. The decision on the optimal approach will eventually depend on the manipulations required to induce differentiation of non-β cells into surrogate β cells. Manipulations that can be performed in vivo will increase the attractiveness of autologous cells. In contrast, the need for genetic manipulations, which cannot be safely performed in vivo, and may compromise the chromosomal integrity of the cells even when performed ex vivo, will increase the appeal of a universal donor allograft, which can be thoroughly characterized in tissue culture, banked to serve a large number of recipients, and be more readily rejected in case of a failure. Finally, if the manipulations involve complex gene transfer and quality-control procedures, their application to cells from each patient may be prohibitively difficult and expensive.

Although much work clearly remains to be done, the potential of generating insulin-producing cells from various tissues has already been established. This approach is likely to advance the prospects of cell therapy for type 1 diabetes in the not too distant future.

Acknowledgment

Work in my laboratory was funded by the Israel Science Foundation, the National Institutes of Health, and the Juvenile Diabetes Research Foundation International.

References

1. Shapiro AM, Lakey JR, Ryan EA, et al. Islet transplantation in seven patients with type 1 diabetes mellitus using a glucocorticoid-free immunosuppressive regimen. N Engl J Med 2000;343:230–238.
2. Milo-Landesman D, Berkovich I, Surana M, et al. Correction of hyperglycemia in diabetic mice transplanted with reversibly-immortalized pancreatic β cells

controlled by the tet-on regulatory system. Cell Transplant 2001;10:645–650.
3. de la Tour D, Halvorsen T, Demeterco C, et al. Beta-cell differentiation from a human pancreatic cell line in vitro and in vivo. Mol Endocrinol 2001;5:476–483.
4. Bonner-Weir S, Taneja M, Weir GC, et al. In vitro cultivation of human islets from expanded ductal tissue. Proc Natl Acad Sci USA 2000;97:7999–8004.
5. Ramiya VK, Maraist M, Arfors KE, et al. Reversal of insulin-dependent diabetes using islets generated in vitro from pancreatic stem cells. Nat Med 2000;6:278–282.
6. Rooman I, Lardon J, Bouwens L. Gastrin stimulates beta-cell neogenesis and increases islet mass from transdifferentiated but not from normal exocrine pancreas tissue. Diabetes 2002;51:686–690.
7. Abraham EJ, Leech CA, Lin JC, Zulewski H, Habener JF. Insulinotropic hormone glucagon-like peptide-1 differentiation of human pancreatic islet-derived progenitor cells into insulin-producing cells. Endocrinology 2002;143:3152–3161.
8. Dor Y, Brown J, Martinez OI, Melton DA. Adult pancreatic β-cells are formed by self-duplication rather than stem-cell differentiation. Nature 2004;429:41–46.
9. Thomson JA, Itskovitz-Eldor J, Shapiro SS, et al. Embryonic stem cell lines derived from human blastocysts. Science 1998;282:1145–1147.
10. Wagers AJ, Weissman IL. Plasticity of adult stem cells. Cell 2004;116:639–648.
11. Tosh D, Slack JM. How cells change their phenotype. Nat Rev Mol Cell Biol 2002;3:187–194.
12. Wagers AJ, Weissman IL. Plasticity of adult stem cells. Cell 2004;116:639–648.
13. Fuchs E, Tumbar T, Guasch G. Socializing with the neighbors: stem cells and their niche. Cell 2004;116:769–778.
14. Soria B, Roche E, Berna G, Leon-Quinto T, Reig JA, Martin F. Insulin-secreting cells derived from embryonic stem cells normalize glycemia in streptozotocin-induced diabetic mice. Diabetes 2000;49:157–162.
15. Assady S, Maor G, Amit M, Itskovitz-Eldor J, Skorecki KL, Tzukerman M. Insulin production by human embryonic stem cells. Diabetes 2001;50:1691–1697.
16. Lumelsky N, Blondel O, Laeng P, Velasco I, Ravin R, McKay R. Differentiation of embryonic stem cells to insulin-secreting structures similar to pancreatic islets. Science 2001;292:1389–1394.
17. Segev H, Fishman B, Ziskind A, Shulman M, Itskovitz-Eldor J. Differentiation of human embryonic stem cells into insulin-producing clusters. Stem Cells 2004;22:265–274.
18. Blyszczuk P, Czyz J, Kania G, et al. Expression of Pax4 in embryonic stem cells promotes differentiation of nestin-positive progenitor and insulin-producing cells. Proc Natl Acad Sci USA 2003;100:998–1003.
19. Miyazaki S, Yamato E, Miyazaki J. Regulated expression of pdx-1 promotes in vitro differentiation of insulin-producing cells from embryonic stem cells. Diabetes 2004;53:1030–1037.
20. Osawa M, Hanada K, Hamada H, Nakauchi H. Long-term lymphohematopoietic reconstitution by a single CD34-low/negative hematopoietic stem cell. Science 1996;273:242–245.
21. Gage FH. Mammalian neural stem cells. Science 2000;287:1433–1438.
22. Prockop DJ. Marrow stromal cells as stem cells for nonhematopoietic tissues. Science 1997;276:71–74.
23. Watt FM. Stem cell fate and patterning in mammalian epidermis. Curr Opin Genet Dev 2001;11:410–417.
24. Weissman IL. Translating stem and progenitor cell biology to the clinic: barriers and opportunities. Science 2000;287:1442–1446.
25. Harley CB, Futcher AB, Greider CW. Telomeres shorten during ageing of human fibroblasts. Nature 1990;345:458–460.
26. Bodnar AG, Ouellette M, Frolkis M, et al. Extension of life-span by introduction of telomerase into normal human cells. Science 1998;279:349–352.
27. Vaziri H, Benchimol S. Reconstitution of telomerase activity in normal human cells leads to elongation of telomeres and extended replicative life span. Curr Biol 1998;8:279–282.
28. Yang J, Chang E, Cherry AM, et al. Human endothelial cell life extension by telomerase expression. J Biol Chem 1999;274:26141–26148.
29. Jiang XR, Jimenez G, Chang E, et al. Telomerase expression in human somatic cells does not induce changes associated with a transformed phenotype. Nat Genet 1999;21:111–114.
30. Morales CP, Holt SE, Ouellette M, et al. Absence of cancer-associated changes in human fibroblasts immortalized with telomerase. Nat Genet 1999;21:115–118.
31. Harley CB. Telomerase is not an oncogene. Oncogene 2002;2:494–502.
32. Huang HP, Tsai MJ. Transcription factors involved in pancreatic islet development. J Biomed Sci 2000;7:27–34.
33. Kim SK, MacDonald RJ. Signaling and transcriptional control of pancreatic organogenesis. Curr Opin Genet Dev 2002;12:540–547.
34. Servitja JM, Ferrer J. Transcriptional networks controlling pancreatic development and beta cell function. Diabetologia 2004;47:597–613.
35. Noguchi H, Kaneto H, Weir GC, Bonner-Weir S. PDX-1 protein containing its own antennapedia-like protein transduction domain can transduce pancreatic duct and islet cells. Diabetes 2003;52:1732–1737.
36. Suzuki A, Zheng YW, Kaneko S, et al. Clonal identification and characterization of self-renewing pluripotent stem cells in the developing liver. J Cell Biol 2002;156:173–184.
37. Yang L, Li S, Hatch H, Ahrens K, et al. In vitro transdifferentiation of adult hepatic stem cells into pancreatic endocrine hormone-producing cells. Proc Natl Acad Sci USA 2002;99:8078–8083.
38. Ferber S, Halkin A, Cohen H, et al. Pancreatic and duodenal homeobox gene 1 induces expression of insulin genes in liver and ameliorates streptozotocin-induced hyperglycemia. Nat Med 2000;6:568–572.
39. Horb ME, Shen CN, Tosh D, Slack JM. Experimental conversion of liver to pancreas. Curr Biol 2003;13:105–115.
40. Kojima H, Fujimiya M, Matsumura K, et al. NeuroD-betacellulin gene therapy induces islet neogenesis in the liver and reverses diabetes in mice. Nat Med 2003;9:596–603.
41. Malhi H, Irani AN, Gagandeep S, Gupta S. Isolation of human progenitor liver epithelial cells with extensive replication capacity and differentiation into mature hepatocytes. J Cell Sci 2002;115:2679–2688.

42. Wege H, Le HT, Chui MS, et al. Telomerase reconstitution immortalizes human fetal hepatocytes without disrupting their differentiation potential. Gastroenterology 2003;124:432–444.
43. Zalzman M, Gupta S, Giri R, et al. Reversal of hyperglycemia in mice by using human expandable insulin-producing cells differentiated from fetal liver progenitor cells. Proc Natl Acad Sci USA 2003;100:7253–7258.
44. Kojima H, Nakamura T, Fujita Y, et al. Combined expression of pancreatic duodenal homeobox 1 and islet factor 1 induces immature enterocytes to produce insulin. Diabetes 2002;51:1398–1408.
45. Yoshida S, Kajimoto Y, Yasuda T, et al. PDX-1 induces differentiation of intestinal epithelioid IEC-6 into insulin-producing cells. Diabetes 2002;51:2505–2513.
46. Suzuki A, Nakauchi H, Taniguchi H. Glucagon-like peptide 1 (1-37) converts intestinal epithelial cells into insulin-producing cells. Proc Natl Acad Sci USA 2003;100:5034–5039.
47. Jiang Y, Jahagirdar BN, Reinhardt RL, et al. Pluripotency of mesenchymal stem cells derived from adult marrow. Nature 2002;418:41–49.
48. Kojima H, Fujimiya M, Matsumura K, et al. Extrapancreatic insulin-producing cells in multiple organs in diabetes. Proc Natl Acad Sci USA 2004;101:2458–2463.
49. Ianus A, Holz GG, Theise ND, Hussain MA. In vivo derivation of glucose-competent pancreatic endocrine cells from bone marrow without evidence of cell fusion. J Clin Invest 2003;111:843–850.
50. Hess D, Li L, Martin M, et al. Bone marrow-derived stem cells initiate pancreatic regeneration. Nat Biotechnol 2003;21:763–770.
51. Choi JB, Uchino H, Azuma K, et al. Little evidence of transdifferentiation of bone marrow-derived cells into pancreatic beta cells. Diabetologia 2003;46:1366–1374.
52. Lechner A, Yang YG, Blacken RA, Wang L, Nolan AL, Habener JF. No evidence for significant transdifferentiation of bone marrow into pancreatic beta-cells in vivo. Diabetes 2004;53:616–623.
53. Tang DQ, Cao LZ, Burkhardt BR, et al. In vivo and in vitro characterization of insulin-producing cells obtained from murine bone marrow. Diabetes 2004;53:1721–1732.
54. Oh SH, Muzzonigro TM, Bae SH, LaPlante JM, Hatch HM, Petersen BE. Adult bone marrow-derived cells trans-differentiating into insulin-producing cells for the treatment of type I diabetes. Lab Invest 2004;84:607–617.
55. Efrat S. Cell replacement therapy for type 1 diabetes. Trends Mol Med 2002;8:334–339.
56. Duvivier-Kali VF, Omer A, Parent RJ, O'Neil JJ, Weir GC. Complete protection of islets against allorejection and autoimmunity by a simple barium-alginate membrane. Diabetes 2001;50:1698–1705.

22

Generation of Islets from Pancreatic Progenitor Cells

Susan Bonner-Weir, Tandy Aye, Akari Inada, Elena Toschi, and Arun Sharma

Diabetes, whether autoimmune type 1 or type 2, results from an inadequate supply of insulin-producing β cells. Transplantation of islets isolated from cadaver pancreata has become more successful with new protocols and immunosuppressive drugs.[1,2] However, new sources of insulin-producing cells must become available to extend β-cell replacement therapy to more of the thousands of patients with diabetes. Because the β cell is the cell lacking in diabetes, it is generally assumed that the replacement of just the β cell may be sufficient, but clear evidence is still lacking.

As late as two decades ago, it was still commonly thought that one was born with all the β cells that one ever had; however, it has become clear that the mass of pancreatic β cells is dynamic and is regulated in an effort to maintain euglycemia.[3–5] A number of in vivo models have provided evidence that there is a cell renewal process (both replication and neogenesis) that occurs at low levels in normal adult rodents and can be stimulated greatly by experimental conditions. This latter case is what should be considered regeneration; it is likely, but still needs rigorous evidence, that normal growth and regeneration in response to injury or to increased stimulation involve the same progenitor cells and the same pathways. Understanding the regulation of the normal process may lead to new therapies for diabetes that involve generation of new islets either in vitro for transplantation or in vivo by stimulation of the endogenous pancreas. We will use replication to indicate the mitotic division of a cell already with a β cell phenotype and neogenesis to indicate the formation of new β cells from either progenitor or stem cells.

Normal Growth

Islet mass increases more than 20-fold from the newborn to the adult, but the volume of islet tissue relative to that of the pancreas decreases from birth to adulthood.[6,7] The relation of β cell mass and age through life in the Sprague-Dawley rat can be represented by a simple mass model equation.[7] The β cell mass is linearly correlated with body weight from 4 weeks to 6 months of age in male mice.[8] The slope of the linear regression varies with mouse strain. In our compilation of data from different aged Sprague-Dawley rats, it was clear that β cell mass increased with age in the adult rat because of increases in cell number. At any one time, the number of β cells is determined by the balance of cell renewal and cell loss.

The mechanisms to achieve a dynamic state of β cell mass include changes in new cell formation both by replication and by differentiation of new islets (neogenesis), changes in individual cell size/volume (atrophy to hypertrophy), and changes in cell loss or death rates.[7] All of these mechanisms have been shown in adult rodents.[9] When there is an increase in β cell mass, the cell renewal rate must be greater than that of cell loss. Loss of β cells has been shown to occur in normal conditions both in vitro and in vivo during the involution of the β cell mass in the postpartum pancreas[9] and in the normal neonatal rat.[10] In the neonatal period in rodents, there is a remodeling of the endocrine pancreas that is characterized by very active β-cell replication and neogenesis and an increase in β-cell apoptosis near the time of weaning.[10] In a longitudinal study,[11] the β cell mass increased throughout the life of the male Lewis rat: Initially by an increase in cell number, and then from 15 months onward by an increase in cell size or hypertrophy of the β cell. In addition, β-cell hypertrophy has been reported in rats during glucose infusions,[12] pregnancy,[9] and partial pancreatectomy (Px).[13] Neogenesis is responsible for most of the islet growth during the fetal stage, with replication being high in the perinatal period. In rats, we have found two waves of neogenesis during the neonatal period: One immediately after birth and the second around weaning. Using data from our longitudinal study of the β cell mass and its determinants,[10] we estimate that more than 30% of the β cells seen at day 31 could not be accounted for by replication of preexisting β cells. However, with the natural turnover of cells, a gradual but complete replacement of the β-cell population should occur over time. Thus, the endocrine pancreas should be considered a slowly renewed tissue.

Experimental evidence from rodents shows that there is a substantial compensatory effort by the β cells to maintain normal glycemic levels in the face of obesity and insulin resistance. Two types of compensation can occur: A functional one in which each β cell secretes more insulin, and a second in which there is an increase in β cell mass. Functional adaptations include changes in threshold for glucose-induced insulin secretion that occur during pregnancy[14] and glucose-induced increases in glucokinase activity.[15] Nonetheless, the β cell mass itself is the major factor that determines the amount of insulin that can be secreted. Mice with genetically induced peripheral insulin resistance have an up to 30-fold larger β cell mass, compared with normal mice.[16]

There is also evidence from human autopsied pancreata to suggest a compensatory growth of the β cell mass in obesity. A small but careful study of autopsied pancreata from patients with type 2 diabetes and nondiabetic subjects showed that the β cell mass of obese subjects was approximately 40% larger than that of lean subjects.[6] This compensatory growth of the human β cell mass with obesity was recently confirmed using many more pancreata.[17,18]

What Is the Origin of New β Cells?

Although it is clear that new β cells are formed in the adult pancreas, the source of these new β cells continues to be a matter of debate. Suggestions for the origin of new β cells include: 1) Replication of preexisting β cells[19]; 2) differentiation from another islet cell or an intraislet stem cell[20,21]; 3) transdifferentiation from acinar cells; and 4) differentiation from a cell within the duct epithelium[5,22] (Figure 22.1). More than one mechanism may be involved in new β-cell formation after birth, and normal growth and regeneration or response to injury may occur through different mechanisms. For example, replication of hepatocytes accounts for most of liver growth and regeneration, but the oval cells retain a bipotential capacity to form either new hepatocytes or bile duct epithelium. In aiming to expand the β cell mass either in vivo or in vitro for therapeutic purposes, the main criterion is that the cells of origin have the capacity to expand the functional β cell number.

Replication

Many scientists were mistakenly led to think that β cells did not replicate because of the low observed replication rate of β cells and the concept that terminally differentiated cells do not replicate. Yet the enlarged islets and increased β cell mass seen in obesity and insulin resistance supported replication. Replication was easily verified by incorporation of labeled thymidine or its analog bromodeoxyuridine (BrdU) into new DNA, immunostaining of cell cycle-specific proteins, or the presence of mitotic figures. In adult mice, β cell compensation as the result of pregnancy or response to insulin resistance occurs predominantly by replication, with little neogenesis.[23,24] Using various morphometric analyses, the increase in β cell mass in these

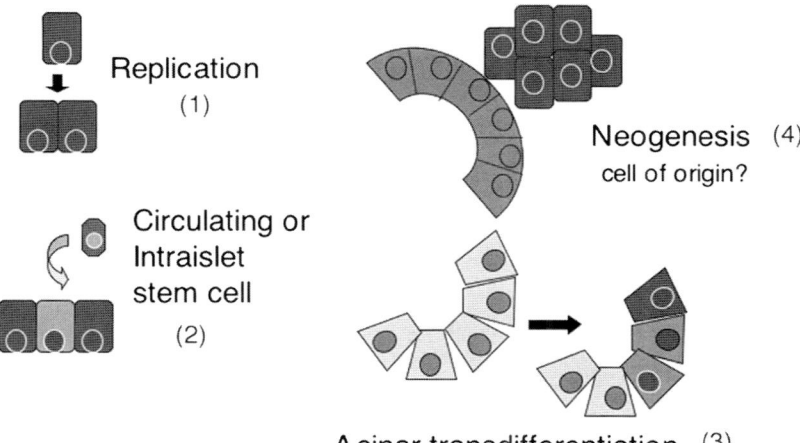

Figure 22.1. Possible sources of cells that can give rise to new insulin-producing β cells. New β cells are found in the pancreas after birth. The origin of new β cells may include: 1) Replication of preexisting β cells; 2) differentiation from another islet cell or an intraislet stem cell; 3) transdifferentiation from acinar cells; and 4) differentiation from a cell within the duct epithelium.

studies was shown to result predominantly from an increase in islet size, not islet number. A recent study using lineage-tracing techniques confirmed the major role of replication in the normal adult mouse.[19]

Replication is also a major response during the regeneration after partial Px. At 3 and 7 days after a 90% Px in the adult rat, both the β cells and exocrine cells have mitotic indices three- to fourfold higher than that of the sham animals.[25] At 14 days, the exocrine cells have only a slightly increased mitotic index, whereas that of the β cells remains double that of the sham animals even at 3 weeks. Because glucose is a powerful mitogenic stimulus for β cells, the continued enhancement of β-cell replication probably results from the mild hyperglycemia seen in these animals. Replication makes a significant contribution to the increase in β cell mass in these Px animals by increasing the number of β cells in the islets. Islets of equivalent size from 4-week Px and sham-operated animals have similar amounts of RNA, but the proportion of β cells is increased in the Px islets.[26]

Intraislet Stem or Progenitor Cells

Some studies have made a case for progenitor cells residing within the islets. In streptozotocin-treated rats, cells that stained for both insulin and somatostatin were suggested as intraislet progenitor or stem cells that regenerated into β cells.[21] Treatment with betacellulin after streptozotocin led to an increase in the number of insulin-positive cells, as well as BrdU-labeled somatostatin-positive cells, providing support for the intraislet progenitor concept.[27] This hypothesis was also favored in a cell-lineage tracing study which labeled cells expressing neurogenin 3, a transcription factor active in islet development, in adult pancreas.[28] Twenty-four hours after the labeling pulse, the few labeled cells were found only in islets; the simplest explanation was that there were progenitor cells within the islet. Another cell type, the nestin-positive, hormone-negative cell grown from isolated islets, has been suggested as an in vitro islet progenitor cell.[29] These studies are provocative and potentially important, but more work is needed to understand whether these cells contribute significantly to in vivo β-cell growth or regeneration.

Acinar Cell Transdifferentiation

It has been difficult to prove that differentiated adult pancreatic acinar cells are converted to insulin-producing cells. The term transdifferentiation is often used to describe the process.[30] A likely scenario is that the acinar cells regress to a duct-like phenotype, and these cells then function as progenitors. Duct-like "tubular complexes" have been reported in various diseases such as chronic pancreatitis, pancreatic adenocarcinoma and cystic fibrosis,[31,32] pancreatitis after ductal ligation,[33,34] and in regeneration of exocrine pancreas after experimentally induced acute pancreatitis.[33,34] The origin of these structures has been debated, with suggestions ranging from proliferation or reduplication of intralobular ducts[35] to dedifferentiation of acinar tissue into duct-like structures.[33,34] In ductal ligation studies, it is clear that there is replication of ductal cells, increased number of hormone-positive cells budding from ducts, and initially increased β cell mass; however, it is unclear if these replicating ducts originate from acinar or duct tissue.[33,34,36,37] A rat duct ligation model in which gastrin was infused produced changes consistent with transdifferentiation of acinar cells to duct cells and subsequent β-cell neogenesis.[38] A similar pathway leading to β-cell neogenesis has been postulated in rats receiving glucose infusions.[39]

Interestingly, these tubular complexes resemble the focal regions of regeneration seen in the Px model. Data from this latter model supports a regenerative origin of these focal regions: 1) The BrdU data show expansion of the ductal tree and then further proliferation of branching ductules; 2) the coincidence of the appearance and disappearance of the focal regions with the marked growth of the pancreatic remnant; and 3) the continuum of differentiation from ductal epithelium to islets and acini.

Neogenesis

Replication is clearly a pathway for new β cells in adult rodents, but neogenesis is also seen. The process of neogenesis in the adult pancreas closely resembles embryonic new islet formation [Figure 22.2 (see color section)].[40] In both, hormone-containing cells are seen first within the basement membrane of the duct epithelium and then the islet cells delaminate and coalesce. Adult duct tissue retains the ability to differentiate into islet cells. When adult ductal epithelium was wrapped in fetal mesenchyme and implanted in nude mice, approximately 20% of the grafts resulted in budding of islet-like clusters that had islet hormone immunostaining.[41,42]

Whereas replication is easy to verify, measurement of neogenesis has been less direct or definitive. There are no good markers for it yet, and increased hormone staining within the ducts has been considered indicative of neogenesis. In normal adult rodent pancreas, occasional (1 in 1000) cells within the ductal epithelium immunostain for an islet hormone,[43] but neogenesis is seen experimentally with dietary treatment with soybean trypsin inhibitors,[44] overexpression of interferon (IFN)-γ in the β cells of transgenic mice,[45] overexpression of transforming growth factor (TGF)-α,[46] after partial pancreatectomy,[47] after cellophane wrapping of the head of the pancreas,[48] after treatment with exendin 4[49,50] or betacellulin,[51] and clinically with recent onset of type 1 diabetes and severe liver disease.[52,53] In humans, neogenesis seems to have a more important role in the compensation of the β cell mass in obesity, compared with replication. In the samples from the Butler-Mayo collection[17] as well as from the more than 100 human organ donations to the Harvard Islet Transplantation program, neogeneic regions of ductal profiles and hormone-positive cells budding from these ducts are more common than enlarged islets that would be seen with enhanced replication. The dominance of the replicative pathway in adult mice may reflect their long telomeres such that telomere shortening is not limiting,[54] whereas in humans, in whom telomere shortening is limiting and the rate of β-cell replication appears very low,[55] neogenesis may be more important.

Models of Neogenesis

In rodents, there is considerable evidence of neogenesis in a number of models, but no lineage-tracing evidence is available as yet. Dor et al.[19] recently found no evidence of neogenesis in mice after a 70% partial Px using lineage tracing. However, one must realize that it is always difficult to show the absence of an event. Additionally, this work raised a number of experimental concerns, particularly regarding the possibility that the sampling was inadequate.[56] In contrast, other studies show strong, albeit circumstantial evidence, of islet neogenesis in the adult.

The ductal ligation models mentioned above showed increases of ductal replication, islet neogenesis, and β cell mass.[33,34,36,37,57] An important unanswered question is whether the acinar tissue mainly dies and the ductal component proliferates or, alternatively, the acinar phenotype is lost (transdifferentiates or dedifferentiates) to become a ductal phenotype. In either case, the budding of islet tissue from ductal structures is well documented.

In the RIP-IFN-γ transgenic mice, newly formed islets were often seen bulging within the lumen of the ducts, suggesting their origin from ducts.[3,45,58] Intriguingly, occasional cells that express intestinal or hepatocyte markers were also seen budding from the ducts, implying plasticity. Initially, it was thought that the insulitis seen in this model may have triggered the neogenesis, but similar duct proliferation and islet neogenesis were observed with this transgene on an immunocompromised background. In the RIP-IFN-γ transgenic mice, PDX1 protein, a transcription factor important for both pancreas development and β-cell function, is seen in proliferating ducts from which there is budding of new islets; additional transcription factors known to be involved in the differentiation of islets were expressed in these areas,[59,60] again suggesting active new islet formation.

The cellophane-wrapped pancreas of Syrian golden hamster resulting in partial duct obstruction has been studied by the groups of Rosenberg and Vinik.[48,61–64] This model differs from the ductal ligation model because there is no obvious acinar degeneration reported. In the original study, half of the streptozotocin-induced diabetic animals became euglycemic after cellophane wrapping, with the restoration thought to be the result of new islet formation rather than replication.[64] Even though the early studies defining the time course of euglycemia restoration after the surgery are incomplete, and the model is only reported in the hamster, this model has led to the identification of a putative factor that initiates islet neogenesis, INGAP (islet neogenesis associated protein), a member of the pancreatitis-associated peptide family.[61] More work is needed to determine if this protein can stimulate neogenesis in other models and species.

In the 90% Px rat model, a well-defined remnant of 10% of the weight and of islet mass left in a young adult rat regenerates to 27% of the weight of the sham-operated pancreas with 45% of the sham islet mass by 4 weeks after surgery.[49,65,66] The regeneration occurs in this model both by replication of preexisting differentiated acinar and β cells and by neogenesis, resulting in the rapid formation of whole new lobes.[66] At 72 hours after surgery, small clumps of branching ductal structures project from the common pancreatic duct. In sections, these clumps are seen as focal regions of proliferating ductules. These regions comprise 10%–15% of the volume of the remnant pancreas, but by 7 days after Px, most of these regions have differentiated into new pancreatic lobes with a normal composition of exocrine and endocrine cells.

Oval Cells as Possible Pancreatic Islet Progenitors

Because neogenesis implies the formation of new islets from the ducts, one must consider which cells are the actual progenitors. By ultrastructural analysis in both embryonic[40] and postnatal pancreas, hormone-positive cells are seen within the basement membrane of the ductal epithelium, therefore circulating or stromal cells can be ruled out as progenitors for the bulk of new islet formation. Another possibility may be the pancreatic equivalent of "oval cells" found in the liver.[67,68] After liver injury from carcinogenic agents, there seems to be proliferation of small (7 μm), oval cells just at the periductular junction; these cells have the potential to differentiate into bile duct epithelium or hepatocytes.[69] In this schema, pancreatic oval cells would proliferate, delaminate from the epithelium with disruption of the plasma membrane, and coalesce into islets. Ultrastructural analysis of the common pancreatic duct of adult rats shows rare (1 in 100–200 cells) basal cells that are small and ovoid with fairly undifferentiated cytoplasm; these cells resemble liver oval cells.[5] When Px rats were given colchicine in order to arrest mitosis at 20 hours after surgery, there was no evidence of an amplification of a small population of putative stem cells/oval cells, with all the arrested cells being columnar epithelial cells. Even so, in the liver, the oval cells are not the usual mechanism for regeneration but rather a backup one.

Additionally, estimates of the number of progenitor cells needed for formation of a new islet are not consistent with a progenitor role for these "oval cells" in the Px model. After partial Px in rats, fully formed new islets can be seen by 72 hours after surgery, each consisting of 1000–1500 cells. No increased replication in the pancreas is seen about 24 hours after surgery, so the islets must form within 48 hours. With cell-cycle times in rodents being 10–20 hours, 16 starting cells with a doubling time of 10 hours (five doublings over 48 hours) would be required to make 1000 cells or one islet. If the doubling time were 12 hours, then 64 cells would be required. Because there are so few nonduct cells found ultrastructurally within the basement membrane of the duct epithelium, these calculations favor the possibility that the duct epithelial cells themselves are the progenitor cells.

Ductal Epithelial Cells as Pancreatic Progenitors

Another schema would have the ductal epithelial cells regress to a less differentiated stage after replication, and then in a dedifferentiated state function as progenitor cells.[22] This hypothesis allows for both a lifetime supply and a large number of potential progenitor cells. External signals can then direct differentiation of these multipotent cells to endocrine, acinar, or mature duct phenotypes. This hypothesis is consistent with data from many models and the estimated number of cells needed for each new islet described above. Lineage tracing experiments using a duct promoter are in process and should address this question directly.

Data from the regenerating rat pancreas after partial Px favor this hypothesis. After partial Px, ductal cells rapidly replicate and dedifferentiate with a marked increase in PDX1 protein. PDX1 protein is normally expressed in pancreatic ducts until shortly before birth; others have suggested it as a marker for the adult progenitor cells.[59,70,71] The return to a more embryonic phenotype precedes the formation of whole new lobes of pancreas.[22] A wave of DNA synthesis (as seen by BrdU incorporation) passes through the ductal tree. Whereas little to no PDX1 protein was detected in the epithelium of the quiescent common pancreatic duct from unoperated or sham-operated animals 24 hours after Px, most of the ductal epithelial cells were BrdU$^+$ PDX1$^-$ or BrdU$^+$ PDX1$^+$ in the Px animals. Then by 3 days after Px, few cells of the common pancreatic duct epithelium were BrdU$^+$ but most cells still expressed PDX1 protein. Addition of PDX1 protein, which has a protein transduction domain that allows the protein to enter cells, to cultured ductal cells induced mRNA of PDX1, insulin, and several other β-cell genes, supporting the origin of the new islets from duct cells themselves.[72]

The MT-TGF-α transgenic mouse supports the concept of ductal cells as the islet progenitor cells. In this mouse, the pancreas has uncontrolled ductular proliferation resulting in metaplastic ductules, increased fibrosity, and interstitial cellularity.[73] PDX1 expression was seen in the metaplastic ductal epithelium, as well as focally expressed PAX6.[71] The data from both MT-TGF-α and RIP-IFN-γ mice on the expression of PDX1 protein after replication of the ductal cells are consistent with regression of the duct cells to a more embryonic state. In the MT-TGF-α transgenic mice, 6% of the epithelial cells in the metaplastic ducts expressed low levels of insulin, with 1% showing strong staining and presence of insulin granules,[46] again suggesting the transition from duct to islet phenotype.

The marked change in composition of porcine neonatal pancreatic cell clusters transplanted under the kidney capsule of immunodeficient mice adds even further support.[74] When transplanted, the majority of cells can be stained with the duct marker cytokeratin 7, but, after several months, 94% of the cells were β cells. During this engraftment, as well as in intact neonatal pancreas, cells costained for both insulin and cytokeratin 7 are found, suggesting residual expression of duct markers as duct cells become β cells. This finding is extended by gene profiling with microarrays of new versus mature islets 7 days after partial Px in rats.[75] The β cells of new islets, which can be identified in the new lobes, express a variety of duct markers at both the mRNA and protein level, also supporting the duct progenitor hypothesis.[22]

Recent Evidence for Pancreatic Progenitor Cells with Limited Clonal Expansion

Two recent articles[76,77] reported isolation of cells from whole mouse pancreas that can be expanded clonally and express low levels of insulin and other pancreatic markers. These cells were rare (one in several thousand) and not yet localized within the pancreas. Although it is not clear yet that these cells can differentiate to fully functional islet cells, their potential is very exciting, and further studies on such cells are eagerly awaited.[78]

Implications of In Vivo Data for Formation of New β Cells for Therapy

Understanding the regulation of the normal process may lead to new therapies for diabetes that involve generation of new islets either in vitro for transplantation or in vivo by stimulation of the endogenous pancreas. β cells are formed after birth from several different origins or pathways. Data support occurrence of β-cell replication, and differentiation from a pancreatic stem cell/progenitor within the islet or within the duct, or from a duct-like structure that was previously a mature duct or acinar cell, or a combination of these pathways. In each model, more than one pathway may be involved. In fact, the data suggest that different states (injury versus normal growth) or different species favor one or another pathway. An important issue is how this knowledge can be used to generate new islets for therapeutic replacement.

In vitro replication of β cells has been studied for many years.[79-81] It is clear from these studies that the conditions used in vitro do not yet match those found in vivo because it has not been possible to even double the number of β cells in vitro. Under conditions favoring substantial expansion, using growth factors and matrices or oncogene expression, the β-cell phenotype is lost[82-84] but there has been question whether the proliferation of contaminant ductal cells diluted out the β cells.[85] Reaggregation of the expanded cells did lead to some reexpression of islet mRNAs, but more work is needed to improve the expansion of primary β cells. Studies manipulating the culture further may eventually yield conditions for expansion and then redifferentiation of β cells; this is an area of great importance.

Several groups have been studying the potential of non–islet pancreatic tissue for in vitro generation of islets. Human duct-cell-rich fractions remaining after islet isolation and purification have been cultured and shown to form new islets after exposure to growth factors and matrix.[86,87] Over 3–4 weeks of culture, the insulin content per flask increased 10- to 15-fold as the DNA content increased up to 7-fold. The cultivated human islet buds, shown by immunofluorescence to consist of cytokeratin 19-positive duct cells and hormone-positive islet cells, were glucose responsive. With semiquantitative multiplex reverse transcriptase-polymerase chain reaction, transcription factors known to be involved in islet development, such as Ngn3 and Pax4, which were not detected in initial cells, adult islets, or acinar fractions, were evident in final differentiated cultures. The finding that transcription factors important to embryonic islet development are involved in islet differentiation from adult human pancreatic cells suggests an active differentiation process. The efficiency of differentiation is at present inadequate to render this process clinically useful. Work continues to increase the new islet formation in vitro. The cells that give rise to the new islets in this heterogeneous cell population have not been identified as yet, although they have been shown to be initially in the epithelial component and thought to be ductal.[87] Their ductal origin is supported by other studies that have manipulated in culture the human pancreatic duct PANC1 cell line,[88] or cells expanded from mouse pancreatic duct cells to give islet hormone-expressing cells.[89] In the latter report, the cells were able to reverse diabetes in mice, but concerns have been raised about compatibility of these results with the very low insulin content of the cells.[90] However, Bouwens and colleagues[91-94] have shown that both human and rat acinar tissue in culture can become duct-like or even hepatocyte-like, depending on the culture conditions, suggesting that at least some of the cells from the human cultures may have been acinar cells previously. Some acinar cells clearly die when cultured but some may lose their acinar phenotype and regress to a duct-like progenitor as we have suggested for the mature ducts.

Other approaches to enhance islet neogenesis are being investigated using signaling molecules that have been reported to stimulate β cell growth or differentiation. These molecules, including exendin 4/GLP-1,[49,50,95,96] betacellulin,[27] EGF/gastrin,[97-99] tungstate,[100] INGAP,[61] and conophylline,[101] are being tested in vivo as well as in culture. Identification of the progenitor cells by lineage tracing from cells with acinar or ductal phenotype, or localization of cells that have clonal expansion and differentiative capacities, will also be critical to this field. The importance of identifying these cells is further highlighted by recent results suggesting that in humans neogenesis may have a more important role in increasing β cell mass than replication. Thus, for the purpose of therapeutically expanding the human β cell mass, the main criterion should be to identify progenitor cells that have the capacity to expand, either in vitro or in vivo, the functional β cell number. Hence, to achieve the therapeutic goal, a continued interest in the process of neogenesis of β cells from progenitors is necessary and will require many different avenues to study the regulation of its normal process. This, we suggest, would lead to new therapies for diabetes that involve generation of new islet tissue, either in vivo by stimulation of the endogenous pancreas or in vitro for transplantation.

References

1. Shapiro AM, Lakey JR, Ryan EA, et al. Islet transplantation in seven patients with type 1 diabetes mellitus using a glucocorticoid-free immunosuppressive regimen. N Engl J Med 2000;27:230–238.
2. Ryan EA, Lakey JR, Paty BW, et al. Successful islet transplantation: continued insulin reserve provides long-term glycemic control. Diabetes 2002;51:2148–2157.
3. Gu D, Sarvetnick N. A transgenic model for studying islet development. Recent Prog Horm Res 1994;49: 161–165.
4. Bonner-Weir S. Life and death of the pancreatic beta cells. Trends Endocrinol Metab 2000;11:375–378.
5. Bonner-Weir S, Sharma A. Pancreatic stem cells. J Pathol 2002;197:519–526.
6. Kloppel G, Lohr M, Habich K, Oberholzer M, Heitz PU. Islet pathology and the pathogenesis of type 1 and type 2 diabetes mellitus revisited. Surv Synth Pathol Res 1985;4:110–125.
7. Finegood DT, Scaglia L, Bonner-Weir S. Dynamics of β-cell mass in the growing rat pancreas: estimation with a simple mathematical model. Diabetes 1995;44: 249–256.
8. Bonner-Weir S. Islet growth and development in the adult. J Mol Endocrinol 2000;24:297–302.
9. Scaglia L, Smith FE, Bonner-Weir S. Apoptosis contributes to the involution of β cell mass in the post partum rat pancreas. Endocrinology 1995;136: 5461–468.
10. Scaglia L, Cahill CJ, Finegood DT, Bonner-Weir S. Apoptosis participates in the remodeling of the endocrine pancreas in the neonatal rat. Endocrinology 1997;138:1736–1741.
11. Montanya E, Nacher V, Biarnes M, Soler J. Linear correlation between beta cell mass and body weight throughout life in Lewis rats: role of beta cell hyperplasia and hypertrophy. Diabetes 2000;49: 1341–1346.
12. Bonner-Weir S, Deery D, Leahy JL, Weir GC. Compensatory growth of pancreatic B-cells in adult rats after short-term glucose infusion. Diabetes 1989;38:49–53.
13. Jonas J-C, Sharma A, Hasenkamp W, et al. Chronic hyperglycemia triggers loss of pancreatic β cell differentiation in an animal model of diabetes. J Biol Chem 1999;274:14112–14121.
14. Parsons JA, Brelje TC, Sorenson RL. Adaptation of islets to pregnancy: increased islet cell proliferation and insulin secretion correlates with the onset of placental lactogen secretion. Endocrinology 1992;130:1459–1466.
15. Chen C, Hosokawa H, Bumbalo LM, Leahy JL. Regulatory effects of glucose on the catalytic activity and cellular content of glucokinase in the pancreatic B cell. J Clin Invest 1994;94:1616–1620.
16. Bruning JC, Winnay J, Bonner-Weir S, Taylor SI, Accili D, Kahn CR. Development of a novel polygenic model of NIDDM in mice heterozygous for IR and IRS-1 null alleles. Cell 1999;88:561–572.
17. Butler AE, Janson J, Bonner-Weir S, Ritzel R, Rizza RA, Butler PC. Beta-cell deficit and increased beta-cell apoptosis in humans with type 2 diabetes. Diabetes 2003;52:102–110.
18. Yoon KH, Ko SH, Cho JH, et al. Selective β-cell loss and α-cell expansion in patients with type 2 diabetes mellitus in Korea. J Clin Endocrinol Metab 2003;88:2300–2308.
19. Dor Y, Brown J, Martinez OI, Melton DA. Adult pancreatic beta-cells are formed by self-duplication rather than stem-cell differentiation. Nature 2004;429:41–46.
20. Fernandes A, King LC, Guz Y, Stein R, Wright CV, Teitelman G. Differentiation of new insulin-producing cells is induced by injury in adult pancreatic islets. Endocrinology 1997;138:1750–1762.
21. Guz Y, Nasir I, Teitelman G. Regeneration of pancreatic beta cells from intra-islet precursor cells in an experimental model of diabetes. Endocrinology 2001;142:4956–4968.
22. Sharma A, Zangen DH, Reitz P, et al. The homeodomain protein IDX-1 increases after an early burst of proliferation during pancreatic regeneration. Diabetes 1999;48:507–513.
23. Parsons JA, Bartke A, Sorenson RL. Number and size of islets of Langerhans in pregnant human growth hormone-expressing transgenic, and pituitary dwarf mice: effect of lactogenic hormones. Endocrinology 1995;136:2013–2021.
24. Bock T, Pakkenberg B, Buschard K. Increased islet volume but unchanged islet number in ob/ob mice. Diabetes 2003;52:1716–1722.
25. Brockenbrough JS, Weir GC, Bonner-Weir S. Discordance of exocrine and endocrine growth after 90% pancreatectomy in rats. Diabetes 1988;37:232–236.
26. Zangen DH, Bonner-Weir S, Lee CH, et al. Reduced insulin, GLUT2, and IDX-1 in B-cells after partial pancreatectomy. Diabetes 1997;46:258–264.
27. Li L, Seno M, Yamada H, Kojima I. Betacellulin improves glucose metabolism by promoting conversion of intraislet precursor cells to beta-cells in streptozotocin-treated mice. Am J Physiol Endocrinol Metab 2003;285:E577–583.
28. Gu G, Brown JR, Melton DA. Direct lineage tracing reveals the ontogeny of pancreatic cell fates during mouse embryogenesis. Mech Dev 2003;120:35–43.
29. Zulewski H, Abraham EJ, Gerlach MJ, et al. Multipotential nestin-positive stem cells isolated from adult pancreatic islets differentiate ex vivo into pan-

creatic endocrine, exocrine, and hepatic phenotypes. Diabetes 2001;50:521–533.
30. Bouwens L. Transdifferentiation versus stem cell hypothesis for the regeneration of islet beta-cells in the pancreas. Microsc Res Tech 1998;43:332–336.
31. Bockman DE, Black O Jr, Mills LR, Webster PD. Origin of tubular complexes developing during induction of pancreatic complexes during induction of pancreatic adenocarcinoma by 7,12-dimethylbenz(a) antracene. Am J Physiol 1978;90:645–651.
32. Porta EM, Stein AA, Patterson P. Ultrastructural changes of the pancreas and liver in cystic fibrosis. Am J Clin Pathol 1964;42:451–465.
33. Willemer S, Elsasser HP, Kern HF, Adler G. Tubular complexes in cerulein- and oleic acid-induced pancreatitis in guts: glycoconjugate pattern, immunocytochemical and ultrastructural findings. Pancreas 1987;2:669–675.
34. DeLisle RC, Grendel JH, Williams JA. Growing pancreas acinar cells (post pancreatitis and fetal) express a ductal antigen. Pancreas 1990;5:381–388.
35. Dreiling DA, Bordalo OR, Noronha M, Greenstein R. Update: big duct, little duct or toxic metabolic pathogenesis of pancreatitis. Am J Gastroenterol 1979;71:424–426.
36. Edstrom C. Further quantitative structural studies of the pancreatic islet parenchyma in rats with duct ligation. Acta Soc Med Ups 1971;76:127–138.
37. Hultquist GT, Karlsson U, Hallner ACH. The regenerative capacity of the pancreas in duct-ligated rats. Exp Pathol 1979;17:44–52.
38. Rooman I, Lardon J, Bouwens L. Gastrin stimulates beta-cell neogenesis and increases islet mass from transdifferentiated but not from normal exocrine pancreas tissue. Diabetes 2002;51:686–690.
39. Lipsett M, Finegood DT. Beta-cell neogenesis during prolonged hyperglycemia in rats. Diabetes 2002;51:1834–1841.
40. Pictet R, Rutter WJ. The endocrine pancreas. In: Steiner D, Freinkel N, eds. Handbook of Physiology. Baltimore: Williams & Wilkins; 1972:25–66.
41. Dudek RW, Lawrence IE Jr. Morphologic evidence of interactions between adult ductal epithelium of pancreas and fetal foregut mesenchyme. Diabetes 1988;37:891–900.
42. Dudek RW, Lawrence IE Jr, Hill RS, Johnson RC. Induction of islet cytodifferentiation by fetal mesenchyme in adult pancreatic ductal epithelium. Diabetes 1991;40:1041–1048.
43. Madden ME, Sarras MP Jr. The pancreatic ductal system of the rat: cell diversity, ultrastructure, and innervation. Pancreas 1989;4:472–485.
44. Weaver CV, Sorenson RL, Kaung HC. Immunocytochemical localization of insulin-immunoreactive cells in the ducts of rats treated with trypsin inhibitor. Diabetologia 1985;28:781–785.
45. Gu D, Sarvetnick N. Epithelial cell proliferation and islet neogenesis in IFN-γ transgenic mice. Development 1993;118:33–46.
46. Wang TC, Bonner-Weir S, Oates PS, et al. Pancreatic gastrin stimulates islet differentiation of transforming growth factor α-induced ductular precursor cells. J Clin Invest 1993;92:1349–1356.
47. Bonner-Weir S, Baxter LA, Schuppin GT, Smith FE. A second pathway for regeneration of the adult exocrine and endocrine pancreas: a possible recapitulation of embryonic development. Diabetes 1993;42:1715–1720.
48. Rosenberg L, Vinik AI, Fittenger GL, Rafaeloff R, Duguid WP. Islet-cell regeneration in the diabetic hamster pancreas with restoration of normoglycemia can be induced by local growth factors. Diabetologia 1996;39:256–262.
49. Xu G, Stoffers DA, Habener JF, Bonner-Weir S. Exendin-4 stimulates both β-cell replication and neogenesis, resulting in increased β-cell mass and improved glucose tolerance in diabetic rats. Diabetes 1999;48:2270–2276.
50. Stoffers DA, Kieffer TJ, Hussain MA, et al. Insulinotropic glucagon-like peptide 1 agonists stimulate expression of homeodomain protein IDX-1 and increase islet size in mouse pancreas. Diabetes 2000;49:741–748.
51. Yamamoto K, Miyagawa J, Waguri M, et al. Recombinant human betacellulin promotes the neogenesis of beta-cells and ameliorates glucose intolerance in mice with diabetes induced by selective alloxan perfusion. Diabetes 2000;49:2021–2027.
52. Gepts W. Contribution a l'etude morphologique des ilots de Langerhans au cours du diabete. Ann Soc R Sci Med Nat Brux 1957;10:105–108.
53. Gepts W. Pathological anatomy of the pancreas in juvenile diabetes. Diabetes 1965;14:619–633.
54. Forsyth NR, Wright WE, Shay JW. Telomerase and differentiation in multicellular organisms: turn it off, turn it on, and turn it off again. Differentiation 2002;69:188–197.
55. Tyrberg B, Ustinov J, Otonkoski T, Andersson A. Stimulated endocrine cell proliferation and differentiation in transplanted human pancreatic islets: effects of the ob gene and compensatory growth of the implantation organ. Diabetes 2001;50:301–307.
56. Bonner-Weir S, Toschi E, Inada A, et al. The pancreatic duct epithelium serves as a potential pool of progenitor cells. Pediatr Diabetes 2004;5(Suppl 2):16–22.
57. Rooman I, Lardon J, Bouwens L. Gastrin stimulates beta-cell neogenesis and increases islet mass from transdifferentiated but not from normal exocrine pancreas tissue. Diabetes 2002;51:686–690.
58. Sarvetnick NE, Gu D. Regeneration of pancreatic endocrine cells in interferon-gamma transgenic mice. Adv Exp Med Biol 1992;321:85–89.
59. Kritzik MR, Jones E, Chen Z, et al. PDX-1 and Msx-2 expression in the regenerating and developing pancreas. J Endocrinol 1999;163:523–530.
60. Kritzik MR, Krahl T, Good A, et al. Transcription factor expression during pancreatic islet regeneration. Mol Cell Endocrinol 2000;164:99–107.
61. Rafaeloff R, Pittenger GL, Barlow SW, et al. Cloning and sequencing of the pancreatic islet neogenesis associated protein (INGAP) gene and its expression in islet neogenesis in hamsters. J Clin Invest 1997;99:2100–2109.
62. Rosenberg L, Duguid WP, Vinik AI. The effect of cellophane wrapping of the pancreas in the Syrian golden hamster: autoradiographic observations. Pancreas 1989;4:31–37.
63. Rosenberg L, Vinik AI. Trophic stimulation of the ductular-islet cell axis: a new approach to the treatment of diabetes. Adv Exp Med Biol 1992;321:95–104.

64. Rosenberg LA, Brown RA, Duguid WP. A new approach to the induction of duct epithelial hyperplasia and nesidioblastosis by cellophane wrapping of the hamster pancreas. J Surg Res 1983;35:63–72.
65. Bonner-Weir S, Trent DF, Weir GC. Partial pancreatectomy in the rat and subsequent defect in glucose-induced insulin release. J Clin Invest 1983;71:1544–1553.
66. Bonner-Weir S, Stubbs M, Reitz P, Taneja M, Smith FE. Partial pancreatectomy as a model of pancreatic regeneration. In: Sarvetnick N, ed. Pancreatic Growth and Regeneration. Basel, Switzerland: Karger Landes Systems; 1997:138–153.
67. Farber E. The multistep nature of cancer development. Cancer Res 1984;44:4217–4223.
68. Evarts RP, Nagy P, Marsden E, Thorgeirsson SS. A precursor-product relationship exists between oval cells and hepatocytes in rat liver. Carcinogenesis 1987;8:1737–1740.
69. Germain L, Blouen MJ, Marceau N. Biliary epithelial and hepatocyte cell lineaged relationships in embryonic rat liver. Cancer Res 1988;48:4909–4918.
70. Bouwens L, De Blay E. Islet morphogenesis and stem cell markers in rat pancreas. J Histochem Cytochem 1996;44:947–951.
71. Song SY, Gannon M, Washington MK, et al. Expansion of Pdx1-expressing pancreatic epithelium and islet neogenesis in transgenic mice overexpressing transforming growth factor α. Gastroenterology 1999;117:1416–1426.
72. Noguchi H, Kaneto H, Weir GC, Bonner-Weir S. PDX-1 protein containing its own antennapedia-like protein transduction domain can transduce pancreatic duct and islet cells. Diabetes 2003;52:1732–1737.
73. Jhappan C, Stahle C, Harkins RN, Fausto N, Smith GH, Merlino GT. TGFα overexpression in transgenic mice induces liver neoplasia and abnormal development of the mammary gland and pancreas. Cell 1990;61:1137–1146.
74. Yoon K-H, Quickel RR, Tatarkiewicz K, et al. Differentiation and expansion of beta cell mass in porcine neonatal pancreatic cell clusters transplanted into nude mice. Cell Transplant 1999;8:673–689.
75. Toschi E, Aye T, Fuller A, et al. Gene expression profiling of new β cells: evidence for differentiating β cells passing through a ductal phenotype. Diabetes 2004;53(suppl 2):1613.
76. Suzuki A, Nakauchi H, Taniguchi H. Prospective isolation of multipotent pancreatic progenitors using flow-cytometric cell sorting. Diabetes 2004;53:2143–2152.
77. Seaberg RM, Smukler SR, Kieffer TJ, et al. Clonal identification of multipotent precursors from adult mouse pancreas that generate neural and pancreatic lineages. Nat Biotechnol 2004;22:1115–1124.
78. Weir GC, Bonner-Weir S. Beta-cell precursors: a work in progress. Nat Biotechnol 2004;22:1095–1096.
79. Hellerstrom C, Swenne I, Andersson A. Islet cell replication and diabetes. In: Lefebvre PJ, Pipeleers DG, eds. The Pathology of the Endocrine Pancreas in Diabetes. Heidelberg: Springer-Verlag; 1988:141–170.
80. Chick WL. Beta cell replication in rat pancreatic monolayer cultures: effects of glucose, tolbutamide, glucocorticoid, growth hormone and glucagon. Diabetes 1973;22:687–693.
81. Brelje TC, Scharp DW, Lacy PE, et al. Effect of homologous placental lactogens, prolactins, and growth hormones on islet B-cell division and insulin secretion in rat, mouse and human islets: implication for placental lactogen regulation of islet function during pregnancy. Endocrinology 1993;132:879–887.
82. Halvorsen TL, Beattie GM, Lopez AD, Hayek A, Levine F. Accelerated telomere shortening and senescence in human pancreatic islet cells stimulated to divide in vitro. J Endocrinol 2000;166:103–109.
83. Beattie GM, Cirulli V, Lopez AD, Hayek A. Ex vivo expansion of human pancreatic endocrine cells. J Clin Endocrinol Metab 1997;82:1852–1856.
84. Beattie GM, Itkin-Ansari P, Cirulli V, et al. Sustained proliferation of PDX-1+ cells derived from human islets. Diabetes 1999;48:1013–1019.
85. Lefebvre VH, Otonkoski T, Ustinov J, Huotari MA, Pipeleers DG, Bouwens L. Culture of adult human islet preparations with hepatocyte growth factor and 804G matrix is mitogenic for duct cells but not for beta-cells. Diabetes 1998;47:134–137.
86. Bonner-Weir S, Taneja M, Weir GC, et al. In vitro cultivation of human islets from expanded ductal tissue. Proc Natl Acad Sci USA 2000;97:7999–8004.
87. Gao R, Ustinov J, Pulkkinen MA, Lundin K, Korsgren O, Otonkoski T. Characterization of endocrine progenitor cells and critical factors for their differentiation in human adult pancreatic cell culture. Diabetes 2003;52:2007–2015.
88. Hardikar AA, Marcus-Samuels B, Geras-Raaka E, Raaka BM, Gershengorn MC. Human pancreatic precursor cells secrete FGF2 to stimulate clustering into hormone-expressing islet-like cell aggregates. Proc Natl Acad Sci USA 2003;100:7117–7122.
89. Ramiya VK, Marraist M, Arfors KE, Schatz DA, Peck AB, Cornelius JC. Reversal of insulin dependent diabetes using islets generated in vitro from pancreatic stem cells. Nat Med 2000;6:278–282.
90. Sachs DH, Bonner-Weir S. New islets from old. Nature 2000;6:278–282.
91. Rooman I, Heremans Y, Heimberg H, Bouwens L. Modulation of rat pancreatic acinoductal transdifferentiation and expression of PDX-1 in vitro. Diabetologia 2000;43:907–914.
92. Heimberg H, Bouwens L, Heremans Y, Van De Casteele M, Lefebvre V, Pipeleers D. Adult human pancreatic duct and islet cells exhibit similarities in expression and differences in phosphorylation and complex formation of the homeodomain protein Ipf-1. Diabetes 2000;49:571–579.
93. Lardon J, De Breuck S, Rooman I, et al. Plasticity in the adult rat pancreas: transdifferentiation of exocrine to hepatocyte-like cells in primary culture. Hepatology 2004;39:1499–1507.
94. Lardon J, Huyens N, Rooman I, Bouwens L. Exocrine cell transdifferentiation in dexamethasone-treated rat pancreas. Virchows Arch 2004;444:61–65.
95. Wang Y, Perfetti R, Greig N, et al. Glucagon-like peptide-1 can reverse the age-related decline in glucose tolerance in rats. J Clin Invest 1997;99:2883–2889.
96. Zhou J, Wang X, Pineyro MA, Egan JM. Glucagon-like peptide 1 and exendin-4 convert pancreatic AR42J cells into glucagon- and insulin-producing cells. Diabetes 1999;48:2358–2366.
97. Brand SJ, Tagerud S, Lambert P, et al. Pharmacological treatment of chronic diabetes by stimulating pancreatic beta-cell regeneration with systemic co-administration of EGF and gastrin. Pharmacol Toxicol 2002;91:414–420.

98. Rooman I, Bouwens L. Combined gastrin and epidermal growth factor treatment induces islet regeneration and restores normoglycaemia in C57Bl6/J mice treated with alloxan. Diabetologia 2004;47:259–265.
99. Rooman I, Lardon J, Flamez D, Schuit F, Bouwens L. Mitogenic effect of gastrin and expression of gastrin receptors in duct-like cells of rat pancreas. Gastroenterology 2001;121:940–949.
100. Fernandez-Alvarez J, Barbera A, Nadal B, et al. Stable and functional regeneration of pancreatic beta-cell population in nSTZ-rats treated with tungstate. Diabetologia 2004;47:470–477.
101. Ogata T, Li L, Yamada S, et al. Promotion of β-cell differentiation by conophylline in fetal and neonatal rat pancreas. Diabetes 2004;53:2596–2602.

23

Embryonic Stem Cells as a Source of Pancreatic Precursors and Islet Cells In Vitro

Victoria L. Browning, Brenda W. Kahan, and Jon S. Odorico

The generation of unlimited supplies of islet stem cells or β cells from an abundant, renewable, and readily accessible source for transplantation would probably render current transplantation therapies obsolete. Although this ultimate goal is on the distant horizon, recent progress, representing the first step, has been made in identifying pancreatic precursor cells and differentiated islet cells generated from both mouse and human embryonic stem (ES) cells. The next hurdle, achieving enrichment of these cell types from ES cell cultures and isolating purified populations for functional testing, may be a more challenging step. It is becoming clear that a better understanding of the sequential genetic and epigenetic signals occurring during normal mouse and human development will be necessary. Particularly relevant is the need to understand the nature and identity of true embryonic pancreatic precursor cells and islet progenitor cells, and to identify conditions that allow their efficient, large-scale isolation. An ES cell-based in vitro differentiation system can facilitate these goals by providing a straightforward means to select and purify progenitor cells, and to investigate conditions that promote their expansion and differentiation ex vivo. Specifically, a human ES cell-based in vitro model system would be invaluable for studying human islet development and for providing cells for transplantation.

The Clinical Problem

It is estimated that by 2010, more than 220 million people worldwide will be diagnosed with diabetes,[1] of which approximately 10% will have the type 1 form characterized by profound insulin deficiency, requiring lifelong insulin injections. Although administration of exogenous insulin remains a viable therapy for the disease, inadequate glycemic control results in significant morbidity and premature mortality. For some patients, vascularized pancreas transplants or infusions of isolated islets of Langerhans can eliminate or greatly reduce the amount of exogenous insulin required to maintain euglycemia, resulting in a reduction in long-term complications caused by repeated blood glucose excursions. However, cadaver donor shortages greatly limit the number of transplants that can be performed: Fewer than 100 islet cell transplants and approximately 2000 pancreas transplants are performed annually in the world.[2] Even with substantial efforts to increase donation rates, it is unlikely that the supply will ever meet the demand. Thus, glucose-responsive, insulin-secreting β cells generated from a renewable source would be an ideal alternative to tissue procured through organ donation. Based on their unique capacities for self-renewal and multilineage differentiation, human ES cells may be such a source.[3-6]

ES Cells as Potential Therapy for Diabetes

ES cells are derived from the inner cell mass of a blastocyst, an embryo that is less than 1 week old. For derivation of human ES cell lines, the typical starting materials are discarded blastocyst-stage embryos from in vitro fertilization clinics; after the completion of in vitro fertilization procedures, residual embryos are donated by couples for ES cell derivations after informed consent.[3] Because the derivation process renders the embryo nonviable, ethical questions surrounding the use of human ES cell lines have arisen. However, the great promise of ES cell therapies is a mitigating factor in the minds of many. This promise lies in the unique biology of ES cells: They have both the capacity to replicate indefinitely in an undifferentiated state, and the ability to give rise to daughter cells capable of differentiating into any cell type of the body, a potential that has been demonstrated conclusively in vivo for murine ES cells,[7] and at least partially for both murine and human cells in vitro. It is thus the hope of scientists and nonscientists alike that vast quantities of specialized cells, such as β cells, can be generated from ES cells and used to treat a variety of diseases.

Differentiating in culture, ES cells can recapitulate many aspects of normal embryonic development, including the initial specification of lineage-restricted progenitor cells that can grow and differentiate into specialized postmitotic cell types including neurons, glia, chondrocytes, adipocytes, osteoclasts, endothelial cells, hematopoietic cells, muscle lineages, keratinocytes, melanocytes, yolk sac, as well as endoderm-derived lineages such as hepatocytes and cells reminiscent of pancreatic β cells, among others.[8–31] In order for ES cells to reach their full potential as therapeutic agents, protocols must be established that direct their differentiation into homogenous populations of specific cell types. This is important both to maximize efficiency and also to prevent unwanted cell types and potentially tumorigenic undifferentiated cells from being transplanted into patients. One approach to create enriched populations of specific cell types is to create culture conditions in vitro that mimic the embryonic environment in which the specific cell types develop. This strategy has been used to generate cells of hematopoietic lineage,[28] cardiomyocytes,[32] and motor neurons.[18] For this approach to work for creation of pancreatic β cells in culture, an understanding of signals and cues that promote pancreas development in the embryo is required. Recent studies have advanced our understanding of the progressive stepwise commitment of endoderm to pancreatic epithelial progenitors, and then to islet-restricted progenitors ultimately leading to the formation of the four endocrine cell types of mature islets. Here, we will first review pancreaticogenesis and how islets form in the mouse embryo. In this context, we will then discuss the current state of research on the generation of pancreatic islet cells from murine and human ES cells in vitro and how our understanding of islet ontogeny might help achieve directed differentiation to pancreatic lineages in a more efficient manner.

Pancreaticogenesis

Pancreas formation is initiated as two distinct outgrowths of the foregut endoderm, starting first with the dorsal anlage at embryonic day (e) 9.5–10 in the mouse, and followed by the ventral bud approximately 1 day later. Shortly thereafter, rapid growth and branching morphogenesis begin, and subsequently the ventral bud rotates and fuses with its dorsal counterpart, forming a single gland. Branching morphogenesis culminates in ductal differentiation and the formation of acini composed of digestive enzyme- and bicarbonate-secreting cells. Early endocrine cells expressing glucagon alone or glucagon and insulin can be found at approximately e9.5–10.5 within the early pancreatic duodenal homeobox 1-positive ($PDX1^+$) pancreatic epithelium but these cells do not appear to be the lineage precursors of mature islet endocrine cells. Later in development, individual endocrine cells (α, β, δ, and PP) arising within the epithelium from neurogenin 3-positive ($NGN3^+$) islet progenitors eventually migrate from the epithelium into the stroma of the gland and aggregate to form intact islets. Shortly after birth, the pancreas is able to secrete insulin when stimulated by glucose.

Numerous studies demonstrate that the exocrine and endocrine compartments are derived from the embryonic endoderm. Although the full complement of signals involved in the early formation of endoderm is currently unknown, several key transcription factors have emerged, including Sox17 and Mixl1. First identified as determinants of endoderm in Xenopus and zebrafish, inactivation of the murine homologs of Sox17 and Mixl1 demonstrate phenotypes consistent with their roles in development of the endoderm.[33,34] In addition, Nodal, a transforming growth factor β family member, which is expressed before and during gastrulation, is critically required for the formation of mesoderm and endoderm in mammals.[35] The forkhead box factor Foxa2 is essential for the development of anterior endoderm from which the pancreas and liver are formed.[36,37]

Once formed, the commitment of the endoderm toward a pancreatic fate is thought to occur as the result of expression of a particular combination of transcription factors, growth factors and growth factor receptors, and signaling molecules and their receptors, by the cells within a specific region of anterior embryonic endoderm. To better understand the molecular events that initiate this patterning, researchers have used tissue induction experiments to begin to define the embryonic tissue interactions that may guide pancreatic specification from the prepatterned endoderm. These studies suggest that factors derived from the notochord, such as fibroblast growth factor (FGF) 2 and activin βB are involved in the initial repression of Sonic hedgehog (Shh),[38,39] a protein whose expression must be down-regulated in the presumptive dorsal pancreatic endoderm for correct development of the organ to ensue.[40] In addition to the permissive signals from the notochord, the prepancreatic epithelium appears to respond to vascular epithelium and vascular endothelial growth factor, as determined through coculture studies with dissected dorsal aortae.[41,42] Other adjacent tissues, such as the lateral plate mesoderm (LPM) may also be involved. The LPM appears to be competent to signal endoderm not fated to become pancreas to initiate a pancreatic differentiation program, including expression of pdx1.[43] Bone morphogenetic protein (BMP)4, BMP7, and activin A are apparently capable of inducing expression of pdx1 in anterior chick endoderm when combined with the appropriate mesoderm, suggesting that perhaps these molecules are sufficient to mediate the inductive signals of the LPM.

After specification of the endoderm, proper signaling between the mesenchyme and the epithelium is also required for normal pancreatic development. For instance, FGF10, which is normally expressed in the pancreatic mesenchyme, may mediate inductive interactions.[44] Norgaard and colleagues[45] showed that ectopic expression of FGF10 in the foregut epithelium resulted in an increased proliferation of undifferentiated cells that went on to adopt a pancreatic fate, leading to a hyperplastic pancreas. These studies provide insights into the early steps of embryonic endoderm patterning required for pancreas development.

In addition, the study of "knock-out" mice has revealed valuable information about the roles of a variety of transcription factors involved in pancreatic development[46-48] (reviewed in Edlund[49]). For example, it is known that pdx1 (alias Ipf1) is absolutely required for pancreas development, although in its absence, pancreatic bud formation is initiated.[50,51] Animals missing NGN3 lack mature endocrine cells, whereas exocrine development proceeds normally,[52] placing NGN3 at an important branchpoint for pancreas development. Lineage tagging studies have also been used to determine which adult pancreatic cell types are formed from cells expressing certain gene products during development.[53-55] Together, these studies demonstrate the provenance of mature endocrine cells: They are derived from NGN3$^+$ progenitors present within the early pancreatic epithelium.

Although the roles of these and other important pancreatic transcription factors (Nkx6.1, Nkx2.2, Ptf1a, HNF6, among others) have been described recently, their precise functions, i.e., interactions with other transcription factors and target genes, known and unknown, remain to be elucidated. In addition, how these key transcription factor proteins achieve tissue-specific functions, and exactly why cells in different positions in the embryo that express these proteins develop into distinctive tissue types, are questions that have not yet been answered. Furthermore, the precise complement of homeobox transcription factors involved in the specification of pancreatic fate from uncommitted endoderm is not known. Lastly, characterization of unique cell surface markers of islet progenitors would aid in their efficient large-scale isolation from embryos or ES cells and would facilitate their identification in adult tissues. Although significant insights into pancreas development have been achieved, it is clear we are far from a complete understanding of mammalian pancreaticogenesis. Yet, studies to date provide a rich framework of knowledge to begin to design experiments to more efficiently direct differentiation of ES cells to pancreatic lineages.

Pancreatic Lineage Specification in ES Cell Cultures

Although it was known that, in the context of whole animal development, murine ES cells were capable of differentiation into functional pancreatic cell types, many initial studies were aimed at determining whether the same was true for ES cells differentiating in vitro. We[19] and others[56] demonstrated that ES cells grown under nonselective conditions have the ability to differentiate into lineages of the endocrine pancreas (Figure 23.1). Our protocol includes a period of embryoid body (EB) formation. When ES cells are removed from conditions that prevent their differentiation and permit their growth under nonadherent conditions, they form multicellular aggregates of differentiated cells that are called EBs. To a certain extent, the initial morphogenesis of EB formation mimics that of morula- and blastula-stage embryos in vivo. After several days in culture, a layer of columnar epithelium ectoderm forms beneath the primitive endoderm, which often surrounds a fluid-filled cavity resembling a blastocoele. At this point, EBs begin to express genes of primitive extraembryonic endoderm,[10,30] ectoderm,[20,57] and mesoderm lineages.[31,58] The cell–cell interactions afforded by EB formation may promote inductive signals required for the formation of certain cell types or lineages. Our preliminary results suggest that, when grown under nonselective conditions, EBs express markers of definitive embryonic endoderm such as Sox17, Foxa2, and Pdx1. We also observed that under these conditions endoderm formation is greatly enhanced when a period of EB formation is included (unpublished results).

In studies of murine ES cells, we discovered that a culture protocol including a 5- to 7-day period of EB formation followed by further differentiation in the presence of fetal bovine serum after plating was sufficient to produce foci of cells expressing markers of pancreatic lineages. These include PDX1, a homeodomain protein that is absolutely required for development of the pancreas in humans and mice[50,51,59]; peptide YY, a marker of early endocrine cells; and insulin, glucagon, and somatostatin, hormones produced by the islet endocrine cells [Figure 23.2 (see color section)].[19]

In addition, it appears that these culture conditions provide an environment that facilitates the recreation of some classical developmental stages of islet cytodifferentiation, especially with regard to the timing of specific cell types that emerge in culture. Although lineage tracing experiments have yet to be performed, a series of cultures examined at different time points suggest that the primary to secondary transition that is seen during mouse development in vivo is recapitulated in vitro, because there are cells that are double-positive for both insulin and

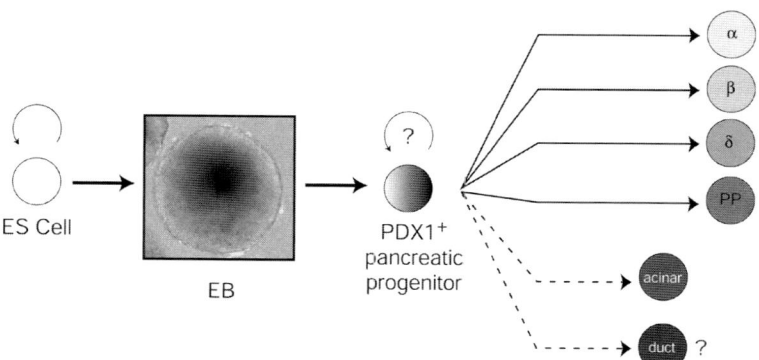

Figure 23.1. Schematic diagram of in vitro ES cell differentiation focused on pancreatic lineage cells. The culture of both murine and human ES cells under conditions that permit the formation of embryoid bodies (EBs) result in a proportion of cells adopting a pancreatic fate. Pancreatic progenitor cells, which are PDX1+, as well as cells with the hallmarks of islet endocrine cells (α, β, δ, and PP) cells, have been identified (solid arrows). Other nonislet functional lineages of the pancreas, such as acinar tissue and ductal cells, are generally not found in serum-containing, non-growth factor supplemented cultures. Curved arrows denote cell division without further differentiation.

glucagon in early stage cultures that appear to be replaced by single hormone-positive cells found in later cultures. At late stages, cells with characteristics similar to true β cells can be identified.[19] We have obtained similar results differentiating human ES cells under nonselective conditions including an EB phase (unpublished results). As in the mouse cultures, discrete foci of PDX1+ cells arise within the cultures during the EB stage and persist after plating. At later stages, hormone-positive cells can be identified.

It is important to note that although apparent pancreas progenitor cells can develop within the cultures grown under nonselective culture conditions, the conditions do not appear to promote growth of this cell type. Indeed, less than 0.1% of the cells in culture adopt a pancreas-specific fate, as judged by immunostaining with antibodies to PDX1, peptide YY, and/or insulin [Figure 23.2 (see color section)]. An obvious question is: Why are pancreatic lineage cells so rare in ES cell cultures? Although not precisely known, the answer may lie in the fact that islet endocrine cells are rare cell types in mammals that do not fully develop until late in gestation. Islet endocrine cells are believed to constitute only approximately 1% of the cellular mass of the pancreas. In adult mammals, the functioning endocrine cells of the islet maintain glycemic control. In the fetus, however, glycemic control is primarily regulated by the mother, and the embryo's islet endocrine axis does not become functional until early postnatal development. Another explanation for the low numbers of pancreas lineage cells observed in vitro is simply the nonselective conditions in which the cells were cultured. Clearly, culture conditions used to date do not precisely recapitulate the temporally and spatially restricted developmental cues that occur in the embryo. Therefore, it is not unexpected that such cell types, although they arise under these conditions, do not dominate the cultures, nor do they preferentially expand or grow over time.

Indeed, it has proven to be a challenge to achieve directed differentiation of any specific cell lineage from ES cells in culture such that homogeneous populations of cells are generated. Several reports have emerged claiming to achieve directed differentiation of ES cells toward pancreatic β cells based on protocols that promote enrichment of nestin+ neuronal precursors.[60–62] The expression of many neuronal cell markers in islet cells, such as synaptophysin and neuron-specific enolase, had led previously to the hypothesis that islets of Langerhans were of a neuroectodermal origin, and thus the idea that nestin might mark islet progenitor cells was put forth.[63] In 2001, Zulewski et al.[64] reported that nestin-positive cells derived from the adult rat pancreas could be expanded in vitro and had the apparent capability to differentiate into cells that expressed insulin, glucagon, and PDX1. Researchers in several groups then used protocols that were originally designed to enrich for neural precursors to differentiate ES cells through a nestin-positive step and into pancreatic β cells.[60–62,65] These protocols typically involved growing cells in serum-free media containing a mixture of insulin, transferrin, selenium, and fibronectin (often abbreviated ITSFn). After this, and depending on the specific protocol, cells were exposed to bFGF, N2 medium, B27 medium, nicotinamide, and/or phosphoinositol-3 kinase inhibitors to first expand pancreatic progenitor cells, and then prompt their final differentiation. Although cells resulting from this type of culturing did often stain with anti-insulin antibodies, the cells typically functioned abnormally in in vitro glucose release assays, and failed to restore euglycemia is streptozotocin-treated animals after transplantation.

Further experimentation with protocols designed to enrich for nestin-positive cells demonstrated that the ES cell-derived clusters did not actually express insulin, but rather had taken up insulin from the medium.[66] Cells derived through such protocols did not robustly synthesize insulin or pdx1 gene products,[60,67] nor did they stain with antibodies specific for C-peptide, a protein generated when proinsulin is cleaved to the functional insulin molecule.[68,69] Furthermore, many of the cells grown under these serum-free conditions that apparently stained with antibodies to insulin appeared to be undergoing apoptosis, as examined through a caspase-3 immunostaining[68] and TUNEL staining.[67,68] In addition, recent lineage-tracing experiments suggest that the endocrine pancreas is not composed of cells that express nestin during their course of development.[70–73] Thus, there is no current evidence that selection of differentiated ES cells that express nestin will result in a population of glucose-responsive insulin-secreting β-like cells.

Enhancement of Islet Differentiation from ES Cells by Lineage Selection and/or Reestablishment of Developmental Pathways

The heterogeneity of differentiating ES cell cultures has hindered researchers' abilities to study the function of ES cell-derived cells and tissues. Therefore, a major goal of ES cell research is to generate purified populations of a desired cell type, in this case, pancreatic progenitors and/or β cells. To achieve this goal, some investigators have taken advantage of the relative ease with which ES cells can be genetically manipulated to create selection strategies. One strategy is to integrate lineage-specific promoter-driven fluorescent transgenes and then select marked cells by flow cytometric cell sorting.[74–77] An alternate approach is to express a drug resistance gene under control of the chosen lineage-specific promoter. In either case, when the promoter is activated in a subset of cells among differentiating ES cell progeny, it is an indication that those cells have adopted the cell fate of interest. Cells activating the lineage-specific promoter can then be selected by virtue of their fluorescence or drug resistance. This technique has now been used to select for neural precursors,[78] cardiomyocytes,[79] and insulin-producing cells.[80,81]

To purify insulin-producing cells derived from murine ES cells, Soria and colleagues[80] generated a cell line in which the βgeo fusion protein (β-galactosidase fused with neomycin resistance gene)[82] was driven by the human insulin promoter. The ES cells were differentiated through a period of EB formation, and then cells that had activated the insulin promoter were selected by addition of G418 to the media. Selected cells were then grown in a low glucose environment (5 mM) for 5 days in the presence of nicotinamide, after which the resulting cell clusters were analyzed in vitro and in vivo. In vitro, the cells appeared to respond appropriately in insulin secretion assays. When transplanted into diabetic mice to assess their ability to normalize hyperglycemia, the cells rescued several animals for a period of up to 16 weeks after transplantation. These successes are promising, although some questions regarding the nature of the selected cells and their phenotypic stability remain. In addition, it is not clear that the animals were cured as a direct result of their ES cell-derived graft as the donor cells (R1 line, 129 hybrid, primarily H-2^b) were allogeneic to the recipients (OF1, outbred) and should have been rejected, and studies to confirm that reversal of diabetes was dependent on the infused cells were not performed. In addition, euglycemia was not durable in a significant proportion of animals for reasons that remain unclear. Nonetheless, this study in murine ES cells is the single study to date that demonstrates significant in vitro and in vivo function from ES cell-derived insulin-producing tissue.

An alternate, or complementary, strategy to achieve enhanced islet differentiation is to modify culture conditions in order to mimic the in vivo growth environment and recapitulate normal developmental pathways in vitro. If embryonic inductive signals could be precisely reestablished, and the correct embryonic microenvironment provided to differentiating ES cells, directed differentiation into large numbers of PDX1-positive pancreatic progenitor cells and ultimately endocrine cells might be achieved. To begin to reconstruct pancreatic lineage differentiation from ES cells in culture, one needs to consider how this tissue forms in the embryo. Because the pancreas and islets are endoderm derived, it might be important to enrich for endodermal precursors by either selecting for cells that express genes required for endoderm development, such as Nodal, or overexpressing these genes in ES cell progeny. Then, to pattern the ES cell-derived endoderm and induce pancreas specification in a large proportion of cells, it might be important to inhibit the function of key developmental signaling molecules, such as Shh, which is normally down-regulated in the region of foregut endoderm that is specified to become pancreas.

Reconstructing combinations of intrinsic and extrinsic signals may also be important. Overexpressing one or more key pancreatic transcription factor genes that are typically expressed in early committed pancreatic epithelium or are necessary for β cell formation may lead to a greater proportion of cells differentiating into endocrine cells or β cells. Indeed, early studies focusing on the overexpression of PDX1 and PAX4 in murine ES cell cultures suggest this strategy may be useful.[65,83] It is important to note, however, that simply because a transcription factor is expressed in a specific tissue at a particular time in development and is required for normal development does not necessarily imply that this protein will *direct* differentiation. In addition, our knowledge of the cellular context in which these critical transcription factors act may be incomplete, but is undoubtedly important. Therefore, it may be difficult to recapitulate the actions of these genes precisely in ES cell progeny.

Mesenchymal-to-epithelial signaling, also critically important for proper growth and maturation and of the pancreatic epithelium, could be recapitulated by adding specific growth factors, such as BMP4 or FGF10, or by coculturing ES cells with stromal cell lines[28,84,85] or embryonic tissues. By providing the proper developmental signals, it may be possible to promote the differentiation of a proliferative precursor population that could be isolated and expanded. However, some growth factors have pleiotropic effects or can function in multiple tissues. Therefore, one needs to consider the context in which the cytokine is acting. The effect of growth factors in mixed populations of ES cell progeny may be unpredictable and not specific to the lineage of interest.[86] In addition, the presence of varied cell types may lead to unpredictable cell–cell interactions that could inhibit endoderm formation and/or pancreatic specification.

The correct cues for differentiating progenitors into postmitotic, single hormone-expressing differentiated islet cells or β cells remain to be determined. Also, little is known about the regulation of the later stages of islet development, including terminal differentiation, migration of islet endocrine cells from the epithelium into the acinar lobules, or the mechanisms regulating their aggregation into micro-organs. Growth factors that have been shown to accelerate the functional maturation of human fetal pancreas tissue may be worthwhile to test in the ES cell differentiation system at these late stages. Clearly, the development of robust methods for enrichment of islet progenitor cell types and β cells from ES cells remains an important goal.

Our current knowledge of developmental mechanisms can be directly applied to ES cells as they differentiate in culture to promote lineage-specific differentiation. This framework serves as a useful starting point. For example, building on prior in vivo developmental studies, Wichterle et al.[18] demonstrated robust, directed differentiation of motor neurons from mouse ES cells. This, and other studies,[87] demonstrates how applying known developmental cues to ES cells can direct differentiation to a desired phenotype and recapitulate normal ontogeny. As gaps in our knowledge of pancreatic islet development are filled in, we will be better able to faithfully reestablish important developmental signals in ES cell cultures.

Remaining Questions

In the quest to generate robustly functional insulin-producing cells from ES cells, numerous questions remain to be answered. For example, i) How do we determine if an insulin-staining cell is a true β cell, and what functional measures should be used? ii) Are all ES cell-derived insulin-staining cells equally mature or does a subpopulation retain a fetal phenotype? iii) Are β cells alone sufficient for normal glucose-responsive insulin secretion in vivo, or are other islet cell types required? iv) Are human ES cell-derived insulin-producing cells able to secrete insulin in a glucose-responsive manner? These questions will be addressed below.

What should the benchmarks be for a "real" β cell? Not only is it important to correctly identify cells, but one needs to consider the fact that cells from a variety of tissues induced in ES cultures can potentially synthesize insulin, including extraplacental membranes[88] and neuronal cells,[89,90] among others.[91,92] Additionally, β cells at various stages of functional maturity might be expected to exist in ES cell cultures, because the differentiation process may be interrupted because of environmental deficiencies. Indeed, the response of islet tissue in standard assays may differ depending on the developmental stage.[93] Consequently, it will be important to evaluate function by a variety of parameters including studies at the single cell level.

Are other islet endocrine cell types, in addition to β cells, necessary for optimal function? It has been suggested that all islet subtypes are required to achieve regulated functionality in normal in situ conditions[94,95] although there is some evidence that β cells alone can rescue streptozotocin-induced diabetes in mice.[96] The answer to this question may be different depending on the species and cause of diabetes.

Normal β-cell function has not yet been convincingly demonstrated for *human* ES-derived cells, and this should be carefully evaluated with dynamic in vitro perifusion assays once enriched populations of insulin-producing tissue are reliably generated. Ultimately, it is hoped that increased numbers of functional β cells can be obtained through a combination of new selective techniques and better culture conditions.

Acknowledgments

The authors thank Kathy Worrall for technical assistance in preparing the manuscript and Nick Weber for helping with production of the figures. This project was generously supported by grants from the NIH-Beta Cell Biology Consortium (U19-DK61244 and subcontract to Vanderbilt University U19-DK42502), JDRF (2001-191, 2004-145), and Roche Organ Transplant Research Foundation (221283847). This work was also supported in part from a grant to the University of Wisconsin Medical School under the Howard Hughes Medical Institute Research Resources Program for Medical Schools.

References

1. Zimmet P, Alberti KG, Shaw J. Global and societal implications of the diabetes epidemic. Nature 2001;414:782–787.
2. Gruessner AC, Sutherland DE. Pancreas transplant outcomes for United States (US) and non-US cases as reported to the United Network for Organ Sharing (UNOS) and the International Pancreas Transplant Registry (IPTR) as of May 2003. Clin Transpl 2003: 21–51.
3. Thomson JA, Itskovitz-Eldor J, Shapiro SS, et al. Embryonic stem cell lines derived from human blastocysts. Science 1998;282:1145–1147.
4. Odorico JS, Kaufman DS, Thomson JA. Multilineage differentiation from human embryonic stem cell lines. Stem Cells 2001;19:193–204.
5. Reubinoff BE, Pera MF, Fong CY, Trounson A, Bongso A. Embryonic stem cell lines from human blastocysts: somatic differentiation in vitro. Nat Biotechnol 2000;18:399–404.
6. Pera MF, Reubinoff B, Trounson A. Human embryonic stem cells. J Cell Sci 2000;113(pt 1):5–10.
7. Nagy A, Gocza E, Diaz EA, et al. Embryonic stem cells alone are able to support fetal development in the mouse. Development 1990;10:815–821.
8. Doetschman TC, Eistetter H, Katz M, Schmidt W, Kemler R. The in vitro development of blastocyst-derived embryonic stem cell lines: formation of visceral yolk sac, blood islands and myocardium. J Embryol Exp Morphol 1985;87:27–45.
9. Zhang SC, Wernig M, Duncan ID, Brustle O, Thomson JA. In vitro differentiation of transplantable neural precursors from human embryonic stem cells. Nat Biotechnol 2001;19:1129–1133.
10. Levinson-Dushnik M, Benvenisty N. Involvement of hepatocyte nuclear factor 3 in endoderm differentiation of embryonic stem cells. Mol Cell Biol 1997;17:3817–3822.
11. Yamashita J, Itoh H, Hirashima M, et al. Flk1-positive cells derived from embryonic stem cells serve as vascular progenitors. Nature 2000;408:92–96.
12. Levenberg S, Golub JS, Amit M, Itskovitz-Eldor J, Langer R. Endothelial cells derived from human embryonic stem cells. Proc Natl Acad Sci USA 2002;99:4391–4396.
13. Yamane T, Hayashi S, Mizoguchi M, Yamazaki H, Kunisada T. Derivation of melanocytes from embryonic stem cells in culture. Dev Dyn 1999;216:450–458.
14. Yamada T, Yoshikawa M, Takaki M, et al. In vitro functional gut-like organ formation from mouse embryonic stem cells. Stem Cells 2002;20:41–49.
15. Yamane T, Kunisada T, Yamazaki H, Era T, Nakano T, Hayashi SI. Development of osteoclasts from embryonic stem cells through a pathway that is c-fms but not c-kit dependent. Blood 1997;90:3516–3523.
16. Xu C, Police S, Rao N, Carpenter MK. Characterization and enrichment of cardiomyocytes derived from human embryonic stem cells. Circ Res 2002;91:501–508.
17. Wobus AM, Guan K, Yang HT, Boheler KR. Embryonic stem cells as a model to study cardiac, skeletal muscle, and vascular smooth muscle cell differentiation. Methods Mol Biol 2002;185:127–156.
18. Wichterle H, Lieberam I, Porter JA, Jessell TM. Directed differentiation of embryonic stem cells into motor neurons. Cell 2002;110:385–397.
19. Kahan BW, Jacobson LM, Hullett DA, Oberley TD, Odorico JS. Pancreatic precursors and differentiated islet cell types from murine embryonic stem cells: an in vitro model to study islet differentiation. Diabetes 2003;52:2016–2024.
20. Bain G, Kitchens D, Yao M, Huettner JE, Gottlieb DI. Embryonic stem cells express neuronal properties in vitro. Dev Biol 1995;168:342–357.
21. Green H, Easley K, Iuchi S. Marker succession during the development of keratinocytes from cultured human embryonic stem cells. Proc Natl Acad Sci USA 2003;100:15625–15630.
22. Sottile V, Thomson A, McWhir J. In vitro osteogenic differentiation of human ES cells. Cloning Stem Cells 2003;5:149–155.
23. Reubinoff BE, Itsykson P, Turetsky T, et al. Neural progenitors from human embryonic stem cells. Nat Biotechnol 2001;19:1134–1140.
24. Rambhatla L, Chiu CP, Kundu P, Peng Y, Carpenter MK. Generation of hepatocyte-like cells from human embryonic stem cells. Cell Transplant 2003;12:1–11.
25. Perlingeiro RC, Kyba M, Daley GQ. Clonal analysis of differentiating embryonic stem cells reveals a hematopoietic progenitor with primitive erythroid and adult lymphoid-myeloid potential. Development 2001;128:4597–4604.
26. Okabe S, Forsberg-Nilsson K, Spiro AC, Segal M, McKay RD. Development of neuronal precursor cells and functional postmitotic neurons from embryonic stem cells in vitro. Mech Dev 1996;59:89–102.
27. Mujtaba T, Piper DR, Kalyani A, Groves AK, Lucero MT, Rao MS. Lineage-restricted neural precursors can be isolated from both the mouse neural tube and cultured ES cells. Dev Biol 1999;214:113–127.
28. Kaufman DS, Hanson ET, Lewis RL, Auerbach R, Thomson JA. Hematopoietic colony-forming cells derived from human embryonic stem cells. Proc Natl Acad Sci USA 2001;98:10716–10721.

29. Dani C. Embryonic stem cell-derived adipogenesis. Cells Tissues Organs 1999;165:173–180.
30. Abe K, Niwa H, Iwase K, et al. Endoderm-specific gene expression in embryonic stem cells differentiated to embryoid bodies. Exp Cell Res 1996;229:27–34.
31. Baker RK, Lyons GE. Embryonic stem cells and in vitro muscle development. Curr Top Dev Biol 1996;33:263–279.
32. Wobus AM, Kaomei G, Shan J, et al. Retinoic acid accelerates embryonic stem cell-derived cardiac differentiation and enhances development of ventricular cardiomyocytes. J Mol Cell Cardiol 1997;29:1525–1539.
33. Kanai-Azuma M, Kanai Y, Gad JM, et al. Depletion of definitive gut endoderm in Sox17-null mutant mice. Development 2002;129:2367–2379.
34. Hart AH, Hartley L, Sourris K, et al. Mixl1 is required for axial mesendoderm morphogenesis and patterning in the murine embryo. Development 2002;129:3597–3608.
35. Conlon FL, Lyons KM, Takaesu N, et al. A primary requirement for nodal in the formation and maintenance of the primitive streak in the mouse. Development 1994;120:1919–1928.
36. Ang SL, Wierda A, Wong D, et al. The formation and maintenance of the definitive endoderm lineage in the mouse: involvement of HNF3/forkhead proteins. Development 1993;119:1301–1315.
37. Weinstein DC, Ruiz IAA, Chen WS, et al. The winged-helix transcription factor HNF-3 beta is required for notochord development in the mouse embryo. Cell 1994;78:575–588.
38. Hebrok M. Hedgehog signaling in pancreas development. Mech Dev 2003;120:45–57.
39. Hebrok M, Kim SK, St. Jacques B, McMahon AP, Melton DA. Regulation of pancreas development by hedgehog signaling. Development 2000;127:4905–4913.
40. Hebrok M, Kim SK, Melton DA. Notochord repression of endodermal Sonic hedgehog permits pancreas development. Genes Dev 1998;12:1705–1713.
41. Lammert E, Cleaver O, Melton D. Induction of pancreatic differentiation by signals from blood vessels. Science 2001;294:564–567.
42. Yoshitomi H, Zaret KS. Endothelial cell interactions initiate dorsal pancreas development by selectively inducing the transcription factor Ptf1a. Development 2004;131:807–817.
43. Kumar M, Jordan N, Melton D, Grapin-Botton A. Signals from lateral plate mesoderm instruct endoderm toward a pancreatic fate. Dev Biol 2003;259:109–122.
44. Bhushan A, Itoh N, Kato S, et al. Fgf10 is essential for maintaining the proliferative capacity of epithelial progenitor cells during early pancreatic organogenesis. Development 2001;128:5109–5117.
45. Norgaard GA, Jensen JN, Jensen J. FGF10 signaling maintains the pancreatic progenitor cell state revealing a novel role of Notch in organ development. Dev Biol 2003;264:323–338.
46. Edlund H. Transcribing pancreas. Diabetes 1998;47:1817–1823.
47. Madsen OD, Jensen J, Petersen HV, et al. Transcription factors contributing to the pancreatic beta-cell phenotype. Horm Metab Res 1997;29:265–270.
48. Sander M, German MS. The beta cell transcription factors and development of the pancreas. J Mol Med 1997;75:327–340.
49. Edlund H. Pancreatic organogenesis: developmental mechanisms and implications for therapy. Nat Rev Genet 2002;3:524–532.
50. Jonsson J, Carlsson L, Edlund T, Edlund H. Insulin-promoter-factor 1 is required for pancreas development in mice. Nature 1994;371:606–609.
51. Offield MF, Jetton TL, Labosky PA, et al. PDX-1 is required for pancreatic outgrowth and differentiation of the rostral duodenum. Development 1996;122:983–995.
52. Gradwohl G, Dierich A, LeMaur M, Guillemot F. Neurogenin 3 is required for the development of the four endocrine cell lineages of the pancreas. Proc Natl Acad Sci USA 2000;97:1607–1611.
53. Gu G, Dubauskaite J, Melton DA. Direct evidence for the pancreatic lineage: NGN3+ cells are islet progenitors and are distinct from duct progenitors. Development 2002;129:2447–2457.
54. Gu G, Brown JR, Melton DA. Direct lineage tracing reveals the ontogeny of pancreatic cell fates during mouse embryogenesis. Mech Dev 2003;120:35–43.
55. Herrera PL. Adult insulin- and glucagon-producing cells differentiate from two independent cell lineages. Development 2000;127:2317–2322.
56. Assady S, Maor G, Amit M, Itskovitz-Eldor J, Skorecki KL, Tzukerman M. Insulin production by human embryonic stem cells. Diabetes 2001;50:1691–1697.
57. Liu S, Qu Y, Stewert TJ, et al. Embryonic stem cells differentiate into oligodendrocytes and myelinate in culture and after spinal cord transplantation. Proc Natl Acad Sci USA 2000;97:6126–6131.
58. Robertson SM, Kennedy M, Shannon JM, Keller G. A transitional stage in the commitment of mesoderm to hematopoiesis requiring the transcription factor SCL/tal-1. Development 2000;127:2447–2459.
59. Stoffers DA, Zinkin NT, Stanojevic V, Clarke WL, Habener JF. Pancreatic agenesis attributable to a single nucleotide deletion in the human IPF1 gene coding sequence. Nat Genet 1997;15:106–110.
60. Lumelsky N, Blondel O, Laeng P, Velasco I, Ravin R, McKay R. Differentiation of embryonic stem cells to insulin-secreting structures similar to pancreatic islets [erratum appears in Science 2001;293(5529):428]. Science 2001;292:1389–1394.
61. Hori Y, Rulifson IC, Tsai BC, Heit JJ, Cahoy JD, Kim SK. Growth inhibitors promote differentiation of insulin-producing tissue from embryonic stem cells. Proc Natl Acad Sci USA 2002;99:16105–16110.
62. Segev H, Fishman B, Ziskind A, Shulman M, Itskovitz-Eldor J. Differentiation of human embryonic stem cells into insulin-producing clusters. Stem Cells 2004;22:265–274.
63. Hunziker E, Stein M. Nestin-expressing cells in the pancreatic islets of Langerhans. Biochem Biophys Res Commun 2000;271:116–119.
64. Zulewski H, Abraham EJ, Gerlach MJ, et al. Multipotential nestin-positive stem cells isolated from adult pancreatic islets differentiate ex vivo into pancreatic endocrine, exocrine, and hepatic phenotypes. Diabetes 2001;50:521–533.
65. Blyszczuk P, Czyz J, Kania G, et al. Expression of Pax4 in embryonic stem cells promotes differentiation of nestin-positive progenitor and insulin-producing cells. Proc Natl Acad Sci USA 2003;100:998–1003.

66. Rajagopal J, Anderson WJ, Kume S, Martinez OI, Melton DA. Insulin staining of ES cell progeny from insulin uptake. Science 2003;299:363.
67. Sipione S, Eshpeter A, Lyon JG, Korbutt GS, Bleackley RC. Insulin expressing cells from differentiated embryonic stem cells are not beta cells. Diabetologia 2004;47:499–508.
68. Hansson M, Tonning A, Frandsen U, et al. Artifactual insulin release from differentiated embryonic stem cells. Diabetes 2004;53:2603–2609.
69. Odorico JS, Kahan BW, Hullett DA, Jacobson LM, Browning VL. Modeling islet development with embryonic stem cells. In: Odorico JS, Pedersen RA, Zhang SC, eds. Human Embryonic Stem Cells. Oxford: Garland Science/BIOS Scientific; 2004.
70. Treutelaar MK, Skidmore JM, Dias-Leme CL, et al. Nestin-lineage cells contribute to the microvasculature but not endocrine cells of the islet. Diabetes 2003;52:2503–2512.
71. Humphrey RK, Bucay N, Beattie GM, et al. Characterization and isolation of promoter-defined nestin-positive cells from the human fetal pancreas. Diabetes 2003;52:2519–2525.
72. Delacour A, Nepote V, Trumpp A, Herrera PL. Nestin expression in pancreatic exocrine cell lineages. Mech Dev 2004;121:3–14.
73. Esni F, Stoffers DA, Takeuchi T, Leach SD. Origin of exocrine pancreatic cells from nestin-positive precursors in developing mouse pancreas. Mech Dev 2004;121:15–25.
74. Meyer N, Jaconi M, Landopoulou A, Fort P, Puceat M. A fluorescent reporter gene as a marker for ventricular specification in ES-derived cardiac cells. FEBS Lett 2000;478:151–158.
75. Roy NS, Wang S, Harrison-Restelli C, et al. Identification, isolation, and promoter-defined separation of mitotic oligodendrocyte progenitor cells from the adult human subcortical white matter. J Neurosci 1999;19:9986–9995.
76. Hawley TS, Telford WG, Hawley RG. "Rainbow" reporters for multispectral marking and lineage analysis of hematopoietic stem cells. Stem Cells 2001;19:118–124.
77. Meyer K, Irminger JC, Moss L, et al. Sorting human beta-cells consequent to targeted expression of green fluorescent protein. Diabetes 1998;47:1974–1977.
78. Li M, Pevny L, Lovell-Badge R, Smith A. Generation of purified neural precursors from embryonic stem cells by lineage selection. Curr Biol 1998;8:971–974.
79. Klug MG, Soonpaa MH, Koh GY, Field LJ. Genetically selected cardiomyocytes from differentiating embryonic stem cells form stable intracardiac grafts. J Clin Invest 1996;98:216–224.
80. Soria B, Roche E, Berna G, Leon-Quinto T, Reig JA, Martin F. Insulin-secreting cells derived from embryonic stem cells normalize glycemia in streptozotocin-induced diabetic mice. Diabetes 2000;49:157–162.
81. Leon-Quinto T, Jones J, Skoudy A, Burcin M, Soria B. In vitro directed differentiation of mouse embryonic stem cells into insulin-producing cells. Diabetologia 2004;47:1442–1451.
82. Friedrich G, Soriano P. Promoter traps in embryonic stem cells: a genetic screen to identify and mutate developmental genes in mice. Genes Dev 1991;5:1513–1523.
83. Miyazaki S, Yamato E, Miyazaki J. Regulated expression of pdx-1 promotes in vitro differentiation of insulin-producing cells from embryonic stem cells. Diabetes 2004;53:1030–1037.
84. Kitajima K, Tanaka M, Zheng J, Sakai-Ogawa E, Nakano T. In vitro differentiation of mouse embryonic stem cells to hematopoietic cells on an OP9 stromal cell monolayer. Methods Enzymol 2003;365:72–83.
85. Buttery LD, Bourne S, Xynos JD, et al. Differentiation of osteoblasts and in vitro bone formation from murine embryonic stem cells. Tissue Eng 2001;7:89–99.
86. Schuldiner M, Yanuka O, Itskovitz-Eldor J, Melton DA, Benvenisty N. Effects of eight growth factors on the differentiation of cells derived from human embryonic stem cells. Proc Natl Acad Sci USA 2000;97:11307–11312.
87. Kyba M, Perlingeiro RC, Daley GQ. HoxB4 confers definitive lymphoid-myeloid engraftment potential on embryonic stem cell and yolk sac hematopoietic progenitors. Cell 2002;109:29–37.
88. Giddings SJ, Carnaghi L. Rat insulin II gene expression by extraplacental membranes. A non-pancreatic source for fetal insulin. J Biol Chem 1989;264:9462–9469.
89. Devaskar SU, Giddings SJ, Rajakumar PA, Carnaghi LR, Menon RK, Zahm DS. Insulin gene expression and insulin synthesis in mammalian neuronal cells. J Biol Chem 1994;269:8445–8454.
90. Rulifson EJ, Kim SK, Nusse R. Ablation of insulin-producing neurons in flies: growth and diabetic phenotypes. Science 2002;296:1118–1120.
91. Giddings SJ, Carnaghi LR. Selective expression and developmental regulation of the ancestral rat insulin II gene in fetal liver. Mol Endocrinol 1990;4:1363–1369.
92. Goldfine ID, German MS, Tseng H-C, et al. The endocrine secretion of human insulin and growth hormone by exocrine glands of the gastrointestinal tract. Nat Biotechnol 1997;15:1378–1382.
93. Hullett DA, MacKenzie DA, Alam T, Sollinger HW. Preparation of fetal islets for transplantation: importance of growth factors. In: Peterson CM, Jovanovic-Peterson L, Formby B, eds. Fetal Islet Transplantation. New York: Plenum Press; 1995:27–36.
94. Schuit FC, Pipeleers DG. Regulation of adenosine 3′,5′prime-monophosphate levels in the pancreatic B cell. Endocrinology 1985;117:834–840.
95. Tourrel C, Bailbe D, Meile MJ, Kergoat M, Portha B. Glucagon-like peptide-1 and exendin-4 stimulate beta-cell neogenesis in streptozotocin-treated newborn rats resulting in persistently improved glucose homeostasis at adult age. Diabetes 2001;50:1562–1570.
96. Pericin M, Althage A, Freigang S, et al. Allogeneic beta-islet cells correct diabetes and resist immune rejection. Proc Natl Acad Sci USA 2002;99:8203–8206.

Section 7

Hematology

Section 7

Hematology

Arnon Nagler

Allogeneic hematopoietic stem cell transplantation (alloSCT) is an effective established curative treatment of genetic and malignant hematologic disorders. Moreover, recent clinical trials are evaluating the potential therapeutic role of alloSCT in patients with solid tumors and autoimmune disorders. Preliminary results of alloSCT for the later indications are encouraging. However, the procedure suffers from two main limitations: 1) Only one of four patients that need alloSCT has a human leukocyte antigen (HLA) full-matched sibling donor; the other three patients therefore need an alternative donor, and 2) high-dose chemoradiotherapy with alloSCT is associated with significant morbidity and mortality because of the toxicity of the preparative regimen. Moreover, the transplant-related organ toxicity increases with advanced age, concurrent medical problems, or extensive prior therapy. These two major obstacles limited, up to now, this potentially curative procedure to only a minority of the patients with malignancies, mainly young patients (less than 40 years of age) with hematologic malignancies and a full-matched sibling donor. Recent advances in alloSCT in the last decade almost revolutionized the field. It is now possible to perform alloSCT in the vast majority of patients in need including medically infirm patients and to perform successful alloSCT from alternative (nonsiblings or non-HLA-matched) donors. These achievements are mainly the result of: 1) The development of relatively nontoxic and tolerable preparative regimens based on intelligent immune manipulations and posttransplantation immunotherapy (namely, reduced-intensity and nonmyeloablative protocols), 2) the possibility of performing HLA mismatched allogeneic transplantation from peripheral blood of related donors (haploidentical alloSCT) or from HLA mismatched human umbilical cord blood. We will detail this outstanding progress in the next three chapters. Shimoni and Nagler will discuss "Nonmyeloablative Stem Cell Transplantation in the Treatment of Hematologic Malignancies." Leiba and Nagler will discuss "Hematopoietic Stem Cell Transplantation from HLA Haploidentical Donor," and Goldstein et al. will discuss "Human Umbilical Cord Blood Transplantation: A Viable Option for Stem Cell Graft."

24

Human Umbilical Cord Blood Transplantation: A Viable Option for Stem Cell Graft

Gal Goldstein, Amos Toren, and Arnon Nagler

Introduction

During the last decades, allogeneic SCT has become an important lifesaving procedure for malignant and nonmalignant disorders. Most patients do not have a human leukocyte antigen (HLA)-matched donor. Although HLA-identical sibling BMT remains the main strategy, there is an increasing interest among transplantation teams in using alternative sources and donors for transplants. CBSC has established itself as an important source for transplantations.

The first successful umbilical CBT (UCBT) was performed by Gluckman and colleagues in 1988.[1] CB of a female newborn was collected and cryopreserved in the United States. It was transfused later in Paris, to her 5-year-old brother, who had Fanconi anemia. In 1996, the first report of a UCBT in an adult recipient was published.[2] Since then, it is estimated that more then 3500 CB units were transplanted worldwide from related and UDs, for the treatment of various malignant and nonmalignant disorders. The International Bone Marrow Transplant Registry had estimated that 20% of all allogeneic SCTs in young patients were CBTs.[3]

CB Banking

The first CB bank was established at the Indiana School of Medicine. The first CBTs were performed using units from this bank.[4] At the beginning of the third millennium, more than 80,000 units CB were being kept in European CB banks, about 70,000 in the United States, 10,000 in Asia, and a similar number in Australia. Private CB banking for autologous or related transplantations began in 1992.

Collection of CB

The collection process is being done by a special team of the CB bank, or delivery room crew. The CB is being collected before, or after, the expulsion of the placenta, from the umbilical vein. Collection could also be done in Cesarean deliveries. CB with a similar quality has also been collected from small for gestational age or preterm newborns. Median volume of collection is 73 ± 23 mL, with each mL containing $10–15 \times 10^6$ NCs.[5,6]

Cryopreservation and Thawing

CB banks confront several challenges, such as limited storage volume and cryopreserving and thawing techniques, which might affect the number of NCs and their viability.

Many units are needed in each bank, in order to offer a wide range of CB units. Availability of storage volume is limited. This has prompted banks to use several techniques to freeze only a small volume, containing NCs, separated from red blood cells (RBCs). One of the most used techniques for volume reduction is the one reported by Rubinstein et al.[7] After using electric potential in hydroxyethyl starch gel and soft centrifugation, RBCs are removed, leaving a 20-mL unit, and 5 additional mL of cryopreservative solution.

Whether the above methods could harm the graft is unclear, but the separation process joins the cryopreserving and thawing processes that every graft undergoes. Questions have been asked if the route CB grafts are being taken could not be one of the explanations for late recovery of neutrophils and platelets in CBT. According to Rubinstein and Stevens,[5] their technique does not cause significant delay in engraftment time, compared with non-volume reduced units.

However, Xu et al.[8] have demonstrated that megakaryocytes in CB units are more sensitive to stresses caused by freezing, thawing, and washing. They suggested that these processes contribute to the slow recovery of thrombocytes.

HLA and RBC Typing, and Infectious Agents Testing

Banked CB units are being tested for RBC and HLA types, and for infectious agents, as well as for the biological quality of the blood. The limited volume of each CB unit poses another problem to CB bankers. Efforts are being made to utilize molecular methods for class I and II HLA typing, using small amounts of CB. But the balance between the importance of precision of HLA typing and the clinical need for it is not clear. The optimal degree of resolution affecting engraftment had not yet been determined.

Ethical Issues in CBT

During the last two decades, CBT has caused several unique ethical concerns of interest clinicians.

Ownership

CB collection is done after the consent of the laboring mother has been given. The question is who owns the CB unit once the newborn becomes an adult. BM donations from children are being given after their parents have given consent for it, but such dilemma does not exist in this type of donation, because these units are not cryopreserved.

Consent

Information regarding the exact purposes for which every unit will be used should be given to each family. Collection is not painful and can almost never cause harm to the laboring women or to the newborn. This might make collection teams over-enthusiastic in expanding CB banks, and skip the important stage of consent giving. The disclosure should be done before the onset of labor and in a manner that allows the family to exercise effectively their right to grant or refuse informed consent. The family must agree to donate the unit to anyone who might need it, to disclose any medical information of the mother or the father, whether by an interview, or by tests, and to allow the CB bank team to inform them, or their physician, of the results of the test that were done.

Availability

Concern regarding private CB banks had emerged as soon as the financial potential of CB private banking gave rise to several companies dealing with the collection of CB. Questions about the need for the availability of this resource for the entire population are being asked. Apart from the lack of evidence in favor of cryopreserving CB for the potential future use for an autologous transplantation, this action denies potential recipients from finding it in public, nonprofit CB banks. Whether this growing trend will make CB donation for public banks an act unique to the low socioeconomic population is to be determined.

Table 24.2. Related donor umbilical cord blood transplantations

Reference	Gluckman et al.[35]	Rocha et al.[27]	Wagner and Kurtzberg[36]
No. of patients	78	113	74
HLA loci disparity (%)			
0	60	100	56
1	3		
2	5		18
3	9	0	
4	1		0
Engraftment (median day)			
ANC ≥500/μL	30	26	22
PLT ≥20,000/μL	49	44	NA
PLT ≥50,000/μL	NA	NA	51
Neutrophil recovery (%)	82	89	91

Table 24.3. Unrelated donor umbilical cord blood transplantations: patient and graft characteristics

			Median cell dose		HLA loci disparity (%)			
Reference	No. of patients	Median age (yr)	NCs ×10⁷/kg	CD34+ ×10⁵/kg	0	1	2	≥3
Pediatric series								
Wagner et al.[37]	102	7.4 (0.2–57)	3.1 (0.7–57)	2.8 (0.4–39.1)	14	43	41	2
Ohnuma et al.[38]	Malig	3.1 (0.5–28)	4.2 (1.4–10.6)	NA	Serology only			
	37	Other	4.1 (0.3–16)	6.2 (2.1–13.1)	0	62	38	0
Gluckman et al.[39]	291	5.0 (0.2–15)	5.6 (n = 261) (0.8–60)	1.9 (n = 190) (0.6–78)	17			83
Locateili et al.[40]	60	5.5 (1.7–14)	5.0 (1.5–46.5)	1.8*(0.1–78)	10	45	37	8
Michel et al.[41]	95	6.0 (0.3–16)	4.4 (0.4–36)	1.4 (NA)	8	46	33	13
Rubinstein and Stevens[5]	861	<2 = 20% 2–5 = 22% 6–11 = 23% 12–18 = 14% >18 = 21%	≥10 = 15% 5–9.9 = 22% 2.5–4.9 = 34% < 2.5 = 29%	NA	6	39	48	7
Styczynski et al.[42]	29	9.0 (0.5–20)	3.8 (1.1–11)	2.3 (0.2–9.9)	7	17	76	0
Staba et al.[43]	20	1.3 (0.16–2.7)	10.5 (3.3–23)	2.5 (0.6–104)	5	55	30	10
Thomson et al.[44]	27	4.8 (0.4–17)	4.4 (1.2–20.6)	1.5 (0.05–7)	10	57	33	0
Adult series								
Gluckman et al.[39]	108	26 (15–53)	2.2 (1.2–7.3)	0.8 (0.01–8.9)	6		94	
Sanz et al.[45]	22	29 (18–46)	2.5 (1.5–6.9)	NA	5	59	36	0
Iseki et al.[46]	30	38 (NA)	2.4 inf. (NA)	NA				NA
Laughlin et al.[47]	68	31 (18–58)	2.1 (1–6.3)	1.2 (0.2–16.7)	3	26	54	17
Cornetta et al.[48]	34	34.5 (18–55)	1.7 in. (1.1–3.7)	NA	3	29	68	0
Long et al.[49]	57	31 (18–58)	2.12 (1.1–4.4)	1.37 (0.02–12.4)	4	14	77	5
Takahashi et al.[50]	68	36 (16–53)	2.47 (1.1–5.29)	0.9 (0.2–9.0)	0	21	54	25

New York Blood Center.[5] Clinical series reporting preliminary results of UD-CBT have demonstrated hematopoietic recovery and sustained engraftment in the majority of pediatric and adult CBTs.

In the pediatric series, rates of myeloid engraftment ranged from 63% to 100%, with lower rates among nonmalignant disease patients, as will be discussed later.

Engraftment

Concerns about the ability of CB to produce sustained hematologic engraftment have proved to be wrong. Engraftment rates in these trials are comparable to BMT, especially with respect to the high proportion of HLA disparate transplantations.

Cell Dose

These reports have established the importance of NC dose in engraftment and survival. The debate about the minimal cell dose has not finished. Several studies have suggested that a dose of 2×10^7 NCs/kg is the threshold for producing reasonable engraftment rates. The Eurocord trial

Table 24.4. Unrelated donor umbilical cord blood transplantations: outcome

Reference		Hematopoietic recovery Median day		Neutrophil recovery (%)	AGVHD (III–IV) / chronic (%)	Relapse rate, % (yr)	TRM, % (yr)	Survival, % (yr)	EFS, % (yr)
		ANT ≥500	PLT ≥50,000						
Wagner et al.[37]		23	86	88	11/9	37 (2)	30 (1)	47 (2)	NA
Ohnuma et al.[38]	Malig.	28	54 (>20,000)	82.3	13/17	28 (3)	43 (1)	51.9 (3)	51.4 (3)
	Other	22		66.7	0/0	NA	22 (1)	64.2 (3)	37.5 (3)
Gluckman et al.[39]		29	NA	82	39/NA		NA	AA 21 Gen. 51 Malig. 36	
Locatelli et al.[40]		33	85*	79	23/12	40	52	NA	30
Michel et al.[41]		NA	NA	78	35†/15 (2)	29 (2)	20 (2)	45 (2)	42 (2)
Rubinstein and Stevens[5]		23 28	Matched 75 Mismatched 94	92.7	24/31	56.8‡	56.8 (1)	EFS (OS-NA) Gen. 48 Malig. 27 Acq. 29 (2)	
Styczynski et al.[42]		28	NA	53	20/3	NA	NA	46 (1)	NA
Staba et al.[43]		24	56	85	11/11	NA	10	85 (2.4)	85 (2.4)
Thomson et al.[44]		27	75	100	8.8/0	33 (5)	20 (1)	40 (5)	49.6 (1)
Adult series									
Gluckman et al.[39]		32	NA	81	38†/NA	NA	54 (100 d)	27 (1)	21 (1)
Sanz et al.[45]		22	105	100	32/90	NA	43 (100 d)	NA	53 (1)
Iseki et al.[46]		22	38	NA	3/NA	13	NA	76 (3)	76 (1)
Laughlin et al.[47]		27	99	90	20/36	5.9 (1)	51	28 (3.3)	26 (3.3)
Cornetta et al.[48]		28.5	NA	100	18/NA	NA	53	30 (0.5)	NA
Long et al.[49]		26	84 (≥20,000)	71	16/32	15.7	50	19 (3)	15 (3)
Takahashi et al.[50]		22	48	88	7/77	16 (2)	9 (1)	NA	74 (2)

*Including related and unrelated donor cohorts.
†Above grade II.
‡Transplant related episodes – autologous reconstitution, receiving another transplant, death.
NA, not available; EFS, event-free survival; OS, overall survival; malig., malignant diseases; inf., infused; AA, aplastic anemia; gen., genetic diseases; ANC, absolute neutrophil count.

has shown association between dose of 3.7×10^7 NCs/kg and more and faster time to neutrophil engraftment.[39] In the New York Blood Group report, a correlation between myeloid recovery and NC dose was seen. It was suggested that doses above 2.5×10^7 NCs/kg correlate with sustained myeloid engraftment. Interestingly, Rubinstein and Stevens[5] did not demonstrate such a correlation when doses continued to escalate above this threshold. It is probably agreed that the minimal acceptable threshold of NCs/dose should be 1.5×10^7 NCs/kg.

Median cell doses in the pediatric series ranged from 3.1 to 10.5×10^7 NCs/kg. These doses provide good chances for myeloid engraftment and low rates of TRM and high rates of overall survival (OS).

Which Cell Should Be Counted?

Because counting NCs involves many cells that are not contributing to the engraftment potential, it has been suggested that CD34+ cell count, as in BMT, is an important factor. And indeed, Wagner et al.[37] have shown correlation between CD34+ dose of 1.7×10^5 cells/kg and higher to rapid neutrophil engraftment and probability of engraftment. It is still debated whether CD34+ counts should be done on a regular basis before cryopreserving CB units. For now, the only standardized counts that are done before freezing are the NC counts. It should be mentioned that according to the Eurocord data, there is a correlation between high CD34+ counts and the probability of grade III–IV acute GVHD, but this had not been confirmed in other studies.[39]

HLA Disparity

HLA-matched donors were found in 0%–17% of the pediatric series. HLA disparity of 2–3 alleles comprised the majority of matching in these trials, and was found in 79%–100% of the CBTs.

The impact of HLA disparity on the outcome of UD-CBT is controversial. Contrary to results obtained in smaller studies, Rubinstein and Stevens[5] had reported that HLA disparity does have a negative impact on engraftment kinetics. In HLA-matched CBTs, median time for myeloid recovery was faster than in mismatched CBTs (23 versus 28 days). However, there was no significant difference in the time of engraftment for a single allele mismatch versus greater than one mismatch.

Graft-Versus-Host Disease

The probability of acute and chronic GVHD was lower than might be expected in a UD-BMT. Grade III and higher acute GVHD occurred in 0%–38% of the patients in the pediatric series. Regimens for GVHD prophylaxis varied among studies. The large trial of Rubinstein et al. did not provide the information about these regimens. In almost all of the other reports, cyclosporine A was the backbone of the prophylactic strategy. It was used alone, or in combination with steroids, mycophenolate, or in some cases methotrexate.

Survival

OS rates for malignant diseases achieved in pediatric series ranged from 38% (at 2 years) to 52% (at 3 years). Considering the type of diseases and the proportion of high-risk patients, these results are acceptable. In several studies there was correlation between status of disease at transplantation and survival.[34,40,41] In the University of Minnesota study, survival of high-risk acute lymphocytic leukemia was 32%, 55% for standard risk, and 33% for acute myeloid leukemia.[37]

Some authors stated other factors as contributing to OS such as cytomegalovirus seronegativity.[39]

Treatment-Related Mortality

Most authors defined TRM as nonrelapse death. The high rates of TRM in UD-CBT remains a major disadvantage of these procedures. Although lower than seen in adult patients, in pediatric series, TRM rates ranged from 10% to 56% at 1–2 years, with most studies in the range of 20%–40%. TRM was related to disease status at transplantation, cell dose (mostly NCs, but in some trials CD34+ doses), to severe GVHD, and in the Rubinstein et al. study, to HLA mismatch.[5,37,39]

Relapse

As stated earlier, occurrence of GVHD was shown to have a negative impact on malignant disease relapse. Concerns were raised whether lower rates of GVHD in CBT could result in high rates of relapse.

Wagner et al.[37] and Locatelli et al.[40] could not find any correlation between relapse and GVHD. Interestingly, Rubinstein did find such a negative correlation. Occurrence of GVHD and stage of disease at the time of transplantation were independently associated with rates of relapse.[5] In a multicenter retrospective analysis comparing the outcome of UD-CBT to UD-BMT in children with acute leukemia, no difference in the relapse rates was seen between the groups.[40]

Nonmalignant Diseases

Most of the experience with CBT for nonmalignant diseases is with children. Although this procedure has proved to be a feasible one for many nonmalignant diseases, some disadvantages of CBT in these disease settings should be remembered. From the data published so far, it seems that CBT is an acceptable alternative for nonmalignant diseases, with the exception of bone marrow failure syndrome. Although limited, we have gained some experience with several bone marrow failure syndromes, for example, Fanconi anemia.[51] We observed high rates of event-free survival (EFS), especially in children who received a matched family donor transplant (Tables 24.5 and 24.6). A novel strat-

Table 24.5. Cord blood stem cell transplantation, Safra Children's Hospital 1996–2004: Characteristics of recipients and donors

Patient No.	Diagnosis	Age at transplantation (yr)	Donor	HLA mismatch	Conditioning protocol	No. of Nucleated cells $\times 10^7$/kg Cryopreserved	No. of Nucleated cells $\times 10^7$/kg Infused	No. of CD34 $\times 10^5$/kg
1	Severe combined immune deficiency	0.25	MRD	0	None	87.2	50	65
2	Thalassemia	14	MRD	0	Bu/CY/ATG	2.9	0.87	0.004
3	Fanconi anemia	9	MRD	0	Bu/CY/ATG	4.1	3.1	13.9
4	Hurler	1.75	MRD	0	Bu/CY/ATG	1.8	2.1	NE
5	Fanconi anemia	10	MRD	0	Fluda/CY	2.1	0.65	NE
6	Fanconi anemia	3.5	MRD	0	Fluda/CY	10	7.6	2.3
7	Congenital amegakaryocytic thrombocytopenia	2.5	URD	2/10	Fluda/CY/Bu/ATG	10.9	9.5	9.1
8	Acute lymphoblastic leukemia, Ph+	14.5	URD	2/10	Fluda/CY/Bu/ATG	6.2	3.0	0.9
9	Acute lymphoblastic leukemia relapse	10.5	MRD	0	TBI/VP	2.7	1.3	3.4
10	Wiskott-Aldrich syndrome	0.5	URD	3/10	Bu/Fluda/ATG	30.9	2.2	32
11	Myelodysplastic syndrome	6.5	URD	5/10	Bu/CY/ATG	8.8	3.9	8
		Median age, 6.5 (0.25–14.5) yr	MRD-7 URD-4			Median no., 6.2 (1.8–87)	Median no., 3.0 (0.65–50)	Median no., 1.5 (0.004–65)

MRD, matched related donor; NE, not evaluated; CY, cyclophosphamide; fluda, fludarabine; URD, unrelated donor; BU, busulfan; ATG, anti-thymocytic globuline; TBI, total body irradiation.

Table 24.6. Cord blood stem cell transplantation, Safra Children's Hospital 1996–2004: engraftment, chimerism, incidence of GVHD, and outcome

Patients No.	Neutrophil engraftment*	Platelet engraftment*	Chimerism 100 d (%)	Chimerism 1 yr (%)	Acute GVHD Grade	Chronic GVHD Site	Day of discharge	Follow-up (mo)	Outcome	
1	Nonconditioning protocol		80	80	0		No	64	93	Alive and well
2	11	14	100	100%	0		No	33	73	Alive and well
3	13	34	100	100	0		No	20	72	Alive and well
4	43	No	NE		II	Skin, GIT	No			Died (2), TRM
5	15	28	100	100	II	Skin, liver	Limited	38	30	Alive and well
6	14	37	100	98.6	0		No	21	25	Alive and well
7	Autologous reconstitution							72		Autologous reconstitution. Underwent 2nd BMT
8	12	34	100	100	0		No	37	15	Alive
9	24	67	100	NE	0		No	NE		Died (4), relapse
10	15	68	100	100	0		No	39	11	Alive and well
11	Not engrafted									Died (1), TRM
	Median 14.5 (11–43)	Median 34 (14–68)	Median 100	Median 100	2 (II)	1 (limited)		Median 38 (20–72)	Median 45 (11–93)	

*Days posttransplantation.
NE, not evaluated; TRM, treatment-related mortality.

egy of preimplantation genetic diagnosis was used successfully for one of the patients.[52]

CB offers a good solution for these patients because of the low weight of most pediatric patients, the low rates of GVHD, and the availability of the units, especially for patients for whom their siblings might carry a high risk for the same disease.

It seems that UD-CBT is a less attractive solution for bone marrow failure syndromes, and especially in Fanconi anemia, because of the tendency toward graft failure. In 19 patients with bone marrow failure syndromes that were given related donor grafts, the probability of neutrophil recovery at day 60 and EFS at 1 year, were 81% and 67%, respectively. However, 14 children with similar diseases who were treated with UD-CBT had a 36% probability of engraftment, and 13 of them died within 1 year.[53] Only 33% of the Fanconi anemia patients engrafted.

Locatelli et al. had reported results of related CBT in 44 children with hemoglobinopathies (thalassemia and sickle cell disease), and showed that this procedure is feasible, and high rates of engraftment (89% at day 60) and EFS (79% for thalassemia and 90% for sickle cell disease) could be achieved. In our series, we have performed a successful CBT from a related donor (Table 24.5).

The use of methotrexate in the prophylactic regimen for GVHD, together with a conditioning regimen of busulfan and cyclophosphamide, were both related to lower probability of myeloid recovery and EFS. Contrary to other CBT reports, cell dose did not correlate with outcome.[54]

The results of UD-CBT for primary immune deficiencies are comparable to those obtained in UD-BMT. OS at 2 years has been reported as 69%.[55,56]

As for CBT in inborn errors of metabolism, Staba et al.[43] had reported impressive results in children with Hurler syndrome who were given UD grafts. Although 19 of the 20 patients received mismatched grafts, cell doses were relatively high (median of 10.5×10^7 NCs/kg), which might explain the high rates of engraftment (at 2.4 years follow-up 85%). All 17 patients who were alive also had normal peripheral blood α-L-iduronidase activity.[45]

Adult Series of CBT

Approximately 30% of UD-CBTs were done in adults. In this subset of patients, lack of a matched related donor in 30% of cases, together with the urgent need to manage aggressive malignant diseases, make this HSC source very appealing. Most adult patients enter CBT studies at advanced stages of their disease, a fact that must be kept in mind when analyzing the results of these trials. Several series of more than 20 patients have been published, four multicenter studies,[34,47-51] and three from a single institution.[45,46,50]

Patients' Ages and Diagnoses

All seven studies enrolled patients at relatively similar ages, at a range of 15–58 years. Hematologic malignancies comprised most cases. Three diseases encompassed the majority of the diagnoses: Chronic myelogenous leukemia at different stages of the disease, relapsed or high-risk acute myeloid leukemia, and acute lymphocytic leukemia. Other diagnoses were MDS, NHL, CLL, and refractory Hodgkin's disease. Some patients already had an autologous BMT.

Patients with nonmalignant diseases were included in three series, comprising only 4% of the total number of patients, indicating that malignancies, mainly hematologic, are the main indications for UD-CBT in adults. The small group of nonmalignant diseases comprised mainly of bone marrow failure syndrome, and several inborn error of metabolism syndromes. Most of the nonmalignant diseases were reported in the Laughlin et al. study.[39,45-50]

Cell Dose

Most groups reported similar NCs/kg and CD34+/kg median doses, ranging from 1.7 to 2.5×10^7, and 0.8 to 1.37×10^5, respectively. As expected, median NC and CD34+ doses for children were reported to be much higher.

HLA Disparity

Matched UDs were scarce. In all the trials, matched transplants comprised not more than 6% of the units, whereas 2–3 allele disparities comprised 75%–95% of them. However, higher rates of fully matched donors were reported in the pediatric studies. A reasonable explanation for this might be the fact that it is easier to find a matched UD unit with adequate NC dose for a small child than for a heavier adult.

Conditioning Regimens

All patients in the seven trials received myeloablative regimens, based on total body irradiation (TBI), busulfan, or both. Cyclophosphamide, fludarabine, and thiotepa were added in different combinations. Anti-thymocytic globulins were also given in several studies. Less aggressive protocols were used for Fanconi anemia patients.

Engraftment

Despite initial concern, adult patients do engraft CB. Sustained short- and long-term hematopoietic recovery was demonstrated in adult CBT trials.

Median day of engraftment ranged from 22 to 28.5, similar to the results obtained in pediatric UD-CBT; 71%–100% of patients showed myeloid engraftment, which is a better result than in most children's series. This phenomenon might be explained by the larger proportion of nonmalignant diseases, mainly bone marrow failure diseases, in children studies, a group of patients with a tendency toward graft failure.

Median day of platelet engraftment occurred at a range of 38 to 105, again, similar to the results in pediatric series.

Graft-Versus-Host Disease

The variability in different studies regarding the incidence of GVHD is remarkable. Rates of 3%–32% in the occurrence of grade III–IV acute GVHD were reported. Chronic GVHD rates ranged from 32% to 90%.

GVHD prophylaxis regimens varied among the different trials. Most of them consisted of different protocols with cyclosporine A together with steroids. In one study, tacrolimus was given to some of the patients. The use of methotrexate was limited, probably because of concern of the impact of engraftment and the expected low risk for GVHD. It is interesting that Iseki et al.[48] reported that only 1 of 30 patients developed acute GVHD after receiving a prophylactic regimen of cyclosporine and methotrexate. This regimen did not have a negative effect on engraftment, although relatively high NC doses (median 2.4×10^7/kg) were used in this trial.

Treatment-Related Mortality

Excluding one study, rates of TRM probability ranged from 43% to 54% at 100 days. These rates are higher than TRM in the children's series. This could reflect the poorer general condition and prior exposure to higher doses of chemotherapy of most adult patients compared with children. Interestingly, in the large multicenter study of Eurocord, low TRM rates were related to the chronic phase of diseases, or remission, number of infused NCs more than 2×10^7/kg, and transplantation that was performed after January 1998.[39]

Methods Aiming to Lower Treatment Mortality Rates of CB

NC dose in CB units is a major factor influencing recovery of neutrophils and platelets, and therefore the outcome of CBT.[57] This is true especially in adult patients. Realizing that, basic and clinical research for finding methods to overcome this obstacle is underway.

Several strategies are used to minimize TRM. First, an attempt to improve engraftment kinetics is being done by the use of cytokines in vivo, ex vivo expansion, the use of multiple stem cell units, by trying to improve CB collection, or to select the larger units, and by using different routes for transfusion of the graft. Second, new techniques are being explored to use different regimens with lower rates of toxicity (Table 24.7).

Ex Vivo Expansion

Because CBSCs have the ability to proliferate rapidly and indefinitely, attempts were made to expand their number in several ways. In 1998, Koller and colleagues[58,59] reported that CB HSCs could be expanded in a media-rich automated perfusion culture system, which was originally used for BM HSC expansion. On the basis of these experiments, several attempts were made to define the optimal composition of the media. It became clear that cytokines not only contribute to the accelerated proliferation of stem cells, but also to their commitment and differentiation. Some of the cytokines (e.g., stem cell factor, thrombopoietin, Flt3-ligand, interleukin-6) are considered to have mainly a proliferative effect on cells, whereas others accelerate differentiation (e.g., interleukin-3, granulocyte colony-stimulating factor, erythropoietin).[60–62] Concern has risen whether the long-term marrow repopulating cells are also being expanded, or if only committed progenitors are being expanded. There is a considerable amount of data that support the correlation between the CD34+ cells and colony-forming unit of granulocyte-macrophage (CFU-GM) cell doses, and the rate of hematopoietic recovery. The latter trait has usually been evaluated in a model known as a NOD-SCID mouse repopulating cell (SRC) assay, or the long-term culture-initiating cells (LTC-ICs).

The combination of cytokines and chemokines has produced remarkable expansion of CFU-GM, LTC-ICs, together with maintenance of SRCs.[63–65]

But despite the impressive effect seen in vitro, the clinical benefit of ex vivo expansion is yet to be proved. Two clinical studies and one case report of ex vivo-expanded CB transplantation have been published. According to these studies, the transplantation of unmanipulated CB with expanded CB is feasible, but so far it does not alter the engraftment kinetics.[66–70]

Ex vivo expansion can only be done in parallel with the transplantation itself. Because CB units can be thawed only once, a fragment of the

Table 24.7. Different strategies for overcoming high rates of early posttransplantation complications and graft failure in CBT

Method	Results	Reference
Ex vivo expansion (ex. ep.)		
Ex. ep. using different combinations of cytokines and chemokines	Feasible, but improvement in engraftment kinetics had not been shown in clinical studies.	66–68
Ex. ep. using differentiation blocking agents	Increased in vitro expansion and repopulating of murine model. Promising technique, which is currently in clinical trials.	69–72
Ex. ep. using knocked-out gene of cell cycle regulator	Increase in in vitro proliferation of HSCs, with functional compromise in murine model.	76
Ex. ep. using different cells as feeder layer	Impressive expansion and repopulating of murine model.	77,78
Selection of specific cells for ex. ep.	In vitro expansion of noncommitted hematopoietic stem cells.	81
Two-step harvesting ex vivo expansion	Increased in vitro expansion and differentiation of SCs and MK.	79,80
In vivo manipulation (IVM)		
IVM up-regulation of adhesion molecules	Enhancement of HSCs in murine model.	82
Co-transplantation		
Cotransplantation of several CB units	Stable double chimerism, without improvement in engraftment kinetics in clinical trials.	85–87
Cotransplantation with haploidentical donor	Early recovery of neutrophils, low rates of TRM, and low rates of GVHD in a clinical trial.	88,89
Cotransplantations with mesenchymal cells	Improves engraftment kinetics in murine model	101
Cotransplantations of two CB units and mesenchymal cells from third party	Improves engraftment kinetics in murine model, and alleviates single donor predominance	102
Intraosseous/intravenous cotransplantations	Improved engraftment kinetics in murine model. Feasible in BMT.	91–93
Reduced-intensity transplantations	Feasible, sustained engraftment, low rates of early TRM. Longer follow-up needed.	93–100

total volume is taken to the expansion laboratory, while the main portion is being transfused.

With the completion of the process, 10–14 days later, the expanded cells are added. Obviously, this schedule minimizes the potential to demonstrate the effect on engraftment kinetics.

Ex Vivo Expansion Using Differentiation Blocking Agents

A complementary measure directed to enhance cell proliferation without driving the cells into differentiation imposes maturation arrest. Relying on the important role of copper in differentiation of hematopoietic cells, Peled et al.[64–72] have used copper chelator [tetraethylenepentamine (TEPA)] to reduce intracellular copper content. With this manipulation, an enhancement of the long-term CD34+ cells, the short-term committed progenitors, and also SRCs, was seen. Following large-scale experiments, this promising approach has been introduced into the clinic in phase I trials. The same concept was behind the experiment conducted by Nolta et al.,[73] who cocultured primitive CBSCs (CD34+ CD38−) together with a feeder layer of immortalized murine stromal cell-line AFT024. This method has yielded high rates of myeloid and lymphoid engraftment in a NOD/SCID mouse xenograft model.[73] Other differentiation blocking agents that might serve for ex vivo expansion are the Gfi-1 and some of the Notch ligand protein family. These molecules have major roles in differentiation of hematopoietic cells and might be used in the future for ex vivo expansion of CB.[74–76]

Ex Vivo Expansion Using Different Cells as Feeder Layer

Not only has the question regarding the optimal composition for the media of the culture had not been solved, but it had been suggested that coculturing might give better conditions for ex vivo expansion. Coculturing of CB cells with placental-derived mesenchymal progenitor cells as a feeder layer had succeeded in expanding CD34+, CFU-GM, and LTC-ICs by 14.89, 36.73, and 7.43, respectively,[77] and when human brain endothelial cells were used as feeder layer, neutrophil engraftment and long-term repopulating capacity were superior compared with liquid suspension-cultured CD34+ cells.[78]

Two-Step Harvesting Ex Vivo Expansion

This is an additional investigational strategy aiming to optimize the expansion process and to harvest a greater dose of cells. It is done by harvesting the stem cells in two steps, using the same media.[79,80]

Selection of Cells for Ex Vivo Expansion

Positive or negative selection could be used as a method to refine the expanded cell population to the most primitive ones. This might help to maintain the long-term repopulating ability of CBSCs. It has been suggested that negative selection of the known lineage markers enrich CB with the most primitive stem cells (Lin−, CD34+/−, CD133+/−) that also had been found to express surface markers involved in HSC homing to the BM.[81]

In Vivo Up-Regulation of Adhesion Molecules

This investigational method has been applied in in vivo all-trans retinoic acid in order to stimulate CBSCs to up-regulate the expression of intercellular adhesion molecule-1 and vascular adhesion molecule-1.[82]

Cotransplantations

Multiple Units of CBT

The rationale behind cotransplantations is to augment the infused cell dose. As performed in BMT, double units of CBT were studied in an effort to improve hematologic recovery. Several reports have been published after high-risk adult patients received two mismatched CB units. In most cases, stable double chimerism was observed.

One of the encouraging results in this field is the fact that mutual tolerance between the mismatched units was seen. Hematologic recovery was not accelerated by this strategy.[83–88]

Cotransplantations with Haploidentical Donor

Another measure aiming to improve engraftment kinetics is a supportive cotransplantation of a low number of highly purified peripheral blood CD34+ cells from an HLA-haploidentical donor. Because a haploidentical donor is available for almost every patient, it was used as a source for additional stem cells to the CB graft. Fernandez et al.[89] reported early recovery of neutrophils using this technique in 11 high-risk adults with acute leukemia. In seven patients, a prompt recovery of the absolute neutrophil count (ANC) (9–17 days, median 10) was noted, as well as low rates of early posttransplantation toxicity. Analysis of DNA polymorphism showed initial predominance of the haploidentical genotype in granulocytes and in mononuclear and gradual replacement by cells of the CB genotype, until final complete CB chimerism was achieved by patients who survived for sufficient periods of time. Although survival within this high-risk patient group was relatively low (40% at 42 months), death was not attributed to early posttransplantation complications. Acute GVHD rates were also not higher than might have been expected in a single CB transplantation. These results are encouraging, and could help in reducing early posttransplant complications.[89]

Intraosseous Transplantations

The possibility of transplantation of CBSCs directly into the bone marrow has been suggested, but so far no data exist regarding this technique in human CBT. It has been shown that human CBSCs that were injected into

NOD/SCID mouse bones had better engraftment kinetics. In those studies, the cells engrafted distant skeletal sites. The feasibility of intra-bone marrow HSC transplantation was shown in 1998 by Hagglund, who transplanted 39 adults with this method. The suggested reasons for the accelerated engraftment were fewer cell losses in the microenvironment of the bone during homing and the lack of homing adhesion molecules in the most primitive subset of stem cells. Time will tell if intraosseous transplantation could shorten the way for CBSCs into the bone marrow, and by this improve time to engraftment.[89–91]

Reduced-Intensity Transplantations

RIC, or nonmyeloablative regimens, for BM transplantations had emerged as a necessity in transplantations for the older and the sicker patients, or heavily treated ones. The concept behind these conditioning protocols was that the immune effect of the transplant against the malignancy is more important than the conditioning effect, and engraftment occurs even without complete destruction of the recipient's bone marrow. This approach was based on the assumption that these attenuated regimens would decrease mucosal and tissue damage, minimize the release of inflammatory cytokines, decrease the incidence of infections, reduce the incidence of GVHD, and allow alloimmune responses to eradicate disease progression, whereas minimize treatment-related toxicities.

Because CBT in heavier and sicker patients poses them in a greater risk for early treatment-related morbidity and mortality, RIC has emerged as a plausible alternative. Experience with BMT using RIC, although follow-up time is still short, has shown encouraging results. Adult patients with high-risk refractory malignancies (especially CLL, low-grade lymphoma, and multiple myeloma) gained reasonable rates of survival, with lower treatment-related morbidity and mortality. The main problems with this strategy are high rates of GVHD, low probability of engraftment, and high risk for relapses.

In the CB setting, RIC seems to be a tempting possibility. It was postulated that these regimens might offer the opportunity for CBT in older, sicker, and heavier patients, who may not have a suitable donor. The first report of RIC in two adult high-risk lymphoma patients was published by Rizzieri et al.[106] Both had 100% donor engraftment and remained in remission for 6 and 12 months.

Four major studies of RIC in adult and pediatric patients have been published since then. Table 24.8 summarizes the results of these reports. Whether RIC could be an alternative for CBT in adults and children, by decreasing treatment-related toxicities, is yet to be proven. The major conclusion that could be redrawn from these series is that RIC is feasible in CBT. Graft rejection, a major concern, had not occurred in most of the patients. Although survival rates were low, it must be emphasized that most studies included mainly high risk, heavily treated patients. GVHD rates correlated, and were even lower than UD-BMT. Another encouraging finding is the lower than expected rate of TRM at 100 days posttransplantation. Because of the small number of patients, and diversity of methods, conclusions regarding the optimal nonmyeloablative conditioning regimen, or the GVHD prophylaxis, cannot be gained. It is definitely too early to recruit patients for RIC CBTs outside clinical trials for selected patients; this protocol could offer an alternative for several groups of patients.[93–100]

Conclusions

CBT has earned its place among SCT techniques. Almost two decades after the first successful CBT, this procedure has proved to be feasible in a variety of malignant and nonmalignant diseases, in children and adult patients. From the reports published, it is clear today that CB has some advantages over marrow HSCs. Collection of CB is safer and simpler, its availability for immediate transplantation is greater, more varied ethnic groups are represented among donors, and the risk of acute and chronic GVHD is lower, expanding potential donor pools. The major setback of CBT is the prolonged time to myeloid recovery, with its implications on transplantation outcome. This obstacle is more pronounced in the adult patient population, a reflection of the impact of cell dose infused on these parameters.

Understanding these problems, several strategies were sought to achieve low TRM rates. By

Table 24.8. Reduced-intensity conditioning for CBT

Reference	Barker et al.[100]	Chao et al.[97]	Del Toro et al.[96]	Miyakoshi et al.[95]	
No. of patients	43	13	14	30	
Median age (yr)	49.5	49	NA, children	58	
Cell dose, median (range)	Bu/Flu/TBI	Cy/Flu/TBI			
NCs ($\times 10^7$/kg)	3.3	4.0	2.07 (inf.)	4.3	3.1 (inf.)
CD34+ ($\times 10^5$/kg)	3.7	4.3	1.3	1.9	0.74
Engraftment %/median day of ANC >500	76/26	94/9.5	41/12	79/18	87/17.5
PLT recovery, days to >20,000/μL	NA	NA	14	31	39
GVHD, % acute II–IV/chronic	44/21 (1 yr)		20/10	NA	
TRM at day 100 (%)	48	28	7.6	NA	27
Overall survival (%)	39 (1 yr)		23 (5 mo)	NA	

selecting the better expected units, improving collection, cryopreserving, volume reduction, and thawing techniques, better doses of stem cells could be obtained for every transplantation. Ways to deal with the relatively low number of cells in CB units included many investigational methods. None of these has proved to lower the rates of treatment toxicities. These strategies include in vivo cytokine manipulation, ex vivo expansion alone, or in combination with cytokines, differentiation blocking agents, cotransplantation of two CB units or one unit with a haploidentical donor unit. Another promising way to detour the impact of cell dose in CBT is RIC transplantations. At present, the last method has proven to lower TRM in small series of high-risk patients. As in other SCT techniques, it is difficult to have a controlled trial, and most of the data regarding new methods arrives from limited numbers of patients, mostly high-risk ones.

CB is still considered a second choice for most patients who need transplantation, but as more experience is gained and better results are reported, many advocate a parallel search in BM and CB banks.

A well-coordinated and carefully planned data collecting system among CB banks and transplantation centers around the world is a true necessity for accelerating the continuous progress in this field.

References

1. Gluckman E, Broxmeyer HA, Auerbach AD, et al. Hematopoietic reconstitution in a patient with Fanconi's anemia by means of umbilical-cord blood from an HLA-identical sibling. N Engl J Med 1989;321:1174–1178.
2. Laporte JP, Gorin NC, Rubnstein P, et al. Cord-blood transplantation from unrelated donor in an adult with chronic myeloid leukemia. N Engl J Med 1996;335:167–170.
3. International Bone Marrow Transplant Registry/Autologous Blood and Marrow Transplant Registry IBMTR/ABMTR Newsletter 2003;10;1–12.
4. Broxmeyer HE. Introduction: the past, present, and future of cord blood transplantation. In: Broxmeyer HE, ed. Cellular Characteristics of Cord Blood and Cord Blood Transplantation. Bethesda, MD: AABB Press; 1988:1–9.
5. Rubinstein P, Stevens CE. Placental blood for bone marrow replacement: the New York Blood Center's program and clinical results. Baillieres Best Pract Res Clin Haematol 2000;13:565–584.
6. Elchalal U, Fasouliotis SJ, Shtockheim D, et al. Postpartum umbilical cord blood collection for transplantation: a comparison of three methods. Am J Obstet Gynecol 2000;182:227–232.
7. Rubinstein P, Dobrila L, Rosenfield RE, et al. Processing and cryopreservation of placental/umbilical cord blood for unrelated bone marrow reconstitution. Proc Natl Acad Sci USA 1995;92:10119–10122.
8. Xu Y, Kashiwakura I, Takahashi TA. High sensitivity of megakaryocytic progenitor cells contained in placenta/umbilical cord blood to stresses during cryopreservation. Bone Marrow Transplant 2004;34(6):537–543.
9. Sugarman J, Kaalund V, Kodish E, et al. Ethical issues in umbilical cord blood banking. Working Group on ethical issues in umbilical cord blood banking. JAMA 1997;278:938–943.
10. Mayani H, Landsrop PM. Biology of human umbilical cord blood-derived hematopoietic stem/progenitor cells. Stem Cells 1998;16:153–165.
11. Lewis I, Vefaillie CM. Multi-lineage expansion potential of primitive hematopoietic progenitors. Superiority of umbilical cord blood compared to mobilized peripheral blood. Exp Hematol 2000;28:1087–1095.
12. Nagler A, Peacock M, Tantoco M, et al. Red blood cell depletion and enrichment of CD34+ hematopoietic progenitor cells from human umbilical cord blood using soybean agglutinin and CD34 immunoselection. Exp Hematol 1994;12:1134–1140.

13. Tsafrir A, Brautbar C, Nagler A, et al. Alloreactivity of umbilical cord blood mononuclear cells: specific hyporesponse to noninherited maternal antigens. Hum Immunol 2000;61:548–554.
14. Toren A, Einat M, Fabian I, et al. Human umbilical cord blood myeloid progenitor cells are relatively chemoresistant: a potential model for autologous transplantations in HIV-infected newborns. Am J Hematol 1997;56:161–167.
15. Risdon G, Gaddy J, Stehman FB, Broxmeyer HE. Proliferative and cytotoxic responses of human cord blood T lymphocytes following allogeneic stimulation. Cell Immunol 1994;154:14–24.
16. Risdon G, Gaddy J, Horie M, Broxmeyer HE. Alloantigen priming induces a state of unresponsiveness in human cord blood T cells. Proc Natl Acad Sci USA 1995;92:2413–2417.
17. Roncarolo MG, Bigler M, Martino S, Ciuti E, Tovo PA, Wagner J. Immune functions of cord blood cells before and after transplantation. J Hematother 1996;5:157–160.
18. Cohen SB, Madrigal JA. Immunological and functional differences between cord and peripheral blood. Bone Marrow Transplant 1998;21(suppl 3):S9–S12.
19. Garderet L, Dulphy N, Douay C, et al. The umbilical cord blood alphabeta T-cell repertoire: characteristics of a polyclonal and naive but completely formed repertoire. Blood 1998;91:340–346.
20. Leung W, Ramirez M, Mukherjee G, Perlman EJ, Civin CL. Comparisons of alloreactive potential of clinical hematopoietic grafts. Transplantation 1999;68:628–635.
21. Kedereit S, Mohammad SF, Miller RE, et al. Reduced NFATl protein expression in human umbilical cord blood T lymphocytes. Blood 1999;94:3101–3107.
22. Sorg RV, Kogler G, Wernet P. Functional competence of dendritic cells in human umbilical cord blood. Bone Marrow Transplant 1998;22(suppl 1):S52–54.
23. Canque B, Camus S, Dalloul A, et al. Characteristic of dendritic cell differentiation pathway from cord blood CD34(+)CD7(+)CD45(+) hematopoietic progenitors cells. Blood 2000;96:3748–3756.
24. Phillips JH, Hori T, Nagler A, et al. Ontogeny of human natural killer (NK) cells: fetal NK cells mediate cytolytic function and express cytoplasmic CD3 epsilon, delta proteins. J Exp Med 1992;175:1055–1066.
25. Liu E, Law HK, Lau YL. Tolerance associated with cord blood transplantation may depend on the state of host dendritic cells. Br J Haematol 2004;126:517–526.
26. Rocha V, Cornish J, Sievers EL, et al. Comparison of outcomes of unrelated bone marrow and umbilical cord blood transplants in children with acute leukemia. Blood 2001;97:2962–2971.
27. Rocha V, Wagner JE, Sobocinski KA, et al. Graft-versus-host disease in children who have received a cord-blood or bone marrow transplant from HLA-identical sibling. N Engl J Med 2000;342:1846–1854.
28. Thomson BG, Robertson KA, Gowan D, et al. Analysis of engraftment, graft-versus-host disease, and immune recovery following unrelated cord blood transplantation. Blood 2000;96:2703–2711.
29. Locatelli F, Maccario R, Comoli P, et al. Hematopoietic and immune recovery after transplantation of cord blood progenitor cells in children. Bone Marrow Transplant 1996;18:1095–1101.
30. Giraud P, Thuret I, Reviron D, et al. Immune reconstitution and outcome after unrelated cord blood transplantation: a single paediatric institution experience. Bone Marrow Transplant 2000;25:53–57.
31. Nihues T, Rocha V, Fillipovich AH, et al. Factors affecting lymphocyte subset reconstitution after either related or unrelated cord blood transplantation in children: a Eurocord analysis. Br J Haematol 2001;114:42–48.
32. Moretta A, Maccario R, Fagioli F, et al. Analysis of immune reconstitution in children undergoing cord blood transplantation. Exp Hematol 2001;29:371–379.
33. Talvensaari K, Clave E, Douay C, et al. A broad T-cell repertoire diversity and an efficient thymic function indicate a favorable long-term immune reconstitution after cord blood stem cell transplantation. Blood 2002;99:1458–1464.
34. Grewal SS, Kahn JP, MacMillan ML, et al. Successful hematopoietic stem cell transplantation for Fanconi anemia from an unaffected HLA-genotype-identical sibling selected using preimplantation genetic diagnosis. Blood 2004;103:1147–1151.
35. Eurocord Transplant Group and the European Blood and Marrow Transplantation Group, Gluckman E, Rocha V, Boyer-Commard A, et al. Outcome of cord-blood transplantation from related and unrelated donors. N Engl J Med 1997;337:373–381.
36. Wagner JE, Kurtzberg J. Allogeneic umbilical cord blood transplantation. In: Broxmeyer HE, ed. Cellular Characteristics of Cord Blood and Cord Blood Transplantation. Bethesda, MD: AABB Press; 1998:113–146.
37. Wagner JE, Barker JN, Defor TE, et al. Transplantation of unrelated donor umbilical cord blood in 102 patients with malignant and nonmalignant diseases: influence of CD34 cell dose and HLA disparity on treatment-related mortality and survival. Blood 2002;100:1611–1618.
38. Ohnuma K, Isoyama K, Nishihira H. Cord blood transplantation from HLA-mismatched unrelated donor. Leuk Lymphoma 2002;43:1029–1034.
39. Gluckman E, Rocha V, Chevret S. Results of unrelated umbilical cord blood hematopoietic transplantation. Rev Clin Exp Hematol 2002;5:87–99.
40. Locatelli F, Rocha V, Chastang C, et al. Factors associated with outcome after cord blood transplantation in children with acute leukemia. Blood 1999;93:3662–3671.
41. Michel G, Rocha V, Arcese W, et al. Unrelated cord blood donor transplantation for children with AML. Blood 2002;100. Abstract 145.
42. Styczynski J, Cheung YK, Garvin J, et al. Outcome of unrelated cord blood transplantation in pediatric recipients. Bone Marrow Transplant 2004;34:129–136.
43. Staba SL, Escolar ML, Poe M, et al. Cord-blood transplants from unrelated donors in patients with Hurler's syndrome. N Engl J Med 2004;350:1960–1969.
44. Thomson BG, Robertson KA, Gowan D, et al. Analysis of engraftment, graft-versus-host disease, and immune recovery following unrelated donor cord blood transplantation. Blood 2000;96:2703–2711.
45. Sanz GF, Saavedra S, Planelles D. Standardized, unrelated donor cord blood transplantation in adults with hematologic malignancies. Blood 2001;98:2332–2338.
46. Iseki T, Ooi J, Tomonari A. Unrelated donor cord blood transplantation in adult patients hematological

malignancy: a single institution experience. Blood 2001;98. Abstract 2789.
47. Laughlin MJ, Barker J, Bambach B, et al. Hematopoietic engraftment and survival in adult recipients of umbilical cord blood from unrelated donors. N Engl J Med 2001;344;1815–1822.
48. Cornetta K, Laughlin MJ, Carter S, et al. Umbilical cord blood transplantation in adults: results of a prospective, multi-institutional, NHBLI sponsored trial. Blood 2002;100. Abstract 146.
49. Long GD, Laughlin M, Madan B, et al. Unrelated umbilical cord blood transplantation in adult patients. Biol Blood Marrow Transplant 2003;9:772–780.
50. Takahashi S, Iseki T, Ooi J, et al. Single institute comparative analysis of unrelated bone marrow transplantation and cord blood transplantation for adult patients with hematological malignancies. Blood 2004;104(12):3813–3820.
51. Aker M, Varadi G, Slavin S, et al. Fludarabine-based protocol for human umbilical cord blood transplantation in children with Fanconi anemia. J Pediatr Hematol Oncol 1999;21:237–239.
52. Bielorai B, Hughes MR, Auerbach AD, et al. Successful umbilical cord blood transplantation for Fanconi anemia using preimplantation genetic diagnosis for HLA-matched donor. Am J Hematol. In press.
53. Rocha V, Chastang C, Pasquini R, et al. Cord blood transplant in patients with bone marrow failure syndromes. Blood 1998;92(suppl 1):136a.
54. Locatelli F, Rocha V, Reed W, et al. Related umbilical cord blood transplant in patient with thalassemia and sickle cell disease. Blood 2003;101:2137–2143.
55. Howrey RP, Martin PL, Ciocci G, et al. Unrelated cord blood transplantation for correction of genetic disease. Blood 1998;921a.
56. Ortega J, Yaniv L, Rocha V, et al. Cord blood transplantation for inborn errors. Blood 1998;92(suppl 1):291a.
57. Gluckman E, Rocha V, Arcese W, et al., on behalf of Eurocord Group. Factors associated with outcomes of unrelated cord blood transplant. Guidelines for donor choice. Exp Hematol 2004;32:397–407.
58. Koller MR, Palsson MA, Manchel I, Palsson BO. Long-term culture-initiating cell expansion is dependent on frequent medium exchange combined with stromal and other accessory cell effects. Blood 1995;86:1784–1793.
59. Koller MR, Manchel I, Maher RJ, Goltry KL, Armstrong RD, Smith AK. Clinical-scale human umbilical cord blood cell expansion in a novel automated perfusion culture system. Bone Marrow Transplant 1998;21:653–663.
60. Bruno S, Gammaitoni L, Gunetti M, et al. Different growth factor requirements for the ex vivo amplification of transplantable human cord blood cells in a NOD/SCID mouse model. J Biol Regul Homeost Agents 2001;15:38–48.
61. Piacibello W, Gammaitoni L, Bruno S, et al. Negative influence of IL3 on the expansion of human cord blood in vivo long-term repopulating stem cells. J Hematother Stem Cell Res 2000;9:945–956.
62. Kohler T, Plettig R, Wetzstein W, et al. Defining optimum conditions for the ex vivo expansion of human umbilical cord blood cells. Influences of progenitor enrichment, interference with feeder layers, early-acting cytokines and agitation of culture vessels. Stem Cells 1999;17:19–24.
63. Lewis ID, Verfaillie CM. Differential culture requirements for the expansion of umbilical cord and mobilized blood myeloid and lymphoid progenitors. Exp Hematol 2000;28:1087–1095.
64. Gupta P, Dudek A, Slungaard A, Oegema T, Verfaillie CM. 6-O-Sulphated heparin enhances IL3+KIP-mediated expansion of LTC-IT in stroma free cultures. Blood 2001;95:147–155.
65. Lewis ID, Du J, Almeida-Porada G, Zanjani ED, Verfaillie CM. Long-term repopulating cord blood stem cells are preserved after ex-vivo culture in a non-contact system. Blood 2001;97:3441–3449.
66. Shapal EJ, Quinones R, Giller R, et al. Transplantation of ex vivo expanded cord blood. Biol Blood Marrow Transplant 2002;8:368–376.
67. Jaroscak J, Goltry K, Smith A, et al. Augmentation of umbilical cord blood (UCB) transplantation with ex-vivo expanded UCB cells: results of a phase I trial using the AastromReplicell System. Blood 2003;101:5061–5067.
68. Pecora AL, Stiff P, Jennis A, et al. Prompt and durable engraftment in two adult patients with high risk chronic myelogenous leukemia (CML) using ex-vivo expanded and unmanipulated unrelated umbilical cord blood. Bone Marrow Transplant 2000;25:797–799.
69. Peled T, Landau E, Mandel J, et al. Linear polyamine copper chelator tetraethylenepentamine augments long-term ex vivo expansion of cord blood-derived CD34+ cells and increases their engraftment potential in NOD/SCID mice. Exp Hematol 2004;32:547–555.
70. Peled T, Rubinstein P, Kurtzberg J, et al. TEPA augments ex-vivo and in-vivo potential of cord blood derived CD34+ cells: from basic science to clinical trials. Blood 2004;111. Abstract 3581.
71. Peled T, Mandel J, Goudsmid RN, et al. Pre-clinical development of cord blood-derived progenitor cell graft expanded ex vivo with cytokines and polyamine copper chelator tetraethylenepentamine. Cytotherapy 2004;6:344–355.
72. Peled T. Blood. ASH 2004 Abstract.
73. Nolta JA, Thiemann FT, Arakawa-Hoyt J, et al. The AFT024 stromal cell line supports long term ex-vivo maintenance of engrafting multipotent human hematopoietic progenitors. Leukemia 2002;16:352–361.
74. Lauret E, Catalain C, Titeux M, et al. Membrane-bound delta-4 notch ligand reduces the proliferative activity of primitive human hematopoietic CD34+CD38low cell while maintaining their LTC-IC potential. Leukemia 2004;4:788–797.
75. Masuya M, Katayama N, Hoshino N, et al. The soluble Notch ligand, Jagged-1, inhibits proliferation of macrophage progenitors. Int J Hematol 2002;3:269–276.
76. Hock H, Hamblen MJ, Rooke HM, et al. Gfi-1 restricts proliferation and preserves functional integrity of hematopoietic stem cells. Nature 2004;431:1002–1007.
77. Zhang Y, Li C, Jiang X, et al. Human placental-derived mesenchymal progenitor cells support expansion of long-term culture-initiating cells from cord blood CD34+ cells. Exp Hematol 2004;32:657–664.
78. Chute JP, Muramoto G, Fung J, Oxford C. Quantitative analysis demonstrates expansion of SCID-repopulating cells and increased engraftment capacity in human brain endothelial cells. Stem Cells 2004;22:202–215.
79. McNiece I, Kubegov D, Kerzic P, Shapal EJ, Gross S. Increased expansion and differentiation of cord blood

79. products using a two-step expansion culture. Exp Hematol 2000;41:1567–1576.
80. Pick M, Nagler A, Grisaru D, Eldor A, Deutsch V. Expansion of megakaryocyte progenitors from human umbilical cord using a new two-step separation procedure. Br J Haematol 1998;103:639–650.
81. Forraz N, Pettengell R, McGuckin CP. Characterization of a lineage-negative stem-progenitor cell population optimized for ex vivo expansion and enriched for LTC-IC. Stem Cells 2004;22:100–108.
82. Huang SL, Mai HR, Fang JP, et al. All-trans-retinoic-acid upregulates ICAM-1 expression and enhances engraftment of hematopoietic stem cells in murine model for unrelated umbilical cord transplantation. Blood 2001;98. Abstract 727.
83. Barker JN, Weisdorf DJ, Wagner JE. Creation of a double chimaera after transplantation of umbilical-cord blood from two partially matched unrelated donors. N Engl J Med 2001;344:1870–1871.
84. De Lima M, St. John LS, Wieder ED, et al. Double-chimaerism after transplantation of two human leucocyte antigen mismatched, unrelated cord blood units. Br J Haematol 2002;119:773–776.
85. Barker JN, DeFor T, Davies S, Verfaillie C, Weisdorf D, Wagner J. Impact of multiple unit unrelated donor umbilical cord transplantation in adults: preliminary analysis of safety and efficacy. Blood 2001;98:666a.
86. Gryn J, Harris DT, Shadduck RK, et al. Multiple unmatched umbilical cord units (MUCs) for adult allogeneic transplantation. ASH 2001. Abstract 2792.
87. Barker JN, Weisdorf DJ, Defor TE, et al. Multiple unit unrelated donor umbilical cord transplantation in high risk adults with hematologic malignancies: impact on engraftment and chimerism [abstract]. Blood 2002;100:41a.
88. Fernandez MN, Regidor C, Cabrera R, et al. Cord blood transplants: early recovery of neutrophils from co-transplanted sibling haploidentical progenitor cells and lack of engraftment of cultured cord blood cells, as ascertained by analysis of DNA polymorphisms. Bone Marrow Transplant 2001;28:355–363.
89. Fernandez MN, Regidor C, Cabrera R, et al. Unrelated umbilical cord transplants in adults: early recovery of neutrophils by supportive co-transplantation of a low number of highly purified peripheral blood CD34+ cells from an HLA-haploidentical donor. Exp Hematol 2003;31:535–544.
90. Yahata T, Ando K, Sato T, et al. A highly sensitive strategy for SCID-repopulating cell assay by direct injection of primitive human hematopoietic cells into NOD/SCID mice bone marrow. Blood 2003;101:2905–2913.
91. Wang J, Kimura T, Asada R, et al. SCID-repopulating cell activity of human cord blood-derived CD34− cells assured by intra-bone marrow injection. Blood 2003;101:2924–2931.
92. Hagglund H, Ringden O, Agren B, et al. Intraosseous compared to intravenous infusion of allogeneic bone marrow. Bone Marrow Transplant 1998;21:331–335.
93. Miyakoshi S, Yuji K, Kami M, et al. Successful engraftment after reduced-intensity umbilical cord blood transplantation for adult patients with advanced hematological disease. Clin Cancer Res 2004;10:3586–3592.
94. Del Toro G, Satwani P, Harrison L, et al. Pilot study of reduced intensity conditioning and allogeneic stem cell transplantation from unrelated cord blood and matched family donors in children and adolescent recipients. Bone Marrow Transplant 2004;33:613–622.
95. Chao NJ, Koh LP, Long GD, et al. Adult recipients of umbilical cord transplants after nonmyeloablative preparative regimens. Biol Blood Marrow Transplant 2004;10:569–575.
96. McSweeney PA, Bearman SI, Jones RB, et al. Nonmyeloablative hematopoietic cell transplant using cord blood [abstract]. Blood 2001;98:666a.
97. Cairo M, Harrison L, Wolownick K, et al. Reduced intensity (RI) allogeneic stem cell transplantation (AlloSCT) from related and unrelated donors in children and adolescents with malignant and non-malignant disease. Exp Hematol 2002;30(suppl):74.
98. Barker JN, Weisdorf DJ, DeFor TE, et al. Rapid and complete donor chimerism in adult recipients of unrelated donor umbilical cord transplantation after reduced intensity conditioning. Blood 2003;102:1915–1919.
99. Ballen KK, Becker PS, Emmons RV, et al. Low-dose total body irradiation followed by allogeneic lymphocyte infusion may induce remission in patients with refractory hematologic malignancy. Blood 2002;100:442–450.
100. Noort WA, Kruisselbrink AB, Anker S, et al. Mesenchymal stem cells promote engraftment of umbilical cord blood-derived CD34+ cells in NOD/SCID mice. Exp Hematol 2002;30:870–878.
101. Kim DW, Chung YJ, Kim YL, Oh IH. Cotransplantation of third party mesenchymal stromal cells can alleviate single-donor predominance and increase engraftment from double cord transplantation. Blood 2004;103:1941–1948.
102. Gluckman E, Rocha V, Boyer-Chammard A, et al. Outcome of cord-blood transplantation from related and unrelated donors. N Engl J Med 2004;337:373–381.
103. Bittencourt H, Rocha V, Chevret S, et al Association of CD34+ cell dose with hematopoietic recovery, infections, and outcomes, after HLA-identical sibling bone marrow transplantation. Blood 2002;99:2726–2733.
104. Bensinger WI, Martin PJ, Storer B, et al. Transplantation of bone marrow as compared with peripheral blood cells from HLA-identical relatives in patients with hematologic cancers. N Engl J Med 2001;344:175–181.
105. Forraz N, Pettengell R, McGuckin CP. Characterization of a lineage-negative stem-progenitor cell population optimized for ex vivo expansion and enriched for LTC-IC. Stem Cell 2004;22:100–108.
106. Rizzieri DA, Long GD, Vredenburgh JJ, et al. Successful allogeneic engraftment of mismatched unrelated cord blood following a nonmyeloablative preparative regimen. Blood 2001;98:3486–3488.
107. Gluckman E, Rocha V. Cord blood transplant: strategy for alternative donor search. Springer Semin Immunopathol 2004;26(1–2):143–154.

25

Nonmyeloablative Stem Cell Transplantation in the Treatment of Hematologic Malignancies

Avichai Shimoni and Arnon Nagler

Allogeneic hematopoietic stem cell transplantation (SCT) is an effective, potentially curative treatment of advanced or high-risk hematologic malignancies.[1] High-dose chemoradiotherapy with allogeneic SCT is associated with significant morbidity and mortality because of the toxicity of the preparative regimen, graft-versus-host disease (GVHD), and the immune-deficiency state that accompanies the procedure. These risks are significantly increased with advanced age, concurrent medical problems, or extensive prior therapy, limiting standard SCT to younger patients in good medical condition. Hematologic malignancies are more common and have a worse prognosis in the elderly. Additionally, disease and prior therapy may result in comorbidities precluding further intensive therapy. Thus, many patients with hematologic malignancies who could benefit from SCT were often deferred from a potentially curative approach. Extensive research has been directed toward the development of safer and less toxic approaches to allogeneic SCT. The introduction of nonmyeloablative and reduced-intensity conditioning regimens is a major step toward extension of allogeneic SCT to a much wider patient population by reducing transplant-related complications.[2] Much experience has been gained with the clinical use of this novel approach over the last decade. In this chapter, we discuss the rationale for nonmyeloablative stem cell transplantation (NST), and the use of immune therapeutic interventions with NST as the curative approach. We discuss how NST reduces some, but not all transplant-related complications, and our personal approach in selecting patients for NST.

Rationale for NST

SCT was initially developed as a means to deliver high-dose chemotherapy and radiation for elimination of the underlying disorder. Escalation of treatment doses results in better tumor kill but leads to irreversible myelosuppression. SCT was viewed as a supportive-care modality to restore hematopoiesis after treatment. However, it has subsequently become apparent that high-dose chemoradiotherapy does not eradicate the disease in many patients and that much of the therapeutic benefit of SCT relates to an associated, immune-mediated, graft-versus-leukemia (GVL) or graft-versus-malignancy (GVM) effect. Extensive experimental and clinical data support the presence of this GVL effect.[2] Higher relapse rates were observed after syngeneic and T cell-depleted transplants whereas patients having acute or chronic GVHD have a reduced relapse risk suggesting the importance of T cell-mediated immunity in eliminating the malignancy and the association of this GVL effect with GVHD. Perhaps the most direct evidence for GVL/GVM was the ability to restore remissions in patients relapsing after SCT by infusion of donor lymphocytes with no additional chemotherapy. The discovery of the curative potential of the immune-mediated GVL/GVM effect has led to a novel therapeutic approach. Low-dose, relatively nontoxic and tolerable conditioning regimens have been designed, not to eradicate the malignancy, but rather to provide sufficient immunosuppression to achieve donor cell engraftment and to allow induction of GVL as the primary treatment.[2-4]

NST does not eliminate all host hematopoiesis and often leads to a state of mixed chimerism (MC). MC describes persistence of donor cells with either normal host hematopoietic cells and/or cells of the underlying malignancy (Figure 25.1). Stable long-lived MC has been reported in animal models and in patients having NST for nonmalignant disorders. However, in patients with malignancies, MC is most often transient and conversion to complete chimerism (CC), autologous reconstitution, or relapse occurs either spontaneously or after immune manipulations within the first few months after NST.[5] The initial nonmyeloablative treatment is expected to produce only transient suppression of the underlying malignancy, but it allows time for the immune GVM effect to develop. This effect may result in gradual elimination of the malignancy and spontaneous delayed achievement of complete remission (CR), over a few months, especially in indolent malignancies. However, patients with MC or with detectable residual malignancy after NST may require additional immune-therapeutic approaches. Immunosuppressive therapy given post-SCT for prevention of GVHD can also suppress the GVL effect.[6] Early withdrawal of immunosuppressive therapy allows the occurrence of potent graft-versus-hematopoietic tissue effect that can potentially eliminate both residual disease and host hematopoiesis producing CC and CR (Figure 25.1). If this does not occur, donor lymphocyte infusions (DLIs) may harness this effect and switch the balance toward CC/CR. The GVL and graft-versus-hematopoietic tissue effects are highly associated with GVHD although may also occur in its absence. The initial NST and donor cell engraftment thus serve as a platform for additional allogeneic cellular therapy.

NST Regimens

NST regimens comprise a spectrum of regimens with different immunosuppressive and myelosuppressive properties. The kinetics of engraftment, chimerism, and eradication of residual disease differ accordingly.[5] Conditioning regimens have been referred to as nonmyeloablative if they do not completely eradicate host hematopoiesis and immunity.[2] A few of these regimens have been given as chemotherapeutic regimens with no stem cell support and allow relatively prompt hematologic recovery. Autologous reconstitution of hematopoiesis is expected if the allograft is rejected. These nonmyeloablative regimens have potent immunosuppressive effects. They are only mildly myelosuppressive and often result in induction of MC. The Seattle regimen consisting of low-dose total body irradiation (TBI, 200 cGy) with (or initially without) fludarabine and intensive pre- and posttransplant immunosuppression is the prototype of these regimens.[7] Other examples are the combinations of fludarabine and cyclophosphamide (FC) and the Flag/Ida regimen developed initially at the MD Anderson for

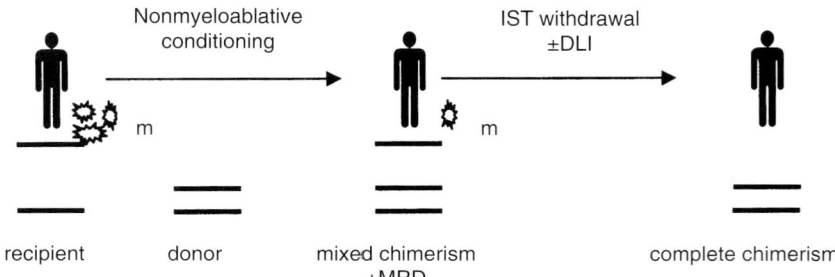

Figure 25.1. NST program: The initial NST regimen induces MC with persistence of both donor and recipient hematopoietic cells. The underlying malignancy (m) is suppressed but not completely eliminated. In the second phase, immune-therapeutic interventions, e.g., withdrawal of immunosuppressive therapy (IST) supplemented if necessary by DLI, induce graft-versus-hematopoietic tissue and graft-versus-tumor effects eliminating recipient hematopoiesis and the underlying malignancy and converting to CC.

non-SCT treatment of lymphoid and myeloid malignancies, respectively, and later explored as nonmyeloablative conditioning regimens for SCT.[4,8] These are very tolerable regimens, allowing in some cases ambulatory treatment, and treatment of elderly patients.

More intensive regimens have also been developed. These regimens have been referred to as reduced-intensity conditioning regimens.[2] They have not been given without stem cell support, and autologous recovery after treatment may be slow if at all. These regimens usually combine immunosuppressive agents such as fludarabine with or without serotherapy [with antithymocyte globulin (ATG) or alemtuzumab] and agents with moderate myelosuppressive effects (such as busulfan or melphalan).[3,9,10] The Hadassah group[3] and the MD Anderson group[4] pioneered the use of purine analogs in NST regimens and they emerged as the cornerstone of these regimens. These are well-tolerated agents, with potent immunosuppressive effects, in addition to antitumor activity against a range of hematologic malignancies. They have synergistic effects with alkylating agents and inhibit DNA repair systems responsible for repair of cellular damage induced by these agents. Although these regimens are more intensive than the nonmyeloablative regimens, dose intensity is still reduced compared with standard ablative regimens allowing reduction of toxicity. Reduced-intensity regimens, in similarity to standard myeloablative regimens, rapidly induce CC and antitumor responses, but are more toxic, and associated with a higher risk for GVHD.[5]

A third approach is using a double-step strategy. Initially, high-dose chemotherapy supported by autologous stem cell transplantation is used for cytoreduction and also as an immunosuppressive platform for the second stage of allogeneic SCT with nonmyeloablative or reduced-intensity regimens usually administered 2–3 months later. The separation of high-dose chemotherapy and allogeneic effects results in reduced toxicity and better tolerability than when allogeneic transplantation immediately follows high-dose chemotherapy.[11,12]

A novel approach is to combine nonmyeloablative or reduced-intensity regimens with targeted therapy. Imatinib is being explored as adjuvant to reduced-intensity conditioning both pre-SCT, allowing reduction of conditioning intensity, and post-SCT, to eliminate MRD.[13] Rituximab has been used in conjunction with reduced-dose chemotherapy in lymphoid malignancies, and by us after SCT to target MRD.[14] More recently, radiolabeled immune conjugates are used with SCT. Antibodies such as radiolabeled anti-CD20 monoclonal antibodies may be used with SCT to target lymphoma cells allowing the use of less intensive conditioning. Radiolabeled antibodies such as Bismuth 213 anti-CD45 antibodies can be used with no additional chemotherapy to ablate the marrow and immune system and not specifically tumor cells as reported in preliminary canine models.[15]

NST and Regimen-Related Complications

NST regimens were originally designed to enable treatment of older and medically infirm patients not eligible for standard ablative conditioning and to allow the application of SCT to a much wider patient population. This goal has largely been achieved. Standard ablative regimens are usually limited to patients up to age 55 years. Most NST studies have no upper age limit. Age per se was not found to be an adverse factor for prediction of outcome[16,17] after both related and unrelated donor SCT and is no longer a contraindication for SCT. Standard SCT in certain high-risk settings such as in heavily pretreated patients, patients failing a prior autologous SCT, and in patients with certain diagnoses such as multiple myeloma, Hodgkin's and non-Hodgkin's lymphoma, was associated with unacceptably high treatment-related mortality (TRM) rates, as high as 50%. TRM in the range of 10%–20% can now be observed in these settings using NST regimens. In particular, NST is becoming a common indication for treatment of patients failing a prior autologous SCT,[18,19] and was able to reduce TRM after unrelated donor SCT.[20,21]

Reduction of TRM is largely attributed to reduction in organ toxicity. The Seattle group has shown marked reduction in cardiovascular, gastrointestinal, hepatic, infectious, metabolic, neurologic, and pulmonary toxicity when comparing their low-dose TBI-based nonmyeloablative regimen to ablative regimens.[22] Nonrelapse mortality within the first 100 days was 9% and 21%, respectively. The major therapy-related organ dysfunction syndromes are reduced in incidence. In particular, idiopathic pneumonia syndrome is less frequent after NST, 2.2% versus 8.4% in one study, despite treatment of older patients.[23] Hepatic toxicity may still be substantial, especially after some reduced-intensity regimens.[3,24] However, not all syndromes are reduced. We have shown that thrombotic microangiopathy is a frequent devastating complication after NST, more common in second SCTs and in association with acute GVHD.[25] Diffuse alveolar hemorrhage is also relatively common in this setting. We have hypothesized based on experimental data that fludarabine-related endothelial and pulmonary epithelial toxicity may be associated with this unexpected observation. It was also shown that other hemolytic complications, associated with ABO donor–recipient incompatibility, might be more common after NST.[26] Although direct toxicities of high-dose chemotherapy are reduced with NST, toxicities involving immune mechanisms may not be. Organ toxicities are largely associated with patient comorbidity score before SCT.[27] Further research is required to define the relative organ toxicities in different regimens.

NST is less myelosuppressive than standard conditioning. This results in a shorter duration of neutropenia and less transfusion requirements.[28] Some of the nonmyeloablative regimens result in only minimal neutropenia and can be safely administered in the outpatient setting.[7] Reduced-intensity regimens usually result in more profound cytopenias more similar to ablative conditioning. The reduced duration of neutropenia and the limitation of mucosal injury result in reduced risk for severe infections in the immediate post-SCT period.[29,30] However, the risk for invasive fungal infections is not reduced.[31,32] These infections are usually associated with GVHD and corticosteroid therapy, and represent one of the major causes of TRM after NST. In the Seattle study, invasive fungal infection occurred in 19% of NST recipients, they occurred relatively late in the course, at a median of 107 days, and were the primary cause for 39% of nonrelapse-associated deaths.[31]

NST and GVHD

GVHD is one of the major causes of post-SCT morbidity and mortality. When the nonmyeloablative and reduced-intensity regimens were introduced, it was hoped that GVHD incidence would reduce. Acute GVHD results at least partially from tissue injury and cytokine release secondary to the toxicity of the preparative regimen, amplified by donor immune cells.[33] The use of less toxic conditioning should theoretically limit tissue injury and cytokine release and reduce the incidence and severity of GVHD. Also, MC that is more common after NST allows bilateral transplantation tolerance with graft acceptance and some protection from GVHD.[34] However, host antigen-presenting cells that have a major role in initiation of the GVHD reaction may persist after NST and contribute to GVHD.[35] The duration of immunosuppressive therapy is usually shorter after NST, and immune manipulations are often incorporated into NST programs increasing the likelihood of GVHD although delayed immune manipulations, once the toxicity of conditioning and cytokine release are already resolved, are less likely to produce severe GVHD.[36] The net effect of these differences between NST and ablative SCT on GVHD is still not well established and is controversial. The Seattle group reported that the incidence of acute GVHD grade II–IV after NST was significantly lower than after ablative therapy, reaching 64% and 85%, respectively. However, the incidence of chronic GVHD was approximately 70% in both cohorts. Moreover, the initiation of steroid therapy was delayed from an average of 1 month to 3 months after SCT, corresponding to a "new" syndrome described as late-onset acute GVHD.[37] This study suggests that GVHD is not reduced in incidence with NST, but is only delayed. In another study, Couriel et al.[38] reported an incidence of grade II–IV acute GVHD of 36% after myeloablative regimens (including the reduced-intensity combination of fludarabine and melphalan), but only 12% after truly nonmyeloablative regimens. They also noted reduced incidence of chronic GVHD after NST.[37] Further prospective studies are needed to determine the relative incidence of GVHD. However, Because it is still a major cause of morbidity and mortality after NST, several approaches have been explored to decrease the risk.

Initially, NST regimens called for only a short course of immune suppression and early administration of DLI for disease eradication and conversion to CC. However, these interventions are thought to markedly increase the risk of GVHD. More recently, more careful approaches were introduced. For example, the Seattle group extended the duration of immune suppression, especially after unrelated donor transplantation, up to 6 months. With better understanding of chimerism and MRD kinetics, the indications for DLI have been restricted, trying to reserve it only for patients destined to relapse or reject their graft and reducing the risk of GVHD in all other SCT recipients (see below for further discussion).

Another approach is the use of in vivo T cell depletion. Alemtuzumab (Campath 1-H) has emerged as an effective agent in prevention of GVHD. Alemtuzumab administered during pre-SCT conditioning depletes host T cells thus reducing the risk of graft rejection reported with in vitro T cell depletion techniques. Alemtuzumab persists after SCT and also depletes, at least partially, T cells of the donor, as well as host antigen-presenting cells and thus has been shown to be very effective in prevention of GVHD after reduced-intensity conditioning from both related and unrelated donors. However, patients given alemtuzumab have a higher risk of opportunistic infections, in particular with cytomegalovirus. Moreover, alemtuzumab recipients have a higher risk of MC and residual disease, require more DLIs, such that after DLI, the ultimate net risk of GVHD is not reduced and there is no improvement in survival or TRM.[10] ATG given pre-SCT has the same effects although may be less effective in prevention of GVHD. Studies are being conducted to determine the dose of alemtuzumab or ATG that may result in net effects that would improve survival.

Immune-Therapeutic Intervention after NST

Relapse of the underlying malignancy remains the major cause of treatment failure after ablative SCT and even more so after NST. Most of the data on the safety and efficacy of DLI comes from myeloablative SCT. DLI has been administered after NST in a variety of indications, mostly for conversion of MC to CC and for the treatment of relapse or residual disease.[39] DLI is associated with significant morbidity and mortality, mostly because of complications related to GVHD and marrow aplasia. Marks et al.[39] reported in a large series of DLI after NST that the rate of severe GVHD was 15%, and TRM was 9%; marrow aplasia was rare, suggesting that DLI after NST was safer than what is reported after standard myeloablative SCT. The Seattle group reported similar results.[40] This may represent advances in DLI administration, such as administration in incremental dosing, and at MRD where DLI may also be more effective, and may be given at a lower starting dose. There is also experimental data suggesting that DLI may even be more potent in mixed chimeras because of persistence of host antigen-presenting cells.[40] DLI administered late after SCT has a lower risk of complications[36]; however, the window of opportunities for administration of DLI for prevention of relapse may be short and missed while waiting for a safer time point. Even in programs planning early DLI, on days 60–100 post-SCT, DLI is only administered after cyclosporine withdrawal and many patients are ineligible for prophylactic DLI because of GVHD or rapid progression already occurring before DLI.

As discussed above, initially DLI was incorporated into NST protocols early in the course for conversion of MC to CC.[5] MC may be associated with increased risk for relapse, especially in aggressive malignancies, and may also be associated with MRD. However, as experience with NST was gained, the role of DLI in this setting became more controversial. High-level MC (more than 50%–60% donor chimerism) usually converts to CC spontaneously, whereas patients with low-level donor chimerism (less than 20%–40%) often reject the graft despite DLI. DLI is now administered more carefully for this indication, and patients are followed closely with DLI reserved for impeding graft rejection as evidenced by declining chimerism. In patients with aggressive malignancies, DLI may still be administered early trying to convert to CC and induce GVL rapidly.

The second indication for DLI has been for persistent or progressive disease, with an overall response rate of 25%–45%, depending on the underlying disease.[39,40] DLI has also been explored as prophylactic therapy after NST. Although this approach may reduce relapse risk, responses are often associated with GVHD. Because DLI is still associated with substantial risk, a more rational approach is to try to limit DLI only to those destined to relapse, avoiding unnecessary toxicity from those destined to remain in remission based on determination of MRD after NST.[42]

Significant progress has been achieved in technologies for MRD assessment.[42] Quantitative polymerase chain reaction tests are very sensitive in detecting tumor-associated transcripts, allowing serial monitoring. Threshold levels have been established for some malignancies above which relapse is imminent. Persistent negative tests, low level or decreasing MRD level are consistent with continuous remission, whereas, high-level MRD or increasing levels predict incipient relapse. Patients at high risk for relapse are candidates for additional cellular or targeted therapy.

The optimal time point and cell dose of DLI have not been established. The decision to administer DLI can be based on several factors: The aggressiveness of the underlying malignancy and the risk for rapid progression, the sensitivity of the test used to determine MRD, the expected kinetics of MRD and the trend of MRD in serial quantitative testing, the level of MRD, as well as the SCT regimen used.

In indolent malignancies such as chronic myeloid leukemia (CML), chronic lymphocytic leukemia, follicular lymphoma, and to a lesser extent multiple myeloma, MRD is often detected after SCT, both after ablative conditioning, and even more so after reduced-intensity conditioning. MRD can be followed and no intervention is indicated unless progression or a plateau in response is observed or quantitative MRD is rising. In aggressive malignancies such as acute leukemia and CML in blast crisis, and especially when not in remission at SCT, timing is more crucial. There may not be sufficient time to follow quantitative MRD because the doubling time of MRD may be short and relapse may occur within weeks, whereas effective DLI response may take 2–3 months. Thus, the sensitivity of the test is important. When using very sensitive tests, such as quantitative polymerase chain reaction, when applicable, one can follow MRD very closely, every 1–2 weeks and if MRD is declining, no intervention is needed. The kinetics of MRD in this setting after NST is not well established as after ablative conditioning.[42] The same level of MRD may not necessarily have the same significance. MRD surviving high-dose chemotherapy, and to a lesser extent reduced-intensity conditioning, represent highly resistant malignancy, whereas MRD is expected after NST. MRD remaining after T cell-depletion SCT or the use of alemtuzumab in NST is also highly predictive of relapse.

In the future, tumor-specific lymphocytes, or DLI generated against hematopoietic-specific minor histocompatibility antigens, such as HA-1 and HA-2,[43] may be used to harness antitumor responses without the risk of GVHD, and may follow SCT with T cell-depleted grafts.

Targeted therapy is another option for treatment or control of MRD. Imatinib mesylate is an effective therapy for CML. There is emerging data that imatinib may be effective in salvaging patients with relapse or persistent disease after SCT, either front line, or as second-line therapy after failure of DLI. Imatinib may also have a synergistic effect with DLI.[13] Rituximab is another example. We have used rituximab after SCT in patients with aggressive lymphoma.[14] The reduced risk of relapse in very high-risk patients suggested that rituximab may have eliminated MRD. It may have synergized with the donor immune system providing effectors for antibody-dependent cytotoxicity. The MD Anderson group showed similar effects of rituximab administered for residual chronic lymphocytic leukemia after NST.[44] Future studies may identify other methods to target MRD, trying to reduce relapse risk after SCT.

Selection of Conditioning Regimen

As a general role, myeloablative conditioning is the standard conditioning before SCT, and NST is still considered an experimental therapy, in which the long-term results have not yet been well defined. As a result, NST should be administered in carefully designed clinical studies. NST regimens should be reserved mainly for patients not eligible for standard ablative conditioning on the basis of the criteria discussed above. However, some groups have also explored NST regimens as a means to reduce toxicity even in younger and medically fit patients in some settings.

The selection of the appropriate regimen for a patient depends on several factors including age, general medical condition, immune competence of the recipient, genetic disparity between the patient and donor, and center experience.[2] Perhaps the most important determining factor is the aggressiveness and chemosensitivity of the underlying malignancy and its known susceptibility to the GVL effect.

There is now a spectrum of nonmyeloablative and reduced-intensity regimens with different immunosuppressive and cytoreductive intensity.

The reduced-intensity regimens are a more appropriate approach for aggressive malignancies such as acute leukemia, and especially when not in remission. In this setting, rapid achievement of CC and transient disease control is needed to induce GVL. However, in indolent malignancies, GVM may occur slowly, even in mixed chimeras, and toxicity may be reduced further using nonmyeloablative regimens. More intensive immune suppression is required for engraftment of allografts from unrelated donors and in patients not previously treated with chemotherapy. Less intensive immune suppression is needed in heavily pretreated patients and in particular those with a recent prior autologous SCT.[2]

There is no prospective study comparing the outcomes after different NSTs and reduced-intensity regimens that can show an advantage of one over the others. One analysis showed that reduced-intensity regimens might give better results in disease control than nonmyeloablative conditioning in patients with active or refractory leukemia whereas results were equivalent when the leukemia was in remission at the time of SCT.[45] Among reduced-intensity regimens, we have shown that the use of intravenous busulfan is associated with less regimen-related toxicity that other regimens, after both related and unrelated SCT, similar to what we have shown in ablative conditioning.[17,46] Thus, differences between regimens may be significant and studies comparing them, and then comparing the best regimen to standard ablative regimen, are urgently needed.

CML is the malignancy most sensitive to GVL as evidenced by the high response rates to DLI. There were some concerns of relatively high incidence of graft rejection in patients conditioned with truly nonmyeloablative regimens who had chronic-phase CML and had not been previously treated with intensive chemotherapy.[7] However, consistent engraftment has been achieved with reduced-intensity conditioning. The Hadassah group reported excellent outcomes in CML in the first chronic phase with 85% of patients surviving disease-free.[47] Results in advanced-phase CML are much less favorable. We currently recommend reduced-intensity conditioning even for younger patients with chronic-phase CML; however, it should be appreciated that there are no long-term studies prospectively comparing the two approaches. For advanced-phase CML, we would recommend reduced-intensity conditioning only for those not eligible for ablative conditioning and usually after a trial of remission induction.

Acute leukemia is a more aggressive malignancy, which is less susceptible to DLI. Responses can be achieved; however, they are most often transient. Although there are no randomized trials, emerging data suggest that NST may be equivalent or inferior to ablative therapy.[48,49] However, these comparisons may be biased by the criteria for patient allocation. Reduced-intensity conditioning may have favorable results in patients in remission; however, results have been disappointing in patients with active and refractory leukemia. In these patients, leukemia often recurs shortly after NST outpacing the developing of the GVL response. Acute lymphatic leukemia (ALL) is considered the least responsive disease to immune effects. This is not because ALL is not susceptible to GVL, rather because ALL is a very rapidly growing malignancy outpacing GVL. Thus, NST may be successful in high-risk ALL in remission, but has a limited role in active disease.

Hodgkin's and non-Hodgkin's lymphoma, and multiple myeloma are often treated with autologous SCT. These diseases show moderate susceptibility to GVM effect. When these patients are candidates for allogeneic SCT, they are often heavily pretreated and standard conditioning is associated with unacceptably high TRM rates. NST is becoming the preferred approach in these patients. It is feasible with favorable results in chemosensitive diseases.[50] Multiple myeloma is an incurable disease with standard chemotherapy as well as with autologous SCT. NST is being explored as an approach that may achieve cure. It is now established that relapse rates are very high when NST is given after relapse to prior therapy, but may be lower when NST is given upfront. The auto/allo approach in which autologous SCT is given for cytoreduction and is followed by NST to induce GVM seems promising in this setting.[12]

Chronic lymphatic leukemia and follicular lymphoma have been shown to be very sensitive to immune effects, similar to CML. These are indolent diseases for which standard ablative conditioning have very high TRM rates. Thus, these diseases are reasonable targets for NST, and we currently prefer this approach, especially in patients with chemosensitive disease.[8,44] As discussed above, SCT can also be supplemented with targeted therapy, such as rituximab, both before and after NST in these diseases.

Conclusions

Nonmyeloablative and reduced-intensity conditioning are increasingly being used before allogeneic SCT, in a growing number of indications. It is now well established that the first goal of allowing SCT for elderly and medically infirm patients has been achieved. NST regimens result in consistent engraftment of allografts from related and unrelated donors. TRM rates have been markedly reduced such that SCT can be administered relatively safely with no upper age limit, and after prior autologous SCT, as well as in certain malignancies, such as lymphomas and myeloma where historically TRM rates were exceedingly high. However, toxicity may still be substantial with some regimens and in patients with a high comorbidity score. GVHD continues to be a major cause of morbidity and mortality after NST, and its incidence may not be lower than after ablative SCT. Invasive fungal infections are a second common cause of TRM, which is closely associated with GVHD, and did not reduce in incidence. Novel approaches to further reduce these two complications are required to further improve outcome. In vivo T cell depletion reduces initial rates of GVHD, but because DLI is required more often for increased risk of disease persistence and MC, the ultimate rate of GVHD remains unchanged. With gained experience, DLI is used more carefully after NST, limiting its use to patients with persistent MRD after SCT, or imminent graft rejection, and delaying administration in others, trying to reduce the risk for GVHD. Methods to deliver cellular immune therapy without GVHD would be a major step forward. The development of tumor or minor histocompatibility antigen restricted DLI, and the combination with targeted therapy and tumor vaccines are promising. Currently, despite initial data, there is no firm evidence for advantage of any of the regimens over the others. Although TRM may reduce with NST, theoretically, relapse rates may increase compared with ablative SCT, such that the net effects on disease-free survival are yet to be determined. Prospective comparative studies to determine the best NST regimen and then randomized studies comparing NST and ablative SCT, are urgently required before NST can be accepted as standard therapy, and to better define its role.

References

1. Thomas ED, Storb R, Clift RA, et al. Bone marrow transplantation. N Engl J Med 1975;292:832–843.
2. Champlin R, Khouri I, Shimoni A, et al. Harnessing graft-versus-malignancy: nonmyeloablative preparative regimens for allogeneic haematopoietic transplantation. An evolving strategy for adoptive immunotherapy. Br J Haematol 2000;11:18–29.
3. Slavin S, Nagler A, Naparstek E, et al. Nonmyeloablative stem cell transplantation and cell therapy as an alternative to conventional bone marrow transplantation with lethal cytoreduction for the treatment of malignant and non malignant hematologic diseases. Blood 1998;91:756–763.
4. Giralt S, Estey E, Albitar M, et al. Engraftment of allogeneic hematopoietic progenitor cells with purine analog-containing chemotherapy: harnessing graft-versus-leukemia without myeloablative therapy. Blood 1997;89:4531–4536.
5. Shimoni A, Nagler A. Non-myeloablative stem cell transplantation (NST): chimerism testing as guidance for immune-therapeutic manipulations. Leukemia 2001;15:1967–1975.
6. Bacigalupo A, Van Lint MT, Occhini D, et al. Increased risk of leukemia relapse with high-dose cyclosporine A after allogeneic transplantation for acute leukemia. Blood 1991;77:1423–1428.
7. McSweeney PA, Niederwieser D, Shizuru JA, et al. Hematopoietic cell transplantation in older patients with hematologic malignancies: replacing high-dose cytotoxic therapy with graft-versus-tumor effects. Blood 2001;97:3390–3400.
8. Khouri I, Keating MJ, Korbling M, et al. Transplant lite: induction of graft vs malignancy using fludarabine based nonablative chemotherapy and allogeneic progenitor-cell transplantation as treatment for lymphoid malignancies. J Clin Oncol 1998;16:2817–2824.
9. Giralt S, Thall PF, Khouri I, et al. Melphalan and purine analog-containing preparative regimens: reduced-intensity conditioning for patients with hematologic malignancies undergoing allogeneic progenitor cell transplantation. Blood 2001;97:631–637.
10. Perez-Simon JA, Kottaridis PD, Martino R, et al. Nonmyeloablative transplantation with or without alemtuzumab: comparison between 2 prospective studies in patients with lymphoproliferative disorders. Blood 2002;100:3121–3127.
11. Carella AM, Cavaliere M, Lerma E, et al. Autografting followed by nonmyeloablative immunosuppressive chemotherapy and allogeneic peripheral blood hematopoietic stem-cell transplantation as treatment of resistant Hodgkin's disease and non-Hodgkin's lymphoma. J Clin Oncol 2000;18:3918–3924.
12. Kroger N, Schwerdtfeger R, Kiehl M, et al. Autologous stem cell transplantation followed by a dose-reduced allograft induces high complete remission rate in multiple myeloma. Blood 2002;100:755–760.
13. Shimoni A, Kroger N, Zander AR, et al. Imatinib mesylate (STI571) in preparation for allogeneic hematopoietic stem cell transplantation and donor lymphocyte infusions in patients with Philadelphia-positive acute leukemias. Leukemia 2003;17:290–297.

14. Shimoni A, Hardan I, Avigdor A, et al. Rituximab reduces relapse risk after allogeneic and autologous stem cell transplantation in patients with high-risk aggressive non-Hodgkin's lymphoma. Br J Haematol 2003;122:457–464.
15. Sandmaier BM, Bethge WA, Wilbur DS, et al. Bismuth 213-labeled anti-CD45 radioimmunoconjugate to condition dogs for nonmyeloablative allogeneic marrow grafts. Blood 2002;100:318–326.
16. Corradini P, Zallio F, Mariotti J, et al. Effect of age and previous autologous transplantation on treatment-related mortality and graft-versus-host disease in 110 patients treated with reduced-intensity conditioning and allografting for advanced hematological malignancies [abstract]. Bone Marrow Transplant 2004;33 (suppl 1):S11.
17. Shimoni A, Kroger N, Zander A, et al. Allogeneic stem-cell transplantation with matched unrelated donors in he elderly (age >55). Age is no longer a contraindication when using reduced-intensity conditioning. Leukemia 2004. In press.
18. Nagler A, Or R, Naparstek E, Varadi G, Slavin S. Second allogeneic stem cell transplantation using non-myeloablative conditioning for patients who relapsed or developed secondary malignancies following autologous transplantation. Exp Hematol 2000;28:1096–1104.
19. Feinstein LC, Sandmaier BM, Maloney DG, et al. Allografting after nonmyeloablative conditioning as a treatment after a failed conventional hematopoietic cell transplant. Biol Blood Marrow Transplant 2003;9: 266–272.
20. Nagler A, Aker M, Or R, et al. Low-intensity conditioning is sufficient to ensure engraftment in matched unrelated bone marrow transplantation. Exp Hematol 2001;29:1–9.
21. Maris MB, Niederwieser D, Sandmaier BM, et al. HLA-matched unrelated donor hematopoietic cell transplantation after nonmyeloablative conditioning for patients with hematologic malignancies. Blood 2003;102: 2021–2030.
22. Diaconescu R, Flowers C, Storer B, et al. Morbidity and mortality with nonmyeloablative compared to myeloablative conditioning before hematopoietic cell transplantation from HLA matched related donors. Blood 2004;104:1550–1558.
23. Fukuda T, Hackman RC, Guthrie KA, et al. Risks and outcomes of idiopathic pneumonia syndrome after nonmyeloablative and conventional conditioning regimens for allogeneic hematopoietic stem cell transplantation. Blood 2003;102:2777–2785.
24. Hogan WJ, Maris M, Storer B, et al. Hepatic injury after nonmyeloablative conditioning followed by allogeneic hematopoietic cell transplantation: a study of 193 patients. Blood 2004;103:78–84.
25. Shimoni A, Yeshurun M, Hardan H, et al. Thrombotic microangiopathy following allogeneic stem-cell transplantation in the era of reduced-intensity conditioning: the incidence is not reduced. Biol Bone Marrow Transplant 2004;10:484–493.
26. Worel N, Kalhs P, Keil F, et al. ABO mismatch increases transplant-related morbidity and mortality in patients given nonmyeloablative allogeneic HPC transplantation. Transfusion 2003;43:1153–1161.
27. Sorror ML, Maris M, Storer B, et al. Transplant-related toxicities (TRT) and mortality following HLA-matched unrelated donor hematopoietic cell transplantation (URD-HCT) using nonmyeloablative (NM) compared to myeloablative (M) conditioning: influence of pre-transplant comorbidities. Blood 2004;104:961–968.
28. Weissinger F, Sandmaier BM, Maloney DG, et al. Decreased transfusion requirements for patients receiving nonmyeloablative compared with conventional peripheral blood stem cell transplants from HLA-identical siblings. Blood 2001;98:3584–3588.
29. Busca A, Locatelli F, Barbui A, et al. Infectious complications following nonmyeloablative allogeneic hematopoietic stem cell transplantation. Transpl Infect Dis 2003;5:132–139.
30. Junghanss C, Marr KA, Carter RA, et al. Incidence and outcome of bacterial and fungal infections following nonmyeloablative compared with myeloablative allogeneic hematopoietic stem cell transplantation: a matched control study. Biol Blood Marrow Transplant 2002;8:512–520.
31. Fukuda T, Boeckh M, Carter RA, et al. Risks and outcomes of invasive fungal infections in recipients of allogeneic hematopoietic stem cell transplants after nonmyeloablative conditioning. Blood 2003;102:827–833.
32. Hagen EA, Stern H, Porter D, et al. High rate of invasive fungal infections following nonmyeloablative allogeneic transplantation. Clin Infect Dis 2003;36:9–15.
33. Antin JH, Ferrara JLM. Cytokine dysregulation and acute graft-vs-host disease. Blood 1992;80:2964–2968.
34. Prigozhina T, Gurevitch O, Slavin S. Non-myeloablative conditioning to induce bilateral tolerance after allogeneic bone marrow transplantation in mice. Exp Hematol 1999;27:1503–1510.
35. Shlomchik WD, Couzens MS, Tang CB, et al. Prevention of graft versus host disease by inactivation of host antigen-presenting cells. Science 1999;285:412–415.
36. Naparstek E, Or R, Nagler A, et al. T-cell depleted allogeneic bone marrow transplantation for acute leukemia using Campath-1 antibodies and post-transplant administration of donor's peripheral blood lymphocytes for prevention of relapse. Br J Haematol 1995;89:506–515.
37. Mielcarek M, Martin PJ, Leisenring W, et al. Graft-versus-host disease after nonmyeloablative versus conventional hematopoietic stem cell transplantation. Blood 2003;102:756–762.
38. Couriel DR, Saliba RM, Giralt S, et al. Acute and chronic graft-versus-host disease after ablative and nonmyeloablative conditioning for allogeneic hematopoietic transplantation. Biol Blood Marrow Transplant 2004;10:178–185.
39. Marks DI, Lush R, Cavenagh J, et al. The toxicity and efficacy of donor lymphocyte infusions given after reduced-intensity conditioning allogeneic stem cell transplantation. Blood 2002;100:3108–3114.
40. Bethge WA, Hegenbart U, Stuart MJ, et al. Adoptive immunotherapy with donor lymphocyte infusions after allogeneic hematopoietic cell transplantation following nonmyeloablative conditioning. Blood 2004; 103:790–795.
41. Mapara MY, Kim YM, Wang SP, et al. Donor lymphocyte infusions mediate superior graft-versus-leukemia effects in mixed compared to fully allogeneic chimeras: a critical role for host antigen-presenting cells. Blood 2002;100:1903–1909.
42. Shimoni A, Nagler A. Clinical implications of MRD monitoring for stem-cell transplantation after reduced-intensity and non-myeloablative conditioning. Acta Haematol 2004;112:93–104.

43. Marijt WA, Heemskerk MH, Kloosterboer FM, et al. Hematopoiesis-restricted minor histocompatibility antigens HA-1- or HA-2-specific T cells can induce complete remissions of relapsed leukemia. Proc Natl Acad Sci USA 2003;100:2742–2747.
44. Khouri IF, Lee MS, Saliba RM, et al. Nonablative allogeneic stem cell transplantation for chronic lymphocytic leukemia: impact of rituximab on immunomodulation and survival. Exp Hematol 2004;32:28–35.
45. Shimoni S, Giralt S, Khouri I, Champlin R. Allogeneic hematopoietic transplantation for acute and chronic myeloid leukemia: non-myeloablative preparative regimens and induction of the graft-versus-leukemia effect. Curr Oncol Rep 2000;2:132–139.
46. Shimoni A, Hardan I, Yeshurun M, et al. Intravenous busulfan versus melphalan-based reduced intensity conditioning prior to allogeneic stem cell transplantation: lower TRM and a more favorable toxicity profile [abstract]. Bone Marrow Transplant 2004;33 (suppl 1):S12.
47. Or R, Shapira MY, Resnick I, et al. Nonmyeloablative allogeneic stem cell transplantation for the treatment of chronic myeloid leukemia in first chronic phase. Blood 2003;101:441–445.
48. Alyea EP, Kim HT, Cutler C, et al. AML and MDS treated with nonmyeloablative stem cell transplantation: overall and progression free survival comparable to myeloablative transplantation [abstract]. Blood 2003;102:79a.
49. Fouillard L, Labopin M, Rocha V, et al. Comparison of reduced-intensity conditioning regimen to conventional conditioning regimen in allogeneic haematopoietic stem cell transplantation for acute myeloid leukemia [abstract]. Bone Marrow Transplant 2004;33 (suppl 1):S13.
50. Robinson SP, Goldstone AH, Mackinnon S, et al. Chemoresistant or aggressive lymphoma predicts for a poor outcome following reduced-intensity allogeneic progenitor cell transplantation: an analysis from the Lymphoma Working Party of the European Group for Blood and Bone Marrow Transplantation. Blood 2002;100:4310–4316.

26

Hematopoietic Stem Cell Transplantation from Human Leukocyte Antigen Haploidentical Donor

Merav Leiba and Arnon Nagler

Hematopoietic stem cell transplantation (SCT) from human leukocyte antigen (HLA)-matched siblings has become the treatment of choice for many hematologic, and nonhematologic diseases, but fewer than 40% of patients will have an HLA-matched sibling. Registries of HLA-typed volunteers have been established worldwide to provide HLA-matched unrelated donors for SCT transplantation. The chance of finding an unrelated donor matched for HLA-A, -B, and -DR depends on the HLA diversity of the population, and varies with race, ranging from 75% in white people to less than 50% for ethnic minorities. A limitation in the use of unrelated donors derives from the rather long duration of the search, which may allow disease progression in patients who urgently need transplantation, such as those with acute leukemia. For these reasons, SCT from an HLA-matched sibling or unrelated donor is not feasible for many patients, and other sources of hematopoietic stem cells are sought.

In contrast, a genetically haploidentical donor is readily available for 90% of patients. Experience in children with severe combined immunodeficiency, who underwent haploidentical SCT, has clearly demonstrated the feasibility of such approach.[1]

Over the past decade, significant progress has been made in increasing the feasibility of such transplants, overcoming the two major obstacles: Intractable graft-versus-host disease (GVHD) and graft rejection.[2,3] Until the early 1990s, the efforts and strategies of preventing GVHD were largely offset by the high incidence of graft rejection, mainly in patients with acute leukemia.[4]

The breakthrough was pioneered by Profs. Reisner and Martelli from the Perugia group[5] who used stem cell dose escalation and the megadose concept to overcome rejection of heavily T cell-depleted mismatched graft, by supplementing and eventually replacing the bone marrow (BM) graft with T cell-depleted (CD34 or CD133 purified) granulocyte colony-stimulating factor (G-CSF) mobilized peripheral blood progenitor cells (PBPCs). In so doing, they were able to increase the number of CD34+ cells 10-fold reaching 20×10^6 cells/kg with only 1×10^4 CD3+ T cells/kg. In their reported initial cohort of patients, 41 of 43 patients (95%) achieved primary sustained engraftment and only one developed acute GVHD grade II–IV despite no postgrafting immunosuppression.

Other strategies for haploidentical SCT include T cell costimulatory blockade with soluble CTLA-4Ig (CD152) induction of tolerance by thymic irradiation, in vivo T cell subset monoclonal antibody administration and in vitro T cell depletion of the graft by anti-CD52 monoclonal antibodies (CAMPATH), cotransplantation with mesenchymal cells, and, recently, intraosseous injection of the graft.

Although the problems of graft rejection and GVHD may have been largely overcome, further obstacles remain, primarily the slow immune reconstitution after haploidentical SCT, which puts the patient at risk of infection [mainly viral, cytomegalovirus (CMV), or fungal aspergillus] for significantly longer periods of time compared with matched donor SCT, and high relapse rates because of tolerance induction.[6]

Selecting the haploidentical donor by natural killer (NK) cells with mismatched killing inhibitor receptors (KIRs) and administration of purified mismatched NK cells – plus the administration of specific T cell clones active against typical posttransplantation infections – may serve as promising novel solutions. The current strategies and recent developments in the field of haploidentical SCTs will be reviewed in this chapter.

Strategies to Prevent GVHD in the Haploidentical Setting

The incidence and the severity of GVHD correlate with the degree of HLA disparity. When patients received methotrexate as single agent for GVHD prophylaxis, the incidence of grade II–IV GVHD was 34% for recipients of HLA identical sibling marrows and increased progressively up to 84% for recipients of a three-locus incompatible marrow.[2] Despite posttransplant immunosuppression with cisplatinum and methotrexate, HLA incompatibility has remained an important risk factor for GVHD.[3]

GVHD in this setting is largely mediated by alloreactive donor T cells recognizing mismatched HLA molecule peptide complexes. Methods to prevent the high rate of GVHD have mainly relied on altering the donor graft immunologic capabilities by removal of, or suppressing the function of, all donor T cells (pan T cell suppression or elimination) regardless of their immunologic specificity.[7] The more profound the degree of T cell depletion, the lower the risk for the development of GVHD. Initially, while BM as a stem cell source has been utilized, a variety of negative selection strategies were used, such as soybean lectin agglutination or the use of monoclonal or polyclonal antibodies.[8,9] Since the introduction of PBPCs as the preferred stem cell source, and the large number of PBPCs that are needed to be processed, alternative T cell depletion strategies have been required.[10]

Removal of less than 2 logs T cells from the donor marrow requires, in general, administration of posttransplant immunosuppression for prevention of GVHD.[11] Henslee-Downey et al.[11] achieved partial T cell depletion by ex vivo treatment of donor marrow with anti-T cell receptor monoclonal antibody T10B9 and rabbit complement. Others have used the CD5-specific immunotoxin H65-RTA in combination with anti-thymocyte globulin (ATG) administered in vivo posttransplantation aiming to deplete both host and donor T cells.[11] In a study of 72 patients, most of whom received two or three HLA-mismatched grafts, the probability of engraftment was 88%, and the incidence of grade II–IV acute GVHD was reduced to 16%. The probability of 2-year survival was 55% in low-risk patients versus 27% in high-risk patients ($P = 0.048$).[12] This study demonstrated that partial T cell depletion can be used to prevent GVHD after transplantation of marrow from donors mismatched for one HLA haplotype, and the risk of graft failure is low if postgrafting immunosuppression is administered.

The anti-CD3 monoclonal antibody OKT3 has been tested as well for T cell depletion of HLA-mismatched marrow grafts in a study of 67 pediatric patients. The engraftment rate was as high as 97% and the probability of grade II–IV acute GVHD was only 24%.[13] The 3-year survival was 26%, better in patients with low blood blast count at transplant and with donors younger than 30 years. In patients with acute leukemia refractory to primary induction chemotherapy, the 3-year disease-free survival was only 14%–19%.[14,15]

In the last few years, a positive selection of CD34+ progenitors using a method of high gradient magnetic-activated cell sorting (MACS) has been used as an indirect method for T cell depletion.[16] The T cell depletion obtained with this method is in the range of 4–5 logs, achieving a threshold of $1-5 \times 10^4$/kg CD3+ cells/kg, below which pharmacologic GVHD prophylaxis is not required.[17]

Using this approach based on Milteni technology, the problem of GVHD has been largely overcome, with an extremely low rate of GVHD in large series.[18] However, the rigorous T cell depletion attained by CD34+ selection and the effective introduction of tolerance, occur at the cost of loss of the graft-versus-leukemia (GVL) effect, largely mediated by alloreactive T cells, and delayed immune reconstitution, resulting in high relapse rates and high morbidity and mortality from viral and fungal infection. Novel strategies designed for selective depletion/tolerization of alloreactive T cells causing GVHD is discussed below.

Recently, much attention has focused on immunoregulatory cells including CD4+CD25+ T and NKT cells. In a murine model, CD4+CD25+ originating from the graft resulted in increased incidence of GVHD whereas depletion of CD4+CD25+ cells significantly inhibited GVHD.[19] We have recently demonstrated similar results with NKT cells.[20] The disadvantage of this modality is that the suppression by CD4+CD25+ cells is not specific for alloantigens, so that loss of antiviral and antileukemic responses would be anticipated.

Recent reports have questioned whether the expression of CD34+ is sufficient to characterize the most pluripotent stem cell.[21] Investigators are looking at the selection of more primitive cells using antigens expressed at an earlier developmental stage (e.g., CD133).[21,22] Ongoing studies are comparing clinical-scale CD34 versus CD133 selection for haploidentical transplantation.

An additional approach is negative rather than positive selection of the CD34+CD133+ hematopoietic stem cells by combined B and T cell depletion. This new strategy leaves the NK cells in the haploidentical graft and may reduce relapse rate in high-risk leukemia patients undergoing haploidentical transplants.

Elimination of Graft Rejection in Haploidentical SCT

Functional studies in patients with graft failure have demonstrated that a possible mechanism in graft rejection involves residual host T lymphocytes, which are cytotoxic against donor alloantigens. Alternatively, the patient's serum may be responsible, because it was shown to be active in the antibody-dependent cell-mediated cytotoxicity test against donor cells.[4,23]

In unmanipulated grafts, the presence of donor T cells usually suppresses the residual host immunity, facilitating engraftment and preventing graft failure and or rejection. Such suppression is abolished by profound T cell depletion of graft, and therefore it is not operating in the haploidentical setting. It was originally believed that this barrier to engraftment could be overcome by a global increase in the intensity of the conditioning regimen, especially with higher doses of total body irradiation (TBI)

and or various combinations of high doses of myeloablative and immunosuppressive regimens.[24,25] However, it soon became apparent that such intensive preparative regimens led to major organ toxicity, morbidity, and mortality in the heavily pretreated patients with advanced disease that were referred to haploidentical SCT.

Historically, a more targeted approach to reduce the incidence of graft failure or rejection was a selective myeloablative therapy using drugs that are particularly potent stem cell toxins such as melphalan,[26] busulphan, and thiotepa,[27] in combination with TBI.

Attempts to ameliorate the toxicities of combined myeloablation and immunosuppression have also focused on careful timing of sequential administration of the myeloablative drugs and immunosuppressive therapy. Morbidity and mortality may be reduced if such toxic substances are not given simultaneously. With more than 210 patients reported, the median time to engraftment was 16 days among patients in whom ATG was added to the TBI-based conditioning regimen.

However, in 1999, Sykes et al.[28] found that engraftment of haploidentical BM can be achieved by a nonmyeloablative conditioning regimen and tolerance induction. They studied five refractory lymphoma patients who underwent BM transplantation from haploidentical related donors. The conditioning regimen included: Cyclophosphamide and thymic irradiation before transplantation; antithymocyte globulin before and after transplantation, and cyclosporine after the transplantation. Four of five patients were evaluated and showed engraftment. Mixed hematopoietic chimerism was established.[28] Two patients were GVHD-free and in complete and partial clinical remission at 103 days posttransplantation.[28]

Multiple other alternatives to the conventional conditioning regimen have been studied, all in an attempt to facilitate engraftment without excessive GVHD and without major organ toxicity. These include the use of high-dose methylprednisolone, total nodal irradiation,[29] anti-T cell antibodies,[11] ATG, and fludarabine, a purine analog that inhibits adenosine deaminase and is the backbone for low-intensity conditioning and nonmyeloablative allogeneic SCT from related and unrelated donors.[30,31] Recently, nonmyeloablative conditioning without TBI has been used successfully for haploidentical SCT. In one report, a durable engraftment has been achieved in a child with Fanconi anemia transplanted from a haploidentical donor using a regimen consisting of fludarabine, CAMPATH 1H, and two anti-CD45 antibodies. Similarly, based on their animal studies, O'Donnell et al. reported sustained engraftment of 8 of 10 patients with hematologic malignancies, receiving a partially HLA-mismatched BM transplant using fludarabine (150 mg/m^2), cyclophosphamide (80 mg/m^2), TBI (2 Gy) regimen with tacrolimus/mycophenolate mofetil (FK506/MMF) as posttransplant immunosuppression.[32,33]

Probably the most important development in preventing rejection has been the concept that the stem cell dose directly contributes to the likelihood of establishing engraftment. Increasing the donor stem cell dose may facilitate competition with residual host stem cells. Furthermore, it was realized that cells within the CD34+ compartment possessed potent veto activity, which neutralizes host alloreactive cytotoxic T lymphocytes (CTL), and the greater the number of CD34+ cells, the greater the induction of tolerance.[17,34] The veto activity appears to be mediated by apoptosis of antigen-specific T cells.

In humans, the concept of stem cell dose escalation was tested after hematopoietic growth factors became available, and collection of PBPCs had been applied.[5,31] Large numbers of CD34+ cells (10×10^6/kg) could be administered to patients by collecting PBPCs from donors after mobilization with G-CSF.[5] The Perugia group[28] has successfully developed a megadose haploidentical SCT procedure using a relatively nontoxic conditioning regimen consisting of thiotepa, a single TBI dose of 800 cGy, fludarabine, and ATG, which achieved more than 90% sustained engraftment with 30-day treatment-related mortality of only 10%. This method has now become widely established and probably offers the greatest promise for current and future studies of haploidentical transplantation.[17]

In addition to cells within the CD34+ fraction, including early myeloid progenitors, several other donor cells possessing veto activity have been described, the most potent of which is CTL.[35] However, some of these cells also possess a marked GVH reactivity. To eliminate the GVH activity, investigators have developed new approaches to deplete alloreactive clones directed against the host by stimulating the donor T cells against third-party stimulators in the absence of interleukin (IL)-2. In this approach, only the activated anti-third-party CTLs survive IL-2 starvation in the primary culture, whereas the alloreactive CTLs directed against the host are depleted.[36] In a mouse model, these alloreactive CTLs are endowed with a very potent veto activity that appears mediated through both FasL and CD8-mediated apoptosis.[36]

Obstacles for Successful Haploidentical SCT: Delayed Immune Reconstitution

Having largely overcome the problems of engraftment and GVHD, much of the focus today in haploidentical transplants is centered on the delayed immune reconstitution that follows haploidentical SCT. Several mechanisms underlie slow immunologic reconstitution. These include the profound T and B cell depletion associated with CD34+ selection, ATG in the conditioning regimen, which may antagonize expansion of the residual T lymphocytes, the degree of HLA disparity between the host and donor, and decaying thymic function in adults.[37] This slow recovery places patients at significant risk from posttransplant viral, fungal, and other opportunistic infections[6] and is the most important cause of mortality in adults undergoing haploidentical SCT, reaching as high as 40% in some studies.[30]

Extrathymic pathways of immune reconstitution after transplantation are predominant in adults because thymus function begins to decline relatively early in life, usually before the age of 20 years. Therefore, T cells that repopulate adult transplant recipients are derived predominantly from the relatively small number of mature donor T cells infused with marrow inoculums.[38]

Surprisingly, recent data have demonstrated that the human thymus continues to function at low levels until late in life, providing hope that effective treatment can be developed to restore immunity quickly in T cell-deficient adults.[39] Preclinical data using IL-7 and keratinocyte growth factor to facilitate the recovery of the immune system are promising and can help to overcome this problem. Clinical studies are underway.[40]

Monocyte and dendritic cells, as well as other antigen-presenting cells, are also vital for the antigen-specific immunity. IL-12 is known to be a major cytokine in the initiation of protective T helper 1 (Th-1) immunity against opportunistic infections. The observation that G-CSF, used to hasten neutrophil recovery post-SCT, blocks IL-12 production by antigen-presenting cells prompted the discontinuation of this cytokine posttransplant. Clinical data suggest that as soon as G-CSF is stopped, IL-12 levels return to normal, and CD4 cell number and function markedly improve, at 3 months posttransplantation.[22]

Much attention at present is being focused on the restoration of specific immunity after transplant in order to prevent infections and perhaps also relapse. The potential and clinical use of this approach has been applied to many infections including candida, aspergillus, and toxoplasma.[41] Mencacci et al.[42] generated large numbers of donor T cell clones against Aspergillus fumigatus and CMV antigens, screened them for cross-reactivity to host alloantigens, and infused pooled nonalloreactive clones into adult recipients at a dose of 5×10^5 on day 15 after transplant. All patients developed aspergillus and CMV-specific responses within 3 weeks compared with untreated patients who developed the corresponding pathogen-specific T cell responses more than 9 months posttransplant.

An alternative approach is a selective ex vivo T cell depletion or tolerization, for the prevention of GVHD, while preserving immunologic reconstitution. These involve the coincubation of T cell-repleted donor BM with recipient antigen-presenting cells in the presence of agents that can selectively eliminate or inactivate host reactive T cells. Using this approach, donor T cells were exposed ex vivo to recipient alloantigens and treated with an immunotoxin specific for IL-2 receptor alpha chain.[43] This strategy was effective in selectively eliminating alloreactive T cells but not T cells reactive to third-party antigens. Reinfusion of nonalloreactive T cells into the patients, previously transplanted with T cell-depleted grafts from HLA-mismatched donors, led to immune reconstitution without GVHD.[43]

Extensive preclinical data demonstrated that antigen presentation in the absence of CD28 costimulation induces a state of T cell unresponsiveness (anergy) to antigen restimulation.[44] Based on these preclinical data, Lee Nadler group used host antigen-presenting cells and soluble CTLA-4Ig to present host alloantigen to donor T cells while blocking CD28 costimulatory pathways. This approach resulted in ex vivo donor T cell unresponsiveness to the HLA-mismatched cells of the recipient.[45] Transplantation of marrow repleted with alloantigen unresponsive T cells led to primary engraftment in 9 of the 12 children, and three cases of acute GVHD despite posttransplant immunosuppressive therapy. These investigators are initiating clinical trials with similar antibodies such as anti-B7-1. Quesenberry et al.[46] have shown that a similar approach is feasible in a murine model using blockade of CD40 ligand-mediated costimulation. The problems with this approach are that anergy may not be complete or permanent, resulting in GVHD, and that the anergized cells may have a negative effect on bystander T cells with antiviral and antileukemic activity. Therefore, it will be crucial to assess the reconstitution of viral-specific immunity in further clinical trials using this approach.

A number of groups have targeted surface markers expressed on activated T cells, e.g., CD25 and CD69, using magnetic microbeads or immunotoxins in order to eliminate alloreactive T cells preserving the T cells with antileukemic and antimicrobial activity. Donor T cells expressed activation markers after coculture with recipient Peripheral Blood Monoclonal Cells (PBMCs). This approach has the advantage that alloreactive T cells are permanently removed and cannot influence the function of the remaining T cells.[47]

Another approach currently being evaluated is based on earlier studies that showed that CD8+ CTL clones possess extremely high veto activity.[17] Researchers from the Weizman Institute in Israel depleted such veto cells of alloreactive activity by generating nonalloreactive anti-third-party clones. These cells are then evaluated by their capacity to facilitate engraftment of purified Sca-1+ Lin–hematopoietic progenitors in sublethally irradiated mismatched recipients.[48–50] If successful, such an approach might dramatically reduce the morbidity and mortality from impaired immunity posthaploidentical transplantation and make this transplant approach more common.

GVL Effect Posthaploidentical SCT

Traditionally, T cell depletion matched allogeneic SCT carried a high risk of leukemic relapse attributed mostly to abrogation of the GVL effect. Paradoxically, clinical reports of patients with advanced acute myeloid leukemia (AML) undergoing T cell-depletion haploidentical SCT suggest a relatively low incidence of GVHD and low relapse rate.[19] This clinical observation may be explained by NK rather than T cell-mediated antitumor effect. NK cell alloreactivity has been recently appreciated as an important biologic phenomenon almost unique to HLA-mismatched transplants. Donor NK cell killing inhibitor receptors (KIRs) do not recognize the MHC allotypes of the recipient as "self." In this way, these donor cells lyse the recipient's malignant cells. This process is of vast importance for HLA-mismatched cells, and have a great impact on the clinical outcome of the transplant.[51,52] In vitro assays have demonstrated that alloreactive NK clones have potent cytotoxic activity against leukemic targets from patients with chronic myeloid leukemia and AML, but not against blasts from most patients with acute lymphoblastic leukemia(ALL).[51]

Long-term follow-up of 75 high-risk AML patients who underwent haploidentical SCT showed an impressive effect of NK alloreactivity on subsequent relapses.[19] No relapses occurred among 20 patients transplanted from haploidentical donors with KIR mismatch in the GVL direction. In contrast, 28 of 37 patients relapsed when transplanted with grafts with no potential for NK alloreactivity ($P < 0.01$).[19] This GVL effect was not associated with GVHD. Moreover, KIR-mismatched patients had a significantly lower incidence of significant GVHD.[19]

Thus, these data strongly support the hypothesis that in mismatched transplants, a GVL effect controls leukemia relapse when KIR epitope incompatibility is in the GVHD direction.[53] Furthermore, it has been suggested that donor-versus-recipient NK cell alloreactivity may become a major criteria for donor selection in mismatched hematopoietic stem cell transplants.

In contrast, in a different cohort of patients with less profound T cell depletion, we found that potential NK alloreactivity in the GVHD direction was associated with an increased incidence of severe GVHD and poorer patient survival, but not with nonengraftment, or leukemia relapse.[54] There was no effect in the rejection direction. These findings suggest that lack of extensive T cell depletion in haploidentical transplantation is associated with high GVHD rates and diminishes the benefits of NK cell alloreactivity.

The GVL effect of donor CTLs recognizing mismatched minor histocompatibility, overexpressed myeloid, and leukemic antigens is largely lost in haploidentical SCT, because of the rigorous T cell depletion used. However, strategies aimed at generation of allorestricted CTLs, recognizing hematopoietic antigens such as WT-1, HA-1, and CD45,[55–57] or selective depletion of alloreactive donor T cells with preservation of CTL responses to myeloid tumor antigens,[58] may offer the prospect of restoring a CTL-mediated GVL effect in the haploidentical setting.

Clinical Perspective

Although the performance of matched allogeneic transplantation has increased over the past decades, it still can only be offered to a minority of patients. The majority of individuals do not have an HLA-matched sibling donor. For those subjects who lack an HLA-matched sibling donor, a matched unrelated donor transplant is often performed. Although success rates are increasing,[59–62] this procedure carries with it high long-term morbidity. Furthermore, a patient must survive the rather long waiting period (3–4 months) to eventually allow a donor to be identified, thereby excluding a relatively high number of patients. In addition, for a significant number of patients who come from ethnic minority groups, no closely matched donor can be found (Table 26.1).

Haploidentical SCT offers an attractive alternative to matched unrelated donor transplants for those patients who do not have a timely matched allogeneic donor. Approximately 90% of patients have a suitable haploidentical donor and the procedure can be offered within a very short time (Table 26.1).

A recent report from Perugia, Italy, with a revised transplant protocol including fludarabine, suggests that, in good risk AML patients, the associated morbidity and mortality do not exceed that reported for matched unrelated

Table 26.1. Haploidentical versus matched unrelated allogeneic transplantation

	Donor issues					Transplantation issues		
Access	Availability cost	Engraftment	Immunity GVHD	Rejection	Relapse GVL	Reconstitution	KIR role speed	Unrelated
Slow cells?	60%–70%*	High	Moderate (14–16 d)	Slow	40%–80%	4%	Low	T cells?
Haploidentical Fast High	90%† NK cells ++	High	Fast (12 d)	Very slow	<20%	10%–15%		

*For ethnic minority, 20%.
†Multiple donors, select for gender, age, CMV status.

donor transplants and there is no excessive risk of relapse.[30] In this report, 43 adult patients with high-risk acute leukemia are described. Primary sustained engraftment was achieved in 41 of the 43 patients (95%). Two patients rejected the first graft but engrafted after second transplants. Hematopoietic recovery was rapid. Analysis of DNA polymorphism documented complete donor chimerism of all evaluable patients. The incidence of grade II–IV GVHD was less than 5%. Twelve of the patients were alive, leukemia-free, and with Karnofsky score of 100 after a median follow-up of 18 months (range 8–30). The 2-year disease-free survival was 36% ± 11% for 20 patients with AML and 17% ± 7% for the 23 patients with ALL ($P = 0.052$).

The status of the leukemia and the length and intensity of chemotherapy before transplant influence patient outcome by selecting for resistant leukemia, and decreasing the patient tolerance to transplant therapies and complications. Because only patients with advanced disease have initially been offered transplantation from HLA haplotype mismatched donors, those preexisting risks have undoubtedly confounded the interpretation of clinical results.[63,64] Inclusion of patients with less advanced leukemia in clinical trials has allowed analyzing results according to disease risk at transplantation. Analysis of 65 patients transplanted in Perugia between January 1999 and September 2002 confirmed the very high engraftment rate and low incidence of GVHD. Patients had a median follow-up of 22 month (range 3–45). Even in ALL, where success rates are usually low, disease-free survival was 40% ± 16% for 12 patients transplanted in remission and 13% ± 11% for 10 patients transplanted in relapse, whereas in AML, disease-free survival was 60% ± 11% for 26 patients transplanted in remission and 10% ± 8% for 17 transplanted in relapse. By multivariate analysis, the most significant risk factor for the clinical outcome was the lack of donor-versus-recipient NK alloreactivity: hazard ratio of 6.1 (95% confidence interval, range 2.6–14.9). AML patients who received transplants from donors with NK alloreactivity against recipient cells had a 2-year disease-free survival of 60% versus 5% of those without such donors which is not different from the results with unrelated transplants.[19]

As for technical issues, this same Perugia group has strongly recommended, with the supporting data of reduced transplant-related mortality, the use of the CliniMACS (Miltenyi Biotech, Begish Gladbach, Germany) for positive CD34 cell selection. In sequential studies, using different stem cell columns for CD34+ selection, the transplant-related mortality was 63% using the Isolex (Baxter, Deerfield, IL), 42% with the Ceprate (CellPro, Bothell, WA), and only 20% with the CliniMACS.

However, other centers have reported less enthusiastic results.[65] Larger prospective randomized multicenter trials are in need to address the mode of haploidentical SCT, the optimal strategy for stem cell purification, ways for facilitating immune recovery, and antitumor effects.

Haploidentical Transplantation for Nonmalignant Conditions

The role of haploidentical SCT for the treatment of genetic disease is firmly established. Because of the immediate availability of a donor, haploidentical SCT has been extensively used in severe combined immunodeficiency,[1,66,67] when a matched family donor is not available. The outcome in such transplants has improved dramatically in recent years with more than 75% surviving for a year.[68]

There is a small amount of experience with haploidentical SCT in the nonmalignant hematologic diseases. Elhasid et al.[69] described a child with Fanconi anemia that underwent haploidentical SCT with a favorable outcome. We described haploidentical SCT in a child with Hurler syndrome, depleting the T cells in the graft with anti-CD52 monoclonal antibodies (CAMPATH) with similar results.[70] Recently, a success in haploidentical SCT was achieved in two patients with thalassemia. One patient was a 5-year-old boy and the other was a 4-year-old girl, both of which were diagnosed with thalassemia major. They both were treated with hydroxyurea and azathioprine from day 59 until day 11, fludarabine from day 11, and busulfan starting on day 10 followed by a CD34 T cell-depleted (CliniMACS system), G-CSF mobilized PBSCs and BM from an HLA-mismatched relative. They received cyclosporine after transplant for GVHD prophylaxis. Both patients experienced minimal toxicity, rapid engraftment, no infection, and no GVHD.[71]

Conclusion

Haploidentical SCT is a viable option for high-risk patients with hematologic malignancies who are in need for an allogeneic transplantation and do not have an HLA compatible sibling or unrelated donor. Almost all patients have a genetically haploidentical family member and the procedure can be performed without delay.

Although the clinical experience is limited, recent data are encouraging and suggest that this procedure is an acceptable alternative to matched unrelated donor transplantation. Ongoing registration study of the European Bone Marrow transplantation (EBMT) is currently comparing haploidentical SCT to either allogeneic transplantation from matched unrelated donor or cord blood transplants.

Much progress has been made in the control of GVHD without increasing the rate of nonengraftment.

The most recent advance in HLA-mismatched SCT has been the use of hematopoietic growth factors to mobilize PBSCs and purified CD34+ grafts, which enable the harvesting and transplantation of "mega doses" of stem cells with engraftment of 90% and low risk of GVHD (Table 26.1). Other ways of tolerance induction are being developed.

Of particular note, it seems that in some T cell-depleted haploidentical transplants from KIR-mismatched donors, in patients with AML, an NK-mediated GVL effect may take place, leading to a low rate of relapse. New trials administrating purified CD56 NK cells after haploidentical transplants mediating GVL effect with no risk of GVHD, look interesting.

Posttransplant infectious viral and fungal complications remain the most important barriers yet to be overcome. New directions in the use of adoptive specific cellular immunity seem promising. Preclinical data demonstrating that anti-third-party nonalloreactive cytotoxic T lymphocytes may improve immunologic reconstitution have yet to be reported in humans. Preliminary human data look promising. In the meantime, ongoing research is very likely to improve this treatment modality.

References

1. Reisner Y, Kapoor N, Kirkpatrick D, et al. Transplantation for severe combined immunodeficiency with HLA-A,B,D,DR incompatible parental marrow cells fractionated by soybean agglutinin and sheep red blood cells. Blood 1983;61(2):341–348.
2. Beatty PG, Clift RA, Mickelson EM, et al. Marrow transplantation from related donors other than HLA-identical siblings. N Engl J Med 1985;313(13):765–771.
3. Anasetti C, Beatty PG, Storb R, et al. Effect of HLA incompatibility on graft-versus-host disease, relapse, and survival after marrow transplantation for patients with leukemia or lymphoma. Hum Immunol 1990;29(2):79–91.
4. Kernan NA, Flomenberg N, Dupont B, O'Reilly RJ. Graft rejection in recipients of T-cell-depleted HLA-nonidentical marrow transplants for leukemia. Identification of host-derived antidonor allocytotoxic T lymphocytes. Transplantation 1987;43(6):842–847.
5. Aversa F, Tabilio A, Terenzi A, et al. Successful engraftment of T-cell-depleted haploidentical "three-loci" incompatible transplants in leukemia patients by addition of recombinant human granulocyte colony-stimulating factor-mobilized peripheral blood progenitor cells to bone marrow inoculum. Blood 1994;84(11):3948–3955.
6. Kook H, Goldman F, Padley D, et al. Reconstruction of the immune system after unrelated or partially matched T-cell-depleted bone marrow transplantation in children: immunophenotypic analysis and factors affecting the speed of recovery. Blood 1996;88(3):1089–1097.

7. Ferrara JL, Deeg HJ. Graft-versus-host disease. N Engl J Med 1991;324(10):667–674.
8. Ho VT. Soiffer RJ. The history and future of T-cell depletion as graft-versus-host disease prophylaxis for allogeneic hematopoietic stem cell transplantation. Blood 2001;98(12):3192–3204.
9. Nagler A, Morecki S, Slavin S. The use of soybean agglutinin (SBA) for bone marrow (BM) purging and hematopoietic progenitor cells enrichment in clinical bone marrow transplantation. Mol Biotech 1999;11: 181–194.
10. Soiffer RJ, Mauch P, Fairclough D, et al. CD6+ T cell depleted allogeneic bone marrow transplantation from genotypically HLA nonidentical related donors. Biol Blood Marrow Transplant 1997;3(1):11–17.
11. Henslee-Downey PJ, Parrish RS, MacDonald JS, et al. Combined in vitro and in vivo T lymphocyte depletion for the control of graft-versus-host disease following haploidentical marrow transplant. Transplantation 1996;61(5):738–745.
12. Henslee-Downey PJ, Abhyankar SH, Parrish RS, et al. Use of partially mismatched related donors extends access to allogeneic marrow transplant. Blood 1997; 89(10):3864–3872.
13. Godder KT, Hazlett LJ, Abhyankar SH, et al. Partially mismatched related-donor bone marrow transplantation for pediatric patients with acute leukemia: younger donors and absence of peripheral blasts improve outcome. J Clin Oncol 2000;18(9):1856–1866.
14. Chiang KY, Van Rhee F, Godder K, et al. Allogeneic bone marrow transplantation from partially mismatched related donors as therapy for primary induction failure acute myeloid leukemia. Bone Marrow Transplant 2001;27(5):507–510.
15. Singhal S, Powles R, Henslee-Downey PJ, et al. Allogeneic transplantation from HLA-matched sibling or partially HLA-mismatched related donors for primary refractory acute leukemia. Bone Marrow Transplant 2002;29(4):291–295.
16. Schumm M, Lang P, Taylor G, et al. Isolation of highly purified autologous and allogeneic peripheral CD34+ cells using the CliniMACS device. J Hematother 1999;8(2):209–218.
17. Reisner Y, Martelli MF. Transplantation tolerance induced by "mega dose" CD34+ cell transplants. Exp Hematol 2000;28(2):119–127.
18. Handgretinger R, Klingebiel T, Lang P, et al. Megadose transplantation of purified peripheral blood CD34(+) progenitor cells from HLA-mismatched parental donors in children. Bone Marrow Transplant 2001;27(8):777–783.
19. Ruggeri L, Capanni M, Urbani E, et al. Effectiveness of donor natural killer cell alloreactivity in mismatched hematopoietic transplants. Science 2002;295(55): 2097–2100.
20. Margalit M, Ilan Y, Ohana M, et al. Adoptive transfer of small numbers DX5+ cells alleviates graft versus host disease in a murine model of semiallogeneic bone marrow transplantation: a potential role for NKT lymphocytes. Bone Marrow Transplant 2005; 35(2):191–197.
21. Zanjani ED, Almeida-Porada G, Livingston AG, Flake AW, Ogawa M. Human bone marrow CD34– cells engraft in vivo and undergo multilineage expression that includes giving rise to CD34+ cells. Exp Hematol 1998;26(4):353–360.
22. Yin AH, Miraglia S, Zanjani ED, et al. AC133, a novel marker for human hematopoietic stem and progenitor cells. Blood 1997;90(12):5002–5012.
23. Barge AJ, Johnson G, Witherspoon R, Torok-Storb B. Antibody-mediated marrow failure after allogeneic bone marrow transplantation. Blood 1939;74(5):1477–1480.
24. Soderling CC, Song CW, Blazar BR, Vallera DA. A correlation between conditioning and engraftment in recipients of MHC-mismatched T cell-depleted murine bone marrow transplants. J Immunol 1985;135(2): 941–946.
25. Champlin RE, Ho WG, Mitsuyasu R, et al. Graft failure and leukemia relapse following T lymphocyte-depleted bone marrow transplants: effect of intensification of immunosuppressive conditioning. Transplant Proc 1987;19(1 pt 3):2616–2619.
26. Lapidot T, Terenzi A, Singer TS, Salomon O, Reisner Y. Enhancement by dimethyl myleran of donor type chimerism in murine recipients of bone marrow allografts. Blood 1989;73(7):2025–2032.
27. Terenzi A, Lubin I, Lapidot T, et al. Enhancement of T cell-depleted bone marrow allografts in mice by thiotepa. Transplantation 1990;50(4):717–720.
28. Sykes M, Preffer F, McAfee S, et al. Mixed lymphohaemopoietic chimerism and graft-versus-lymphoma effects after non-myeloablative therapy and HLA-mismatched bone-marrow transplantation. Lancet 1999; 353(9166):1755–1759.
29. Soiffer RJ, Mauch P, Tarbell NJ, et al. Total lymphoid irradiation to prevent graft rejection in recipients of HLA non-identical T cell-depleted allogeneic marrow. Bone Marrow Transplant 1991;7(1):23–33.
30. Aversa F, Tabilio A, Velardi A, et al. Treatment of high-risk acute leukemia with T-cell-depleted stem cells from related donors with one fully mismatched HLA haplotype. N Engl J Med 1998;339(17):1186–1193.
31. Nagler A, Or R, Naparstek E, Varadi G, Slavin S. Second allogeneic stem cell transplantation using non myeloablative conditioning for patients who relapsed or developed secondary malignancies following autologous transplantation. Exp Hematol 2000;28:1096–1104.
32. Luznik L, Slansky JE, Jalla S, et al. Successful therapy of metastatic cancer using tumor vaccines in mixed allogeneic bone marrow chimeras. Blood 2003;101(4): 1645–1652.
33. O'Donnell PV, Luznik L, Jones RJ, et al. Nonmyeloablative bone marrow transplantation from partially HLA-mismatched related donors using posttransplantation cyclophosphamide. Biol Blood Marrow Transplant 2002;8(7):377–386.
34. Reisner Y, Martelli MF. Bone marrow transplantation across HLA barriers by increasing the number of transplanted cells. Immunol Today 1995;16(9):437–440.
35. Sambhara SR, Miller RG. Programmed cell death of T cells signaled by the T cell receptor and the alpha 3 domain of class I MHC. Science 1991;252(5011): 1424–1427.
36. Reich-Zeliger S, Zhao Y, Krauthgamer R, Bachar-Lustig E, Reisner Y. Anti-third party CD8+ CTLs as potent veto cells: coexpression of CD8 and FasL is a prerequisite. Immunity 2000;13(4):507–515.
37. Weinberg K, Blazar BR, Wagner JE, et al. Factors affecting thymic function after allogeneic hematopoietic stem cell transplantation. Blood 2001;97(5):1458–1466.
38. Mackall CL and RE Gress Pathways of T-cell regeneration in mice and humans: implications for bone marrow transplantation and immunotherapy. Immunol Rev 1997;157:61–72.
39. Douek DC, Vescio RA, Betts MR, et al. Assessment of thymic output in adults after haematopoietic stem-cell

40. Fry TJ, Mackall CL. Interleukin-7: from bench to clinic. Blood 2002;99(11):3892–3904.
41. Drobyski WR, Ash RC, Casper JT, et al. Effect of T-cell depletion as graft-versus-host disease prophylaxis on engraftment, relapse, and disease-free survival in unrelated marrow transplantation for chronic myelogenous leukemia. Blood 1994;83(7):1980–1987.
42. Mencacci A, Perruccio K, Bacci A, et al. Defective antifungal T-helper 1 (TH1) immunity in a murine model of allogeneic T-cell-depleted bone marrow transplantation and its restoration by treatment with TH2 cytokine antagonists. Blood 2001;97(5):1483–1490.
43. Andre-Schmutz I, Le Deist F, Hacein-Bey-Abina S, et al. Immune reconstitution without graft-versus-host disease after haemopoietic stem-cell transplantation: a phase 1/2 study. Lancet 2002;360(9327):130–137.
44. Tan P, Anasetti C, Hansen JA, et al. Induction of alloantigen-specific hyporesponsiveness in human T lymphocytes by blocking interaction of CD28 with its natural ligand B7/BB1. J Exp Med 1993;177(1):165–173.
45. Guinan EC, Boussiotis VA, Neuberg D, et al. Transplantation of anergic histoincompatible bone marrow allografts. N Engl J Med 1999;340(22):1704–1714.
46. Quesenberry PJ, Zhong S, Wang H, Stewart M. Allogeneic chimerism with low-dose irradiation, antigen presensitization, and costimulator blockade in H-2 mismatched mice. Blood 2001;97(2):557–564.
47. Koh MB, Prentice HG, Corbo M, Morgan M, Cotter FE, Lowdell MW. Alloantigen-specific T-cell depletion in a major histocompatibility complex fully mismatched murine model provides effective graft-versus-host disease prophylaxis in the presence of lymphoid engraftment. Br J Haematol 2002;118(1):108–116.
48. Bachar-Lustig E, Li HW, Marcus H, Reisner Y. Tolerance induction by megadose stem cell transplants: synergism between SCA-1+ Lin− cells and nonalloreactive T cells. Transplant Proc 1998;30(8):4007–4008.
49. Bachar-Lustig E, Li HW, Gur H, Krauthgamer R, Marcus H, Reisner Y. Induction of donor-type chimerism and transplantation tolerance across major histocompatibility barriers in sublethally irradiated mice by Sca-1(+)Lin(−) bone marrow progenitor cells: synergism with non-alloreactive (host x donor)F(1) T cells. Blood 1999;94(9):3212–3221.
50. Champlin R, Ho W, Gajewski J, et al. Selective depletion of CD8+ T lymphocytes for prevention of graft-versus-host disease after allogeneic bone marrow transplantation. Blood 1990;76(2):418–423.
51. Ruggeri L, Capanni M, Casucci M, et al. Role of natural killer cell alloreactivity in HLA-mismatched hematopoietic stem cell transplantation. Blood 1999;94(1):333–339.
52. Lee LA, Sergio JJ, Sykes M. Natural killer cells weakly resist engraftment of allogeneic, long-term, multilineage-repopulating hematopoietic stem cells. Transplantation 1996;61(1):125–132.
53. Rowe JM, Lazarus HM. Genetically haploidentical stem cell transplantation for acute leukemia. Bone Marrow Transplant 2001;27(7):669–676.
54. Nagler A, Slavin S, Brautbar C, Or R, Shapira M, Bishara A. Killer Inhibitory Receptor (KIR) mismatches correlate with high incidence of transplant related complication post-haploidentical stem cell transplantation (HaploSCT). Bone Marrow Transplant 2001;27(Suppl 1).
55. Amrolia PJ, Reid SD, Gao L, et al. Allorestricted cytotoxic T cells specific for human CD45 show potent antileukemic activity. Blood 2003;101(3):1007–1014.
56. Mutis T, Blokland E, Kester M, Schrama E, Goulmy E. Generation of minor histocompatibility antigen HA-1-specific cytotoxic T cells restricted by nonself HLA molecules: a potential strategy to treat relapsed leukemia after HLA-mismatched stem cell transplantation. Blood 2002;100(2):547–542.
57. Gao L, Bellantuono I, Elsasser A, et al. Selective elimination of leukemic CD34(+) progenitor cells by cytotoxic T lymphocytes specific for WT1. Blood 2000;95(7):2198–2203.
58. Amrolia PJ, Muccioli-Casadei G, Yvon E, et al. Selective depletion of donor alloreactive T cells without loss of antiviral or antileukemic responses. Blood 2003;102(6):2292–2299.
59. Anasetti C. Transplantation of hematopoietic stem cells from alternate donors in acute myelogenous leukemia. Leukemia 2000;14(3):502–504.
60. McGlave P. Hematopoietic stem-cell transplantation from an unrelated donor. Hosp Pract (Off Ed) 2000;35(8):43–46, 49–52, 55; discussion 55–56.
61. Nagler A, Brautbar C, Slavin S, Bishara A. Bone marrow transplantation using unrelated and family related donors-the impact of HLA-C disparity. Bone Marrow Transplant 1996;18:891–897.
62. Bishara A, Amar A, Brautbar C, et al. The putative role of HLA recognition in graft vs. host disease (GVHD) and graft rejection post unrelated bone marrow transplantation (BMT). Exp Hematol 1995;23:1667–1675.
63. Aversa F, Velardi A, Tabilio A, Reisner Y, Martelli MF. Haploidentical stem cell transplantation in leukemia. Blood Rev 2001;15(3):111–119.
64. Kato S, Yabe H, Yasui M, et al. Allogeneic hematopoietic transplantation of CD34+ selected cells from an HLA haplo-identical related donor. A long-term follow-up of 135 patients and a comparison of stem cell source between the bone marrow and the peripheral blood. Bone Marrow Transplant 2000;26(12):1281–1290.
65. Passweg JR, Kuhne T, Gregor M, et al. Increased stem cell dose, as obtained using currently available technology, may not be sufficient for engraftment of haploidentical stem cell transplants. Bone Marrow Transplant 2000;26(10):1033–1036.
66. Buckley RH, Schiff SE, Schiff RI, et al. Hematopoietic stem-cell transplantation for the treatment of severe combined immunodeficiency. N Engl J Med 1999;340(7):508–516.
67. Fischer A, Landais P, Friedrich W, et al. European experience of bone-marrow transplantation for severe combined immunodeficiency. Lancet 1990;336(8719):850–854.
68. Antoine C, Cant MS, Cavazzana-Calvo A, et al. Long term survival & transplantation of haemopoietic stem cells for immunodeficiencies. Lancet 2003;361:553–560.
69. Elhasid R, Ben Arush MW, Katz T, et al. Successful haploidentical bone marrow transplantation in Fanconi anemia. Bone Marrow Transplant 2000;26(11):1221–1223.
70. Kapelushnik J, Mandel H, Varadi G, Nagler A. Fludarabine based protocol for haploidentical peripheral blood stem transplantation in Hurler syndrome. J Pediatr Hematol Oncol 2000;22:433–436.
71. Sodani P, Gaziev D, Polchi P, et al. New approach for bone marrow transplantation in patients with class 3 thalassemic aged younger than 17 years. Blood 2004;104(4):1201–1203.

Section 8

Skin

Section 8

Skin

Nili Grossman

Skin is among the largest tissues in the body that undergoes a continuous expansion and renewal through life. Morphologically and functionally, it is composed of two layers. The epidermis – a stratified squamous epithelium, rich with keratinocytes, that provides a barrier between the outside and the inside of the body preventing moisture loss, and actively protecting against environmental assaults, such as infections, chemicals and ultraviolet irradiation. The dermis – a collagen-rich underlying layer, provides a support and nourishes the epidermis, and is responsible for the elasticity and mechanical integrity of the skin. Skin may be covered with hairs, which were proved to be important for both its self-renewal and differentiation, and contribute to the wound-healing process.

The last 30 years have been marked with advances in various disciplines such as histology, biochemistry, and cellular and molecular biology. Numerous experiments conducted in in vivo and in vitro rodent and human models culminated in three major achievements regarding skin regeneration: (a) A better understanding of skin biology and the cellular, molecular, and biochemical basis of the wound-healing process; (b) development of clinically effective skin substitutes; (c) identification, localization, and characterization of adult and embryonic stem cells, and elucidation of their role in skin regeneration and wound healing. Analyses of these studies reveal that these were achieved concomitantly and complemented each other. The recently applied gene-manipulation techniques in various skin models implicate their future gene-based therapeutic use in the clinic.

The paradigm of skin regeneration is the wound-healing process, as presented and discussed in the first chapter in this section by Singer and Simon (Stoneybrook, NY).

This complex process requires the collaborative efforts of many cell lineages: Hemopoietic cells (such as platelets, macrophages, neutrophiles, and lymphocytes), ectodermal (keratinocytes), and mesodermal cells (fibroblasts). All secrete and respond to growth factors and matrix signals that contribute to the phases of normal wound healing: Inflammation, proliferation, migration, matrix synthesis, maturation, and remodeling, thus restoring the function and esthetics of skin.

Damage to the skin barrier, for example, large body surface area burns, and the need of skin cover as a lifesaving technique, promoted the use and development of skin substitutes for grafting. These include temporary and permanent products: Biological-based, cultured cells (cellular), synthetic, acellular, and composite skin substitutes. Most are available commercially, or provided by skin bank laboratories. Many of those products were inspired by the pioneering studies from the Boston area: Howard Green et al. who were the first to report the isolation, and propagation of human keratinocytes (1975), and participated in its first clinical application using autologous cultured keratinocytes for grafting large burn areas; Bell – designing composite substitutes of neonatal epidermal keratinocytes overlaying collagen seeded with neonatal dermal fibroblasts (1980), and Yannas, Burk et al., who engineered a synthetic skin substitute based on the current structure and function of skin (1980).

Back in the 1970s and the 1980s, the concept that basal layer epidermal keratinocytes differed in their growth capability was established (Potten and Barrandon, respectively). Keratinocytes termed as "holoclones" had the extensive growth potential (130 divisions) and thus were termed "stem cells," whereas "paraclones," transient amplification cells, were committed to terminal differentiation and underwent a maximum of 15 divisions. The "meroclones" were an intermediate type.

Currently, it is accepted that the adult epidermis is sustained by multipotent stem cells, which give rise to cells of different fates including those forming hair follicles, interfollicular epidermis, and sebaceous glands. This is presented and discussed in the second chapter in this section, by Turksen and Troy (Ottawa, Canada), on the identification of epithelial multipotent embryonic and adult stem cells, and their contribution to our understanding of skin regeneration.

The main storage of these epidermal stem cells seems to be located in the bulge of hair follicles. However, it was hypothesized that the follicular stem cells may not participate in the renewal of epidermis under normal conditions, and might serve as a reservoir and be recruited and migrate when the epidermis is damaged. Stem cell fate determination has been envisioned to depend on tissue response and to be regulated by specific signaling molecules and pathways. However, as yet, this important question is still unsolved.

A second type of epidermal stem cell, unipotent, is located in the basal layer of the interfollicular epidermis. These cells undergo a short-term self-renewal and give rise to keratinocytes that are committed to terminal differentiation, an intrinsic decision of this cell lineage. The latter are being pushed up toward the skin outer surface, resulting in keratin-containing scale-like structures, devoid of nucleus and cytoplasm, and form the cornified layer.

The advances in skin regeneration during the last 30 years, discussed in this section, with the recently employed gene-based studies, might yield to new clinical tools of lifesaving procedures and cell therapy. In addition, it is envisioned that new model systems might be elucidated, leading to a better understanding of processes involved in aging, and various hyperproliferative skin diseases as psoriasis and cancer.

# 27

Wound Healing and Skin Substitutes

Adam J. Singer and Marcia Simon

A variety of insults can result in injury to the skin including mechanical, thermal, chemical, nuclear, and infectious. In all cases, the injury to the skin triggers a response aimed at restoring the integrity and function of the skin. Wound healing is a dynamic process that involves a complex and closely orchestrated interaction between blood cells, cutaneous parenchymal cells, soluble factors, and the extracellular matrix (ECM). Although considerable overlap exists among the various stages of wound healing, it is helpful to divide the healing process into three classical stages: Inflammation, tissue formation, and tissue remodeling. The goals of wound healing include rapid wound closure with restoration of its barrier function, avoiding infection, and achieving an optimal aesthetic and functional result. Increased understanding of the molecular and cellular pathophysiology of wound healing over the last decade has led to the development of new healing devices and dressings. Skin substitutes that contain various combinations of epidermal and/or dermal components are now commercially available. The current chapter will review the biology of healing and discuss the various skin substitutes available for treating wounds.

The skin is the largest organ in the human body. Although it has multiple functions, its primary role is to serve as a barrier to the external environment. Other functions of the skin include fluid homeostasis, thermoregulation, immune surveillance, and sensory detection. A variety of insults can result in injury to the skin including mechanical, thermal, chemical, nuclear, and infectious. In all cases, the injury to the skin triggers a response aimed at restoring the integrity and function of the skin.

Cutaneous wounds, both acute and chronic, are very common. Each year there are more than 8 million traumatic lacerations[1] and 1 million burns treated in the United States alone.[2] In addition, up to 90 million surgically induced incisions are created each year.[3] Chronic wounds, such as diabetic ulcers, decubitus ulcers, and venous stasis ulcers are also quite common with more than 6 million ulcers reported annually.[4] Chronic ulcers are especially problematic because they tend to affect the most vulnerable populations, such as the elderly, the diabetic, and the physically debilitated.

Wound healing is a dynamic process that involves a complex and closely orchestrated interaction between blood cells, cutaneous parenchymal cells, soluble factors, and the ECM.[5] Although considerable overlap exists among the various stages of wound healing, it is helpful to divide the healing process into three classical stages: Inflammation, tissue formation, and tissue remodeling. The goals of wound healing include rapid wound closure with restoration of its barrier function, avoiding infection, and achieving an optimal aesthetic and functional result. Increased understanding of the molecular and cellular pathophysiology of wound healing over the last decade has led to the development of new healing devices and dressings. The current chapter will review the biology of healing and discuss the various skin substitutes available for treating wounds.

Growth Factors and Cytokines

Because cytokines and growth factors have such a central role in regulating wound healing, a brief description of the origins and actions of some of the most common ones follows (Table 27.1). Cytokines and growth factors are members of a large group of regulatory polypeptides that are secreted by many different cell lines, which act through autocrine and paracrine mechanisms to affect other cells.[6] In general, growth factors refer to polypeptides that regulate cell maturation whereas cytokines are important for host defense. Although essential for wound healing and host defense, in excess, cytokines and growth factors may also be responsible for poor healing and scarring. Most cytokines and growth factors are produced by more than one type of cell and have multiple pleiotropic functions. Considerable overlap and redundancy are also common among these substances, ensuring that wound healing proceeds even when any individual cytokine or growth factor is absent. Individual growth factors do not act alone but in concert, and the overall effect is determined by their relative concentration and timing.

The biological effects of the growth factors and cytokines are mediated by interacting with cell surface receptors. In turn, interaction with these receptors results in the formation of secondary messengers that affect the cell's structure or function. Although the exact molecular pathways that lead to alterations in function are not completely understood, several have been elucidated. Many of the recognized intracellular signal transduction pathways act through activation of a host of tyrosine kinases.[7] In contrast, the effects of TGF-β are propagated via a signal transduction network involving receptor serine/threonine kinases at the cell surface and their substrates, the SMAD proteins.[8,9]

Platelet-derived growth factor (PDGF) is first released from platelet α granules resulting in recruitment and activation of immune cells and fibroblasts.[10] Later, PDGF is released by macrophages and stimulates the production of collagen and proteoglycan. There are three different isoforms of PDGF including AA, AB, and BB that are named after the arrangement of two polypeptide chains, A and B. All three isoforms influence wound healing. Topical application of recombinant PDGF has resulted in increased wound breaking strength and faster healing in both animals and humans.[11-13] To date, PDGF is the only Food and Drug Administration-approved growth factor for clinical use.

Table 27.1. Cytokines and growth factors that have a role in wound healing

Mediator	Origin	Major Actions
PDGF	Platelets, macrophages, epidermal cells	Fibroblast proliferation and chemoattraction, macrophage chemoattraction and activation
FGF-1 and -2	Macrophages, endothelial cells	Angiogenesis and fibroblast proliferation
KGF-1	Fibroblasts	Keratinocyte proliferation and motility, production of granulation tissue
KGF-2	Fibroblasts	Fibroblast migration and granulation tissue formation
EGF	Platelets, macrophages	Reepithelialization, angiogenesis, ECM formation
TGF-β1 and -β2	Platelets, macrophages	Epidermal cell motility, chemotaxis of macrophages and fibroblasts, ECM synthesis
TGF-β3	Macrophages	Anti-scarring effects
TGF-α	Macrophages, keratinocytes	Reepithelialization
VEGF	Epidermal cells, macrophages	Angiogenesis, increased vascular permeability
IGF	Fibroblasts, epidermal cells	Reepithelialization and granulation tissue formation
TNF-α	Monocytes	Neutrophil chemotaxis and activation, mitogenic activity in fibroblasts, pleiotropic expression of growth factors
IL-1	Neutrophils, lymphocytes, keratinocytes, macrophages	Neutrophil chemotaxis, fibroblast and ECM proliferation
IL-6	Keratinocytes, macrophages, fibroblasts	Major mediator of acute phase response
IL-8	Keratinocytes,	Neutrophil chemoattraction, reepithelialization, angiogenesis

Transforming growth factor (TGF)-β is released by platelets, macrophages, and fibroblasts resulting in fibroblast migration, maturation, and ECM formation.[14] TGF-β exists in three isoforms – TGF-β1, TGF-β2, and TGF-β-3. Although essential for wound healing, the potent fibrogenic effects of TGF-β have been implicated in several fibroproliferative conditions, including scleroderma, keloids, and hypertrophic scarring.[15,16] In contrast, low levels of TGF-β in the fetus are partially responsible for their ability to heal without scar formation. Whereas TGF-β1 and TGF-β2 promote ECM formation and scarring, TGF-β3 may prevent scarring. Shah et al.[17,18] have shown that administration of TGF-β1 and TGF-β2 neutralizing antibodies reduce scarring as does administration of TGF-β3.

The fibroblast growth factor (FGF) family consists of 22 related proteins that regulate cellular proliferation, differentiation, migration, and/or survival of a variety of cells, mostly fibroblasts and endothelial cells.[19] In contrast, FGF-7 and FGF-10 [also known as keratinocyte growth factors (KGFs) 1 and 2] mostly affect keratinocytes.[20] The most recent addition to this family is FGF-22, which has also been implicated in reepithelialization.[21] Basic FGF and acidic FGF (aFGF or FGF-2) are released by macrophages and endothelial cells and stimulate the proliferation and migration of keratinocytes and fibroblasts. Basic FGF also stimulates the growth and migration of endothelial cells and has an important role in wound contraction and remodeling.[22]

KGF belongs to the FGF family and contains two isomers that share the same receptor.[23] Whereas KGF is secreted by fibroblasts and endothelial cells (of mesenchymal origin), its receptors are only located on epithelial cells of ectodermal origin. Thus, KGF may have a key role in the epidermal–dermal interaction. KGF is an important regulator of keratinocyte proliferation and maturation.[24] KGF may also stimulate epithelial cells to release other growth factors such as PDGF, TGF, and FGF. Administration of KGF-1 or KGF-2 in animal wound models has resulted in improved reepithelialization, collagen content, and wound breaking strength.[25]

Epidermal growth factor (EGF) is secreted by keratinocytes and acts locally through an autocrine function to direct reepithelialization.[26] EGF also stimulates the secretion of fibroblast collagenases that are important in wound remodeling. Whereas topical application of EGF to human skin donor sites accelerated healing in one study,[27] another study showed no difference in healing rates between split thickness skin wounds treated with EGF or silver sulfadiazine.[28]

Vascular endothelial growth factor (VEGF) is primarily released by keratinocytes but also by macrophages and fibroblasts.[29] VEGF is one of the most potent stimulators of angiogenesis and is induced by local hypoxia, high lactate levels, and nitric oxide production.[30,31] Topical administration of VEGF has resulted in increased granulation tissue formation in normal and hypoxic experimental wound models.[32] VEGF is also responsible for increasing vascular permeability at the wound site.

Insulin-like growth factor (IGF) exists as 2 isoforms – IGF-1 and IGF-2 (also known as somatomedins). IGF is primarily produced by hepatocytes and skeletal muscle, but also by wound fibroblasts, neutrophils, and macrophages.[33] IGF stimulates the proliferation of fibroblast and keratinocytes as well as collagen synthesis. IGF is reduced in diabetic and steroid-dependent animals and its administration has improved wound healing in diabetic and steroid-dependent animals.[34]

Early after injury, interleukin (IL)-1 and tumor necrosis factor (TNF)-α are released and chemoattract multiple inflammatory cells and stimulate them to produce additional growth factors and cytokines.[35] IL-8, which has been shown to enhance reepithelialization,[36] is also released secondary to the actions of IL-1.[37] Fibroblast proliferation and angiogenesis are also under the influence of IL-1 and IL-2, respectively.

Hemostasis

Injury to the skin usually results in disruption of the vascular integrity and the extravasation of blood and its products into the site of injury. To stop blood loss, the injured vessels undergo vasospasm and platelets adhere to the injured vessels. After their adherence, platelets are activated and release a host of factors that participate in the wound healing process. Additionally, the injury results in the release of tissue factor by endothelial cells.[38] Exposure of subendothelial collagen and the release of extrinsic tissue factor activate the coagulation system through the intrinsic and extrinsic pathways in an attempt to stop the bleeding by forming a clot.

The coagulation system is composed of a complex enzyme cascade in which the components are activated by proteolysis. The end result of coagulation is the formation of fibrin, which forms the backbone of the clot. Other components of the clot include ECM proteins such as fibronectin, vitronectin, and thrombospondin.

In addition to plugging the defect, the aggregated platelets serve as a surface for formation and activation of the blood clot.[39] This blood clot not only helps stop bleeding and provides a barrier to microbial invasion, but also serves as the provisional matrix for invading cells and as a reservoir of growth factors. Activation of the coagulation system also results in activation of the complement system,[40,41] another plasma proteinase cascade system that generates several chemotactic agents, such as C5-derived monocyte chemotactic factor C5a.[42] The role of the coagulation system in wound healing is further demonstrated by the ability of factor XIII to modulate tissue remodeling and repair by mediating interaction between platelets and endothelial cells.[43] Degranulation of platelet α-granules results in the release of multiple cytokines including PDGF, and TGF-β that stimulate chemotaxis of neutrophils, monocytes, and lymphocytes and enhance their proliferation.[39]

The Inflammatory Phase

Injury to the skin results in the release of multiple inflammatory mediators that initiate the inflammatory response.[35] Substances released from the complement system and platelets results in the chemotaxis of inflammatory cells such as the neutrophils and monocytes.[23] These processes are also enhanced by the release of histamines, bradykinins, and leukotrienes from adjacent mast cells.[44] The adherence and passage of neutrophils into the wound site through the injured blood vessels is mediated through adhesion molecules that are expressed on the endothelial cells, partially in response to TGF-α.[45] The release of mediators such as PDGF, TGF-β, FGF, and EGF by platelets also helps recruit and activate inflammatory cells.

The main function of the infiltrating neutrophils is to engulf and destroy any bacteria, foreign debris, or necrotic tissue in the wound area. The neutrophils also produce angiogenic factors (VEGF, TNF-α, and IL-1) and proteinases that are necessary in degrading the matrix of the wound bed. Whereas most of the neutrophils are shed with the wound eschar over the first few days after injury, the entrance of monocytes that are stimulated by monocyte-specific chemoattractants continues for longer periods. Upon entry to the wound, the monocytes are transformed into macrophages that release a large number and amount of growth factors and cytokines such as PDGF, TGF-α, TGF-β, IGF-1, VEGF, and TNF-α.[46] Thus, macrophages become the predominant leukocyte in the wound by day 3 after injury. Maturation of monocytes into macrophages is regulated by IL-2, TNF-α, and interferon-γ that are secreted by T lymphocytes as well as by PDGF.

The fibrin-rich provisional wound matrix of the resolving clot also has an important role in wound healing and the inflammatory response.[47] It serves as a protein reservoir by binding cytokines and growth factors and amplifies their chemotactic properties by increasing local mediator concentration and directing cellular migration through its scaffold by the specific expression of integrins that are recognized by the various cells in the wound.[48]

Although inflammation is an essential component of wound healing, excessive inflammation can result in impaired healing, such as in chronic, nonhealing ulcers. Persistent accumulation of neutrophils in chronic ulcers results in the release of large amounts of proteolytic enzymes that degrade connective tissue matrix[49] and growth factors.[50] Furthermore, prolonged inflammation resulting in high prostaglandin levels may result in fibroblast proliferation and excessive collagen production.[51,52] Indeed, pharmacologic reduction of the early inflammatory phase by topical application of a cyclooxygenase-2 inhibitor has been shown to reduce scar formation in full-thickness murine wounds.[53]

Reepithelialization

Reepithelialization is one of the earliest and most important stages of wound healing aimed at restoring the barrier function of the skin.[54] With healing by primary intention, in which the divided wound edges are approximated, the process of reepithelialization is completed within 48–72 hours of injury. With healing by secondary intention, this process is more prolonged, requiring dermal reconstitution before being completed. Reepithelialization and epidermal maturation is delayed in the presence of infection.[55]

In order for reepithelialization to proceed, the well-differentiated keratinocytes at the wound edges and within the epidermal appendages of the dermis must detach from their neighboring cells and basement membrane, migrate over the wound defect, and proliferate. Separation of keratinocytes from neighboring cells occurs after breakdown of the hemidesmosomes that connect neighboring cells.[56] Shedding of the keratinocyte cell–cell adhesion molecules is aided by the presence of multiple growth factors such as EGF, TGF-α, TGF-β, granulocyte-macrophage colony-stimulating factor, and FGFs. Changes in the keratinocyte cytoskeleton occur that result in the exposure of lamellipodia and filopodia, which are structures that adhere to surrounding integrins (structures that allow cell–matrix and cell–cell interaction and adhesion), resulting in forward movement of the cells.[57] To facilitate keratinocyte migration, the expression of integrins on the cell surface is also altered.[58,59] Movement of the keratinocytes through the ECM is further aided by the secretion of proteolytic enzymes, the matrix metalloproteinases (MMPs), which are expressed and secreted from the keratinocytes, helping to pave a pathway for the migrating cells.[60–62] Collagen types I and IV, fibronectin, and vitronectin, which are components of the ECM, also facilitate keratinocyte migration.[63–65] Additionally, the MMPs are probably required to detach the keratinocytes from the ECM to allow their forward movement. The direction of cellular migration is further dictated by the presence of chemotactic factors.[57] Cytokines such as TGF-α, TGF-β, IL-1, and IL-8, also have an important role in mediating keratinocyte migration.[66–69]

Although the exact mechanisms responsible for signal transduction in the keratinocytes are still under investigation, several processes have been elucidated. After injury, rapid activation of various transcription factors [such as activated protein (AP)-1] occurs, probably through increased levels of intracellular Ca^{2+} and mitogen activated protein kinase.[70] Increases in the intracellular Ca^{2+} levels probably result from direct stimulation of the injured cells as well as from paracrine signals from surrounding uninjured cells. AP-1 in turn is known to stimulate downstream genes involved in keratinocyte migration and proliferation, such as genes for collagenase, stromelysin, and gelatinase B, that facilitate cell migration through the provisional ECM. AP-1 also regulates genes encoding for cell adhesion molecules such as integrins and laminins that allow migrating cells to attach to and crawl over the provisional matrix. Increased proliferation of basal keratinocytes at the wound edges is also thought to be regulated by AP-1. Other transcription factors, such as nuclear factor-κB also have a role in regulating keratinocyte migration.[71]

As the epidermal integrity is restored, the basement membrane proteins reappear in a highly organized, zipper-like manner.[72] The epidermal cells then revert to their original phenotype and become firmly attached to their underlying dermis.

Angiogenesis

Angiogenesis, or the process of forming new blood vessels, is critical to wound healing, because it allows the delivery of vital cells and nutrients to the wound.[73] Angiogenic factors that have an important role in neovascularization include FGF-1,[74] TGF-β,[75] PDGF-BB,[76] and VEGF.[77,78] Other angiogenic agents include angiogenin,[79] angiopoietin,[80] and human mast cell tryptase.[81] Of the angiogenic factors, VEGF has a central role. Under hypoxic conditions, hypoxia-inducible factor-1 activates the VEGF gene.[82] Furthermore, the beneficial effects of hyperbaric oxygen on wound healing[83] have been attributed to up-regulation of VEGF.[84] Nitric oxide (NO) also has a key role in angiogenesis.[85] Indeed, blockage of endothelial NO synthase that produces NO in endothelial cells results in impaired healing.[86] Many of the actions of VEGF are dependent on NO, and expression of VEGF by keratinocytes is increased by NO.[87]

The process of neovascular formation is tightly regulated by a set of antiangiogenic factors such as endostatin[88] and the thrombospondins.[89] Disruption of parenchymal cells such as keratinocytes and fibroblast results in the release of potent angiogenic factors such as VEGF and FGF-1, respectively. Additionally, macrophages are a major source of angiogenic factors. The release of VEGF is also induced by tissue hypoxia and lactic acid.[90]

One of the critical phases of angiogenesis is the dissolution of the endothelial cell basement membrane. This process is mediated by MMPs (mostly MMP-9 and MMP-2) that normally are not present in the skin.[91] Fibroblasts express MMP-9 at wound sites within 1–4 days of injury resulting in secretion of large amounts of MMP-9 that helps dissolve the basement membrane of vessel walls.[92] Fibroblasts also enhance angiogenesis by secreting a host of mediators (such as VEGF, bFGF, PDGF, IL-1β, and granulocyte colony-stimulating factor) that stimulate endothelial cell proliferation.[93] Fragmentation of the basement membrane allows the sprouting of capillary buds that migrate into the injured area in response to FGF-1 and VEGF. The endothelial cells at the tips of the capillary buds express specific integrins such as $\alpha v\beta 3$[94] that enable attachment to the fibronectin in the basement membrane and the ECM. This integrin also mediates endothelial cell migration.[95] The expression of these integrins is also regulated by the fibrin and fibronectin in the provisional ECM[96] further demonstrating the importance of cell–matrix interactions in the healing process. Endothelial cell proliferation is stimulated by FGF and VEGF whereas the secretion of fibronectin and proteoglycan by these cells is stimulated by TGF-β. Under the influence of factors such as VEGF, FGF, and mast cell tryptase, the capillary sprouts branch and join to form capillary networks allowing the restoration of blood flow. As the ECM matures and is replaced by scar tissue, the endothelial cells undergo apoptosis and degenerate,[97] which explains why the color of the scar fades with time.

The Proliferative Phase

During the proliferative phase of wound healing, there is an increase in the number of fibroblasts and blood vessels in the wounded area. The granular appearance of this tissue is the source of its name. The fibroblasts invade the wound in response to a number of chemoattractants and growth factors.[92] Their entry into the wound is aided by the presence of extracellular proteins within the matrix (such as fibrin, fibronectin) that help guide the motion of the fibroblast. The expression of ECM receptors by fibroblasts is further regulated by the ECM proteins themselves.[98] This complex interaction between cells and the ECM has been coined "dynamic reciprocity."[99] Once in the wound, the fibroblasts begin to produce new matrix in the form of collagen and glycosaminoglycans. With the arrival of fibroblasts, the wound content of collagen, especially collagen type I, increases. Transcription of collagen mRNA is followed by hydroxylation of proline and lysine residues within the polyribosomes of the endoplasmic reticulum.[100] Formation of a triple-helical structure and glycosylation of the collagen is followed by secretion of procollagen into the extracellular space. Further processing of the collagen includes cleavage of the procollagen N and C-terminal peptides and action by the enzyme lysyl oxidase that helps form stable crosslinks.

Wound Remodeling

In response to TGF-β that is secreted during the early and middle phases of wound healing, the fibroblasts differentiate into "myofibroblast-like" cells that express α-smooth muscle actin.[101] This enables the cells to exhibit a contractile force in vivo that results in a reduction in the size of the wound that is critical to wound repair.[102,103]

Wound remodeling is a highly organized process that includes regulation of both the production of new ECM and its degradation by proteases (primarily MMPs). The degradation of the ECM is further controlled by the tissue inhibitors of metalloproteinases that inhibit the action of the proteinases.[104] By 3 weeks after injury, the production of collagen is matched by its degradation and restructuring and remodeling of the ECM is the primary mode of increased wound strength. As the collagen matures, the number of intramolecular and intermolecular crosslinks increases, giving collagen its strength and stability over time.[105] In normal tissue, the collagen fibers form a highly organized basket-weave architecture. In contrast, the collagen fibers in scar tissue are smaller, thinner, and randomly arranged, making scar tissue weaker than normal. In fact, even when fully healed, wounds have a tensile strength that is only 70%–80% of the skin's original strength.[106]

Apoptosis and Wound Healing

Apoptosis, or programmed cell death, is an active physiologic process that is critical to all stages of wound healing.[97,107] This process is distinctly different from necrosis, which represents passive cell death. Apoptosis is highly regulated and results in formation of nuclear and plasma membrane blebs, loss of cell volume, detachment from cellular matrixes, and structural changes in organelles.[108] Resolution of the inflammatory response in the healing wound is critical to wound healing[109] and is regulated in part by TGF-β that induces apoptosis through mitochondrial signaling.[110] Apoptosis is also important in wound maturation and remodeling and is responsible for the removal of the myofibroblasts.[111] Indeed, excessive scarring in keloids may be the result of abnormal control of apoptosis in fibroblasts.[112,113] Integrins at the leading edge of the wound may also have an important role in effecting apoptosis.[114,115] Enhanced epithelial cell apoptosis may have a role in chronic wounds such as gastric ulcers.[116] The ability of growth factors such as PDGF to prevent apoptosis[117] may help explain its beneficial effects in chronic ulcers.[11]

The Therapeutic Role of Growth Factors

Treatment of wounds with exogenous growth factors or cytokines has been shown to accelerate healing, especially in chronic wounds. For example, Steed[13] conducted a clinical trial involving patients with diabetic foot ulcers and demonstrated accelerated healing after treatment with recombinant PDFG-BB. Similar results were demonstrated by Robson et al.[11] for pressure ulcers. Other growth factors that have resulted in accelerated healing include bFGF with pressure ulcers, KGF-2 with venous stasis ulcers, and TGF-β1 for diabetic foot ulcers.[118] Unfortunately, clinical experience with these growth factors has been very disappointing. One possible explanation for the lack of dramatic clinical benefit using these agents is the presence of bacteria and bacterial proteases that degrade both the growth factors and their receptors.[6] Several methods that may overcome the local degradation of growth factors include sustained release of these agents from a delivery system or introduction of genetic material that results in transient local production of cytokines. Carboxymethylcellulose suspensions improve the handling and delivery of growth factors to open wounds, but are cumbersome and unreliable. Fibrin-based carriers can improve growth factor delivery, but act as mechanical barriers to wound healing. Delayed-release polymers aid in the delivery and handling of growth factors.

Priming of wounds with growth factors has been shown to reduce the lag period required prior to increased levels of fibroproliferative growth factors such as TGF-β, thus shifting the wound healing trajectory in a leftward direction. Recently, Robson et al.[119] demonstrated reduced rates of incisional hernias in rodents pretreated with TGF-β2, bFGF, and IL-1β. Thus, priming of acute wound sites with growth factors before injury can result in earlier activation of the repair process. This method may prove to be useful in patients undergoing repair of abdominal incisions for which the rates of hernia formation are especially high.

The development of gene therapy offers the potential to enhance or inhibit the gene expression of specific cytokines and extracellular molecules.[120] Because gene therapy generally results in only transient gene expression, it is especially well suited for wound healing that is temporary in itself.

Fetal Wound Healing

During the early phases of gestation, the fetus has the extraordinary capacity to heal without scarring.[121] Increasing understanding of the differences between fetal and adult wound healing that are responsible for scarless healing in the fetus is likely to result in knowledge that may ultimately lead to the development of novel therapies aimed at reduced scarring.

In the fetus, reepithelialization occurs by the action of actin fibers within the epidermal cells that draws the wound edges together similar to the function of a purse string.[122] In contrast, epidermal cells in the adult resurface the wound by crawling across it.

Several notable differences between fetal and adult wound healing may be responsible for the reduced tendency to form scars. First, lack of proinflammatory signals may limit the amount of inflammation during the early phases of healing.[123] The reduction in inflammation in turn reduces the stimulus for fibroblast proliferation and collagen production. Second, fetal fibroblasts have the capacity to produce collagen in a more rapid and orderly manner than in adults. Also, more collagen type III than type I is produced in the fetus.[124] Because type III collagen fibers are smaller and finer than type I fibers, the higher proportion of type III fibers in the fetus may result in a more reticular pattern of fiber distribution. Furthermore, the highly hydroscopic, hyaluronic acid-rich environment characteristic of the fetus may help proliferating cells avoid inhibitory signals.[125] Third, reduced expression of TGF-β1 and increased expression of TGF-β3 reduce the amount of scar tissue formation.[126] Other growth factors, such as PDGF and FGF-2 also differ between the fetus and the adult.[127] Fourth, in the fetus, there is an altered balance between the MMPs and their inhibitors that favors rapid turnover of the ECM that is required for scarless healing.[128] Finally, there is now evidence that differences in gene expression and cell signaling in the fetus may also be responsible for the reduced tendency for scarring.[129]

Tissue Engineering and Skin Biology

The genesis of tissue engineered products as skin substitutes began more than 20 years ago with improved culture methods for the growth keratinocytes, and the production of natural and synthetic matrices used either as delivery systems for cells or cell products. The goal is the recapitulation of normal skin and normal skin function. Any epidermal replacement must restrict transepidermal water loss, limit bodily damage induced by environmental chemical and physical insults, and minimize microbial load. Any dermal replacement must provide epidermal support, neovascularization, and functional pliability.

Normal epidermis turns over once a month during which time cells from the outermost layer are sloughed. This necessitates a lifelong process of self-renewal fueled presumably by keratinocyte stem cells, which by definition are capable of both self-maintenance and of production of differentiated cells.[130] We might therefore view our normal physiologic state as one of subclinical wound healing in which stem cells are accessed to support tissue maintenance. To obtain the requisite cell numbers while limiting the accumulation of replicative errors in the stem cell population, stem cells give rise to progeny, transit amplifying cells, that undergo rapid cell division and then terminally differentiate.[131-137]

Access to populations of keratinocytes that can be grown and expanded in vitro, and still serve as stem cells subsequent to transplant is a requirement for producing epidermal skin substitutes. This is independent of whether the cultures are to be used as epidermal replacements, biologic dressings, or genetically modified epithelia that deliver therapeutically required factors. It has therefore been of interest to isolate and identify stem cell populations. To date, the identity and genetic signature of epidermal stem cells have remained elusive. It is generally agreed that they have a high nucleus/cytoplasmic ratio and can be enriched by density gradient centrifugation or by their rapid adherence to a variety of ECMs.[138-140] They have been reported to either express high levels of integrin β1[140] or alternatively to express high levels of integrin α6 coupled with low levels of transferrin receptors.[141] Among other markers, stem cells have been associated with localized keratin 19 expression,[142,143] reduced connexin 43 expression with decreased gap junction function[144] (see, however, Bjerknes et al.[145]), and, under certain circumstances, associated with keratin 15 expression.[146] The actual complexity of the genetic signature is undoubtedly greater, as has been indicated by the detection of clusters of genes correlating stem cell functions and their modulation by environmental cues.[147] The location of the stem cell population has also been a matter of contention. Putative stem cell populations have been identified in the bulge of the pilosebaceous unit,[148] in the region below the bulge,[149] both in the follicular and interfollicular epidermis,[150] and in the eccrine duct.[151,152] Whereas these differences may simply distinguish differences in the endpoint assays or model systems used, they may reflect the inherent plasticity of the keratinocyte. In the context of wound healing, it is fortunate that follicular keratinocytes can be accessed for reepithelialization,[153] that interfollicular keratinocytes can give rise to follicular and sebaceous gland elements,[154-157] and that transit amplifying cells can exhibit stem cell functions.[137,156,157]

Epidermal Substitutes: Delivering Autologous Epithelial Tissue

The extensive capacity for keratinocyte in vivo proliferation predicts that, with proper signals, the proliferative potential of keratinocytes might be accessed in vitro. The first report validating this prediction appeared in the mid-1970s. In this early work, Rheinwald and Green[158] described a technique using serum-containing medium together with lethally irradiated 3T3 cells to serially cultivate human keratinocytes. With continued growth, individual keratinocytes produce colonies that fuse (confluence) and form a multilayered epithelium, containing differentiated cell layers suprabasal to a proliferative cell layer adherent to the surface of the culture dish; the irradiated 3T3 cells are displaced and removed during successive feedings. The discovery that incubation of confluent keratinocyte cultures with Dispase II results in detachment of an intact epithelial tissue from the surface of the culture vessel[159] promoted the use of epithelial sheets for treatment of burn injury.[160,161] By 1988, cultured epithelial autografts (CEA) were being commercialized with indications for deep partial-thickness injury, full-thickness burn injury, and congenital nevi.

The long-term persistence of grafted CEA indicative of functional stem cell transfer has been demonstrated in two types of studies. The first followed patients who had received CEA comprising plantar-derived keratinocytes grafted onto nonpalmoplantar surfaces. The grafted areas were found to contain cells with plantar keratinocyte specific markers[162,163]; similar graft maintenance was later demonstrated using human xenografts on athymic mice.[164] In the second type of study, telomere length was compared in keratinocytes isolated from engrafted CEA with those isolated from engrafted split-thickness skin grafts (STSG). It was found that the CEA contained cells with shortened telomeres.[165] Although these observations are consistent with CEA persistence, some concern is raised as to the remaining lifespan of the engrafted CEA. However, whereas the telomere length in the CEA was typical of aged epidermal keratinocytes, this cell type has an extraordinary proliferative potential that extends beyond the requirements for lifelong tissue maintenance. The clinical significance of these findings is not yet known.

Despite the demonstrated lifesaving potential of CEA and the relatively high percentage of engraftment (60%–65%) reported in a large multicenter and a large single center study,[166,167] and although CEA may be the preferred therapeutic option in certain clinical settings, three factors place this product as an adjunct therapy rather than as a replacement for split-thickness grafting. First, reports from the late 1980s and through the late 1990s document large variations in the percentage engraftment ("take").[168] The variations were observed even in studies in which wound beds were prepared with de-epidermized dermis to promote engraftment and that excluded patients whose wounds contained excessive microbial loads.[169-172] Second, during the first 2 weeks posttransplant, the grafts are delicate and particularly sensitive to loss because of infection. Lastly, using the suggested 2-cm^2 skin biopsies, the time between biopsy and graft production is 14–21 days, dependent on donor and surface area to be covered. Although larger biopsies can be used to decrease the production time, the first cell expansion requires 7–10 days. Obviously, with early excision, more rapid coverage is preferable. In an effort to speed CEA production, consideration has been given to the use of allogeneic-syngeneic cultures.[173] However, there have not been multicenter trials to demonstrate safety and efficacy. CEA are currently marketed as Epicel™ (Genzyme Biosurgery) and can be used in conjunction with de-epidermized cadaveric skin, with Alloderm® and with Integra® (see below).

Epidermal Substitutes: Delivery of Autologous Epithelia Before Tissue Formation

To shorten the time between biopsy and transplantation of autologous epithelia, two additional approaches have been evaluated. One utilizes keratinocytes grown on matrices that do not require enzymatic release from the culture surface to allow culture transplant before the keratinocyte confluence. Autologous keratinocytes that have been grown on perforated matrices of benzyl esterified hyaluronic acid, currently marketed as Laserskin™ (Fidia Advanced Biopolymers), have been used to heal diabetic foot ulcers,[174] and those grown on fibrin glue have been used to successfully treat deep partial and full-thickness burn injuries.[175–177] Histologically normal epidermis has been shown to develop in situ.

A second approach utilizes keratinocyte cell suspensions delivered directly to the wound bed. Keratinocytes delivered within a fibrin spray have been shown to promote wound closure of deep partial and full-thickness burns, and of chronic wounds; the fibrin helps secure even placement of the keratinocytes.[178–182] The requirement for fibrin is therefore dependent on the architecture of the wound.[183,184] The preclinical investigations of these alternative approaches to delivering autologous keratinocytes have been reviewed elsewhere.[185] The keratinocyte spray technology is being commercialized for human use pending clinical trials and regulatory approvals (ReCell®, CellSpray®, CellSpray®XP; see also Grant et al.[186]

Epidermal Dressings: Use of Cultured Epithelial Allografts

Because keratinocytes can also serve as a source of growth factors and specific matrix molecules, cultured epithelial allografts (CEAllo) have been evaluated for their ability to promote the healing of donor sites, leg ulcers, and partial-thickness burn wounds. The preparation of grafts with allogeneic material avoids the delays inherent in autologous graft production, whereas serial cultivation attenuates the expression of the MHC class I and II antigens in keratinocytes.[187,188] Typically, allogeneic keratinocytes are replaced rather than rejected.[189–196] Using CEAllo, the time required for reepithelialization of donor sites was reduced 18%–52% in studies described for both pediatric and geriatric burns. Healing times for the control groups ranged from 9.2 to 15.3 days, whereas healing times in the treatment groups ranged from 6.2 to 8.4 days.[197–201] Comparative evaluations between Op-site and CEAllo have alternatively demonstrated significant improvement with CEAllo or no difference.[202,203]

Similar to the early reports using autologous keratinocytes,[204] results on the treatment of venous ulcers and diabetic leg ulcers with allogeneic keratinocytes have shown promise.[205] Complete reepithelialization has been noted in some patients,[206,207] and most patients have experienced reductions in wound size because of healing from the indolent edges.[208–215] Efficacy has been reported to be independent of whether CEAllo have been prepared immediately before use or have been cryopreserved,[210–212] frozen,[213,214] or lyophilized.[215] Freshly prepared and banked CEAllo have also shown promise for treatment of partial-thickness burn injury presumably by promoting reepithelialization from the wound edges and remaining epidermal appendages. Time to wound closure was reduced by 18%–60%.[216–220] Despite these successes, CEAllo are not yet commercially available.

Dermal Substitutes: Acellular Dermal Matrices

Acellular dermal substitutes have been evaluated for their ability to jump start neodermis formation, limit wound contracture associated with deep dermal injuries, and to provide a matrix compatible with reepithelialization and neovascularization.[221] Currently, there are two types of acellular materials available that fulfill at least some of these requirements. The first material, de-epidermized dermis, is structurally identical to dermis but requires cellular repopulation. Although a variety of methods are available to produce the material, an "off-the shelf" form, sold as Alloderm®, is available. The product is decellularized to limit antigenicity and subsequently preserved by freeze-drying. It can be used in conjunction with either STSG or CEA. It is often meshed to allow release of exudates and development of granulation tissue within the interstices. De-epidermized dermis offers the advantage of being able to support engraftment of thin rather than thick STSG. This is particularly useful for repair of extensive full-thickness burn injuries that may require repeated harvesting of donor sites. In addition, the presence of an intact, organized basement membrane predicts better adhesion of CEA with rapid deposition of laminin 5 and hemidesmosome formation.[222,223] Successful use of the commercial product has been reported for patients with burn injuries and with cutis aplasia.[224–227] The second type of dermal substitute comprises dermal matrix molecules, but extensive remodeling is required to achieve a normal dermal structure. The material, sold as Integra®, is composed of collagen-chondroitin-6-sulfate covered by a nonporous protective silastic layer.[228-231] The pore size of the matrix is designed to be sufficient to allow fibroblast and endothelial cell migration to occur, and for the product to be remodeled by invading host cells.[232] Neodermis is formed in about 3 weeks, at which time the silastic layer readily detaches. As with de-epidermized dermis, to achieve permanent wound closure, the treated area must be grafted with either a thin STSG or with CEA. In multicenter clinical trials with more than 200 burn patients, it was found that Integra® was both safe and effective, and that the neodermis formed within 2–3 weeks of application was capable of supporting the "take" of STSG.[233,234]

Dermal Substitutes: Fibroblast-Containing Matrices

Dermal matrices have also been generated that incorporate dermal fibroblasts as a source of cytokines, growth factors, and matrix molecules all of which can reciprocally modulate other skin cells and which can potentially augment tissue repair.[235] The results of clinical evaluations of products containing metabolically viable and nonviable fibroblasts are consistent with critical differences between the needs of acute wounds and chronic ulcers. Thus, distinct fibroblast-containing products are indicated for different wound types. For example, Transcyte® is indicated for the treatment of deep partial-thickness burns and excisional wounds, but not for venous ulcers. This product is a temporary dressing that contains human neonatal fibroblasts cultured on a bovine collagen-coated nylon mesh bonded to silicone. During production, the fibroblasts secrete new matrix molecules and cytokines; cell viability is lost during a subsequent freezing process. It is assumed that fibroblast-derived factors promote the observed healing of partial-thickness burn injuries and excisional wounds.[236-240] As a temporary dressing, it differs from the acellular dermal products that become engrafted and are modified by host cells. A second product produced by the same manufacturers, Dermagraft®, contains viable fibroblasts on a bioabsorbable fiber. It is indicated for use on chronic ulcers, and has been found effective when used in combination with standard of care for diabetic wounds.[241,242]

Because chronic wounds may have aberrations in both the resident matrix and cellularity, fibroblast viability and continued cytokine production may be significant factors in clinical outcome.[243,244]

Composite Skin Substitutes and Skin Replacements

In 1983, Eugene Bell and colleagues[245] described construction of a human "living skin equivalent" (LSE) comprising a fibroblast-contracted collagen gel overlaid with keratinocytes. Cultures require a number of different media formulations and placement of the construct at the air–liquid interface for final epithelial maturation. The system has been optimized for neonatal keratinocytes and fibroblasts and has been subject to multiple improvements.[246-248] Although it resembles skin having dermal and epidermal components, it is allogeneic and is not used as a permanent wound covering but as a biologic dressing that promotes wound healing.[249] To date, "LSE" has been used effectively as treatment for chronic ulcers[250-253] and is marketed under the name of Apligraf® (formerly called Grafskin®) for that purpose. A second allogeneic product, OrCel®, uses a collagen sponge with keratinocytes and fibroblasts seeded on opposite faces. Although initially used for the treatment of mitten formation in patients with epidermolysis bullosa, it is also used on donor sites.[254]

Use of autologous fibroblasts and keratinocytes together with capillary-forming endothelial cells has been proposed.[255] Such changes could potentially transform the LSE from a biologic dressing into a skin substitute. Other promising modifications include a new skin equivalent combining de-epidermized dermis with a fibroblast-populated collagen matrix as a support for epidermal production.[256]

An autologous composite skin substitute, composed of a stratified epithelium produced on a fibroblast-containing matrix of collagen and glycosaminoglycan (GAG), was first described in the late 1980s. It has demonstrated sufficient "take" to help reduce requirements for harvesting of donor skin.[257,258] Although it appears to provide an epidermal replacement, de novo dermal formation is required because the construct's matrix is lost within 2 weeks of transplant.[249] How this autologous skin substitute will compare to others awaits clinical trial.

Future Perspectives

New tissue engineering materials and advances in stem cell biology will undoubtedly result in an even greater choice of biologic and nonbiologic skin substitutes. The best treatment modality will have to be determined by comparative evaluations of available products. Although increasing infrastructure costs can limit the number of clinical trials used to make such determinations, the newer and highly sensitive technologies for assessing wound status may offset these costs and lead to improved patient care. Our apologies are given to those investigators whose novel approaches or product variations might not have been mentioned.

Acknowledgment

The authors thank Abha Kochhar for her assistance in the preparation of the manuscript.

References

1. Singer AJ, Thode HC Jr. National epidemiology of lacerations [abstract]. Ann Emerg Med 2002;40:S41.
2. US Markets for Current Emerging Wound Closure Technologies 2001. Tustin, CA: MedTech Insight; August 2002.
3. Brigham PA, McLoughlin E. Burn incidence and medical care use in the United States: estimate, trends, and data sources. J Burn Care Rehabil 1996;17:95–107.
4. US Markets for Wound Management Products. Irvine, CA: Medical Data International; August 1997.
5. Singer AJ, Clark AF. Cutaneous wound healing. N Engl J Med 1999;341:738–746.
6. Cross KJ, Mustoe TA. Growth factors in wound healing. Surg Clin North Am 2003;83:531–545.
7. Friesel RE, Maciag T. Molecular mechanisms of angiogenesis: fibroblast growth factor signal transduction. FASEB J 1995;9:919–925.
8. Schiller M, Javelaud D, Mauviel A. TGF-β-induced SMAD signaling and gene regulation: consequences for extracellular matrix remodeling and wound healing. J Dermatol Sci 2004;35:83–92.
9. Qiu P, Feng XH, Li L. Interaction of Smad3 and SRF-associated complex mediates TGF-β1 signals to regulate SM22 transcription during myofibroblast differentiation. J Mol Cell Cardiol 2003;35:1407–1420.
10. Pierce GF, Mustoe TA, Altrock BW, et al. Role of platelet-derived growth factor in wound healing. J Cell Biochem 1991;45:319–326.
11. Robson MC, Phillips LG, Thomason A, et al. Platelet-derived growth factor BB for the treatment of chronic pressure ulcers. Lancet 1992;339:23–25.
12. Mustoe TA, Cutler NR, Allman RM, et al. A phase II study to evaluate recombinant platelet-derived growth factor-BB in the treatment of stage 3 and 4 pressure ulcers. Arch Surg 1994;129:213–219.
13. Steed DL. Clinical evaluation of recombinant human platelet-derived growth factor for the treatment of lower extremity diabetic ulcer. Diabetic Ulcer Group. J Vasc Surg 1995;21:71–81.
14. Shah M, Rorison P, Ferguson MWJ. The role of transforming growth factors-beta in cutaneous scarring. In: Garg HG, Longaker MT, eds. Scarless Wound Healing. New York: Marcel Dekker; 2000:213–326.
15. Wang R, Ghahary A, Shen Q, et al. Hypertrophic scar tissues and fibroblast produce more transforming growth factor-beta1 mRNA and protein than normal skin and cells. Wound Rep Reg 2000;8:128–137.
16. Chin GS, Liu W, Peled Z, et al. Differential expression of transforming growth factor-beta receptors I and II and activation of Smad 3 in keloids fibroblasts. Plast Reconstr Surg 2001;108:423–429.
17. Shah M, Foreman DM, Ferguson MW. Control of scarring in adult wounds by neutralizing antibody to transforming growth factor beta. Lancet 1992;339:213–214.
18. Shah M, Foreman DM, Ferguson MWJ. Neutralisation of TGF-β1 and TGF-β2 or exogenous addition of TGF-β3 to cutaneous rat wounds reduces scarring. J Cell Sci 1995;108:985–1002.
19. Ornitz DM, Itoh N. Fibroblast growth factors. Genome Biol 2001;2:1–12.
20. Werner S. Keratinocyte growth factor: a unique player in epithelial repair process. Cytokine Growth Factor Rev 1998;2:153–165.
21. Beyer TA, Werner S, Dickson C, et al. Fibroblast growth factor 22 and its potential role during skin development and repair. Exp Cell Res 2003;287:228–236.
22. Bernardini G, Ribatti D, Spinetti G, et al. Analysis of the role of chemokines in angiogenesis. J Immunol Methods 2003;273:83–101.
23. Werner S, Grose R. Regulation of wound healing by growth factors and cytokines. Physiol Rev 2002;83:835–870.
24. Xia YP, Zhao Y, Marcus J, et al. Effects of keratinocyte growth factor-2 (KGF-2) on wound healing in an ischaemia-impaired rabbit ear model and on scar formation. J Pathol 1999;188:431–438.
25. Werner S, Smola H, Liao X, et al. The function of KGF in morphogenesis of epithelium and reepithelialization of wounds. Science 1994;266:819–822.
26. Nanney LB, King LE Jr. Epidermal growth factor and transforming growth factor-α. In: Clark RAF, ed. The Molecular and Cellular Biology of Wound Repair. 2nd ed. New York: Plenum Press; 1996:427–474.
27. Brown GL, Nanney LB, Griffen J, et al. Enhancement of wound healing by topical treatment with epidermal growth factor. N Engl J Med 1989;321:76–79.
28. Cohen KI, Crossland MC, Garrett A, et al. Topical application of epidermal growth factor onto partial-thickness wounds in human volunteers does not enhance reepithelialization. Plast Reconstr Surg 1999;96:251–254.
29. Brown DL, Yeo KT, Berse B, et al. Expression of vascular permeability factor (vascular endothelial growth

29. factor) by epidermal keratinocytes during wound healing. J Exp Med 1995;176:1375–1379.
30. Shweiki D, Itin A, Soffer D, et al. Vascular endothelial growth factor induced by hypoxia-initiated angiogenesis. Nature 1992;359:843–845.
31. Corral CJ, Siddiqui A, Wu L, et al. Vascular endothelial growth factor is more important than basic fibroblast growth factor during ischemic wound healing. Arch Surg 1999;134:200–205.
32. Galiano RD, Tepper O, Pelo CR, et al. Topical vascular endothelial growth factor accelerates diabetic wound healing through increased angiogenesis and by mobilizing and recruiting bone marrow-derived cells. Am J Pathol 2004;164:1935–1947.
33. Edmondson SR, Thumiger SP, Werther GA, et al. Epidermal homeostasis: the role of growth hormone and insulin-like growth factor systems. Endocr Rev 2003;24:737–764.
34. Nakamura M, Kawahara M, Morishige N, et al. Promotion of corneal epithelial wound healing in diabetic rats by the combination of a substance P-derived peptide (FLGM-NH2) and insulin-like growth factor-1. Diabetologia 2003;46:839–842.
35. Henry G, Garner WL. Inflammatory mediators in wound healing. Surg Clin North Am 2003;83:483–507.
36. Rennekampff HO, Hansbrough JF, Kiessig V, et al. Bioactive interleukin-8 is expressed in wounds and enhances wound healing. J Surg Res 2000;93:41–54.
37. Gillitzer R, Goebler M. Chemokines in cutaneous wound healing. J Leukoc Biol 2001;69:513–521.
38. Slupsky JR, Kalbas M, Willuweit A, et al. Activated platelets induce tissue factor expression on human umbilical vein endothelial cells by ligation of CD40. Thromb Hemost 1998;80:1008–1014.
39. Heldin C-H, Westmark B. Role of platelet derived growth factor in vivo. In: Clark RAF, ed. The Molecular and Cellular Biology of Wound Repair. 2nd ed. New York: Plenum Press; 1996:249–273.
40. Okamoto M, Yamamoto T, Matsubara S, et al. Factor XIII-dependent generation of 5th complement component (C5)-derived monocyte chemotactic factor coinciding with plasma clotting. Biochim Biophys Acta 1992;1138:53–61.
41. Ghebrehiwet B, Silverberg M, Kaplan AP. Activation of the classical compliment pathway by Hageman factor fragment. J Exp Med 1981;153:665–667.
42. Piccolo MT, Wang Y, Verbrugge S, et al. Role of chemotactic factors in neutrophil activation after thermal injury in rats. Inflammation 1999;23:371–385.
43. Dardik R, Shenkman B, Tamarin I, et al. Factor XIII mediates adhesion of platelets to endothelial cells through alpha(v)beta(3) and glycoprotein IIb/IIIa integrins. Thromb Res 2002;105:317–323.
44. Artuc M, Hermes B, Steckelings UM, et al. Mast cells and their mediators in cutaneous wound healing: active participants or innocent bystanders? Exp Dermatol 1999;8:1–16.
45. Arturson G. Pathophysiology of the burn wound and pharmacological treatment. The Rudi Hermans Lecture, 1995. Burns 1996;22:255–274.
46. Riches DWH. Macrophage involvement in wound repair, remodeling and fibrosis. In: Clark RAF, ed. The Molecular and Cellular Biology of Wound Repair. 2nd ed. New York: Plenum Press; 1996:95–141.
47. Bosman FT, Stamenkovic I. Preface to extracellular matrix and disease. J Pathol 2003;200:421–422.
48. Train KT, Giffith L, Wells A. Extracellular matrix signaling through growth factor receptors during wound healing. Wound Rep Reg 2004;12:262–268.
49. Nwomeh BC, Liang HG, Diegelmann RF, et al. Dynamics of the matrix metalloproteinases MMP-1 and MMP-8 in acute open dermal wounds. Wound Rep Reg 1998;6:127–134.
50. Yager DR, Zhang LY, Liang XH, et al. Wound fluids from human pressure ulcers contain elevated matrix metalloproteinase level and activity compared to surgical wound fluids. J Invest Dermatol 1996;107:743–748.
51. Talwar M, Moyana TN, Bharadwaj B, et al. The effect of a synthetic analogue of prostaglandin E2 on wound healing in rats. Ann Clin Lab Sci 1996;26:451–457.
52. Lupulescu A. Effects of prostaglandins on protein, RNA, DNA, and collagen synthesis in experimental wounds. Prostaglandins 1975;10:573–579.
53. Wilgus TA, Vodovotz Y, Vittadini E, et al. Reduction of scar formation in full-thickness wounds with topical celecoxib treatment. Wound Rep Reg 2003;11:25–34.
54. Coulombe PA. Towards a molecular definition of keratinocyte activation after acute injury to stratified epithelia. Biochem Biophys Res Commun 1997;236:231–238.
55. Singer AJ, McClain SA. Persistent wound infection delays epidermal maturation and increases scarring in thermal burns. Wound Rep Reg 2002;10:372–377.
56. Borradori L, Sonnenberg A. Structure and function of hemidesmosomes: more than simple adhesion molecules. J Invest Dermatol 1999;112:411–418.
57. Garrett B. The proliferation and movement of cells during re-epithelialisation. J Wound Care 1997;6:174–177.
58. Larjava H, Salo T, Haapasalmi K, et al. Expression of integrins and basement membrane components by wound keratinocytes. J Clin Invest 1993;92:1425–1435.
59. Clark RAF, Ashcroft GC, Spencer MJ, et al. Re-epithelialization of normal human excisional wounds is associated with a switch from $\alpha v \beta 5$ to $\alpha v \beta 6$ integrins. Br J Dermatol 1996;135:46–51.
60. Agren MS. Matrix metalloproteinases (MMPs) are required for re-epithelialization of cutaneous wounds. Arch Dermatol Res 1999;291:583–590.
61. Piltcher BK, Wand M, Qin XG, et al. Role of matrix metalloproteinases and their inhibition in cutaneous wound healing and allergic hypersensitivity. Ann NY Acad Sci 1999;878:12–24.
62. Parks WC. Matrix metalloproteinases in repair. Wound Rep Reg 1997;7:423–432.
63. O'Keefe EJ, Payne RE Jr, Russel N, et al. Spreading and enhanced motility of human keratinocytes on fibronectin. J Invest Dermatol 1985;85:125–130.
64. Kim JP, Zhang K, Chen JD, et al. Vitronectin-driven human keratinocytes locomotion is mediated by the alpha v beta 5 integrin receptor. J Biol Chem 1994;269:26926–26932.
65. Brown C, Stenn KS, Falk RJ, et al. Vitronectin: effects on keratinocytes motility and inhibition of collagen induced motility. J Invest Dermatol 1991;96:724–728.
66. Cha D, O'Brien P, O'Toole EA, et al. Enhanced modulation of keratinocyte motility by transforming growth factor alpha (TGF-α) relative to epidermal growth factor. J Invest Dermatol 1996;106:590–597.

67. Garlick JA. Effect of TGF-β1 on re-epithelialization of human keratinocytes in-vitro: an organotypic model. J Invest Dermatol 1994;103:554–559.
68. Chen JD, Lapiere JC, Saunder DN, et al. Interleukin-1 alpha stimulates keratinocyte migration through an epidermal growth factor/transforming growth factor-alpha-independent pathway. J Invest Dermatol 1995;104:729–733.
69. Michel G, Kemeny L, Peter RU, et al. Interleukin-8-receptor mediated chemotaxis of normal human epidermal cells. FEBS Lett 1992;305:241–243.
70. Yates S, Rayner TE. Transcription factor activation in response to cutaneous injury: role of AP-1 in reepithelialization. Wound Rep Reg 2002;10:5–15.
71. Takao J, Yudat T, Das A, et al. Expression of NF-kappaB in epidermis and the relationship between NF-kappaB activation and inhibition of keratinocyte growth. Br J Dermatol 2003;148:680–688.
72. Clark RAF, Lanigan JM, DellaPelle P, et al. Fibronectin and fibrin provide a provisional matrix for epidermal cell migration during wound reepithelialization. J Invest Dermatol 1982;79:264–269.
73. Tonnesen MG, Feng X, Clark RAF. Angiogenesis in wound healing. J Invest Dermatol Symp Proc 2000;5:40–46.
74. Folkman J, Klagsbrun M. Angiogenic factors. Science 1987;235:442–448.
75. Yang EY, Moses HL. Transforming growth factor-β1-induced changes in cell migration, proliferation, and angiogenesis in chicken chorioallantoic membrane. J Cell Biol 1990;111:731–741.
76. Battegay EF, Rupp J, Iruela-Arispe L, et al. PDGF-BB modulates endothelial proliferation and angiogenesis in vitro via PDGF β-receptors. J Cell Biol 1994;125:917–928.
77. Keck PJ, Hauser SD, Krivi G, et al. Vascular permeability factor, an endothelial cell mitogen related to PDGF. Science 1989;246:1309–1313.
78. Dvorak HF, Brown LF, Detmar M, et al. Vascular permeability factor/vascular endothelial growth factor: microvascular permeability and angiogenesis. Am J Pathol 1995;146:1029–1039.
79. Vallee BL, Riordan JF. Organogenesis and angiogenin. Cell Mol Life Sci 1997;53:803–815.
80. Suri C, Jones PF, Patan S, et al. Requisite role of angiopoietin-1, a ligand for the TIE2 receptor, during embryonic angiogenesis. Cell 1996;87:1171–1180.
81. Blair RJ, Meng H, Marchese MJ, et al. Human mast cells stimulate vascular tube formation. Tryptase is a novel, potent angiogenic factor. J Clin Invest 1997;99:2691–2700.
82. Forsythe JA, Jiang BH, Iyer NV, et al. Activation of vascular endothelial growth factor gene transcription by hypoxia inducible factor 1. Mol Cell Biol 1996;16:4609–4613.
83. Tandara AA, Mustoe TA. Oxygen in wound healing: more than a nutrient. World J Surg 2004;28: 294–300.
84. Sheikh AY, Gibson JJ, Rollins MD, et al. Effect of hyperoxia on vascular endothelial growth factor levels in a wound model. Arch Surg 2000;135:1293–1297.
85. Schwentker A, Biliar TR. Nitric oxide and wound repair. Surg Clin North Am 2003;83:521–530.
86. Konturek SJ, Brzozwski T, Majka J, et al. Inhibition of nitric oxide synthase delays healing of chronic gastric ulcers. Eur J Pharmacol 1993;239:215–217.
87. Frank S, Stallmeyer B, Kampfer H, et al. Nitric oxide triggers enhanced induction of vascular endothelial growth factor expression in cultured keratinocytes (HaCaT) during cutaneous wound repair. FASEB J 1999;13:2002–2014.
88. O'Reilly MS, Boehm T, Shing T, et al. Endostatin: an endogenous inhibitor of angiogenesis and tumor growth. Cell 1997;88:277–285.
89. Adams JC, Lawler J. The thrombospondins. Int J Biochem Cell Biol 2004;36:961–968.
90. Trabold O, Wagner S, Wicke C, et al. Lactate and oxygen constitute a fundamental regulatory mechanism in wound healing. Wound Rep Reg 2003;11:504–509.
91. Agren MS. Gelatinase activity during wound healing. Br J Dermatol 1994;131:634–640.
92. Metz CN. Fibrocytes: a unique cell population in wound healing. Cell Mol Life Sci 2003;60:1342–1350.
93. Hartlapp I, Abe R, Saeed R, et al. Fibrocytes induce an angiogenic phenotype in cultured endothelial cells and promote angiogenesis in vivo. FASEB J 2001; 15:2215–2224.
94. Cheresh DA. Human endothelial cells synthesize and express an Arg-Gly-Asp-directed adhesion receptor involved in attachment to fibrinogen and von Willebrand factor. Proc Natl Acad Sci USA 1987;84: 6471–6475.
95. Leavesly DI, Schwartz MA, Rosenfeld M, et al. Integrin β-1 and β-3 mediated endothelial cell migration is triggered through distinct signaling mechanisms. J Cell Biol 1993;121:163–170.
96. Feng X, Clarg RAF, Galanakis D, et al. Fibrin and collagen differentially regulate human dermal vascular endothelial cell integrins: stabilization of $\alpha v\beta 3$ mRNA by fibrin. J Invest Dermatol 1999;113:913–919.
97. Greenhalgh DG. The role of apoptosis in wound healing. Int J Biochem Cell Biol 1998;30:1019–1030.
98. Xu J, Clark RAF. Extracellular matrix alters PDGF regulation of fibroblast integrins. J Cell Biol 1996;132: 239–249.
99. Bissell MJ, Hall HG, Parry G. How does the extracellular matrix direct gene expression? J Theor Biol 1982;99:31–68.
100. Peterofsky B. Ascorbate requirement for hydroxylation and secretion of procollagen: relationship to inhibition of collagen synthesis in scurvy. Am J Clin Nutr 1991;54:1135S.
101. Arora PD, McCulloch CA. Dependence of collagen remodeling on alpha-smooth muscle actin expression by fibroblast. J Cell Physiol 1994;159:161–175.
102. Hinz B, Celetta G, Tomasek JJ, et al. Alpha-smooth muscle actin expression upregulates fibroblast contractile activity. Mol Biol Cell 2001;12:2730–2741.
103. Hinz B, Gabbiani G. Cell-matrix and cell-cell contacts of myofibroblasts: role in connective tissue remodeling. Thromb Haemost 2003;90:993–1002.
104. Lambert E, Dasse E, Hayne B, et al. TIMPs as multifactorial proteins. Crit Rev Oncol Hematol 2004;49: 187–198.
105. Hornstra IK, Birge S, Starcher B, et al. Lysl oxidase is required for vascular and diaphragmatic development in mice. J Biol Chem 2003;278:14387–14393.
106. Levenson SM, Geever EF, Crowley LV, et al. The healing of rat skin wounds. Ann Surg 1965;161:293–308.
107. Gastman BR, Futrell JW, Manders EK. Apoptosis and plastic surgery. Plast Reconstr Surg 2003;111:1481–1496.

108. Maruyama W, Irie S, Sato TA. Morphological changes in the nucleus and actin cytoskeleton in the process of Fas-induced apoptosis in Jurkat T cells. Histochem J 2000;32:495–503.
109. Edwards M, Jones D. Programmed cell death in human cutaneous wounds. J Cutan Pathol 2001;28:151–155.
110. Chipuk J, Bhat M, Hsing AY, et al. Bcl-xL blocks transforming growth factor beta 1-induced apoptosis by inhibiting cytochrome c release and not by directly antagonizing Apaf-1-dependent caspase activation in prostate epithelial cells. J Biol Chem 2001;276:26614–26621.
111. Desmouliere A, Redard M, Darby I, et al. Apoptosis mediates the decrease in cellularity during the transition between granulation tissue and scar. Am J Pathol 1995;146:56–66.
112. Luo S, Benethan M, Raffoul W, et al. Abnormal balance between proliferation and apoptotic cell death in fibroblasts derived from keloid lesions. Plast Reconstr Surg 2001;107:87–96.
113. Sayah DN, Soo C, Shaw WW, et al. Down regulation of apoptosis-related genes in keloid tissues. J Surg Res 1999;87:209–216.
114. Shaw LM, Rabinovitz I, Wang HH, et al. Activation of phosphoinositide 3-OH kinase by alpha6beta4 integrin promotes carcinoma invasion. Cell 1997;91:949–960.
115. Zhang Z, Vuoi K, Reed JC, et al. The alpha 5 beta 1 integrin supports survival of cells on fibronectin and upregulates Bcl-2 expression. Proc Natl Acad Sci USA 1995;92:6161–6165.
116. Slomiani BL, Piotrowski J, Slomiani A. Role of fibroblast growth factor in the suppression of apoptotic caspse-3 during chronic gastric ulcer healing. J Physiol Pharmacol 1998;49:489–500.
117. Yao R, Cooper GM. Requirement for phosphatidylinositol-3 kinase in the prevention of apoptosis by nerve growth factor. Science 1995;267:2003–2006.
118. Robson MC, Steed DL, McPherson JM, et al. Use of transforming growth factor-β2 (TGF-β2) in the treatment of chronic foot ulcers in diabetic patients. 3rd Joint Meeting of the European Tissue Repair Society and Wound Healing Society. Bordeaux, France, August 23–7, 1999.
119. Robson MC, Dubay DA, Wang X, et al. Effect of cytokine growth factors on the prevention of acute wound failure. Wound Rep Reg 2004;12:38–43.
120. Petrie NC, Yao F, Eriksson E. Gene therapy in wound healing. Surg Clin North Am 2003;83:597–616.
121. Bullard KM, Longaker MT, Lorenz HP. Fetal wound healing: current biology. World J Surg 2003;27:54–61.
122. Martin P, Lewis J. Actin cables and epidermal movement in embryonic wound healing. Nature 1992;360:179–183.
123. Azdick NS, Harrison MR, Glick PL. Comparison of fetal, newborn, and adult wound healing by histologic, enzyme-histochemical and hydroxyproline determinations. J Pediatr Surg 1985;2:315–319.
124. Lovvorn HH, Cheung DT, Nimni ME, et al. Relative distribution and crosslinking of collagen distinguish fetal from adult sheep wound repair. J Pediatr Surg 1999;34:218–223.
125. Estes JM, Azdick N, Harrison MR, et al. Hyaluronate metabolism undergoes and ontogenic transition during fetal development: implications for scar-free wound healing. J Pediatr Surg 1993;28:1227–1231.
126. Dang C, Beanes R, Soo C, et al. A high ratio of TGF-β3 to TGF-β1 expression in wounds is associated with scarless repair [abstract]. Wound Rep Reg 2001;9:153.
127. Whitby DJ, Ferguson MWJ. Immunohistochemical studies in fetal and adult wound healing. In: Azdick NS, Longaker MT, eds. Fetal Wound Healing. New York: Elsevier; 1992:161–176.
128. Lorenz HP, Soo C, Beanses SR, et al. Differential expression of matrix metalloproteinases and their tissue-derived inhibitors in scarless fetal wound healing. Surg Forum 2001;52:397–401.
129. Stelnicki EJ, Komuves LG, Holmes D, et al. The human homeobox genes MSX-1, MSX-2, and MOX-1 are differentially expressed in the dermis and epidermis of the fetal and adult skin. Differentiation 1997;62:33–41.
130. Lajtha LG. Stem cell concepts. Differentiation 1979;14(1–2):23–34.
131. Potten CS. Stem Cells: Their Identification and Characterization. Edinburgh: Churchill Livingston; 1983:200–232.
132. Morris RJ, Fischer SM, Slaga TJ. Evidence that the centrally and peripherally located cells in the murine epidermal proliferative unit are two distinct cell populations. J Invest Dermatol 1985;84:277–281.
133. Mackenzie IC, Bickenbach JR. Label-retaining keratinocytes and Langerhans cells in mouse epithelia. Cell Tissue Res 1985;242:551–556.
134. Potten CS. Cell cycles in cell hierarchies. Int J Radiat Biol Relat Stud Phys Chem Med 1986;49:257–278.
135. Bickenbach JR, McCutcheon J, Mackenzie IC. Rate of loss of tritiated thymidine label in basal cells in mouse epithelial tissues. Cell Tissue Kinet 1986;19:325–333.
136. Cairns J. The Leeuwenhoek Lecture, 1978. Bacteria as proper subjects for cancer research. Proc R Soc Lond B Biol Sci 1980;208:121–133.
137. Potten CS, Loeffler M. Stem cells: attributes, cycles, spirals, pitfalls and uncertainties. Lessons for and from the crypt. Development 1990;110:1001–1020.
138. Watt FM, Green H. Involucrin synthesis is correlated with cell size in human epidermal cultures. J Cell Biol 1981;90:738–742.
139. Watt FM, Kubler MD, Hotchin NA, et al. Regulation of keratinocyte terminal differentiation by integrin-extracellular matrix interactions. J Cell Sci 1993;106:175–182.
140. Jones PH, Watt FM. Separation of human epidermal stem cells from transit amplifying cells on the basis of differences in integrin function and expression. Cell 1993;73:713–724.
141. Tani H, Morris RJ, Kaur P. Enrichment for murine keratinocyte stem cells based on cell surface phenotype. Proc Natl Acad Sci USA 2000;97:10960–10965.
142. Commo S, Gaillard O, Bernard BA. The human hair follicle contains two distinct K19 positive compartments in the outer root sheath: a unifying hypothesis for stem cell reservoir? Differentiation 2000;66:157–164.
143. Michel M, Torok N, Godbout MJ, et al. Keratin 19 as a biochemical marker of skin stem cells in vivo and in vitro: keratin 19 expressing cells are differentially localized in function of anatomic sites, and their number varies with donor age and culture stage. J Cell Sci 1996;109:1017–1028.

144. Matic M, Evans WH, Brink PR, et al. Epidermal stem cells do not communicate through gap junctions. J Invest Dermatol 2002;118:110–116.
145. Bjerknes M, Cheng H, Erlandsen S. Functional gap junctions in mouse small intestinal crypts. Anat Rec 1985;212:364–367.
146. Gambardella L, Barrandon Y. The multifaceted adult epidermal stem cell. Curr Opin Cell Biol 2003;15:771–777.
147. Tumbar T, Guasch G, Greco V, et al. Defining the epithelial stem cell niche in skin. Science 2004;303:359–363.
148. Cotsarelis G, Sun TT, Lavker RM. Label-retaining cells reside in the bulge area of pilosebaceous unit: implications for follicular stem cells, hair cycle, and skin carcinogenesis. Cell 1990;61:1329–1337.
149. Rochat A, Kobayashi K, Barrandon Y. Location of stem cells of human hair follicles by clonal analysis. Cell 1994;76:1063–1073.
150. Ghazizadeh S, Taichman LB. Multiple classes of stem cells in cutaneous epithelium: a lineage analysis of adult mouse skin. EMBO J 2001;20:1215–1222.
151. Kamimura J, Lee D, Baden HP, et al. Primary mouse keratinocyte cultures contain hair follicle progenitor cells with multiple differentiation potential. J Invest Dermatol 1997;109:534–540.
152. Miller SJ, Burke EM, Rader MD, et al. Re-epithelialization of porcine skin by the sweat apparatus. J Invest Dermatol 1998;110:13–19.
153. Taylor G, Lehrer MS, Jensen PJ, et al. Involvement of follicular stem cells in forming not only the follicle but also the epidermis. Cell 2000;102:451–461.
154. Reynolds AJ, Jahoda CA. Cultured dermal papilla cells induce follicle formation and hair growth by transdifferentiation of an adult epidermis. Development 1992;115:587–593.
155. Ferraris C, Bernard BA, Dhouailly D. Adult epidermal keratinocytes are endowed with pilosebaceous forming abilities. Int J Dev Biol 1997;41:491–498.
156. Li A, Pouliot N, Redvers R, et al. Extensive tissue-regenerative capacity of neonatal human keratinocyte stem cells and their progeny. J Clin Invest 2004;113:390–400.
157. Merrill BJ, Gat U, DasGupta R, et al. Tcf3 and Lef1 regulate lineage differentiation of multipotent stem cells in skin. Genes Dev 2001;15:1688–1705.
158. Rheinwald JG, Green H. Serial cultivation of strains of human epidermal keratinocytes: the formation of keratinizing colonies from single cells. Cell 1975;6:331–343.
159. Green H, Kehinde O, Thomas J. Growth of cultured human epidermal cells into multiple epithelia suitable for grafting. Proc Natl Acad Sci USA 1979;76:5665–5668.
160. O'Connor NE, Mulliken JB, Banks-Schlegel S, et al. Grafting of burns with cultured epithelium prepared from autologous epidermal cells. Lancet 1981;1:75.
161. Gallico GG 3rd, O'Connor NE, Compton CC, et al. Permanent coverage of large burn wounds with autologous cultured human epithelium. N Engl J Med 1984;311:448–451.
162. Compton CC, Nadire KB, Regauer S, et al. Cultured human sole-derived keratinocyte grafts re-express site-specific differentiation after transplantation. Differentiation 1998;64:45–53.
163. Stoner ML, Wood FM. Cultured epithelial autograft "take" confirmed by the presence of cytokeratin 9. J Invest Dermatol 1999;112:391–392.
164. Kolodka TM, Garlick JA, Taichman LB. Evidence for keratinocyte stem cells in vitro: long term engraftment and persistence of transgene expression from retrovirus-transduced keratinocytes. Proc Natl Acad Sci USA 1998;95:4356–4361.
165. Counter CM, Press W, Compton CC. Telomere shortening in cultured autografts of patients with burns. Lancet 2003;361:1345–1346.
166. Odessey R. Addendum: multicenter experience with cultured epidermal autograft for treatment of burns. J Burn Care Rehabil 1992;13:174–180.
167. Carsin H, Ainaud P, Le Bever H, et al. Cultured epithelial autografts in extensive burn coverage of severely traumatized patients: a five year single-center experience with 30 patients. Burns 2000;26:379–387.
168. Chester DL, Balderson DS, Papini RP. A review of keratinocyte delivery to the wound bed. J Burn Care Rehabil 2004;25:266–275.
169. Heck EL, Bergstresser PR, Baxter CR. Composite skin graft: frozen dermal allografts support the engraftment and expansion of autologous epidermis. J Trauma 1985;25:106–112.
170. Cuono C, Langdon R, McGuire J. Use of cultured epidermal autografts and dermal allografts as skin replacement after burn injury. Lancet 1986;1:1123–1124.
171. Cuono CB, Langdon R, Birchall N, et al. Composite autologous-allogeneic skin replacement: development and clinical application. Plast Reconstr Surg 1987;80:626–637.
172. Teepe RG, Kreis RW, Koebrugge EJ, et al. The use of cultured autologous epidermis in the treatment of extensive burn wounds. J Trauma 1990;30:269–275.
173. Rouabhia M, Germain L, Bergeron J, et al. Allogeneic-syngeneic cultured epithelia. A successful therapeutic option for skin regeneration. Transplantation 1995;59:1229–1235.
174. Lobmann R, Pittasch D, Muhlen I, et al. Autologous human keratinocytes cultured on membranes composed of benzyl ester of hyaluronic acid for grafting in nonhealing diabetic foot lesions: a pilot study. J Diabetes Complication 2003;17:199–204.
175. Ronfard V, Broly H, Mitchell V, et al. Use of human keratinocytes cultured on fibrin glue in the treatment of burn wounds. Burns 1991;17:181–184.
176. Pellegrini G, Ranno R, Stracuzzi G, et al. The control of epidermal stem cells (holoclones) in the treatment of massive full-thickness burns with autologous keratinocytes cultured on fibrin. Transplantation 1999;68:868–879.
177. Ronfard V, Rives JM, Neveux Y, et al. Long-term regeneration of human epidermis on third degree burns transplanted with autologous cultured epithelium grown on a fibrin matrix. Transplantation 2000;70:1588–1598.
178. Kaiser HW, Stark GB, Kopp J, et al. Cultured autologous keratinocytes in fibrin glue suspension, exclusively and combined with STS-allograft (preliminary clinical and histological report of a new technique). Burns 1994;20:23–29.
179. Stark GB, Kaiser HW. Cologne Burn Centre experience with glycerol-preserved allogeneic skin. Part II. Combination with autologous cultured keratinocytes. Burns 1994;20(suppl 1):S34–S38.
180. Bannasch H, Horch RE, Tanczos E, et al. Treatment of chronic wounds with cultured autologous keratinocytes as suspension in fibrin glue. Zentralbl Chir 2000;125(suppl 1):79–81.

181. Horch RE, Bannasch H, Stark GB. Transplantation of cultured autologous keratinocytes in fibrin sealant biomatrix to resurface chronic wounds. Transplant Proc 2001;33:642–644.
182. Kopp J, Jeschke MG, Bach AD, et al. Applied tissue engineering in the closure of severe burns and chronic wounds using cultured human autologous keratinocytes in a natural fibrin matrix. Cell Tissue Bank 2004;5:81–87.
183. Hafemann B, Hettich R, Ensslen S, et al. Treatment of skin defects using suspensions of in vitro cultured keratinocytes. Burns 1994;20:168–172.
184. Currie LJ, Martin R, Sharpe JR, et al. A comparison of keratinocyte cell sprays with and without fibrin glue. Burns 2003;29:677–685.
185. Chester DL, Balderson DS, Papini RP. A review of keratinocyte delivery to the wound bed. J Burn Care Rehabil 2004;25:266–275.
186. Grant I, Warwick K, Marshall J, et al. The co-application of sprayed cultured autologous keratinocytes and autologous fibrin sealant in a porcine wound model. Br J Plast Surg 2002;55:219–227.
187. Morhenn VB, Benike CJ, Cox AJ, et al. Cultured human epidermal cells do not synthesize HLA-DR. J Invest Dermatol 1982;78:32–37.
188. Wikner NE, Huff JC, Norris DA, et al. Study of HLA-DR synthesis in cultured human keratinocytes. J Invest Dermatol 1986;87:559–564.
189. Thivolet J, Faure M, Demidem A, et al. Long-term survival and immunological tolerance of human epidermal allografts produced in culture. Transplantation 1986;42:274–280.
190. Gielen V, Faure M, Mauduit G, et al. Progressive replacement of human cultured epithelial allografts by recipient cells as evidenced by HLA class I antigens expression. Dermatologica 1987;175:166–170.
191. Brain A, Purkis P, Coates P, et al. Survival of cultured allogeneic keratinocytes transplanted to deep dermal bed assessed with probe specific for Y chromosome. BMJ 1989;298:917–919.
192. Burt AM, Pallett CD, Sloane JP, et al. Survival of cultured allografts in patients with burns assessed with probe specific for Y chromosome. BMJ 1989;298: 915–917.
193. Phillips TJ, Bhawan J, Leigh IM, et al. Cultured epidermal autografts and allografts: a study of differentiation and allograft survival. J Am Acad Dermatol 1990;23(2 pt 1):189–198.
194. Roseeuw DI, De Coninck A, Lissens W, et al. Allogeneic cultured epidermal grafts heal chronic ulcers although they do not remain as proved by DNA analysis. J Dermatol Sci 1990;1:245–252.
195. van der Merwe AE, Mattheyse FJ, Bedford M, et al. Allografted keratinocytes used to accelerate the treatment of burn wounds are replaced by recipient cells. Burns 1990;16:193–197.
196. Kaawach WF, Oliver AM, Weiler-Mithoff E, et al. Survival assessment of cultured epidermal allografts applied onto partial-thickness burn wounds. Br J Plast Surg 1991;44:321–324.
197. Teepe RG, Koch R, Haeseker B. Randomized trial comparing cryopreserved cultured epidermal allografts with tulle-gras in the treatment of split-thickness skin graft donor sites. J Trauma 1993;35:850–854.
198. Phillips TJ, Provan A, Colbert D, et al. A randomized single-blind controlled study of cultured epidermal allografts in the treatment of split-thickness skin graft donor sites. Arch Dermatol 1993;129:879–882.
199. Yanaga H, Udoh Y, Yamauchi T, et al. Cryopreserved cultured epidermal allografts achieved early closure of wounds and reduced scar formation in deep partial-thickness burn wounds (DDB) and split-thickness skin donor sites of pediatric patients. Burns 2001;27:689–698.
200. Madden MR, LaBruna AA, Hajjar DP, et al. Transplantation of cryopreserved cultured epidermal allografts. J Trauma 1996;40:743–750.
201. Fratianne R, Papay F, Housini I, et al. Keratinocyte allografts accelerate healing of split-thickness donor sites: applications for improved treatment of burns. J Burn Care Rehabil 1993;14(2 pt 1):148–154.
202. Duinslaeger LA, Verbeken G, Vanhalle S, et al. Cultured allogeneic keratinocyte sheets accelerate healing compared to Op-site treatment of donor sites in burns. J Burn Care Rehabil 1997;18:545–551.
203. Blight A, Fatah MF, Datubo-Brown DD, et al. The treatment of donor sites with cultured epithelial grafts. Br J Plast Surg 1991;44:12–14.
204. Hefton JM, Caldwell D, Biozes DG, et al. Grafting of skin ulcers with cultured autologous epidermal cells. J Am Acad Dermatol 1986;14:399–405.
205. Phillips TJ, Gilchrest BA. Clinical applications of cultured epithelium. Epithelial Cell Biol 1992;1:39–46.
206. Phillips TJ, Kehinde O, Green H, Gilchrest BA. Treatment of skin ulcers with cultured epidermal allografts. J Am Acad Dermatol 1989;21(2 pt 1):191–199.
207. Marcusson JA, Lindgren C, Berghard A, et al. Allogeneic cultured keratinocytes in the treatment of leg ulcers. A pilot study. Acta Derm Venereol 1992;72:61–64.
208. Leigh IM, Purkis PE, Navsaria HA, et al. Treatment of chronic venous ulcers with sheets of cultured allogenic keratinocytes. Br J Dermatol 1987;117:591–597.
209. Beele H, Naeyaert JM, Goetyn M, et al. Repeated cultured epidermal allografts in the treatment of chronic leg ulcers of various origins. Dermatologica 1991;183:31–35.
210. Teepe RG, Koebrugge EJ, Ponec M, et al. Fresh versus cryopreserved cultured allografts for the treatment of chronic skin ulcers. Br J Dermatol 1990;122:81–89.
211. De Luca M, Albanese E, Cancedda R, et al. Treatment of leg ulcers with cryopreserved allogeneic cultured epithelium. A multicenter study. Arch Dermatol 1992;128:633–638.
212. Teepe RG, Roseeuw DI, Hermans J, et al. Randomized trial comparing cryopreserved cultured epidermal allografts with hydrocolloid dressings in healing chronic venous ulcers. J Am Acad Dermatol 1993;29:982–988.
213. Bolivar-Flores YJ, Kuri-Harcuch W. Frozen allogeneic human epidermal cultured sheets for the cure of complicated leg ulcers. Dermatol Surg 1999;25:610–617.
214. Navratilova Z, Slonkova V, Semradova V, et al. Cryopreserved and lyophilized cultured epidermal allografts in the treatment of leg ulcers: a pilot study. J Eur Acad Dermatol Venereol 2004;18:173–179.
215. Harris N, Coady M, Wilson Y. Scalds related to bleeding domestic heating radiators. Burns 1993;19:415–417.
216. Bolivar-Flores J, Poumian E, Marsch-Moreno M, et al. Use of cultured human epidermal keratinocytes for allografting burns and conditions for temporary banking of the cultured allografts. Burns 1990;16:3–8.

217. Soeda J, Inokuchi S, Ueno S, et al. Use of cultured human epidermal allografts for the treatment of extensive partial thickness scald burn in children. Tokai J Exp Clin Med 1993;18:65–70.
218. Brychta P, Suchanek I, Rihova H, et al. Cultured epidermal allografts for the treatment of deep dermal burns. Acta Chir Plast 1995;37:20–24.
219. Braye F, Pascal P, Bertin-Maghit M, et al. Advantages of using a bank of allogenic keratinocytes for the rapid coverage of extensive and deep second-degree burns. Med Biol Eng Comput 2000;38:248–252.
220. Brychta P, Adler J, Rihova H, et al. Cultured epidermal allografts: quantitative evaluation of their healing effect in deep dermal burns. Cell Tissue Bank 2002;3:15–23.
221. Kearney JN. Clinical evaluation of skin substitutes. Burns 2001;27:545–551.
222. Nishiyama T, Amano S, Tsunenaga M, et al. The importance of laminin 5 in the dermal-epidermal basement membrane. J Dermatol Sci 2000;24(suppl 1):S51–S59.
223. Tsunenaga M, Adachi E, Amano S, et al. Laminin 5 can promote assembly of the lamina densa in the skin equivalent model. Matrix Biol 1998;17:603–613.
224. Wainwright DJ. Use of an acellular allograft dermal matrix (AlloDerm) in the management of full-thickness burns. Burns 1995;21:243–248.
225. Wainwright D, Madden M, Luterman A, et al. Clinical evaluation of an acellular allograft dermal matrix in full-thickness burns. J Burn Care Rehabil 1996;17:124–136.
226. Lattari V, Jones LM, Varcelotti JR, et al. The use of a permanent dermal allograft in full-thickness burns of the hand and foot: a report of three cases. J Burn Care Rehabil 1997;18:147–155.
227. Simman R, Priebe CJ Jr, Simon M. Reconstruction of aplasia cutis congenita of the trunk in a newborn infant using acellular allogenic dermal graft and cultured epithelial autografts. Ann Plast Surg 2000;44:451–454.
228. Burke JF, Yannas IV, Quinby WC Jr, et al. Successful use of a physiologically acceptable artificial skin in the treatment of extensive burn injury. Ann Surg 1981;194:413–428.
229. Heimbach D, Luterman A, Burke J, et al. Artificial dermis for major burns. A multi-center randomized clinical trial. Ann Surg 1988;208:313–320.
230. Ryan CM, Schoenfeld DA, Malloy M, et al. Use of Integra artificial skin is associated with decreased length of stay for severely injured adult burn survivors. J Burn Care Rehabil 2002;23:311–317.
231. Pandya AN, Woodward B, Parkhouse N. The use of cultured autologous keratinocytes with Integra in the resurfacing of acute burns. Plast Reconstr Surg 1998;102:825–828; discussion 829–830.
232. Yannas IV, Burke JF, Gordon PL, et al. Design of an artificial skin. II. Control of chemical composition. J Biomed Mater Res 1980;14:107–132.
233. Heimbach DM, Warden GD, Luterman A, et al. Multicenter postapproval clinical trial of Integra dermal regeneration template for burn treatment. J Burn Care Rehabil 2003;24:42–48.
234. Stern R, McPherson M, Longaker MT. Histologic study of artificial skin used in the treatment of full-thickness thermal injury. J Burn Care Rehabil 1990;11:7–13.
235. Kearney JN. Clinical evaluation of skin substitutes. Burns 2001;27:545–551.
236. Purdue GF, Hunt JL, Still JM Jr, et al. A multicenter clinical trial of a biosynthetic skin replacement, Dermagraft-TC, compared with cryopreserved human cadaver skin for temporary coverage of excised burn wounds. J Burn Care Rehabil 1997;18(1 pt 1):52–57.
237. Demling RH, DeSanti L. Management of partial thickness facial burns (comparison of topical antibiotics and bio-engineered skin substitutes). Burns 1999;25:256–261.
238. Noordenbos J, Dore C, Hansbrough JF. Safety and efficacy of TransCyte for the treatment of partial-thickness burns. J Burn Care Rehabil 1999;20:275–281.
239. Lukish JR, Eichelberger MR, Newman KD, et al. The use of a bioactive skin substitute decreases length of stay for pediatric burn patients. J Pediatr Surg 2001;36:1118–1121.
240. Kumar RJ, Kimble RM, Boots R, et al. Treatment of partial-thickness burns: a prospective, randomized trial using Transcyte. ANZ J Surg 2004;74:622–626.
241. Naughton G, Mansbridge J, Gentzkow G. A metabolically active human dermal replacement for the treatment of diabetic foot ulcers. Artif Organs 1997;21:1203–1210.
242. Veves A, Falanga V, Armstrong DG, et al. Graftskin, a human skin equivalent, is effective in the management of noninfected neuropathic diabetic foot ulcers: a prospective randomized multicenter clinical trial. Diabetes Care 2001;24:290–295.
243. Mansbridge J, Liu K, Patch R, et al. Three-dimensional fibroblast culture implant for the treatment of diabetic foot ulcers: metabolic activity and therapeutic range. Tissue Eng 1998;4:403–414.
244. Krejci-Papa NC, Hoang A, Hansbrough JF. Fibroblast sheets enable epithelialization of sounds that do not support keratinocyte migration. Tissue Eng 1999;5:555–562.
245. Bell E, Sher S, Hull B, et al. The reconstitution of living skin. J Invest Dermatol 1983;81(1 suppl):2S–10S.
246. Bell E, Rosenberg M, Kemp P, et al. Recipes for reconstituting skin. J Biomech Eng 1991;113:113–119.
247. Boyce ST, Williams ML. Lipid supplemented medium induces lamellar bodies and precursors of barrier lipids in cultured analogues of human skin. J Invest Dermatol 1993;101(2):180–184.
248. Ponec M, Kempenaar J, Weerheim A, et al. Triglyceride metabolism in human keratinocytes cultured at the air-liquid interface. Arch Dermatol Res 1995;287:723–730.
249. Phillips TJ, Manzoor J, Rojas A, et al. The longevity of a bilayered skin substitute after application to venous ulcers. Arch Dermatol 2002;138:1079–1081.
250. Falanga V, Margolis D, Alvarez O, et al. Rapid healing of venous ulcers and lack of clinical rejection with an allogeneic cultured human skin equivalent. Human Skin Equivalent Investigators Group. Arch Dermatol 1998;134:293–300.
251. Sabolinski ML, Alvarez O, Auletta M, et al. Cultured skin as a 'smart material' for healing wounds: experience in venous ulcers. Biomaterials 1996;17:311–320.
252. Brem H, Balledux J, Sukkarieh T, et al. Healing of venous ulcers of long duration with a bilayered living skin substitute: results from a general surgery and dermatology department. Dermatol Surg 2001;27:915–919.

253. Curran MP, Plosker GL. Bilayered bioengineered skin substitute (Apligraf): a review of its use in the treatment of venous leg ulcers and diabetic foot ulcers. BioDrugs 2002;16:439–455.
254. Still J, Glat P, Silverstein P, et al. The use of a collagen sponge/living cell composite material to treat donor sites in burn patients. Burns 2003;29:837–841.
255. Black AF, Berthod F, L'heureux N, et al. In vitro reconstruction of a human capillary-like network in a tissue-engineered skin equivalent. FASEB J 1998;12:1331–1340.
256. Lee DY, Ahn HT, Cho KH. A new skin equivalent model: dermal substrate that combines de-epidermized dermis with fibroblast-populated collagen matrix. J Dermatol Sci 2000;23:132–137.
257. Hansbrough JF, Boyce ST, Cooper ML, et al. Burn wound closure with cultured autologous keratinocytes and fibroblasts attached to a collagen-glycosaminoglycan substrate. JAMA 1989;262:2125–2130.
258. Boyce ST, Kagan RJ, Yakuboff KP, et al. Cultured skin substitutes reduce donor skin harvesting for closure of excised, full-thickness burns. Ann Surg 2002;235:269–279.

# Skin Regeneration from Multipotent Adult and Embryonic Stem Cells

Kursad Turksen and Tammy-Claire Troy

The epidermis is prone to injury and epithelial cell loss; therefore, it is essential that it be able to maintain and repair itself throughout life from cells quiescent within the epidermal stem cell niche. Although the origin, location, and cellular characteristics of epidermal stem cells are beginning to become clearer, less is known about the genes that are critical for the formation and maintenance of epidermal stem cells as well as the signals that commit specific subpopulations within the epidermal lineages. Nevertheless, recent developments have made epidermal stem cells prime candidates for the development of various therapeutic modalities aimed at regeneration of epidermal tissues. In this review, the current understanding of epidermal stem cell biology from embryonic and adult sources is summarized, as well as their potential for regenerative medicine.

Throughout life, the skin acts as the interface between internal organs and the external environment, providing a physical barrier and first line of response to a variety of environmental insults including physical trauma, ultraviolet irradiation, chemical invasion, and microbial assault.[1] To maintain its physical integrity and function, the epidermis continuously renews itself from a pool of differentiating epidermal cells supplied by the epidermal stem cell niche.[2] Advances in our understanding of the epidermal lineage have been substantial over the last 20 years, and although much remains to be learned, the field is positioned to devise ways to regenerate skin in severe injury situations such as observed in burn victims, patients with diabetic foot ulcers, as well as individuals with congenital or acquired skin blistering diseases. In all such circumstances, the normal cycle of epidermal differentiation is incapable of fulfilling the renewal demands of the epidermis, resulting in epidermal failure with all its life-threatening consequences; thus, the potential of skin regeneration is enormous. To achieve this, however, will require a greater understanding of the self-renewal and directed differentiation of epidermal stem cells as well as the signals and their transduction pathways that govern the proliferation and differentiation of regeneration-competent cells. This review examines our current knowledge of epidermal stem cells and explores their potential use for epidermal regeneration and future clinical stem cell-based treatment regimens for epidermal defects.

Epidermis as a Developmental System

In mouse, the epidermis is derived from primitive ectoderm that gives rise to surface ectoderm during gastrulation at embryonic age E5–E6.[3] After initial cell fate selection, surface ectodermal cells are selected to either the neuronal or epidermal fate.[4] Pluripotent epidermal stem cells give rise to epidermal cells, which go through a complex series of morphogenic steps that give rise to the epidermis, hair follicles, and sebaceous glands where appropriate. From gestational days E8–E12, the putative epidermis is a single layer of proliferating cells (stratum germinativum), which is overlain by the periderm expressing characteristic markers of surface ectodermal cells [keratins 8 and 18 (K8/K18)]. At E12–E14, an intermediate layer of cells (stratum intermedium) develops from the stratum germinativum, and comes to separate it from the periderm. Differentiation to the mature epidermis begins at day E15, with epidermal stratification. At this stage, the stratum germinativum expresses K5/K14 (characteristic of basal cells), whereas the cells in the two layers of the stratum intermedium down-regulate the expression of K8/K18 and the expression of K1/K10 is induced in the suprabasal cells.[5,6] Differentiation of the mouse epidermis into mature structures is completed by E17–E18 with the appearance of the granular and cornified layers of the epidermis[6] giving rise to the insoluble cornified envelope and the completion of epidermal permeability barrier (EPB) formation.[7–12] Similar steps and events in epidermal morphogenesis also take place (in their appropriate timeline) for other mammals.

Epidermis as a Self-Renewing Differentiation System

In response to discrete yet unidentified signals, throughout life, epidermal cells in the basal compartment become irreversibly committed to terminal differentiation and move upward away from the basal layer.[13–16] This process can be very nicely followed by the expression profile of keratins (epidermal structural proteins) as well as other proteins known to be involved in terminal differentiation.[12,17,18] Upon leaving the basal layer, the expression of K5 and K14 is shut down whereas K1 and K10 expression is induced. As these cells progress to the spinous layer, they begin to express involucrin, a protein involved in the eventual formation of the insoluble cornified envelope. Granular cells, which directly follow the spinous cells, are characterized by electron-dense keratohyalin granules containing filaggrin, a protein that facilitates the aggregation of keratin filaments.[19] As the terminally differentiating cells transit from the granular layer to the cornified layer, cornified cells undergo a destruction of their organelles to form the cornified envelope. Cornified envelope proteins include involucrin, loricrin, small proline rich proteins,[20,21] calcium binding S100 proteins, cystatin A (keratolinin), repetin, loricrin,[22] envoplakin,[23–25] sciellin,[26] and late envelope proteins[27] (reviewed in refs. 11, 19, 28). The cornified envelope is constructed through the sequential expression, processing, and deposition of several other distinct proteins that are crosslinked by disulfide and Ne-(g-glutaminyl) lysine isodipeptide bonds, the formation of which is catalyzed by transglutaminase.[29]

Thus, the permeability barrier of the skin is formed in the last stage of epidermal differentiation consisting of corneocytes, an insoluble cornified envelope, and lipid-enriched intercellular domains.[11,30–33] The lipids for barrier function are synthesized in the nucleated epidermal layers, stored in the lamellar bodies, and extruded into the intercellular space during the transition from the stratum granulosum to the stratum corneum forming a system of continuous membrane bilayers.[8,34] Using a qualitative, whole-mount assay for skin permeability, Hardman and colleagues[10] demonstrated that barrier formation is indeed highly patterned during development. Morphologic and biochemical observations have been further corroborated recently by the transepidermal water loss assay as a powerful indicator of barrier function. Quantitative transepidermal water loss assays indicate that the EPB forms rapidly between days 19 and 21 of the 22-day rat gestational period,[35] between days 17 and 19 of the 20-day mouse gestation period,[10] and between weeks 30 and 33 of the 40-week human gestational period.[36] Generally, therefore, mammalian EPB formation is completed just before birth as part of the preparation of the organism for terrestrial living. This barrier provides a first line of defense against bacterial infection, thermoregulation, and dehydration, and the consequences of EPB dysfunction are generally deadly in the environment we occupy.

The histology of the mature epidermis as well as the overall changes in the expression pattern of structural molecules during development and adulthood have been described. However, the patterned expression of signaling molecules thought to be regulating cell fate selection[16,37,38] as well as the epidermal and associated appendage lineages (i.e., hair and sebaceous glands) during embryologic development are slowly beginning to be identified from a series of transgenic mouse studies. These include several transcription factors such as LEF-1/Tcf-3,[39] p63,[40] c-Myc,[40-43] GATA-3,[44] Foxn1 (nude),[45,46] Hairless, RBP-J,[47] and members of several signaling pathways including Wnts,[48] Delta-Notch,[49] sonic hedgehog,[50] fibroblast growth factor (FGF),[51] and bone morphogenetic proteins.[52,53] However, very little is known of the early steps leading to the onset of cell lineage commitment, the allocation and identity of appropriate stem cells, or the control of the developmental program thereafter.

Epidermal Stem Cells and Their Potentiality

Continuous renewal of the epidermis and its appendages throughout life has predicted that there is a stem cell population with characteristics similar to those of other renewing systems.[54-57] Until recently, however, technical difficulties with culturing epidermal cells in vitro and the absence of markers to identify and isolate stem cells, as well as the lack of a biological assay to demonstrate their stem cell-like characteristics, has plagued the epidermal stem cell field; hence, stem cells of the epidermis have not been explored with the same vigor of other lineages (such as hemopoietic cells). The first definitive study addressing the existence and location of putative stem cells in the epidermis was published in the 1980s, when Cotsarelis et al.[58] demonstrated the existence of label-retaining,[59] slowly proliferating cells concentrated in the bulge region of the hair follicle, leading to the concept that these cells could constitute a stem cell pool in a specialized stem cell niche. The demonstration of the true potential of bulge region-derived epidermal stem cells and the ability to measure the frequency of putative stem or more restricted precursor cells in vitro or in vivo have been hampered by the absence of appropriate assay systems and the lack of reliable/specific markers for epidermal stem cells and their immediate progeny. Nevertheless, considerable data have been generated documenting the high proliferative capacity/colony-forming capacity of cells isolated from carefully dissected regions along the hair follicle as well as within the heterogeneous population of basal layer epidermal cells.[60] However, it is important to note that, given the way these experiments were done, it was not possible to address the clonality of the colony-forming precursors. Indeed, the conditions that had been derived for mature keratinocyte growth[61] fail to support growth of the isolated precursor cells at limiting dilution or single cell clonal levels. By the same token, the approaches were also not suitable for attempting to determine lineage relationships and potentiality of putative multipotential epidermal stem cells and their more restricted progeny. Similarly, suitable reconstitution-type biological assays were not available to test the potentiality of putative stem cells in vivo.

Identification of the hair follicle bulge as the likely location of stem cells has allowed identification of a number of potential stem cell markers by region-specific immunohistochemical labeling[62]; these include β-integrin,[63,64] K19,[65,66] K15,[67,68] δ-1,[49] p63,[69] CD34,[70] melanoma-associated CSPG,[67] and Nestin.[71] None of these markers is absolutely specific for putative stem cells nor is use of any one alone sufficient to allow isolation of homogeneous stem or precursor cells from the bulge; however, the markers provide additional support for stem cells and a stem niche in the bulge region. Early attempts to enrich epidermal stem cells was based on the observation that the putative stem cells adhered strongly to basement membranes and exhibited high levels of β1-integrin (surface adhesion proteins).[72,73] Thus, enriched β1-integrin[bright] cells exhibited high proliferative and colony-forming capacity in vitro.[73] Putative epidermal stem cells have also been reported to express not only high levels of β1 but also α6-integrins and low levels of CD71 (transferrin receptor).[74] K19, a tailless keratin molecule, was also reported to be a putative stem cell marker based on its restricted localization to the bulge region of the hair follicle.[66] Another keratin (K15), although associated with various epithelial cells,[75] may also be a good marker of bulge cells in adult epidermis.[76,77]

More recently, the hemopoietic cell marker CD34 has been said to be highly expressed by epidermal stem cells, based on the intense membrane staining on keratinocytes in the bulge region of the mouse hair follicle.[70] In these studies, CD34 expression colocalized with both slowly cycling (label-retaining) cells and K15 expression. When cells were selected with fluorescence-activated cell sorting (FACS) with antibodies against CD34 and α6-integrin in combination, the positively selected cells were found to be predominantly in G0/G1, characteristic of a quiescent or slowly cycling stem or precursor population, in contrast to the CD34– cells which had well-defined G2/M and S phases. Interestingly, the majority of the CD34+ cells (98%) were positive for K6, establishing this population as the basal keratinocytes of follicular origin. Notably, when putative adult epidermal stem cells were labeled with Hoechst 33342 and a side population (SP) was sorted by FACS, the cells within the SP did not exhibit the stem cell-like characteristics that SP cells have been reported to have in other adult stem cell isolates.[78,79] This emphasizes the need for caution in attributing widely accepted stem cell characteristics to all stem cell populations.

Recently, two groups[61,80] independently, and with somewhat different genetic strategies, tracked and isolated a stem cell-like subpopulation of cells from the hair follicle bulge. Based on their assumption that bulge stem cells would uniquely be both slow-cycling and active for a keratinocyte-specific promoter, Fuchs' group[61] engineered transgenic mice to express histone H2B–green fluorescent protein (GFP) controlled by a tetracycline (tet)-responsive regulatory element and crossed them to mice harboring a K5 promoter–tet repressor–VP16 transgene. Four weeks of tet treatment of the double transgenic offspring with tet-controlled regulation restricted to skin epithelium selected for a low frequency (<1%) of slowly cycling bulge cells. Cotsarelis' group,[80] however, used a K15 promoter fragment to target mouse bulge cells with an inducible Cre recombinase construct or with the gene encoding GFP to mark bulge cells for lineage analysis in vivo and isolation, respectively. Further characterization of either of the GFP-positive populations on the basis of a number of phenotypic and functional properties in vitro and in vivo indicate that the cells meet many of the hallmark definitions of stem cells.

The authors of both studies recognized the need to address whether any of the isolated cells are multipotential and generate or regenerate hair follicles and other cutaneous lineages, a feature attributed to bulge stem cells.[81,82] This is key, given that there is evidence both for multipotent cells as well as more restricted progenitor cells (i.e., cells that give rise to only the hair follicle or only the sebaceous gland). By following the fate of marked label-retaining cells in relation to coexpression of a variety of proliferation-associated markers during the normal hair cycle and in response to injury, the Fuchs group concluded that only a few bulge label-retaining cells initiate each new follicle, and that upon exit from the bulge their progeny rapidly proliferate, markedly change their biochemical and gene expression profiles, and regenerate all differentiated cutaneous cell types.[61] Using somewhat different methodologies, including isolated bulge cell cotransplantation with dermal cells, the Cotsarelis group reached similar conclusions. Notably, however, the observations suggest that, although multipotent, under normal circumstances the bulge stem cells have a preference for generating hair follicles over the other cutaneous lineages. Both studies also reported observations suggesting that after exit from the bulge, the progeny of bulge cells retain significant proliferative and multilineage differentiation capacity. This is consistent with numerous previous indications that primitive progenitors for the cutaneous lineages, as for many other lineages, retain extensive proliferative capacity and multipotentiality, and these features alone are insufficient to rigorously define definitive stem cells.

It remains of interest to define the lineage relationships between the putative multipotent stem cells, multipotent progenitors, and/or more restricted unipotent progenitors for any one of the cutaneous lineages, especially when one considers these new data in the context of previous work that suggested the existence of multiple classes of stem cells in the cutaneous epithelium.[83] Ideally, one might attempt to address these latter issues by additional in vitro studies in combination with transplantation assays at single cell and clonal levels. Both the Fuchs and Cotsarelis groups FACS-enriched their marked cells and provided solid evidence that the populations with highest GFP expression were relatively quiescent when isolated but were capable of extensive proliferation in vitro; i.e., the efficiency of large colony formation was higher in their enriched versus nonbulge, basal keratinocytes, or GFP-positive populations with lower fluorescence intensity. They also showed that the most intensely fluorescent-sorted fraction of cells coexpressed other markers associated with bulge stem cells, including β1-integrin and CD34. However, clonal differentiation assays to address self-renewal, multilineage differentiation capacity of single putative stem cells within the FACS-sorted enriched populations, and the detailed lineage relationships mentioned above have not yet been done.

As previously noted, hair follicle and epidermal lineages pose significant problems in this regard. To date, no appropriate conditions have been reported by which primary epidermal cells can be maintained at single cell density in culture, and, based on data reported in recent studies, it seems likely that hair follicle stem cells may be similarly intransigent and require very different conditions than mature epidermal cells. Nevertheless, some hints may come from the gene expression profiling that was done in these studies. Studies from both the Fuchs and Cotsarelis groups include extensive transcriptional profiling of the isolated enriched bulge stem cell populations versus non-stem cell populations as well as, excitingly, other stem cell populations [i.e., hematopoietic, neural, and embryonic stem (ES) cells]. Generally, transcriptional profiling clearly supported other evidence presented that the hair follicle stem cells are quiescent or slowly cycling cells and are distinctly different from the more rapidly proliferating and differentiating progeny in expression of, for example, multiple growth factors and related signaling molecules including FGFs, transforming growth factor (TGF)-β, Wnts, and a variety of other molecular classes (extracellular matrix molecules, transcription factors, etc). In this regard, however, although there was considerable overlap in the stem cell transcriptional profiles reported in the two studies, there were some notable differences that may reflect variations in the homogeneity of the different populations assessed and/or the fact that the follicles compared in the studies were at different stages of the hair cycle. Interestingly, three genes were identified as common to hair follicle, neural, hemopoietic, and ES cells (namely, Eps8, Col18a1, and Pkd2); although it is premature to suggest that these comprise a definitive stem cell signature, the overlap in expression profiles as the transcriptomes of additional purified stem cell populations are compared will be interesting (e.g., ref. 84).

Stem Cell Niche and Regulation of Stem Cell Fate

Most mammalian continuously renewing tissues are maintained by stem cells located within stem cell niches[2,85]; the bulge area fits these criteria in the epidermis. For example, Blanpain et al.[86] showed that within the bulge there are two distinct populations, one of which maintains basal lamina contact and temporally precedes the other, which is suprabasal and arises only after the start of the first postnatal hair cycle. This spatial distinction endows them with discrete transcriptional programs; surprisingly, however, both populations are growth inhibited in the niche, yet can self-renew in vitro and make epidermis and hair when grafted. These findings suggest that the niche microenvironment imposes intrinsic "stemness" features without restricting the establishment of epithelial polarity and changes in gene expression.

The abrupt change in proliferative and biochemical properties when cells exit the bulge as reported in the aforementioned studies from the Fuchs group is consistent with the notion of a distinct stem cell niche in the bulge.[2,61,86] What are the signals that may help to define this niche and what keeps bulge stem cells in a low cycling state but activates them to leave the niche? As just summarized, several different families of growth factors are differentially expressed in bulge cells enriched on the basis of the markers used. One particularly interesting family of candidate molecules is the Wnt family, which has been demonstrated to be involved in stem cell renewal.[87] Defining the mechanism of action of Wnt signaling in epidermal stem cell maintenance in the context of the surrounding microenvironment and determining how this signal may integrate with other niche-derived signals represents the next challenge in epidermal stem cell biology. Regulating these signaling pathways might pave the way for the regeneration of damaged epithelia by stimulating stem cell function and inducing rapid expansion of progenitor cells in tissue regeneration.

Skin and Regenerative Medicine

One successful approach for the treatment of epidermal dysfunction is cellular transplantation, built on the techniques pioneered by Green and colleagues[88,89] more than two decades ago for culturing committed epidermal cells. In this approach, bioengineered skin substitutes created by culturing living cell sheets of human epidermal keratinocytes together with dermal fibroblasts[90-93] have been used successfully, for example, to promote the healing of chronic skin ulcers and to cover full-thickness burns. Although this process allows the replacement of nonfunctional or lost epidermal cells and scar tissue with fully functional epidermal cells, resolving the immediate problem of skin failure (namely, barrier function),[94] its utility has been rather limited.[92] Such problems as: i) lack of long-term integration, ii) incomplete healing/generation of scar tissue, iii) lack of regenerative potential, iv) inadequate appendage contribution, and v) overt rejection, have plagued the approach. Problems are further exacerbated by infection as well as the development of hyperproliferative disorders as a consequence of the immunosuppressive treatments used for modulating rejection. It is also not yet entirely clear what the cellular composition of the grafts is, but likely they comprise heterogeneous and not well-controlled mixtures of already committed mature epidermal cells as well as some progenitors and very few putative stem cells. This may contribute to many of the problems seen, including the lack of long-term regenerative potential, because it seems unlikely that the limited stem cells present would be able to home and reconstitute a stem cell in the disrupted or missing microenvironment of injured areas. Thus, much pressure remains to develop alternative stem cell-based epidermal transplant approaches.

Sources and Potential Usefulness of Stem Cells in Regenerative Medicine

Based on developments in stem cell biology over the last few years, there exist three principal sources of stem cells capable of generating organ-specific cell types: i) ES cells, ii) adult stem cells isolated from the target organ, and iii) adult stem cells from other organs.[95-98] ES cells of the mammalian blastocyst give rise to all the tissue lineages that begin to emerge at gastrulation and they can be propagated in vitro without loss of pluripotency. Many adult tissues also contain adult stem cells, which serve as self-renewing stem cells whose normal fate is to regenerate tissue-specific cells, in response to either physiological cell turnover or damage inflicted by injury or disease. In some cases, adult stem cells thought to be tissue-specific may possess plasticity or developmental potency far greater than their normal lineage-restricted fate (e.g., bone marrow-derived stem cells). The growth potential and pluripotency of ES cells and the developmental plasticity of adult stem cells make them potentially useful for replacing tissues (via transplantation or construction of bioartificial tissues) that either do not regenerate naturally or are damaged beyond their natural capability for regeneration. In addition to these two ways of replacing tissue, a third strategy of regenerative medicine is to stimulate regeneration in vivo from resident stem cells. Thus, the regeneration of epidermal cells can, theoretically, involve ES cells, adult epidermal stem cells, or adult stem cells (including from bone marrow).

ES Cells

The ability to generate differentiated epidermal progeny from a continuously growing stem cell population in vitro would provide a unique system for the study of stem cell/very early progenitor potential.[99] It would also make possible a comprehensive analysis of the underlying molecular mechanisms for the onset of embryonic epidermal commitment and differentiation. In fact, similar in vitro approaches have yielded invaluable information on the mechanism of differentiation of other cell types. In the past, several attempts have been made to conduct similar studies on epidermal differentiation[100,101] (for review, see ref. 102). However, the difficulties encountered in stably maintaining the putative stem cell population in culture limited the usefulness of these systems. Indeed, until recently, even the maintenance of mature epithelial cells in culture has been problematic[103] (for review, see ref. 104).

ES cells have been shown to provide excellent model systems in which to study lineage commitment and progression in vitro. ES cells were initially isolated from mice and more recently from monkeys and humans[105-107] and can be maintained in culture under appropriate conditions in an undifferentiated state, theoretically indefinitely. A switch in culture conditions to induce embryoid body formation (aggregation) leads to spontaneous differentiation; depending on the conditions and factors to which they are exposed, cells representative of all three germ layers can occur. The use of mouse ES cell culture models and more recently human-derived

ES cells has revealed invaluable information concerning the commitment of stem cells to various lineages,[108] including neurons,[109] cardiomyocytes,[110,111] adipocytes[112] as well as osteoclast,[113] epidermal,[114] and hair follicle[115] cells. Compared with certain other lineages, the use of ES cells for studies of the epidermal lineage has been relatively slow to advance. However, studies from three independent groups[13,18,116–118] have indicated that mouse ES cells have the potential to be directed robustly along the epidermal lineage. The protocols for derivation of epidermal cells from murine ES cells were based on exposing ES cells to in vivo-like conditions, including extracellular matrix[13] and bone morphogenetic protein-4 signaling,[119] conditions known to be required for ectodermal lineage commitment.

Proliferating keratinocytes in culture have the ability to undergo terminal differentiation as revealed by the expression of differentiation markers important for the generation, maturation, and maintenance of differentiated epidermal cells (i.e., keratinocytes and hair follicle cells), ultimately forming an epidermis-like tissue. An obvious issue is whether very early multi- or bipotential progenitors can be identified and expanded. In a recent study, the existence of bipotential progenitors expressing K17 has been reported.[118,120] ES-derived epidermal progenitor cells cultured at high density have also been induced to a hair follicle-like phenotype accompanied by the up-regulation of structural hair-cell proteins (keratins and terminal differentiation markers, suggesting that these cultures may indeed contain bipotential or putative epidermal stem cells. However, conditions to generate the sebaceous gland lineage remain to be established.

The ability of stimulated ES cells to produce a stratified epidermal tissue was assayed in an organotypic culture model in which cells were cultured on a cell-free inert filter substrata at the air–liquid interface.[119] Histologic and indirect immunofluorescent staining revealed an artificial skin quite similar to that of mice, in which both epidermal and dermal compartments were formed. In addition, the spatial distribution of differentiation markers was consistent with that seen in vivo with: i) basal cells expressing K14, ii) a basement membrane containing collagen IV and VII, as well as laminin-1, β-integrin, α6 β4, fibronectin, and nidogen,[119] and iii) K1-expressing cells in the suprabasal layer.[119] In all cases reported to date, K14-positive basal epidermal-like cells developed. Importantly, the derived cells function as bone fide early epidermal cells, following lineage progression and exhibiting appropriate markers in a temporal manner; in addition, a subpopulation of these cells retain progenitor characteristics, with the potential to generate epidermal cells in vitro. These studies support the notion that ES cell-derived epidermal stem and/or progenitor cells can be generated and can respond to cues in their local environment to undergo terminal differentiation, faithfully mimicking the developmental program observed in vivo. Although the mouse epidermis is far different than injured or diseased mammalian epidermis, nevertheless, these results are the first successful approach using ES cell-derived epidermal cells to generate epidermis and follow the differentiation program in vitro.

These initial studies convincingly demonstrate the potential of ES cells to commit and differentiate along the epidermal lineage in vitro; however, there remains a considerable amount of work to do to define the conditions necessary to support the generation and expansion of a homogeneous population of ES, progenitor, or even relatively mature cells in vitro. This is crucial because any remaining undifferentiated ES cells injected into an organism have a high capacity for teratoma formation.[121] There are also other challenges to consider; for example, because the dynamics of the in vivo setting are unknown, transplantation of predifferentiated cells (such as epidermal and hair follicle lineage cells) into the hair follicle could act to destabilize the differentiation milieu and lead to defects. Thus, among the technical challenges is the need to improve protocols by which ES cells can be induced to differentiate in a much more directed manner to specific lineages and developmental stages. Developmental studies indicate that several factors alone and/or in combination may be involved in differentiation along the epidermal lineage. These include epidermal growth factor, FGF-2, TGF-β1, platelet-derived growth factor, retinoic acid, vitamin C, as well as a number transcription factors (i.e., KLF-4 and GATA-4).[44,122–124] The one-step coculture protocol recently developed by our laboratory should aid in identifying conditions that support a more efficient and highly enriched culture of ES cell-derived epidermal progenitor cells with controlled progression along the epidermal lineage. The use of growth factors individually in a sequential manner or in combination may provide the conditions needed to enrich and expand epidermal stem and progenitor cells in vitro.

As discussed above, currently there are no markers that can be reliably used in the purification of a homogeneous population of epidermal stem cells. However, one approach to enrich very early progenitor cells in the absence of appropriate markers is to isolate cells using cell-marker/separation techniques. The key to this process is to use a specific marker for the epidermal lineage that is ideally able to distinguish (for instance) hair follicle cells from other epidermal cells. One such method might involve the transfection of ES cells with a fusion gene of a K15 (an adult stem cell marker[77]) or a K17 (a bipotential early progenitor marker[120]) promoter linked to a cDNA encoding aminoglycoside phosphotransferase and an antibiotic resistance gene. After differentiation, antibiotic selection of cells of the epidermal lineage is possible, generating a relatively pure epidermal sample (approximately 99%). To date, this cell-marker/separation technique has been used successfully with an αMHC promoter in the muscle lineage[95,125] as well as with the 2'3'-cyclic nucleotide 3'-phosphodiesterase (CNP) promoter in the oligodendrocyte progenitors.[126] Of course, the ultimate utility of these approaches for regenerative medicine in a clinical setting will require the development of protocols for human ES cells, including the demonstration of the potential, feasibility, and success of human ES cell-derived epidermis formation in vivo.

Recent success in the generation of a number of established human ES cell lines has raised great promise for stem cell and regenerative biology[106,127–129]; however, their isolation and proposed studies thereafter generated a highly controversial social debate of legal and ethical implications. Despite controversy, some studies with human ES cells are underway, although protocols for maintaining undifferentiated cells and controlled differentiation have not been easily achieved. Initial conditions to generate and maintain human ES cells were based on the use of mouse fibroblasts as feeders,[129] a less than ideal protocol for clinical consideration. Some human ES cell lines have been shown to remain undifferentiated when grown in the presence of either human fetal fibroblasts, adult human epithelial cells, foreskin cells, or a matrigel/laminin matrix in medium conditioned by MEFs.[130–132] Unfortunately, these protocols too will be problematic for regulatory agencies.

Adult Epidermal Stem Cells

As summarized, recent advances in identifying adult mouse epidermal stem cells in the hair follicle bulge have generated excitement on the possibility of this adult stem cell source. Of course, the race is on to isolate the human equivalent of these mouse cells. In this regard, one of the most interesting corollaries to the potential clinical use of adult hair follicle stem cells for hair growth is their additional potential as a cell source for other clinically important cellular therapies (e.g., epidermal and hair regeneration in burn patients). Recent studies indicated that the bulge region, as predicted earlier, contains multipotential stem cells that have the potential to contribute to all three lineages of the epidermis. Protocols to isolate, expand, and direct differentiation of human adult epidermal stem cells remain to be devised,[96] but the gene expression profiling done with isolated mouse cells gives some guidance as to potential markers and factors of interest.

Challenges and Summary

There are a number of advantages and disadvantages with the use of adult or ES cells for application in patients; however, for the therapeutic administration of human ES cells to be an option, the rejection of cells by the immune system will have to be addressed. Although the immune response should be less intense than the response to xenotransplants, the major histocompatibility complex differences between human ES cells and a recipient will require immunosuppression (e.g., ref. 133), the extent of which must be determined for the transplantation of cells into the epidermis. It is conceivable that stem cell-based therapy alone will not be the ultimate solution for the treatment of epidermal damage and loss of regeneration, and that therapies of the distant future might be a combination of stem cell transplantation, gene therapy, and drug treatment. Such a combination of therapies will be customized to the particular cellular ailment of the individual patient.

At this point, it is difficult to predict how stem cell-based therapy will be translated into clinical practice for epidermal tissues. Some of the limitations and potential issues regarding ES cell and adult stem cell plasticity have been discussed; nevertheless, the promise is real and basic science advances continue to spur new skin cell biology that holds promise for novel skin cell therapeutics.

Acknowledgments

The authors thank Dr. Jane Aubin for many stimulating discussions on stem cells over the years. Our work has been supported by a grant from the Canadian Institutes of Health Research (CIHR).

References

1. Fitzpatrick TBEA. Dermatology in General Medicine. 4th ed. New York: McGraw-Hill; 1993.
2. Fuchs E, Tumbar T, Guasch G. Socializing with the neighbors: stem cells and their niche. Cell 2004;116(6):769–778.
3. Hanson J. The histiogenesis of the epidermis in the rat and mouse. J Anat 1947;81:174–197.
4. Chang C, Hemmati-Brivanlou A. Cell fate determination in embryonic ectoderm. J Neurobiol 1998;36(2):128–151.
5. Coulombe PA, Kopan R, Fuchs E. Expression of keratin K14 in the epidermis and hair follicle: insights into complex programs of differentiation. J Cell Biol 1989;109(5):2295–2312.
6. Kopan R, Fuchs E. A new look into an old problem: keratins as tools to investigate determination, morphogenesis, and differentiation in skin. Genes Dev 1989;3(1):1–15.
7. Byrne C, Tainsky M, Fuchs E. Programming gene expression in developing epidermis. Development 1994;120(9):2369–2383.
8. Elias PM, Feingold KR. Coordinate regulation of epidermal differentiation and barrier homeostasis. Skin Pharmacol Appl Skin Physiol 2001;14(suppl 1):28–34.
9. Elias PM, Menon GK. Structural and lipid biochemical correlates of the epidermal permeability barrier. Adv Lipid Res 1991;24:1–26.
10. Hardman MJ, Sisi P, Banbury DN, Byrne C. Patterned acquisition of skin barrier function during development. Development 1998;125(8):1541–1552.
11. Kalinin AE, Kajava AV, Steinert PM. Epithelial barrier function: assembly and structural features of the cornified cell envelope. Bioessays 2002;24(9):789–800.
12. Turksen K, Troy TC. Permeability barrier dysfunction in transgenic mice overexpressing claudin 6. Development 2002;129(7):1775–1784.
13. Turksen K, Troy TC. Epidermal cell lineage. Biochem Cell Biol 1998;76(6):889–898.
14. Fuchs E. Epidermal differentiation: the bare essentials. J Cell Biol 1990;111(6 pt 2):2807–2814.
15. Fuchs E. Epidermal differentiation. Curr Opin Cell Biol 1990;2(6):1028–1035.
16. Byrne C. Regulation of gene expression in developing epidermal epithelia. Bioessays 1997;19(8):691–698.
17. Turksen K, Troy TC. Overexpression of the calcium sensing receptor accelerates epidermal differentiation and permeability barrier formation in vivo. Mech Dev 2003;120(6):733–744.
18. Troy TC, Turksen K. In vitro characteristics of early epidermal progenitors isolated from keratin 14 (K14)-deficient mice: insights into the role of keratin 17 in mouse keratinocytes. J Cell Physiol 1999;180(3): 409–421.
19. Presland RB, Dale BA. Epithelial structural proteins of the skin and oral cavity: function in health and disease. Crit Rev Oral Biol Med 2000;11(4):383–408.
20. Cabral A, Voskamp P, Cleton-Jansen AM, South A, Nizetic D, Backendorf C. Structural organization and regulation of the small proline-rich family of cornified envelope precursors suggest a role in adaptive barrier function. J Biol Chem 2001;276(22):19231–19237.
21. Song HJ, Poy G, Darwiche N, et al. Mouse Sprr2 genes: a clustered family of genes showing differential expression in epithelial tissues. Genomics 1999;55(1): 28–42.
22. Hohl D, Mehrel T, Lichti U, Turner ML, Roop DR, Steinert PM. Characterization of human loricrin. Structure and function of a new class of epidermal cell envelope proteins. J Biol Chem 1991;266(10): 6626–6636.
23. Darmstadt GL, Dinulos JG. Neonatal skin care. Pediatr Clin North Am 2000;47(4):757–782.
24. Maatta A, DiColandrea T, Groot K, Watt FM. Gene targeting of envoplakin, a cytoskeletal linker protein and precursor of the epidermal cornified envelope. Mol Cell Biol 2001;21(20):7047–7053.
25. Nakane H, Ishida-Yamamoto A, Takahashi H, Iizuka H. Elafin, a secretory protein, is cross-linked into the cornified cell envelopes from the inside of psoriatic keratinocytes. J Invest Dermatol 2002;119(1):50–55.
26. Champliaud MF, Baden HP, Koch M, Jin W, Burgeson RE, Viel A. Gene characterization of sciellin (SCEL) and protein localization in vertebrate epithelia displaying barrier properties. Genomics 2000;70(2): 264–268.
27. Marshall D, Hardman MJ, Nield KM, Byrne C. Differentially expressed late constituents of the epidermal cornified envelope. Proc Natl Acad Sci USA 2001;98(23):13031–13036.
28. Kalinin A, Marekov LN, Steinert PM. Assembly of the epidermal cornified cell envelope. J Cell Sci 2001;114(pt 17):3069–3070.
29. Hohl D. Cornified cell envelope. Dermatologica 1990;180(4):201–211.
30. Downing DT. Lipid and protein structures in the permeability barrier of mammalian epidermis. J Lipid Res 1992;33(3):301–313.
31. Roop D. Defects in the barrier. Science 1995;267(5197): 474–475.
32. Steinert PM. The complexity and redundancy of epithelial barrier function. J Cell Biol 2000;151(2): F5–8.
33. Steinert PM, Marekov LN. Initiation of assembly of the cell envelope barrier structure of stratified squamous epithelia. Mol Biol Cell 1999;10(12):4247–4261.

34. Menon GK, Feingold KR, Elias PM. Lamellar body secretory response to barrier disruption. J Invest Dermatol 1992;98(3):279–289.
35. Aszterbaum M, Menon GK, Feingold KR, Williams ML. Ontogeny of the epidermal barrier to water loss in the rat: correlation of function with stratum corneum structure and lipid content. Pediatr Res 1992;31 (4 pt 1):308–317.
36. Wilson DR, Maibach HI. Transepidermal water loss in vivo. Premature and term infants. Biol Neonate 1980;37(3–4):180–185.
37. Sengel P. Pattern formation in skin development. Int J Dev Biol 1990;34(1):33–50.
38. Byrne C, Hardman M, Nield K. Covering the limb: formation of the integument. J Anat 2003;202(1): 113–123.
39. Merrill BJ, Gat U, DasGupta R, Fuchs E. Tcf3 and Lef1 regulate lineage differentiation of multipotent stem cells in skin. Genes Dev 2001;15(13):1688–1705.
40. Honeycutt KA, Koster MI, Roop DR. Genes involved in stem cell fate decisions and commitment to differentiation play a role in skin disease. J Investig Dermatol Symp Proc 2004;9(3):261–268.
41. Gandarillas A, Watt FM. c-Myc promotes differentiation of human epidermal stem cells. Genes Dev 1997;11(21):2869–2882.
42. Arnold I, Watt FM. c-Myc activation in transgenic mouse epidermis results in mobilization of stem cells and differentiation of their progeny. Curr Biol 2001;11(8):558–568.
43. Waikel RL, Kawachi Y, Waikel PA, Wang XJ, Roop DR. Deregulated expression of c-Myc depletes epidermal stem cells. Nat Genet 2001;28(2):165–168.
44. Kaufman CK, Zhou P, Pasolli HA, et al. GATA-3: an unexpected regulator of cell lineage determination in skin. Genes Dev 2003;17(17):2108–2122.
45. Lee D, Prowse DM, Brissette JL. Association between mouse nude gene expression and the initiation of epithelial terminal differentiation. Dev Biol 1999; 208(2):362–374.
46. Janes SM, Ofstad TA, Campbell DH, Watt FM, Prowse DM. Transient activation of FOXN1 in keratinocytes induces a transcriptional programme that promotes terminal differentiation: contrasting roles of FOXN1 and Akt. J Cell Sci 2004;117(pt 18):4157–4168.
47. Yamamoto N, Tanigaki K, Han H, Hiai H, Honjo T. Notch/RBP-J signaling regulates epidermis/hair fate determination of hair follicular stem cells. Curr Biol 2003;13(4):333–338.
48. Reddy ST, Andl T, Lu MM, Morrisey EE, Millar SE. Expression of Frizzled genes in developing and postnatal hair follicles. J Invest Dermatol 2004;123(2): 275–282.
49. Lowell S, Jones P, Le Roux I, Dunne J, Watt FM. Stimulation of human epidermal differentiation by delta-notch signalling at the boundaries of stem-cell clusters. Curr Biol 2000;10(9):491–500.
50. Morgan BA, Orkin RW, Noramly S, Perez A. Stage-specific effects of sonic hedgehog expression in the epidermis. Dev Biol 1998;201(1):1–12.
51. Petiot A, Conti FJ, Grose R, Revest JM, Hodivala-Dilke KM, Dickson C. A crucial role for Fgfr2-IIIb signalling in epidermal development and hair follicle patterning. Development 2003;130(22):5493–5501.
52. Kobielak K, Pasolli HA, Alonso L, Polak L, Fuchs E. Defining BMP functions in the hair follicle by conditional ablation of BMP receptor IA. J Cell Biol 2003;163(3):609–623.
53. Andl T, Ahn K, Kairo A, et al. Epithelial Bmpr1a regulates differentiation and proliferation in postnatal hair follicles and is essential for tooth development. Development 2004;131(10):2257–2268.
54. Lajtha LG. Stem cell concepts. Differentiation 1979; 14(1–2):23–34.
55. Alonso L, Fuchs E. Stem cells of the skin epithelium. Proc Natl Acad Sci USA 2003;100(suppl 1):11830–11835.
56. Weissman IL. Stem cells: units of development, units of regeneration, and units in evolution. Cell 2000; 100(1):157–168.
57. Weissman IL, Anderson DJ, Gage F. Stem and progenitor cells: origins, phenotypes, lineage commitments, and transdifferentiations. Annu Rev Cell Dev Biol 2001;17:387–403.
58. Cotsarelis G, Cheng SZ, Dong G, Sun TT, Lavker RM. Existence of slow-cycling limbal epithelial basal cells that can be preferentially stimulated to proliferate: implications on epithelial stem cells. Cell 1989;57(2): 201–209.
59. Braun KM, Watt FM. Epidermal label-retaining cells: background and recent applications. J Investig Dermatol Symp Proc 2004;9(3):196–201.
60. Rochat A, Kobayashi K, Barrandon Y. Location of stem cells of human hair follicles by clonal analysis. Cell 1994;76(6):1063–1073.
61. Tumbar T, Guasch G, Greco V, et al. Defining the epithelial stem cell niche in skin. Science 2004;303(5656): 359–363.
62. Watt FM. The stem cell compartment in human interfollicular epidermis. J Dermatol Sci 2002;28(3):173–180.
63. Jones PH. Epithelial stem cells. Bioessays 1997;19(8): 683–690.
64. Jones PH, Harper S, Watt FM. Stem cell patterning and fate in human epidermis. Cell 1995;80(1):83–93.
65. Commo S, Gaillard O, Bernard BA. The human hair follicle contains two distinct K19 positive compartments in the outer root sheath: a unifying hypothesis for stem cell reservoir? Differentiation 2000;66(4–5): 157–164.
66. Michel M, Torok N, Godbout MJ, et al. Keratin 19 as a biochemical marker of skin stem cells in vivo and in vitro: keratin 19 expressing cells are differentially localized in function of anatomic sites, and their number varies with donor age and culture stage. J Cell Sci 1996;109(pt 5):1017–1028.
67. Ghali L, et al. Epidermal and hair follicle progenitor cells express melanoma-associated chondroitin sulfate proteoglycan core protein. J Invest Dermatol 2004;122(2):433–442.
68. Waseem A, Dogan B, Tidman N, et al. Keratin 15 expression in stratified epithelia: downregulation in activated keratinocytes. J Invest Dermatol 1999;112(3): 362–369.
69. Pellegrini G, Dellambra E, Golisano O, et al. p63 identifies keratinocyte stem cells. Proc Natl Acad Sci USA 2001;98(6):3156–3161.
70. Trempus CS, Morris RJ, Bortner CD, et al. Enrichment for living murine keratinocytes from the hair follicle bulge with the cell surface marker CD34. J Invest Dermatol 2003;120(4):501–511.
71. Li L, Mignone J, Yang M, et al. Nestin expression in hair follicle sheath progenitor cells. Proc Natl Acad Sci USA 2003;100(17):9958–9961.

72. Watt FM. Role of integrins in regulating epidermal adhesion, growth and differentiation. Embo J 2002; 21(15):3919–3926.
73. Jones PH, Watt FM. Separation of human epidermal stem cells from transit amplifying cells on the basis of differences in integrin function and expression. Cell 1993;73(4):713–724.
74. Tani H, Morris RJ, Kaur P. Enrichment for murine keratinocyte stem cells based on cell surface phenotype. Proc Natl Acad Sci USA 2000;97(20):10960–10965.
75. Whitbread LA, Powell BC. Expression of the intermediate filament keratin gene, K15, in the basal cell layers of epithelia and the hair follicle. Exp Cell Res 1998; 244(2):448–459.
76. Lyle S, Christofidou-Solomidou M, Liu Y, Elder DE, Albelda S, Cotsarelis G. The C8/144B monoclonal antibody recognizes cytokeratin 15 and defines the location of human hair follicle stem cells. J Cell Sci 1998;111(pt 21):3179–3188.
77. Liu Y, Lyle S, Yang Z, Cotsarelis G. Keratin 15 promoter targets putative epithelial stem cells in the hair follicle bulge. J Invest Dermatol 2003;121(5):963–968.
78. Triel C, Vestergaard ME, Bolund L, Jensen TG, Jensen UB. Side population cells in human and mouse epidermis lack stem cell characteristics. Exp Cell Res 2004;295(1):79–90.
79. Terunuma A, Jackson KL, Kapoor V, Telford WG, Vogel JC. Side population keratinocytes resembling bone marrow side population stem cells are distinct from label-retaining keratinocyte stem cells. J Invest Dermatol 2003;121(5):1095–1103.
80. Morris RJ, Liu Y, Marles L, et al. Capturing and profiling adult hair follicle stem cells. Nat Biotechnol 2004;22(4):411–417.
81. Taylor G, Nakamura H, Katata T, et al. Involvement of follicular stem cells in forming not only the follicle but also the epidermis. Cell 2000;102(4):451–461.
82. Oshima H, Rochat A, Kedzia C, Kobayashi K, Barrandon Y. Morphogenesis and renewal of hair follicles from adult multipotent stem cells. Cell 2001;104(2):233–245.
83. Ghazizadeh S, Taichman LB. Multiple classes of stem cells in cutaneous epithelium: a lineage analysis of adult mouse skin. Embo J 2001;20(6):1215–1222.
84. Cai J, Weiss ML, Rao MS. In search of "stemness." Exp Hematol 2004;32(7):585–598.
85. Spradling A, Drummond-Barbosa D, Kai T. Stem cells find their niche. Nature 2001;414(6859):98–104.
86. Blanpain C, Lowry WE, Geoghegan A, Polak L, Fuchs E. Self-renewal, multipotency, and the existence of two cell populations within an epithelial stem cell niche. Cell 2004;118(5):635–648.
87. Rattis FM, Voermans C, Reya T. Wnt signaling in the stem cell niche. Curr Opin Hematol 2004;11(2):88–94.
88. Green H, Kehinde O, Thomas J. Growth of cultured human epidermal cells into multiple epithelia suitable for grafting. Proc Natl Acad Sci USA 1979;76(11): 5665–5668.
89. Banks-Schlegel S, Green H. Formation of epidermis by serially cultivated human epidermal cells transplanted as an epithelium to athymic mice. Transplantation 1980;29(4):308–313.
90. Langer R, Vacanti JP. Tissue engineering. Science 1993;260(5110):920–926.
91. Parenteau NL, Nolte CM, Bilbo P, et al. Epidermis generated in vitro: practical considerations and applications. J Cell Biochem 1991;45(3):245–251.
92. Tabata Y. Recent progress in tissue engineering. Drug Discov Today 2001;6(9):483–487.
93. De SK, Reis ED, Kerstein MD. Wound treatment with human skin equivalent. J Am Podiatr Med Assoc 2002;92(1):19–23.
94. Ehrlich HP. Understanding experimental biology of skin equivalent: from laboratory to clinical use in patients with burns and chronic wounds. Am J Surg 2004;187(5A):29S–33S.
95. Strom TB, Field LJ, Ruediger M. Allogeneic stem cells, clinical transplantation and the origins of regenerative medicine. Curr Opin Immunol 2002;14(5): 601–605.
96. Verfaillie CM. Adult stem cells assessing the case for pluripotency. Trends Cell Biol 2002;12(11):502–508.
97. Passier R, Mummery C. Origin and use of embryonic and adult stem cells in differentiation and tissue repair. Cardiovasc Res 2003;58(2):324–335.
98. Hedrick MH, Daniels EJ. The use of adult stem cells in regenerative medicine. Clin Plast Surg 2003;30(4): 499–505.
99. Hall PA, Watt FM. Stem cells: the generation and maintenance of cellular diversity. Development 1989;106(4): 619–633.
100. Potten CS, Morris RJ. Epithelial stem cells in vivo. J Cell Sci Suppl 1988;10:45–62.
101. Barrandon Y, Green H. Cell size as a determinant of the clone-forming ability of human keratinocytes. Proc Natl Acad Sci USA 1985;82(16):5390–5394.
102. Morris RJ, Potten CS. Slowly cycling (label-retaining) epidermal cells behave like clonogenic stem cells in vitro. Cell Prolif 1994;27(5):279–289.
103. Green H. Terminal differentiation of cultured human epidermal cells. Cell 1977;11(2):405–416.
104. Rheinwald JG. Human epidermal keratinocyte cell culture and xenograft systems: applications in the detection of potential chemical carcinogens and the study of epidermal transformation. Prog Clin Biol Res 1989;298:113–125.
105. Evans MJ, Kaufman MH. Establishment in culture of pluripotential cells from mouse embryos. Nature 1981;292(5819):154–156.
106. Thomson JA, Itskovitz-Eldor J, Shapiro SS, et al. Embryonic stem cell lines derived from human blastocysts. Science 1998;282(5391):1145–1147.
107. Reubinoff BE, Pera MF, Fong CY, Trounson A, Bongso A. Embryonic stem cell lines from human blastocysts: somatic differentiation in vitro. Nat Biotechnol 2000;18(4):399–404.
108. Turksen K. Embryonic stem cells, methods and protocols. In: Walker J, ed. Methods in Molecular Biology. Vol 185. Totowa, NJ: Humana Press; 2002.
109. Otero JJ, Fu W, Kan L, Cuadra AE, Kessler JA. Beta-catenin signaling is required for neural differentiation of embryonic stem cells. Development 2004;131(15): 3545–3557.
110. Zandstra PW, Bauwens C, Yin T, et al. Scalable production of embryonic stem cell-derived cardiomyocytes. Tissue Eng 2003;9(4):767–778.
111. Pasumarthi KB, Field LJ. Cardiomyocyte enrichment in differentiating ES cell cultures: strategies and applications. Methods Mol Biol 2002;185:157–168.
112. Dani C. Differentiation of embryonic stem cells as a model to study gene function during the development of adipose cells. Methods Mol Biol 2002;185: 107–116.

113. Yamane T, Kunisada T, Hayashi S. Embryonic stem cells as a model for studying osteoclast lineage development. Methods Mol Biol 2002;185:97–106.
114. Troy TC, Turksen K. Epidermal lineage. Methods Mol Biol 2002;185:229–253.
115. Troy TC, Turksen K. ES cell differentiation into the hair follicle lineage in vitro. Methods Mol Biol 2002;185:255–260.
116. Bagutti C, Wobus AM, Fassler R, Watt FM. Differentiation of embryonal stem cells into keratinocytes: comparison of wild-type and beta 1 integrin-deficient cells. Dev Biol 1996;179(1):184–196.
117. Aberdam D. Derivation of keratinocyte progenitor cells and skin formation from embryonic stem cells. Int J Dev Biol 2004;48(2–3):203–206.
118. Troy TC, Turksen K. Commitment of embryonic stem cells to an epidermal cell fate and differentiation in vitro. Dev Dyn 2005;232(2):293–300.
119. Coraux C, Hilmi C, Rouleau M, et al. Reconstituted skin from murine embryonic stem cells. Curr Biol 2003;13(10):849–853.
120. McGowan KM, Coulombe PA. Onset of keratin 17 expression coincides with the definition of major epithelial lineages during skin development. J Cell Biol 1998;143(2):469–486.
121. Yanai J, Doetchman T, Laufer N, et al. Embryonic cultures but not embryos transplanted to the mouse's brain grow rapidly without immunosuppression. Int J Neurosci 1995;81(1–2):21–26.
122. Peus D, Pittelkow MR. Growth factors in hair organ development and the hair growth cycle. Dermatol Clin 1996;14(4):559–572.
123. Li AG, Koster MI, Wang XJ. Roles of TGFbeta signaling in epidermal/appendage development. Cytokine Growth Factor Rev 2003;14(2):99–111.
124. Segre J. Complex redundancy to build a simple epidermal permeability barrier. Curr Opin Cell Biol 2003;15(6):776–782.
125. Klug MG, Soonpaa MH, Koh GY, Field LJ. Genetically selected cardiomyocytes from differentiating embronic stem cells form stable intracardiac grafts. J Clin Invest 1996;98(1):216–224.
126. Glaser T, Perez-Bouza A, Klein K, Brustle O. Generation of purified oligodendrocyte progenitors from embryonic stem cells. FASEB J 2005;19(1):112–114.
127. Pera MF, Filipczyk AA, Hawes SM, Laslett AL. Isolation, characterization, and differentiation of human embryonic stem cells. Methods Enzymol 2003;365:429–446.
128. Draper JS, Moore HD, Ruban LN, Gokhale PJ, Andrews PW. Culture and characterization of human embryonic stem cells. Stem Cells Dev 2004;13(4):325–336.
129. Reubinoff BE, Itsykson P, Turetsky T, et al. Neural progenitors from human embryonic stem cells. Nat Biotechnol 2001;19(12):1134–1140.
130. Xu C, Inokuma MS, Denham J, et al. Feeder-free growth of undifferentiated human embryonic stem cells. Nat Biotechnol 2001;19(10):971–974.
131. Richards M, Fong CY, Chan WK, Wong PC, Bongso A. Human feeders support prolonged undifferentiated growth of human inner cell masses and embryonic stem cells. Nat Biotechnol 2002;20(9):933–936.
132. Amit M, Margulets V, Segev H, et al. Human feeder layers for human embryonic stem cells. Biol Reprod 2003;68(6):2150–2156.
133. Drukker M. Immunogenicity of human embryonic stem cells: can we achieve tolerance? Springer Semin Immunopathol 2004;26(1–2):201–213.

Index

A

AADC. *See* Amino acid decarboxylase
AAV. *See* Adeno-associated viruses
Aborted embryos
　ethical debate regarding, 82–83
　somatic stem cells in, 210
Acellular tissue matrices
　bladder tissue engineering with, 226
　skin substitutes and, 384–385
Achilles' tendon, 164
ACT. *See* Autologous chondrocyte transplantation
Acute lymphoblastic leukemia
　CBT and, 340
　haploidentical SCT and, 366
　NST and, 357
Acute myeloid leukemia (AML), 366
Acute myocardial infarction (AMI)
　incidence of, 18
　mortality of, 18
　myocardial ischemia and, 27
Acute renal failure, 220
Acute stroke. *See* Stroke
Acute tubular necrosis
　kidney regeneration and, 212
　renal cell replacement and, 220
AD. *See* Alzheimer's disease
Adam, 156
ADAS. *See* Adipose-derived adult stromal cells
Adeno-associated viruses (AAV)
　characteristics of, 136
　gene delivery with, 137–138
Adenoviruses
　characteristics of, 136
　gene delivery with, 137
Adipose-derived adult stromal cells (ADAS), 163
Adipose tissue, 163
Adult neural stem (ANS) cells, 263–264
Adult stem cells
　myocardial tissue repair with, 17–29
　　AMI and, 18
　　ischemic heart disease and, 17–18
　　mechanisms of, 18–19
　PD and, 112–117
　plasticity of, 113
Age-related macular degeneration (AMD), 234

　blindness and, 238
　RPE transplantation and, 271
Aggrecan
　cartilage homeostasis and, 181
　cartilage structure and, 180
Alemtuzumab
　NST and
　　GVHD and, 355
　　reduced-intensity conditioning regimens of, 353
Alginate-gelatin-PEG scaffolds, 7
Alkylating agents, 353
Allogeneic hematopoietic stem cell transplantation (alloSCT), 332
Allograft rejection, 305–306
Allograft transplantation. *See* Organ transplantation
alloSCT. *See* Allogeneic hematopoietic stem cell transplantation
ALS. *See* Amyotrophic lateral sclerosis
ALV. *See* Avian leukosis virus
Alzheimer's disease (AD)
　gene therapy for, 134
　memantine for, 237
　tailored strategies for, 141–142
AMD. *See* Age-related macular degeneration
Amino acid decarboxylase (AADC), 98
Aminoguanidine, 240
AML. *See* Acute myeloid leukemia
Amniotic membrane (AM)
　basement membrane of, 292
　OSR and, 282
Amniotic membrane transplantation (AMT), 285–287
Amyotrophic lateral sclerosis (ALS)
　antioxidants and, 141
　gene therapy for, 134
　Riluzole for, 237
　tailored strategies for, 141
Angina pectoris
　prevalence of, 45
　therapeutic myocardial angiogenesis and, 45
Angiogenesis
　intracoronary cell injections and, 54
　therapeutic myocardial angiogenesis and, 45
ANS cells. *See* Adult neural stem cells
Anticholine esterase compounds, 141–142

Antigens, 254–255. *See also* Human leukocyte antigen
Antioxidant enzymes, 141
Antithymocyte globulin (ATG), 353
Apoptosis
  neuroprotective agents and, 243
  RGCs and, 237–238
  skin wound healing and, 381
  stroke and, 123
Arrhythmia
  myocardial tissue repair and, 20
  skeletal myoblasts and, 8
Arteriogenesis, 45
Ascorbate, 244
Aspartoacylase, 134
ATG. *See* Antithymocyte globulin
Atherosclerotic vascular disease, 45
Autoimmune T cells, 240
Autoimmunity, 253
  antigen-specific T cells and, 254–255
  mechanisms of, 254
  regulatory T cells and, 254
  self-compounds and, 254
Autologous articular chondrocytes, 169
Autologous chondrocyte implantation. *See* Autologous chondrocyte transplantation
Autologous chondrocyte transplantation (ACT)
  cartilage repair and, 184
  clinical research on, 174–176
  disadvantages of, 175–176
  durability of, 174
Autologous perichondrial graft, 184
Automatic defibrillator, 20, 26
Avian leukosis virus (ALV), 135

B

Barbiturates, 244
Basal cells, 282
Basal ganglia, 97
Basic fibroblast growth factor (bFGF), 11
Basic helix-loop-helix (bHLH) transcription factor, 267
β cells, 301–306
  derivation of
    BM cells and, 305
    intestine epithelial cells and, 304–305
    liver cells and, 303–304
    tissue stem cells and, 302–303
  diabetes and, 301
  forced expansion of, 301
  pancreas composition and, 298
  replacement of, 301
  transplantation of, 299
    autoimmune responses and, 305–306
    autologous v. allogeneic, 306
Beta-Glucuronidase, 134
Betaxolol, 240, 242
bFGF. *See* Basic fibroblast growth factor
bHLH transcription factor. *See* Basic helix-loop-helix transcription factor
Biglycan, 180

Bioceramics
  bone reconstruction with, 163
  hydroxyapatite and, 163
Biological pacemaker, 39
Biomaterials
  bladder tissue engineering and
    acellular tissue matrices and, 226
    naturally derived, 226
    synthetic polymers and, 226–227
  myocardial tissue engineering and, 6–7, 12
Biomimetics, 6
Bioreactors
  mechanical signals and, 9
  myocardial tissue engineering and, 9–10
  perfusion and, 9
  spinner flasks and, 9
  tendon repair and, 164–165
Black market, 82
Bladder replacement
  with gastrointestinal segments, 227
  tissue engineering and, 229
Bladder tissue engineering, 225–230
  biomaterials for
    acellular tissue matrices and, 226
    naturally derived, 226
    synthetic polymers and, 226–227
  bladder regeneration and, 227
  bladder replacement with, 229
  cell growth and, 225–226
  ex situ, 229
  stem cells for, 229
Blindness, 234
  causes of, 238
  limbal deficiency and, 284
BM-derived cells
  kidney regeneration and, 220
  types of, 305
BM-derived extrarenal tubular progenitor cells, 212
BM-derived mononuclear cells (BMNC)
  cardiac calcifications and, 8
  therapeutic myocardial angiogenesis and, 54
BM-derived MSCs
  BM cell types and, 305
  bone reconstruction with, 163
  cartilage repair with, 164
  harvest of, 160–161
  immunomodulatory role of, 165
  ligaments repair with, 164–165
  telomere length of, 161
  tendons repair with, 164–165
BMNC. *See* BM-derived mononuclear cells
BMP. *See* Bone morphogenetic proteins
BMSC. *See* Bone marrow stromal cells
BM. *See* Bone marrow
Bone marrow (BM)
  cell types in, 305
  MSCs derivation and, 159
  myocardial tissue repair and, 17
  regeneration vigor of, 156

Bone marrow stem cells
  insulin-producing β cells and, 305
  myocardial tissue engineering and, 4-5
  plasticity of, 210
  types of, 305
Bone marrow stromal cells (BMSC)
  BM cell types and, 305
  bone regeneration and, 197-198
  differentiation of
    dopaminergic lineages and, 102-103
    neural lineages and, 105
  PD and, 98
    gene manipulations and, 114-115
    risks with, 115
    in vitro differentiation and, 113-114
    in vivo differentiation and, 115
  plasticity mechanisms of, 116-117
  remyelination and, 79, 83
  stroke and, 126-127
Bone morphogenesis, 195-205
Bone morphogenetic proteins (BMP)
  bioassays and, 196
  bone regeneration and, 195-197
  cartilage engineering and, 173
  cartilage homeostasis and, 181-182
  cloning of, 196
  embryonic retinal progenitor cells and, 263
  list of, 196
  MSC derivation with, 162
  receptors of, 197
Bone reconstruction
  bioceramic scaffolds and, 163
  BM-derived MSCs and, 163
Bone regeneration, 195-200
  BMPs and, 195-197
  BMSCs and, 197-198
  challenges in, 198-200
  gene therapy and, 198
  morphogens and, 198
Brain-derived neurotrophic factor, 240
Brain tissue salvage, 124
Brimonidine, 240
Bulge stem cells, 397-398

C

CABG. See Coronary artery bypass graft
Cadaveric conjunctival limbal allograft (c-CLAL), 288-291
  allograft rejection and, 289
  bilateral disease and, 288
  cyclosporine and, 289
  keratoepithelioplasty and, 288
  KLAL and, 288
  LKP and, 288
  lr-CLAL and, 288
  OSR and, 285
  patient status and, 289-290
  tissue preparation for, 289
Canadian Cardiovascular Society (CCS), 46
Canavan's disease, 134

Caprolactone-co-L-lactide, 7
Cardiac calcifications, 8
Cardiac progenitor cells, 8
Cardiac regeneration ability, 3
Cardiac stem cell therapy, 2
Cardiac systolic function, 62-63
Cardiogenesis, 36
Cardiomyocytes
  ESC differentiation and, 34
  heart contents of, 40
  heart failure and, 60-61, 62-63
  myocardial tissue engineering and, 7
  myocardial tissue repair and, 19, 27
  myocardium composition and, 3
  porous alginate scaffolds and, 8
  proliferation of, 36
  structural properties of, 34-35
Cardiovascular tissue engineering, 2
  heart muscle cell source for, 3
  heart muscle creation and, 3
Cartilage, 179-189
  function of, 179-180
  homeostasis of, 181-182
  limb morphogenesis and, 182-184
  MSC differentiation and, 183
  repair of, 164
    surgical interventions for, 184
  self-healing ability of, 156, 169, 199
  structure of
    cartilaginous tissues in, 179
    ECM molecules in, 180
    osmotic pressure and, 180
    zonal organization in, 181
Cartilage-derived morphogenetic proteins (CDMP), 195
Cartilage engineering, 169-176, 184-189
  autologous chondrocyte transplantation for
    animal experiments of, 173-174
    cell implantation for, 171
    clinical research on, 174-175
    condensation for, 170
    disadvantages of, 175-176
    gene therapy for, 172
    growth factors for, 172-173
    harvest for, 169-170
    integration after, 171-172
    redifferentiation for, 170-171
    in vitro expansion for, 170
  MSCs and, 186-189
  OA and, 169
Catalase, 141
Cataracts, 238
CAU. See Conjunctival autograft
CBSC. See Cord blood stem cells
CB. See Cord blood
CBT. See Cord blood transplantation
c-CLAL. See Cadaveric conjunctival limbal allograft
CCS. See Canadian Cardiovascular Society
CEA. See Cultured epithelial autografts
CEallo. See Cultured epithelial allografts

Cell painting, 205
Central nervous system (CNS). *See also* Nervous system gene therapy
  diseases of, 72–73
  injuries to, 72
  NSCs in, 99
    adult brains and, 100, 106–107
    embryonic brains and, 99–100
  regeneration of, 72
Cerebellar Bergmann glia, 266
Chlamydia trachomatis, 281
Chondrocytes, 169
Chondrogenesis
  cell integration and, 171
  limb morphogenesis and, 182
Chondroprogenitors, 183–184
Chronic lymphocytic leukemia (CLL)
  immune sensitivity of, 357
  NST and, 356
Chronic myeloid leukemia (CML)
  GVL and, 357
  NST and, 356
Ciliary epithelium-derived stem cells, 264
Ciliary neurotrophic factor (CNTF)
  neurodegenerative disorders and, 134
  retinal repair and, 273–274
Cisplatin, 213
CLAU. *See* Conjunctival limbal autograft
CLL. *See* Chronic lymphocytic leukemia
Cloned cells
  myocardial tissue engineering and, 5
  pancreatic progenitor cell expansion and, 314–315
Cloning, 210
CML. *See* Chronic myeloid leukemia
CNS. *See* Central nervous system
CNS injury
  gene therapy for, 134
  regeneration after, 142
CNS regeneration, 251–255
  macrophages and
    implantation of, 251–252
    innate immune response of, 252
  protective autoimmunity and, 253
    antigen-specific T cells and, 254–255
    mechanisms of, 254
    regulatory T cells and, 254
    self-compounds and, 254
  T cells and
    adaptive immune response of, 252
    MBPs and, 252–253
CNS. *See* Central nervous system
CNTF. *See* Ciliary neurotrophic factor
Collagens
  bladder tissue engineering and, 226
  cartilage structure and, 180
  myocardium composition and, 3
  skin wound strength and, 380
Collagen scaffolds, 7
Collagen synthesis, 4

Collaterogenesis, 45
Computer-assisted design, 199
Congenital amegakaryocytic thrombocytopenia, 340
Conjunctival autograft (CAU), 285
Conjunctival limbal autograft (CLAU)
  OSR and, 285
  technique of, 287
Connexin 43
  heart failure therapy and, 63
  myocardial tissue repair and, 19–20
Contractile phenotype, 62, 64
Cop-1. *See* Copolymer-1
Copaxone, 240, 244
Copolymer-1 (Cop-1), 255
Coral scaffolds, 163
Cord blood (CB)
  banking of, 333
  collection of, 333
  cryopreservation of, 333–334
  SCT with, 333
Cord blood stem cells (CBSC)
  biological properties of, 335
  immune reconstitution of, 336
  SCT with, 333
Cord blood transplantation (CBT)
  adults and, 342–343
  CB banking and, 333
  CB collection and, 333
  CB cryopreservation and, 333–334
  cotransplantations and, 345
  disease transmission and, 335
  ethical issues in
    availability and, 334
    confidentiality and, 335
    consent and, 334
    donor-recipient relationship and, 334
    ownership and, 334
  haploidentical donors and, 345
  HLA typing and, 334
  intraosseous transplantations and, 345–346
  mortality rates in, 333
    strategies for reduction of, 343–345
  nonmalignant diseases and, 340–342
  reduced intensity transplantations and, 346–347
  related donors and, 336–338
  unrelated donors and
    cell count and, 339
    cell dose and, 338–339
    clinical trials on, 336–338
    engraftment and, 338
    GVHD and, 339
    HLA disparity and, 339
    relapse and, 340
    survival rates and, 339
    treatment-related mortality and, 339
Corneal epithelial stem cells, 282
Corneal epithelium
  ocular surface regeneration and, 282–283
  self-renewal of, 282

Corneal limbus, 283
Corneal opacities, 235
Corneal transplantation, 284
Coronary artery bypass graft (CABG)
    clinical studies of, 52–53
    therapeutic myocardial angiogenesis and, 51
Corticosteroids, 240, 241
Creatinine, 218
Crude bone marrow, 5
Crude bone marrow mononuclear cells, 8
Cultured epithelial allografts (CEallo), 384
Cultured epithelial autografts (CEA)
    delivery time of, 383–384
    persistence of, 383
Cyclophosphamide, 352–353
Cyclosporine A, 289
Cyst fluid, 218
Cystic fibrosis, 133
Cytokines, 5
Cytomegalovirus
    haploidentical SCT and, 362
    immune reconstitution and, 365

D

DA. *See* Dopamine agonist
DA neurons, 99
Decorin, 180
Demyelinating disorders, 75–89
    animal models of, 76–77
    cell tracking and, 85–86
    CNS lineages and, 75
    EAE and, 87–88
    list of, 73
    MS and
        animal models and, 88
        current treatment for, 75–76
        myelin regeneration failure in, 77–78
        transplantation candidates for, 88–89
        transplantation site for, 88
    precursor cells and, 77
    remyelination
        BMSCs and, 83
        cell sources for, 79
        embryonic stem cells and, 82–83
        myelinating cell schematic and, 81
        NSCs and, 80–82
        OECs and, 80
        oligodendrocyte lineage cells and, 79
        rationale for, 78
        Schwann cells and, 79–80
    transplantation issues with
        cell delivery route and, 83–85
        cell migration and, 85
        timing of transplantation and, 83
Dermis
    skin composition and, 372
    skin substitutes of
        acellular matrices for, 384–385
        fibroblast-containing matrices for, 385

Dextromethorphan, 240
Diabetes
    β cell function and, 298
    β cell therapies for, 315–316
    ESC therapy and, 321–322
    insulin-producing β cells and, 301, 309
    prevalence of, 321
Diabetic retinopathy, 235, 238
Donor leukocyte infusion (DLI)
    GVHD and, 354–355
    indications for, 355–356
Dopamine agonist (DA)
    biosynthesis of, 98
    pathways of, 98–99
    PD and, 97–99
        nuclear transfer and, 112
        parthenogenesis and, 112
    pharmacologic supplementation of, 97
Dopaminergic cells, 97
Dry bones prophecy, 156
Duchenne muscular dystrophy, 133
Ductal ligation, 313
Dyskinesia
    heart failure therapy and, 64, 66
    PD and, 97

E

EAE. *See* Experimental autoimmune encephalomyelitis
ECM. *See* Extracellular matrix
EGF. *See* Epidermal growth factor
Elastic cartilage, 179
Electroretinography, 238
Embryonic kidney progenitors, 215–219
    gestational window for, 215–216
    host *versus* donor vascularization and, 216–217
    nuclear transfer and, 218–219
    post transplant functionality of, 217–218
    in vitro propagation of, 218
Embryonic neural stem cells (ENS) cells, 262
Embryonic renal progenitor unit, 214
Embryonic retina, 269–270
Embryonic retinal progenitor cells, 263
Embryonic stem cell (ESC), 34–37, 125, 129, 261–262, 321–327, 400–402
Embryonic stem cell-derived cardiomyocytes
    electrophysical characteristics of, 35
    myocardial regeneration and, 34
    potential applications of, 39
    proliferation of, 36
Embryonic stem cells
    differentiation of
        dopaminergic lineages and, 101–102
        insulin-producing β cells and, 302
        neural lineages and, 104–105
    ethical considerations of, 82–83
    heart failure and, 60–61
    immunogenicity of, 40–41
    kidney regeneration with, 214–215
    myocardial regeneration with, 33–41

Embryonic stem cells (*Continued*)
  myocardial tissue engineering and, 5, 7–8
  myocardial tissue repair and, 17
  pancreatic progenitor cells and, 321–322
    developmental pathway recapitulation and, 326–327
    directed differentiation and, 325
    genetic selection strategies and, 326
    lineage specification and, 324–325
    lineage specification of, 324–325
    mesenchymal-to-epithelial signaling and, 327
    nestin-positive cells and, 325
    purification of, 326
  PD and, 107–110
    dopaminergic neuron derivation and, 111
    immunologic concerns and, 111–112
    lineage selection and, 110
    nonhuman primates and, 110
    nuclear transfer and, 112
    parthenogenesis and, 112
    rodents and, 107–110
    TH-positive neuron derivation and, 110
  remyelination and, 79, 82
  retinal repair and, 261–262
  skin regeneration with, 400–402
  stroke and, 125
  teratoma and, 8
Endogenous excitotoxins, 238–239
Endothelial cells, 376
Endothelial progenitor cells (EPC)
  angiogenic properties of, 23
  kidney regeneration and, 211
  myocardial tissue engineering and, 5
  myogenic properties of, 23
  sources of, 21
Endothelium, 211
End-stage renal disease (ESRD)
  kidney regeneration and, 209
  organ transplantation for, 209–210
  renal cell replacement and, 220
ENS. *See* Embryonic neural stem cells
EPC. *See* Endothelial progenitor cells
Epidermal cells, 376
Epidermal growth factor (EGF)
  ENS cells and, 262
  skin wound healing and, 377
Epidermis
  skin composition and, 372
  stem cells in, 373
EPO. *See* Erythropoietin
Erythropoietin (EPO), 11
ESC. *See* Embryonic stem cell
ESRD. End-stage renal disease
Ethidium bromide (EB), 76
ETT. *See* Exercise treadmill test
Euglycemia
  INGAP and, 313
  maintenance of, 309
Eve, 156
EVELAU. *See* Ex-vivo expanded limbal autograft

Exercise treadmill test (ETT), 46
Experimental autoimmune encephalomyelitis (EAE)
  animal models with, 76–77
  pathology of, 76
  stem cell therapy for, 87–88
Extracellular matrix (ECM)
  cartilage structure and, 179–181
  myocardium composition and, 3
Exudative macular degeneration
  retinal regeneration and, 260
  RPE transplantation and, 271
Ex-vivo expanded limbal autograft (EVELAU)
  ocular surface regeneration with, 291
  OSR and, 285
Ezekiel, 156

F

Fanconi anemia
  CBT and, 340
  haploidentical SCT and, 368
Feline immunodeficiency virus (FIV), 135
Fertilized zygote, 210
Fetal brains, 97
Fetal cardiomyocytes, 4–5, 8
Fetal liver cells
  glucose and, 304
  insulin-producing β cells and, 303–304
Fetal wound healing, 381–382
FGF. *See* Fibroblast growth factor
Fibrin, 7
Fibroblast growth factor (FGF). *See also* Basic fibroblast growth factor (bFGF)
  BM-derived MSCs and, 160–161
  cartilage engineering and, 172
  pancreaticogenesis and, 323
  retinal repair and
    cell transplantation and, 273
    ENS cells and, 262
  skin wound healing and, 377
  therapeutic myocardial angiogenesis and, 46, 50
Fibroblasts
  interstitial, 213
  kidney regeneration and, 213–214
  myocardial tissue engineering and, 5, 8
  myocardium composition and, 3
  skin wound healing and, 376, 380
Fibrocartilage, 179–180
Fibromodulin, 180
Fibronectin, 180
FIV. *See* Feline immunodeficiency virus
Flexner-Wintersteiner rosettes, 266
Fludarabine, 352–353
Flunarizine, 240, 242
Flupirtine, 240
Follicular lymphoma
  immune sensitivity of, 357
  NST and, 356
Foreskin-derived fibroblasts, 229
Fovea, 234

Free grafts, 228
Frizzled extracellular domain, 267

G

GAD. *See* Glutamine acid decarboxylase
G-CSF. *See* Granulocyte colony-stimulating factor
GDNF. *See* Glial cell line-derived neurotrophic factor
Gelatin scaffolds, 7
Genesis, 156
Gene therapy
  administration routes for
    intraparenchymal injection and, 143
    intrathecal administration and, 144
    intravascular injection and, 143–144
    intraventricular administration and, 144
    transneuronal transfer and, 144
  bone regeneration and, 198
  cartilage engineering and, 172
  gene expression and, 145–146
  nervous system and, 133–148
    AAVs and, 137–138
    adenoviruses and, 137
    delivery methods and, 135, 143–145
    delivery targeting and, 142
    disease-specific strategies and, 141–142
    gene expression and, 145–146
    HSV-1 and, 138–139
    neuronal cell death and, 141
    nonviral delivery vectors and, 139–140
    postinjury regeneration and, 142
    retroviruses and, 135–137
    safety and, 146–148
    therapeutic approaches for, 134
    viral vectors and, 135–139
  safety of, 146
    immune-mediated damage and, 146–147
    viral vector-related risks and, 147–148
  skin wound healing and, 381
  targeted entry and, 144–145
  targeted expression and, 145
Germline cells, 146
GGF. *See* Glial growth factor
Glaucoma, 234
  blindness and, 238
  neuroprotection and, 239
  neuroprotective agents and, 237
  retinal regeneration and, 260
Glaucomatous neuropathy
  animal models and, 239
  neuroprotective treatment and, 238
Glial cell line-derived neurotrophic factor (GDNF), 134
Glial growth factor (GGF), 78
Glial precursor cells, 75, 79
Glomerular injury, 220
Glomerular mesangial cells, 211–212
Glomerulosclerosis, 212
Glomerulus, 211–212
Glucose, 304
Glutamate, 238–239

Glutamine acid decarboxylase (GAD), 134
Glutathione peroxidase, 141
Graft-*versus*-host disease (GVHD)
  CBT and, 339
    adults and, 343
  haploidentical SCT and, 361
    prevention strategies for, 362–363
  NST and, 351–352, 354–355
Graft-*versus*-leukemia (GVL)
  CML and, 357
  haploidentical SCT and, 366
  NST and, 351–352
Graft-*versus*-malignancy (GVM), 351–352
Granulocyte colony-stimulating factor (G-CSF)
  myocardial tissue engineering and, 11
  myocardial tissue repair and, 28
GVHD. *See* Graft-*versus*-host disease
GVL. *See* Graft-*versus*-leukemia
GVM. *See* Graft-*versus* malignancy

H

Hair follicle bulge, 373, 397–398
Haploidentical SCT
  clinical perspectives on, 366–367
  graft rejection and, 361
    elimination of, 363–364
  GVHD and, 361
    prevention of, 362–363
  GVL and, 366
  HLA matched siblings and, 361
  immune reconstitution and
    extrathymic pathways of, 364
    restoration of specific immunity and, 365
    T cell depletion and, 365
  nonmalignant conditions and, 367–368
  strategies for, 361–362
  unrelated alloSCT and, 367
Heart failure, 59–68
  cell therapy for, 59–66
    cell differentiation and, 62
    cell integration and, 62–63
    cell sources for, 61
    cell survival after, 61–62
    determinants for success of, 60
    graft vascularization and, 63
  left ventricle and, 63–66
    capillary density in, 64
    contractile performance of, 65
    dyskinesia and, 64, 66
    regional myocardial blood flow and, 64
    volume of, 64–65
  models of
    cardiocirculatory, 59
    progressive, 59
  symptoms of, 66–67
  systolic contractile dysfunction and, 67
Heart renovation, 3–13
  myocardial tissue engineering for, 3–13
    beating construct and, 8–9

Heart renovation (*Continued*)
  bioactive molecules and, 11
  biomaterials for, 6–7
  bioreactors and, 9–10
  cell sources for, 4–5, 7–8
  classic paradigm of, 5
  construct transplantation and, 10–11
  construct vascularization and, 11
  direct cell injection and, 6
  injectable biomaterials and, 12
  LV remodeling and, 4
  myocardial infarction and, 4
  myocardial regeneration and, 4
  myocardium composition and, 3–4
  in situ engineering and, 11–12
  summary, 12–13
  tissue engineering v. cellular therapy for, 6
Heart transplantation, 2
Hedgehog, 264. *See also* Sonic hedgehog
Hemangioblasts, 21
Hematopoietic chimerism, 41
Hematopoietic stem cells (HSC)
  angiogenic properties of, 23
  BM cells and, 305
  kidney regeneration with, 220
  myocardial tissue engineering and, 5, 8
  myocardial tissue repair and, 20
    stem cell plasticity and, 17
  myogenic properties of, 23
  stroke and, 126
Hemorrhagic stroke, 123
Hepatocyte growth factor (HGF), 11
Hepatocytes, 303
Herpes simplex virus type 1 (HSV-1)
  characteristics of, 136
  gene delivery with, 138–139
hESCDCM. *See* Human embryonic stem cell-derived cardiomyocytes
HGF. *See* Hepatocyte growth factor
Hippocampal-derived ANS cells, 272–273
HIV. *See* Human immunodeficiency virus
HLA. *See* Human leukocyte antigen
Holoclones, 373
Homer-Wright rosettes, 266
HSV-1. *See* Herpes simplex virus type 1
Human embryonic stem cell-derived cardiomyocytes (hESCDCM), 38–39
Human foamy virus, 135
Human immunodeficiency virus (HIV), 135
Human leukocyte antigen (HLA)
  alloSCT and, 332
  CBT and, 333
    adults and, 342
    disparity and, 339
  myocardial regeneration and, 40
Huntington, 134
Hurler syndrome
  CBT and, 340
  haploidentical SCT and, 368
Hyaline cartilage, 179, 199

Hyaluronan, 180
Hydroxyapatite, 163
Hypoxia, 123

I

ICM. *See* Inner cell mass
IGF. *See* Insulin-like growth factor
Immortalized cell lines. *See also* Mandsley hippocampal stem cell line clone 36; NTerra-2
  experimental data and, 126–127
  stroke and, 125–126
Immunosuppression, 111–112
INGAP. *See* Islet neogenesis associated protein
Inner cell mass (ICM), 261
Insertional mutagenesis, 146, 148
Insulin-like growth factor (IGF)
  cartilage engineering and, 172
  cartilage homeostasis and, 181–182
  myocardial tissue engineering and, 11
  remyelination and, 78–79
  skin wound healing and, 377
Insulin-producing β cells, 301–306
  derivation of
    BM cells and, 305
    intestine epithelial cells and, 304–305
    liver cells and, 303–304
    tissue stem cells and, 302–303
  diabetes and, 301
  forced expansion of, 301
  pancreas composition and, 298
  replacement of, 301
  transplantation of, 299
    autoimmune responses and, 305–306
    autologous v. allogeneic, 306
Interleukin-1
  cartilage homeostasis and, 182
  skin wound healing and, 377
Intestine epithelial cells, 304–305
Intracerebral grafts, 107
Intracerebroventricular injection, 84
Intracoronary injection
  clinical studies of, 52–53
  therapeutic myocardial angiogenesis and, 50, 52–55
Intraocular pressure, 234
Intraparenchymal injection, 143
Intrathecal transplantation
  neurodegenerative disorders and, 144
  remyelination and, 84
Intravascular injection, 143–144
Intravenous injection, 84
Intraventricular transplantation
  neurodegenerative disorders and, 144
  remyelination and, 84
Iris epithelium-derived stem cells, 264
Ischemic heart disease
  interventional treatment of, 2
  pharmacologic treatment of, 2
  prevalence of, 17
  risk factors for, 17–18
Ischemic necrosis, 123

Index

Ischemic optic neuropathy, 238
Ischemic stroke, 123
Islet cell transplants, 321
Islet neogenesis associated protein (INGAP)
  β cell neogenesis and, 313
  in vivo data on, 315
Islets of Langerhans
  diabetes and, 321
  pancreas composition and, 298
Islet stem cells. See β cells

J

Janus phenomenon, 55
Joint replacement, 184

K

Keratinocyte growth factor (KGF), 377
Keratinocytes
  skin wound healing and, 376, 379
  tissue engineering and, 382
Keratoepithelioplasty, 288
Keratolimbal allograft (KLAL), 288–291
  allograft rejection and, 289
  bilateral disease and, 288
  c-CLAL and, 288
  cyclosporine and, 289
  keratoepithelioplasty and, 288
  LKP and, 288
  lr-CLAL and, 288
  OSR and, 285
  patient status and, 289–290
  tissue preparation for, 289
KGF. See Keratinocyte growth factor
Kidney development, 215
Kidney regeneration, 209–220
  endothelial repair and, 211
  fibroblasts and, 213–214
  gestational window and, 215–216
  kidney development and, 215
  mesangial repair and, 211–212
  organ donor demand and, 209–210
  stem cells and, 210
    committed, 214–215
    pluripotent, 214
  teratoma risk and, 216
  tubule regeneration and, 212–213
Kissing lesions, 204
KLAL. See Keratolimbal allograft

L

Lacerations, 375
Lamellar keratoplasty (LKP), 288
Laser abrasion, 184
Laser photocoagulation, 239
Lateral ganglionic eminence cells (LGE), 124
Lavage, 184
Left ventricular (LV) remodeling, 4
Lentiviruses
  biosafety of, 136
  gene delivery with

  characteristics of, 136
  neurodegenerative diseases and, 135–137
Leukemia inhibitory factor (LIF)
  myocardial regeneration and, 34
  myocardial tissue engineering and, 11
Leukocyte, 28. See also Donor leukocyte infusion
Levodopa, 98
LGE. See Lateral ganglionic eminence cells
LIF. See Leukemia inhibitory factor
Ligaments repair, 164–165
Limbal autografts, 282
Limbal stem cell deficiency
  corneal transplantation and, 284
  ocular surface regeneration and, 283–284
Limb fields, 182
Link proteins, 180
Liver cells, 303–304
Living-relative conjunctival allograft (lr-CAL), 285
Living-relative conjunctival limbal allograft (lr-CLAL),
    288–291
  allograft rejection and, 289
  bilateral disease and, 288
  c-CLAL and, 288
  cyclosporine and, 289
  keratoepithelioplasty and, 288
  KLAL and, 288
  LKP and, 288
  OSR and, 285
  patient status and, 289–290
  tissue preparation for, 289
Living-relative ex-vivo expanded limbal allograft
    (lr-EVELAL)
  ocular surface regeneration with, 291
  OSR and, 285
Living skin equivalent (LSE), 385
LKP. See Lamellar keratoplasty
Lomerizine, 242
lr-CAL. See Living-relative conjunctival allograft
lr-CLAL. See Living-relative conjunctival limbal allograft
lr-EVELAL. See Living-relative ex-vivo expanded limbal
    allograft
LSE. See Living skin equivalent
LV. See Left ventricular
Lymphocytes, 376

M

Macrophages
  CNS regeneration with
    implantation for, 251–252
    innate immune response and, 252
  skin wound healing and, 376
Macular edema, 235
Magnetic resonance imaging (MRI)
  cell tracking with, 85–86
  remyelination and, 84
Mandsley hippocampal stem cell line clone 36 (MHP36),
    125–126
MAPC. See Multipotent adult progenitor cells
Marrow-isolated adult multilineage inducible cells
    (MIAMI), 116

Matrigel
    myocardial tissue engineering and, 7
    myocardial tissue repair and, 20
Matrilins, 180
MBP. See Myelin basic protein
MC. See Mixed chimerism
Memantine
    AD and, 237, 240
    neuroprotection with, 240
    PD and, 241
Meroclones, 373
Mesangial cells, 211–212
Mesangium, 211–212
Mesenchymal stem cells (MSC), 159–165
    adipose tissue and, 163
    angiogenic properties of, 23
    BM-derived
        bone reconstruction with, 163
        cartilage repair with, 164
        harvest of, 160–161
        immunomodulatory role of, 165
        ligaments repair with, 164–165
        telomere length of, 161
        tendons repair with, 164–165
    differentiation of
        cartilage development and, 183
    fibroblastic morphology of, 159
    heart failure and, 60–61
    identification of, 186
    immune phenotype of, 21
    kidney regeneration and, 214
        indications for, 220
    lineage potential of, 187
    multipotentiality of, 159–160
    myocardial tissue engineering and, 5, 8
    myocardial tissue repair and, 20
    myogenic properties of, 22–23
    OA and, 203–205
        cell sources and, 204–205
    skeletal muscle and, 162–163
    sources for, 186, 188, 204–205
    sources of, 21
    stroke and, 126
        experimental data and, 127–128
Mesenchymal-to-epithelial signaling
    ESC differentiation and, 327
    pancreaticogenesis and, 323
Metalloproteinases, 181
Metanephric mesenchyme, 214–215
MHP36. See Mandsley hippocampal stem cell line clone 36
MIAMI. See Marrow-isolated adult multilineage inducible cells
Microangiopathy, 235
Microcontact printing, 9
Microfracture
    cartilage repair and, 184
    clinical research on, 175
Microinfarcts, 55
Minocycline, 240
Mixed chimerism (MC), 352

MK-801
    neuroprotection with, 240
    toxicities of, 241
Molecular imprinting, 199
Monocytes, 376
Monogenic inherited disorder, 133
Morphogens, 198
Mosaicplasty, 175
MPS. See Mucopolysaccharidosis
MRI. See Magnetic resonance imaging
MS. See Multiple sclerosis
MSC. See Mesenchymal stem cells
Mucopolysaccharidosis (MPS) VII, 134
Müller cells
    retinal laminar reorganization and, 266
    retinal morphogenesis, 267
    retinal repair and, 263
    retinal structure and, 259
Multiple melanoma, 356
Multiple sclerosis (MS)
    CNS therapy and, 73
    Cop-1 for, 255
    current treatment for, 75–76
    etiology of, 76
    myelin regeneration and, 77–78
    stem cell therapy for
        animal models of, 88
        candidates for, 88–89
        site of, 88
Multipotent adult progenitor cells (MAPC)
    differentiation of, 21
    dopaminergic lineages and, 103
    myocardial tissue repair and, 20
    PD and, 115
MuLV. See Murine leukemia virus
Murine leukemia virus (MuLV), 135
Myelin
    MS and, 77–78
    precursor cells and, 77
Myelin basic protein (MBP), 252–253
Myelodysplastic syndromes, 340
Myocardial ischemia, 45–56
    therapeutic angiogenesis, 45–56
        administration routes for, 50–55
        BM-derived cell-based therapy for, 48–50
        concerns regarding, 55
        FGF trials and, 46
        genes and, 47–48
        growth factor proteins and, 45–47
        VEGF trials and, 46
Myocardial progenitors, 5
Myocardial regeneration, 4, 33–41
    cardiomyocytes and
        electrophysical characteristics of, 35
        generation of, 34
        proliferation of, 36
        structural properties of, 34–35
    ESC differentiation and, 33–34
        cardiomyocyte generation and, 34
        direction of, 36–37

promotion of, 36–37
ESC immunogenicity and, 40–41
genetic engineering and, 40
immunologic tolerance and, 40–41
strategies for
    adult skeletal muscle cells and, 37–38
    bone marrow-derived stem cells and, 37
    cell selection and, 39–40
    hESCDCMs and, 38–39
    organ donation and, 37
tissue engineering and, 40
Myocardial tissue engineering, 3–13
beating construct and, 8–9
bioactive molecules and, 11
biomaterials for, 6–7
bioreactors and, 9–10
cell sources for, 4–5, 7–8
    autologous cells and, 8
    common, 7–8
    optimal, 7
classic paradigm of, 5
    cells and, 5
    cytokines and, 5
    signals and, 5
construct transplantation and, 10–11
construct vascularization and, 11
direct cell injection and, 6
injectable biomaterials and, 12
LV remodeling and, 4
myocardial infarction and, 4
myocardial regeneration and, 4
myocardium composition and, 3–4
in situ engineering and, 11–12
summary, 12–13
Myocardial tissue repair, 17–29
AMI and, 18
animal models and, 23–24
cell mobilization for, 28
cell sources for, 21
cell survival and, 23
clinical application of, 24–28
    CABG operation and, 24, 26
functional effects and, 23–24
ischemic heart disease and, 17–18
mechanisms of, 18–19
progenitor cells and, 19–20
trial designs for, 29
Myocardin, 36–37
Myocardium
composition of, 3–4
infarction of, 4
regeneration of, 4–5
remodeling of, 4
Myofibrillar slippage, 4
Myogenesis, 54
Myotubes, 20

N

Naked matrices, 185
N-cadherin, 63

Neokidneys, 218
Neomycin, 40
Neoplastic disease, 133
Nerve growth factor (NGF), 134
Nervous system gene therapy, 133–149
AAVs and, 137–138
adenoviruses and, 137
approaches of, 134
delivery methods for, 135, 143–145
delivery targeting and, 142
disease-specific strategies for, 141–142
gene expression and, 145–146
HSV-1 and, 138–139
neuronal cell death and, 141
nonviral delivery vectors for, 139–140
postinjury regeneration and, 142
retroviruses and, 135–137
safety of, 146–147
viral vectors for, 135–139
Nestin, 325
Neural progenitor cells (NPC)
demyelinating disorders and, 77
remyelination and, 79–80
retinal repair and, 269
sources of, 124
stroke and, 124
Neural retina, 259
Neural stem cells (NSC). *See also* Adult neural stem cells;
    Embryonic neural stem cells
demyelinating disorders and, 75
remyelination and, 80–82
retinal rosette formation and, 272
sources of, 99
Neuronal cell death, 141
Neuronal injury, 237–238
Neuroprotection
animal models and
    glaucoma and, 239
    optic nerve injury and, 239–240
    retinal exposure to endogenous excitotoxins and, 238
    retinal ischemia and, 238
    retinal laser injury and, 239
history and progress of, 244–245
ophthalmology and, 237–245
Neuroprotective agents
list of, 240
ophthalmology and
    adrenergic agonists/antagonists and, 241–242
    apoptosis preventers, 243
    calcium channel blockers and, 242
    immune-based agents and, 243–244
    neurotrophic factors and, 243
    nitric oxide synthase inhibitors and, 242
    NMDA receptor antagonists and, 240–241
    prednisolone and, 241
stroke and, 124
Neuroretina, 263
Neutrophils, 376, 378
NGF. *See* Nerve growth factor
Nigrostriatal pathway, 99

NMDA. *See* N-methyl-D-aspartate
NMDA receptor antagonists, 240–241
N-methyl-D-aspartate (NMDA), 237–238
Noggin, 264
Nonmyeloablative stem cell transplantation (NST), 351–358
   alloSCT and, 351
   complications with
      GVHD and, 354–355
      organ toxicity and, 353
   DLI and, 354–356
   immune-therapeutic intervention after, 355–356
   MC and, 352
   program of, 352
   rationale for, 351–352
   regimens of
      reduced-intensity, 353
      Seattle, 352–353
      selection of, 356–357
      targeted therapy and, 353
Nonviral vectors, 139–140
NPC. *See* Neural precursor cells
NSC. *See* Neural stem cells
NST. *See* Nonmyeloablative stem cell transplantation
NTerra-2, 125
Nuclear transfer, 112
Nurr1, 100

O

Obesity
   β cells and, 309
   OA and, 203
Ocular surface
   injury to, 281
   structure of, 281
Ocular surface reconstruction (OSR)
   breakthroughs in, 284
   classifications of, 284–285
   corneal epithelial stem cells and, 282
   definition of, 284
   ocular surface regeneration and, 281–282
Ocular surface regeneration, 281–293
   AMT and, 285–287
   corneal epithelium and, 282–283
   corneal limbus and, 283
   limbal allografts and, 288–291
      allograft rejection and, 289
      c-CLAL and, 288
      cyclosporine and, 289
      keratoepithelioplasty and, 288
      KLAL and, 288
      LKP and, 288
      lr-CLAL and, 288
      patient status and, 289–290
      tissue preparation for, 289
   limbal autografts and, 287
   limbal stem cell deficiency and, 283–284
   OSR and, 284–285
   stem cell therapy for, 291–292
   tissue engineering for, 292

   treatment algorithm for, 291
OEC. *See* Olfactory nerve ensheathing cells
Old Testament, 156
Olfactory nerve ensheathing cells (OEC), 79–80
Oligodendrocyte progenitor cells (OPC)
   demyelinating disorders and, 75
   remyelination and, 79
Oligodendrocytes, 77
Oncoretroviruses, 135–136
OPC. *See* Oligodendrocyte progenitor cells
Ophthalmologic neuroprotection
   agents for
      adrenergic agonists/antagonists and, 241–242
      apoptosis preventers, 243
      calcium channel blockers and, 242
      immune-based agents and, 243–244
      neurotrophic factors and, 243
      nitric oxide synthase inhibitors and, 242
      NMDA receptor antagonists and, 240–241
      prednisolone and, 241
   animal models of
      glaucoma and, 239
      optic nerve injury and, 239–240
      retinal exposure to endogenous excitotoxins and, 238
      retinal ischemia and, 238
      retinal laser injury and, 239
   history and progress of, 244–245
Ophthalmology, 234
   retinal protection in, 235
Optic nerve, 234
Optic nerve trauma, 238–240
Optic neuritis, 238
Organ donors
   availability of, 2
   myocardial regeneration and, 37
Organogenesis, 216, 219
Organ printing, 9
Organ transplantation, 209–210
OSR. *See* Ocular surface reconstruction
Osteoarthritis (OA), 158, 203–205
   cartilage engineering and, 169
   incidence of, 184
   MSCs and, 203–204
   pathology of, 203
Osteochondral transplantation, 184
Osteophyte, 205
Osteoprogenitors, 184

P

Pancreas
   composition of, 298
   formation of, 322–324
   immunologic issues of, 299
   transplantation of, 321
Pancreatic duodenal homeobox 1-positive (PDX1+)
   ESC lineage specification and, 324–325
   pancreaticogenesis and, 322
Pancreaticogenesis
   branching morphogenesis and, 322

Index

endoderm commitment and, 323
endoderm formation and, 322–323
foregut endoderm outgrowths and, 322
mesenchymal-to-epithelial signaling and, 323
transcription factors and, 323
Pancreatic progenitor cells, 321–328
  clonal expansion of, 314–315
  compensatory effort of, 310
  diabetes and, 309
    prevalence of, 321
  ductal epithelial cells and, 314
  dynamic state of, 309
  ESCs and, 321–322
    developmental pathway recapitulation and, 326–327
    directed differentiation and, 325
    genetic selection strategies and, 326
    lineage specification of, 324–325
    mesenchymal-to-epithelial signaling and, 327
    nestin-positive cells and, 325
    purification of, 326
  insulin-resistance and, 310
  islets of
    normal growth of, 309
  neogenesis of, 312–313
    ductal ligation model of, 313–313
    INGAP model of, 313
  obesity and, 310
  origin of, 310–313
    acinar cell transdifferentiation and, 311–312
    intraislet progenitor cells and, 311
    neogenesis and, 312–313
    replication and, 310
  oval cells and, 313–314
  pancreaticogenesis and, 322–324
  therapeutic formation of, 315–316
Paraclones, 373
Parkinsonian rats, 111
Parkinson's disease (PD), 97–118
  adult stem cells and, 112–117
    BMSCs and, 113–115
    MAPCs and, 115
    MIAMIs and, 116
  CNS therapy and, 73
  current treatment for, 97
  DA and
    biosynthesis of, 98
    pathways of, 98–99
    pharmacologic supplementation of, 97
  embryonic stem cells and, 107–112
    dopaminergic neuron derivation from, 111
    immunologic concerns with, 111–112
    nonhuman primates and, 110
    nuclear transfer and, 112
    parthenogenesis and, 112
    rodents and, 107–110
    TH-positive neuron derivation from, 110
  fetal brains and, 97
  gene therapy for, 134
  neuroprotection and, 241

NSCs and, 99
  adult brains and, 100, 106–107
  embryonic brains and, 99–100
  neurogenesis after injury and, 106
  neurogenic regions and, 106
pathology of, 97
stem cell differentiation and
  dopaminergic lineages and, 101–103
  neural lineages and, 104–105
tailored strategies for, 141
Parthenogenesis, 112
PDGF. *See* Platelet-derived growth factor
PDGFR. *See* Platelet-derived growth factor receptor
PDR. *See* Proliferative diabetic retinopathy
PD. *See* Parkinson's disease
PDX1+. *See* Pancreatic duodenal homeobox 1-positive
Percoll gradient centrifugation, 40
Pericytes, 162
PERV. *See* Porcine endogenous retrovirus
Phenytoin, 244
Photodynamic therapy, 238
Photophobia, 284
Photoreceptor cells, 269–270
Pigment epithelium-derived factor, 240
Plasma membrane DA transporter, 98
Plasmid DNA, 136
Platelet-derived growth factor (PDGF), 376
Platelet-derived growth factor receptor (PDGFR), 77
Platelets, 376
Pluripotent stem cells, 210
Polyesters, 226–227
Poly-L-lactide-gelatin-PGA, 7
Polymers, 226–227
Polyurethanes, 7
Porcine endogenous retrovirus (PERV), 124
Porcine fetal cells, 124
Porous alginate scaffolds
  cardiomyocyte seeding within, 8
  myocardial tissue engineering and, 7
Prednisolone, 241
Proliferative diabetic retinopathy (PDR), 260
Protective autoimmunity. *See* Autoimmunity

R

RCR. *See* Replication-competent retroviruses
Renal disease
  bioengineering for, 208
  organ donors for, 208
Renal fibrosis, 213
Renal progenitor cells, 213
Renal sepsis, 220
Renal shock, 220
Renal tubule
  acute tubular necrosis and, 212
  BM-derived extrarenal tubular progenitor cells and, 212
  cisplatin and, 213
  regeneration of, 212–213
Replication-competent retroviruses (RCR), 135
Reproductive cloning, 210

Resorbable membranes, 176
Retina, 234
    layers of, 259
    regeneration of, 260
Retinal atrophy, 234
Retinal ganglion cells (RGC)
    adaptive autoimmunity and, 253
    apoptotic death of, 237-238
    neuroprotection and, 237
Retinal laser injury, 239
Retinal pigment epithelium (RPE)
    embryonic retinal cells and, 270-271
    retinal structure and, 259
Retinal repair, 259-274
    cell sources for, 261
        ANS cells and, 263-264
        ciliary epithelium-derived stem cells and, 264
        embryonic retinal progenitor cells and, 263
        ENS cells and, 262
        ESCs and, 261-262
        iris epithelium-derived stem cells and, 264
    NSC neurogenesis and, 264-265
    progenitor cell organization and
        laminar organization and, 266-267
        reaggregation approach to, 266
        rosette occurrence and, 266-267
        signaling molecules and, 267
    retinal regeneration and, 260
    RPE and, 259
    transplantation therapy for, 267-274
        embryonic retina for, 269-270
        growth factor delivery and, 273-274
        progenitor cells for, 267-269
        RPE replacement for, 270-271
        stem cells for, 271-273
Retinal rosettes
    formation of, 270
    NSCs and, 272
    retinal repair and
        progenitor cell organization and, 266-267
        signaling molecules and, 267
Retinitis pigmentosa, 235, 260
Retroviruses
    gene delivery with, 135-137
    replication-competent, 135
RGC. See Retinal ganglion cells
Riluzole
    ALS and, 237
    neuroprotection with, 240
Rosettes. See Retinal rosettes
RPE. See Retinal pigment epithelium

S

SAQ. See Seattle Angina Questionnaire
Scaffolds
    bioceramics for, 163
    cartilage engineering with, 185
    coral and, 163
    hydroxyapatite and, 163

Schwann cells, 79-80
SCID. See Severe combined immunodeficiency
SCT. See Stem cell transplantation
SDF. See Stromal-derived growth factor
Seattle Angina Questionnaire (SAQ), 47
Seattle NST regimen, 352-353
Secondary neuronal degeneration, 237-238
Seizures, 134
Self-compounds, 254
Self-proteins, 255
Severe combined immunodeficiency (SCID)
    CBT and, 340
    haploidentical SCT and, 367-368
Shaving, 184
Shear stress, 45
Shh. See Sonic hedgehog
Simian immunodeficiency virus (SIV), 135
SIV. See Simian immunodeficiency virus
Skeletal muscle, 162-163
Skeletal myoblasts
    angiogenic properties of, 23
    arrhythmia and, 8
    heart failure and, 60-61
    myocardial tissue engineering and, 4-5, 7-8
    myocardial tissue repair and, 19
    myogenic properties of, 23
    sources of, 21
Skeletal tissues
    developmental process of, 157
    regenerative abilities of, 156
    stem cell therapy of
        bone reconstruction with, 163
        cartilage repair with, 164
        ligaments repair with, 164-165
        tendons repair with, 164-165
Skin
    biology of, 382
    composition of, 372
    functions of, 375
    regeneration of, 372
    stem cells in, 373
    tensile strength of, 380
    tissue engineering and, 382
    wounds of
        prevalence of, 375
        tensile strength of, 380
Skin regeneration, 395-403
    cell sources for
        adult epidermal stem cells and, 402
        ESCs and, 400-402
    epidermal stem cells and
        fate regulation for, 399
        hair follicle bulge and, 397-398
        lineage relationships of, 398-399
        potentiality of, 397
    epidermis and
        developmental of, 395-396
        self-renewal of, 396-397
    transplantation for, 399-400

Skin substitutes, 382–386
  composite, 385–386
  dermal
    acellular matrices for, 384–385
    fibroblast-containing matrices for, 385
  epidermal
    CEA for, 383
    CEallo for, 384
    LSE for, 385
  skin regeneration and, 399–400
  tissue engineering and, 382
Skin wound healing, 375–386
  angiogenesis and, 379–380
  apoptosis and, 381
  cytokines for, 376–377
  fetal wounds and, 381–382
  growth factors for, 376–377, 381
  hemostasis and, 377–378
  inflammatory phase of, 378
  proliferative phase of, 380
  reepithelialization and, 378–379
  tissue engineering and, 382
  wound remodeling and, 380
Smooth muscle cells, 5, 8
Somatic cell replication limit, 302
Sonic hedgehog (Shh)
  pancreaticogenesis and, 323
  retinal repair and
    embryonic retinal progenitor cells and, 263
    retinal rosettes and, 267
Spinal ependymal cells, 75
Spinner flask, 9
SPIO. See Superparamagnetic iron oxides
Spumaviruses, 135
Stem cell banking
  CB and, 333
  ethical considerations of, 82–83
Stem cell plasticity, 17
Stem cell transplantation, 332–333
Stevens-Johnson syndrome
  limbal stem cell deficiency and, 283
  ocular surface regeneration and, 281
  OSR and, 284
Stratified nonkeratinizing squamous cells, 282
Stroke, 123–130
  cell replacement therapy for
    clinical trials in, 128–129
    experimental data on, 126–128
  CNS therapy and, 73
  ischemic gradient of, 123
  thrombolytic therapy for, 124
  transplant safety concerns with
    graft rejection and, 124
    PERV and, 124
    preimplantation manipulations and, 129–130
    technical considerations of, 128–129
    teratocarcinoma and, 125, 129
    tumor growth and, 125
  transplant sources for
    BMSCs and, 126–127
    ESCs and, 125
    immortalized cell lines and, 125–126, 126–127
    MSCs and, 127–128
    NPCs and, 124
    porcine fetal cells and, 124
    UCBCs and, 126, 128
  types of, 123
Stromal-derived growth factor (SDF), 11
Superoxide dismutase, 141
Superparamagnetic iron oxides (SPIO), 85–86
Surgical incisions, 375
Syncytium, 62–63
Synovial fluid, 205
Systolic contractile dysfunction, 67

T

T cells
  antigen-specific, 254–255
  CNS regeneration with
    adaptive immune response and, 252
    MBPs and, 252–253
  haploidentical SCT and, 365
  regulatory, 254
Telomerase reverse transcriptase (TERT)
  fetal liver cell propagation and, 303
  somatic cell replication limit and, 302
Tendon repair, 164–165
Teratoma
  ESCs and, 125, 129
  human embryonic stem cells and, 8
  kidney regeneration and, 215–216
TERT. See Telomerase reverse transcriptase
TH. See Tyrosine hydroxylase
Thalassemia
  CBT and, 340
  haploidentical SCT and, 368
Therapeutic cloning
  definition of, 210
  problems of, 210
Therapeutic myocardial angiogenesis, 45–56
  administration route for, 50–55
    CABG approach to, 51
    clinical studies of, 52–53
    intracoronary cell injection approach to, 54–55
    principles of, 50
    transendocardial approach to, 51, 54
  BM-derived cell-based therapy for
    animal models and, 49
    differentiation and, 48, 50
    principles of, 48
    secretory capacity of, 50
  concerns regarding, 55
  FGF trials and, 46
  genes and, 47–48
  growth factor proteins and, 45–47
  VEGF trials and, 46
Thrombolytic therapy, 124
Thrombospondins, 180

Thymosin, 11
Tissue stem cells
    differentiation pathways of, 303
    insulin-producing β cells and, 302–303
TNF. *See* Tumor necrosis factor
Total joint replacement, 184
Totipotent stem cells, 210
Transendocardial injection
    clinical studies of, 52–53
    therapeutic myocardial angiogenesis and, 50–54
Transforming growth factor β (TGF-β)
    cartilage engineering and, 172–173
    cartilage homeostasis and, 181–182
    skin wound healing and, 377
Transient amplifying cells, 283
Transneuronal transfer, 144
Tumor necrosis factor (TNF)
    cartilage homeostasis and, 181–182
    skin wound healing and, 377
Tumors, 55
Tyrosine hydroxylase (TH)
    mesencephalic progenitors and, 100
    PD and, 98, 100
        embryonic stem cells and, 110
        gene therapy for, 134
        symptom alleviation in, 141

U

UCBC. *See* Umbilical cord blood cells
UCBT. *See* Umbilical cord blood transplantation
Ulcers, 375
Umbilical cord blood
    myocardial tissue repair and, 17
    stem cell pool in, 161
Umbilical cord blood cells (UCBC)
    experimental data and, 128
    stroke and, 126
Umbilical cord blood transplantation (UCBT), 333–334
Umbilical cord cells, 5
Universal donor ESC line, 41
Universal somatic stem cells, 21
Unrestricted somatic stem cells (USSC), 161

Urea nitrogen, 218
Ureteric buds, 214
Urothelial cells, 226
USSC. *See* Unrestricted somatic stem cells

V

Vascular epithelial growth factor (VEGF)
    myocardial tissue engineering and, 11
    retinal regeneration and, 260
    skin wound healing and, 377
    therapeutic myocardial angiogenesis and, 46
    BM cell secretions and, 50
Vascular infiltration, 11
VEGF. *See* Vascular epithelial growth factor
Vesicular monoamine transporter 2 (VMAT2), 98
Viral vectors
    AAVs and, 137–138
    adenoviruses and, 137
    cartilage engineering and, 172
    HSV-1 and, 138–139
    nervous system and, 135–139
    retroviruses and, 135–137
Virus-associated gene transfer
    BMSCs and, 114–115
    risks of, 115
Vision, 234
Visual impairment, 234
VMAT2. *See* Vesicular monoamine transporter 2

W

Water, 180
Wild-type virus, 146
Wing cells, 282
Wiskott-Aldrich syndrome, 340
Wnt pathway, 36

X

Xenopus
    retinal repair and, 264
    retinal structure of, 265

Z

Zygote development potential, 210